Blood Groups
in Man

Blood Groups in Man

R.R.RACE

CBE, PhD, FRCP, FRCPath, FRS

Kruis van Verdienst, Royal Netherlands Red Cross
Docteur Honoris Causa de l'Université de Paris
M.D. Honoris Causa of the University of Turku
Member Deutsche Akademie der Naturforscher Leopoldina

Sometime Director, Medical Research Council
Blood Group Unit,
The Lister Institute, London

AND

RUTH SANGER

BSc, PhD, FRS

Director, Medical Research Council
Blood Group Unit,
The Lister Institute, London

WITH A FOREWORD BY

PROFESSOR SIR
RONALD FISHER

FRS

SIXTH EDITION

BLACKWELL SCIENTIFIC PUBLICATIONS

OXFORD LONDON EDINBURGH MELBOURNE

© 1968, 1975 Blackwell Scientific Publications
Osney Mead, Oxford
85 Marylebone High Street, London W1M 3DE
9 Forrest Road, Edinburgh
P.O. Box 9, North Balwyn, Victoria, Australia

ISBN 0 632 00431 2

First published 1950
Second edition 1954
Third edition 1958
Fourth edition 1962
Reprinted 1965
Fifth edition 1968
Reprinted 1970
Sixth edition 1975

Spanish edition 1952
German edition 1958
French edition 1970

Distributed in the United States of America by
J. B. Lippincott Company, Philadelphia
and in Canada by
J. B. Lippincott Company of
Canada Ltd, Toronto

Printed and bound in Great Britain by
William Clowes & Sons Ltd
London, Colchester and Beccles

Foreword

I am extremely glad that Race and Sanger have been induced to undertake the heavy labour of preparing a modern book on the blood groups, giving especial attention to their inheritance. The need for an exact and comprehensive text-book has been increasingly evident during the rapid progress of the last decade, and no authors could be better qualified for the task. Both are, however, fully occupied by new researches in the fields which they themselves have to a great extent opened up, and great self-discipline was surely needed to bring themselves to sacrifice so much of their time as this book needed.

Research people are usually so conscious of how much remains to be done that they sometimes underrate the extent of what has been already accomplished. In particular this seems to be the case with respect to the future use of blood-grouping as the principal tool of a comprehensive study of the human germ plasm. To have established, in a short time, nine usable marked loci is surely to have gone a long way towards establishing that 'basic triangulation' by which in due time the whole will be surveyed. There are in man only twenty-three autosomes, and to have at least one good marker on nine of these puts the future study of the numerous Mendelian factors known in man, through the transmission of rare anomalies, in a position very advantageous compared with that when I left the Galton Laboratory. Many new linkages must be already within reach of detection, when family studies can be combined with comprehensive serological tests.

On matters once controversial (and still so occasionally) the senior author has exercised a commendable restraint. No one would judge from the text how often his personal contributions have been ignored, and when verified have been published without acknowledgement of his priority. Our present understanding of the complex *Rh* situation owes much to the good temper with which, in spite of irritants, he steadily pushed on with his own problems.

It is fortunate that the authors can command a simple and lucid style, for much that is to be expounded is really intricate. Those who have followed the work during its development will often be surprised at the simplicity with which an adequate account can now be given. They may also be amused at the 'evasive action' occasionally taken by the authors when anything heavy in the way of mathematics seems imminent.

R. A. FISHER

Department of Genetics, Cambridge
17 *May* 1950

v

Preface to the Sixth Edition

Here is the last edition of this book: the subject has grown to need more than our two pencils.

In the seven years since the fifth edition the emergence of many more subdivisions of blood group systems and the identification of unlinked inhibitor loci have increased wonder at the antigenic complexity of the red cell surface, if not yet quite confounding all description.

We have included in our account all the subdivisions, the finer niceties of antigenic variety, which cannot be ignored though they need not burden the memory: their existence may be kept at the back of the mind and the details looked up when occasion arises.

The various inhibitor mechanisms herald a deeper understanding of the background of the groups, particularly when they are found to be influencing the antigens of genetically separate systems.

But probably the most fundamental recent advances have come from the biochemists: the discovery of the A, B, H and Le^a glycosyltransferases solved the old puzzle of these antigens being sugar though genes produce protein. Also there has been the gradual recognition that the Rh antigen D is protein and a constituent of the red cell membrane, rather than a surface appendage.

We thank the members of our small Medical Research Council Unit for endless help in the compiling of this book. In quoting our own work, when we say 'we find' we mean 'they found' and Dr Patricia Tippett must be singled out for especial thanks. It is impossible to name here all the friends in this country and abroad who have helped with suggestions, personal communications and papers in the press, but we must mention Dr T.E. Cleghorn, of the North London Blood Transfusion Centre, Dr and Mrs M. Metaxas, of the Swiss Red Cross Blood Transfusion Service, Zurich and Professors W.T.J. Morgan and Winifred M. Watkins, of the Lister Institute.

Mrs Sandra O'Nions for the sixth time, and Mrs Margaret Carey for the second, cheerfully survived the preparation of the manuscript. The skill and good humour of our publishers and printers in tip-toeing through the curious symbols of the blood group fancy continue to astonish us.

The Lister Institute of Preventive Medicine, at Chelsea, is to close towards the end of this its 84th year. Here our Unit has been ideally housed for 29 years and we thank very many past and present members of the Institute for their friendship, their knowledge and their blood. (The future home of the Unit is not decided at the time of returning our page proofs.)

Lister Institute, January 1975

Contents

Chapter 3. The MNSs Blood Groups

Chapter 4. The P Blood Groups

Chapter 5. The Rh Blood Groups

Chapter 6. The Lutheran Blood Groups

Chapter 7. The Kell Blood Groups

Chapter 8. Secretors and Non-secretors

Chapter 9. The Lewis Groups

Chapter 10. The Duffy Blood Groups

Chapter 11. The Kidd Blood Groups

Chapter 12. The Diego Blood Groups

Chapter 13. The Yt Blood Groups

Chapter 14. The Auberger Blood Groups

Chapter 15. The Dombrock Blood Groups

Chapter 16. The Colton Blood Groups

Chapter 17. The Sid Groups

Chapter 18. The Scianna Blood Groups

Chapter 19. Some Very Frequent Antigens

Chapter 20. Some Very Infrequent Antigens

Chapter 21. The I and i Antigens

Chapter 22. The En Blood Groups
and Some Other Phenotypes Affecting the Cell Surface

Chapter 23. Some Other Antigens

Chapter 24. Miscellany

Chapter 25. Blood Groups and Problems of Parentage and Identity

Chapter 26. Blood Groups in Twins and Chimeras

CONTENTS

Chapter 27. Blood Groups and Mapping of the Autosomes

Chapter 28. The Xg Blood Groups

Chapter 29. Xg and X-Chromosome Mapping

Chapter 30. Xg and Sex Chromosome Aneuploidy

Chapter 1
Introduction

BLOOD GROUPS

In 1875 Landois noticed that if red blood cells of an animal of one species were mixed with serum from an animal of another species clumping, or agglutination, of the red cells usually occurred. The phenomenon was recognized as being similar to that which followed the mixing of bacteria with appropriate immune sera. The similarity suggested that the agglutination of the red cells was due, like that of the bacteria, to antigens on their surface uniting with antibodies in the serum. Had there been no knowledge of bacterial immunity already in existence the basic principles of the science of immunology could have been discovered from the behaviour of red cells and serum. As it was, the knowledge of bacterial immunology could be directly applied to the understanding of the nature of red cell agglutination.

The first observation of the agglutination of human red cells by serum belonging to the same species was made by Landsteiner in 1900, when he found that the sera of some of his colleagues agglutinated the red cells of others. Thirty years later he received a Nobel Prize for this discovery of the ABO groups. Until his death in 1943 Landsteiner was the leading figure in this field of biology which he had opened up.

The recognition of the part played by the ABO groups in blood transfusion soon followed and from that time transfusion began to be safe.

The discovery that the blood groups were inherited characters greatly increased their biological interest. Ottenberg and Epstein suggested in 1908 that the groups were inherited, but Bateson writing in 1909 could still say: 'Of Mendelian inheritance of normal characteristics in man there is as yet but little evidence.'

In 1910 von Dungern and Hirszfeld established beyond doubt the Mendelian inheritance of the groups, though it was not till 1924 that a more exact manner of their inheritance was elucidated by the mathematician Bernstein.

The discovery of further systems of blood groups followed that of the ABO by a quarter of a century. In 1927 Landsteiner and Levine discovered the MN system and the P system. These two systems though of genetic and anthropological interest did not influence blood transfusion.

A new and exciting phase in the history of blood groups began when the work of Levine and Stetson, in 1939, and of Landsteiner and Wiener, in 1940, laid the foundations of the vast knowledge of the Rh groups and of their fundamental

1

role in causing a disease called *erythroblastosis foetalis* or *haemolytic disease of the newborn*. Blood groups had now entered the field of scientific medicine.

After 1940 the MN, P and Rh groups were subdivided and many more systems were discovered: a list is given in Table 1 of over 160 of the red cell antigens now identifiable. A notable addition was the antigen Xg^a which, unlike all the others, is X-borne.

Table 1. Blood group antigens in man

System	Antigens detected by	
	positive reaction with specific antibody	positive reaction with one antibody, negative with another*
A_1A_2BO	A_1, B, †H	A_2, A_3, A_x, and other A and B variants
MNSs	M, N, S, s, U, M^g, M_1, M′, Tm, Sj, Hu, He, Mi^a, Vw (Gr), Mur, Hil, Hut, M^v, Vr, Ri^a, St^a, Mt^a, Cl^a, Ny^a, Sul, Far	M_2, N_2, M^c, M^a, N^a, M^r, M^z, S_2
P	P_1, P^k, †Luke	P_2
Rh	D, C, c, C^w, C^x, E, e, e^s (VS), E^w, G, ce(f), ce^s(V), Ce, CE, cE, D^w, E^T, Go^a, hr^s, hr^H, hr^B, $\overline{\overline{R}}{}^N$, Rh33, Rh35, Be^a, †LW	D^u, C^u, E^u, and many other variant forms of D, C and e
Lutheran	Lu^a, Lu^b, Lu^aLu^b (Lu3), Lu6, Lu9, ‡Lu4, Lu5, Lu7, Lu8, Lu10–17	
Kell	K, k, Kp^a, Kp^b, Ku, Js^a, Js^b, Ul^a, Wk^a, K11, ‡KL, K12–16	
Lewis	Le^a, Le^b, Le^c, Le^d, Le^x	
Duffy	Fy^a, Fy^b, Fy3, Fy4	
Kidd	Jk^a, Jk^b, Jk^aJk^b (Jk3)	
Diego	Di^a, Di^b	
Yt	Yt^a, Yt^b	
Auberger	Au^a	
Dombrock	Do^a, Do^b	
Colton	Co^a, Co^b, Co^aCo^b	
Sid	Sd^a	
Scianna	Sc1, Sc2 (Bu^a)	
Very frequent antigens	Vel, Ge, Lan, Gy^a, At^a, En^a, Wr^b, Jr^a, Kn^a, El, Dp, Gn^a, Jo^a, and many unpublished examples	
Very infrequent antigens	An^a, By, Bi, Bp^a, Bx^a, Chr^a, Evans, Good, Gf, Heibel, Hey, Hov, Ht^a, Je^a, Jn^a, Levay, Ls^a, Mo^a, Or, Pt^a, Rl^a, Rd, Re^a, Sw^a, To^a, Tr^a, Ts, Wb, Wr^a, Wu, Zd, and many unpublished examples	
Other antigens	I, i, Bg (HL-A), Chido, Cs^a, Yk^a	
Xg	Xg^a	

* Recognizable only in favourable genotypes.
† A genetically independent part of the system.
‡ Place in system not yet genetically clear.

BLOOD GROUPING

In this section an attempt is made to give those readers who are not serologists a general idea of the tests used in blood grouping. The tests most commonly used are, in principle, very simple, and it is surprising that they have contributed so much to biological knowledge.

The great bulk of the earlier blood group knowledge was gathered from the results of simple agglutination tests. A serum containing a known antibody is added to a saline suspension of red cells. If the cells carry the equivalent antigen they are agglutinated; if no agglutination occurs it is concluded that the cells lack the antigen.

The converse procedure is the identification of the type of antibody present in a serum by adding to the serum different samples of red cells containing various known combinations of antigens. By observing which mixtures show agglutination, the antibody or antibodies present in the serum can be determined by a process of elimination.

A third situation, and much the most exciting, is that which arises when neither the antibody nor the antigen are known. The discovery of the blood group systems Lutheran, Kell, Lewis, Duffy, Kidd, etc., followed the finding of human sera which reacted with certain red cell samples irrespective of their content of known antigens. Other systems such as MN and P were discovered in a more deliberate way. Animals were injected with human red cells in the hope that some of the unknown blood group antigens on the red cell surface would stimulate the production of antibodies in the animal serum; and in the hope that when the immune serum came to be tested against different samples of human red cells only some samples would be found to contain the inciting antigen.

The amount of a particular antibody in different examples of antisera varies considerably. The commonest method of measuring the amount is to *titrate* the antiserum—that is, to make a series of increasingly dilute solutions in saline of the serum; red cells containing the appropriate antigen are added and the serum which causes recognizable agglutination at the greatest dilution is considered to have the most antibody.

The amount of some of the antigens varies in different examples of red cells. This is most notably true of the MN and the Rh antigens. These variations in amount depend on the genetic constitution of the donor. Such differences can be recognized and roughly measured by observing the comparative strengths of the reactions when different cell samples are tested against parallel titrations of the same antisera.

The presence of a particular antigen in a sample of red cells can be recognized in another way. The cells are mixed with the appropriate antiserum and, after an interval, the two are separated by centrifugation and the serum is examined for a fall in antibody content. This *absorption* method is particularly useful in demonstrating that an antiserum contains a mixture of two antibodies; to separate such a mixture cells are added which contain the antigen for only one of the antibodies in the serum.

A similar method can be used to test for blood group antigen in solution, for example, in saliva or seminal fluid. (The antigens of the ABO, Lewis and Sid systems are found in solution.) A mixture is made of antiserum and fluid and after a brief interval the appropriate red cells are added. The red cells act as indicators of the *inhibition* of antibody, which will have occurred if the solution contains the particular antigen.

Blood group antibodies exist which do not agglutinate red cells suspended in saline. These *incomplete* or *blocking* antibodies, as they are called, are of the same specificity as the saline agglutinating antibodies. Let us take as an example a hypothetical blood group system X. The ordinary type of anti-X serum will agglutinate red cells carrying the antigen X when they are suspended in saline: incomplete anti-X will have no effect, visible either to the naked eye or by the microscope, on such cells. We know, nevertheless, that an interaction has occurred between X and incomplete anti-X for four reasons, which are given in the order of their discovery.

1   Red cells of group X treated with incomplete anti-X when suspended in saline are not agglutinated by ordinary anti-X, as are such cells before treatment. Such treated cells are, however, still agglutinated by anti-Y, anti-Z, etc., as before treatment.

2   Incomplete anti-X will agglutinate red cells of group X if they are suspended in a protein medium (e.g. 20% albumin) instead of saline.

3   Red cells of group X exposed to a serum containing incomplete anti-X and then washed free from all serum can be shown to have been sensitized by the anti-X. The sensitization depends on the specific fixation of antibody to antigen which persists in spite of repeated washing of the red cells. The sensitization is demonstrated by the addition of an antiserum made by say, a rabbit, against human globulin: the rabbit antiglobulin serum causes such sensitized red cells to agglutinate.

4   Red cells of group X, after incubation with certain enzymes, become agglutinable in saline by incomplete anti-X.

Blood group antibodies may be able, in some circumstances, to damage red cells carrying the equivalent antigen; the contained haemoglobin escapes and the phenomenon is called *haemolysis*. Haemolysis is not generally used in human blood grouping, for agglutination is more regular in its occurrence and more easily observed. Haemolysis does not normally obscure agglutination for it does not occur in the absence of an entity, present only in fresh serum, called complement. A complement fixation test is beginning to be used to detect certain red cell antigens on white cells and on cultured fibroblasts.

Red cells which have been agglutinated by a blood group antibody, or which have been sensitized by an incomplete antibody, may be made to give up antibody if they are suspended in saline and heated for a few minutes at 56°C. This process, which is called *elution* of the antibody, is often of use in blood group investigations.

Other methods have now been developed which do not involve heating the mixture.

The very sensitive serological phenomenon of *precipitation* is seldom employed in blood group work. When antigen in solution is added to the equivalent antibody a cloudiness may be observed which later settles as a precipitate.

INTRODUCTION TO SOME GENETIC TERMS

We propose to explain in an elementary way some of the genetic terms which recur throughout this book. This is of course quite inadequate as an introduction to human genetics as a whole. To those wishing to learn something of this fascinating subject we recommend four excellent books: *An Introduction to Medical Genetics* by Fraser Roberts[1], *Principles of Human Genetics* by Curt Stern[2] and *Genetics in Medicine* by Thompson and Thompson[3], and the very useful catalogue *Mendelian Inheritance in Man* by McKusick[4], at present in its 4th edition.

At a shallow but convenient level, *genes* may be said to be the units of inheritance. The place of a gene on the chromosome that carries it is called its *locus*. A locus may be occupied by one of several alternative forms of the gene and these alternatives are called *alleles*. If both alleles are the same the owner is said to be *homozygous* in respect of this locus: if different he is said to be *heterozygous*. According to Renwick the usage of the word gene is entirely replaceable by allele.

The difference between one allele and another is the result of *mutation*. Mutation is a rare event which is thought to occur in less than 1 in 100,000 gene generations in man. In species which have been intensively studied, mutations have a constant rate of occurrence though the rate is not the same for all loci.

When two loci are known to be carried on the same chromosome and to be within measurable distance of each other they are said to be *linked*. The nearer their loci are together the closer the linkage. Two alleles whose loci are closely linked may travel together through many generations without being separated. Alleles at loci linked but sited at some distance from each other will often be separated by *crossing-over*. Crossing-over happens at the first meiotic division of gametogenesis. When two loci are known to be on the same chromosome, but whether or not linkage can be directly measured between them, their relationship is described as *syntenic*; for example the *Rh* and the *Duffy* loci are syntenic on chromosome No. 1 but tests for linkage between them are negative. This is another clarification we owe to Renwick.

Alleles at loci which are carried on different chromosomes or at loci far apart on the same chromosome, and whose entry together into a sex cell is a matter of chance, are said to *segregate independently*.

Two useful words are *cis* and *trans*: they have more or less the same meaning as coupling and repulsion. They are particularly useful in the Rh groups and an example may serve to illustrate their meaning: in the heterozygote *CDe/cDE*, *C* and *e* are in *cis* and so are *c* and *E*, but *C* and *E*, and *c* and *e*, are in *trans*.

Loci may be *autosomal*, that is, carried on one of the 22 pairs of autosomes, or they may be X-borne, that is carried on the X chromosome (X-linked is the older name but it is no longer quite appropriate, for the word linkage is reserved for two loci on a chromosome which have been proved to be within measurable distance of each other. For example red-green colour blindness and the blood group Xg are both X-borne, and are therefore syntenic, but their loci being far apart are not linked). The phenomenon of *X-chromosome inactivation* is referred to in Chapter 28. Little is known of loci on the Y.

The aggregate of ordered genes received by a person from his father and mother determines his *genotype*. Sometimes the genotype (in some particular) can be recognized directly; a person of blood group AB must be of the genotype *AB*. Sometimes serological tests and other direct observations cannot distinguish two genotypes such as *AA* and *AO*, which will however behave differently as progenitors: such a class of genotypes is known as a *phenotype*.

A *propositus* is the member of a family through whom the family came to be investigated. It is generally wise to record who is the propositus. In a pedigree this can conveniently be shown by an arrow. We have found it important to record the reason why a particular family has been tested. If, for example, a family is specially investigated because the propositus, perhaps a colleague, is K+, this fact may affect the manner of counting the family when the inheritance of the Kell groups is being studied. If the blood samples of this family are, as a routine, also tested for, say, the Lutheran groups, then the family could be counted without any correction in a study of the inheritance of the Lutheran groups.

Dominant and *recessive* are terms falling out of favour and, as will be seen in the section below, one year's recessive may be the next year's dominant—it all depends on the tests available. But they still can be very useful and to avoid the terms often calls for circumlocution. What we mean when we say a character is dominant is that it is expressed more or less equally when the responsible allele is present in the homozygous or heterozygous state.

Professor J. H. Renwick, who has done much to tighten up the loose phrases we use in human genetics, suggests that the phrase 'is a single-dose condition' could replace 'is a dominant character'.

In some earlier editions we ventured to dip into the subject of *polymorphism* (Ford[5], 1961), but it has now become so mathematical that the best we can do is to refer the reader to the work of Cavalli-Sforza and Bodmer[6] (1971) on the reasons behind 'the occurrence in the same population of two or more alleles at one locus, each with appreciable frequency'.

THE USUAL STEPS IN THE ELUCIDATION OF A BLOOD GROUP SYSTEM

The recognition of most new blood group systems results from the investigation of antibodies caused by blood transfusion or by pregnancy.

First it has to be shown that the immune antibody, say anti-X, is not any of the known antibodies, or mixtures thereof, but is recognizing a new antigen X. The antigen X is then shown almost invariably to be a dominant character and the gene frequency of X is established, together with that of the theoretical and purely negative allele x. The character x, that is the absence of X, then is called recessive. Sometimes the reaction of an antigen is stronger if the corresponding gene is in the double, homozygous, state than if it is in the single, heterozygous, state; but this does not affect the antigen being labelled a dominant character because Mendel's original definition of dominance allowed for such slight quantitative differences which are thought to be the result of gene dosage. The antigen X has to be shown not to be a hitherto unrecognized member of a known system and this can only be done by observing independent segregation in families.

Then, the second step, the antibody anti-x is found, and the antigen x becomes positively detectable and it is realized that the character is not recessive but dominant.

A third stage is that reached by the MNSs, Rh, Lutheran and Kell groups. At this level it is realized that other detectable allelic genes, Y and y etc., are closely associated with X and x.

Yet a further stage is the recognition that a certain independent or 'regulator' gene has to be present before the blood group gene can express itself—a level of knowledge reached in the ABO, P, Rh, Lutheran and Auberger systems.

REFERENCES

1   ROBERTS J.A.F. (1973) *An Introduction to Medical Genetics*, 6th edition, pp. 310, University Press, Oxford.
2   STERN C. (1960) *Principles of Human Genetics*, 2nd edition, pp. 753, Freeman, San Francisco.
3   THOMPSON J.S. and THOMPSON MARGARET W. (1973) *Genetics in Medicine*, 2nd edition, pp. 400, W.B. Saunders, Philadelphia and London.
4   McKUSICK V.A. (1974) *Mendelian Inheritance in Man*, 4th edition, pp. 704, The Johns Hopkins Press, Baltimore and London.
5   FORD E.B. (1961) *Genetics for Medical Students*, 5th edition, pp. 202, Methuen, London.
6   CAVALLI-SFORZA L.L. and BODMER W.F. (1971) *The Genetics of Human Populations*, pp. 965, Freeman, San Francisco.

Chapter 2
The ABO Blood Groups

HISTORY

The observation by Landsteiner that the red cells of some of his colleagues at the pathological anatomy institute of the University of Vienna were agglutinated by the sera of some of the others, the discovery of blood groups, was the beginning of a new branch of human biology. The first, qualified, intimation was in a footnote to a paper[1] published in 1900, but the laureate account[2] appeared in 1901. Incidentally, in this paper[2] possible applications to blood transfusion and criminology were foreseen.

Landsteiner took samples of blood from six colleagues, separated the serum and prepared saline suspensions of the red cells. Each serum was mixed with each cell suspension and in some mixtures the cells were agglutinated, in others they were not. On the basis of the reactions Landsteiner was able to divide human beings into three distinct groups. The fourth and rarest group was discovered by his pupils von Decastello and Sturli[3] in 1902.

Landsteiner saw that only two antigens were needed to explain the four groups of people: those with one (A), those with the other (B), those with both (AB) and those with neither (O). He recognized the reciprocal relationship in a sample blood of the antibodies in the serum to the antigens on the red cells. He showed that a person's serum does not contain the antibody for an antigen present in his own red cells, but that with very rare exceptions anti-A or anti-B (or both) are found in the serum when the red cells do not contain the corresponding antigen. The relationships are shown in Table 2.

Table 2. The ABO blood groups as defined by anti-A and anti-B

Blood groups	Antigens in red blood cells	Antibodies in serum
O	—	anti-A and anti-B
A	A	anti-B
B	B	anti-A
AB	A and B	none

In 1908 Epstein and Ottenberg[9] suggested that the ABO blood groups were inherited and the following two paragraphs are taken from their admirably brief paper:

8

The coincidence of a brother and sister, whose bloods were examined, belonging to the same agglutination group, led the authors to inquire whether this blood characteristic, which from the work of Hektoen and Gay seems to be a permanent characteristic of the individual, is hereditary. Hektoen tested a family, and found that the mother and three of the children belonged to group 1, and the remaining child to group 2. The authors tested two families. In the one the mother and seven children were all found to belong to group 2; the father could not be examined. In another family, mother, father, and four children all belonged to group 3. It seemed probably a coincidence that the father and mother were of the same group, but possibly a matter of heredity that the children were.

Before any definite conclusions can be reached on this point a great deal of careful work must be done, and the authors hope to present further studies later on. It seems, however, from the sharply opposed nature of these blood characteristics that if they are inherited at all they will form a very good example of the Mendelian law of heredity.

Bateson in his book *Mendel's Principles of Heredity*, published in 1909, begins the chapter on 'Evidence as to Mendelian inheritance in man' with the words:

Of Mendelian inheritance of *normal* characteristics in man there is as yet but little evidence. Only a single case has been established with any clearness; namely, that of eye colour.

That the groups were indeed inherited was proved by von Dungern and Hirszfeld[10] in 1910. Opinions of the precise manner of their inheritance varied until, in 1924, Bernstein[11,12] showed that the postulation of three alleles, A, B and O, fitted best the population and family data.

THE $A_1:A_2$ DISTINCTION

The groups A and AB are divided into A_1 and A_2 and A_1B and A_2B. Anti-A sera (from group B donors) contain two antibodies anti-A and anti-A_1; it is generally believed that A_1 has two antigens A, and A_1, while A_2 has only one, A:

		anti-A	
group	antigens	anti-A	anti-A_1
A_1	A A_1	+	+
A_2	A	+	−

It is unfortunate that 'anti-A' is used with two meanings, both for the anti-serum and for one of the antibodies in the serum. And so with the antigens: 'the antigen A' means the blood group antigen of an A_1 or A_2 person and it also means only that part of the whole A antigen which is common to A_1 and A_2. However, anti-A and A are seldom used in their restricted sense and it should be clear from the context when they are so used.

In 1911 von Dungern and Hirszfeld[4] first described subgroups of A, but our present way of looking at them derives from the papers of Thomsen, Friedenreich and Worsaae[5], Friedenreich and Zacho[6] and Friedenreich[7].

Anti-A_1 detectable at room temperature occurs naturally in the sera of 1–2% of A_2 people, and about 26% of A_2B people[8,24]. In Poland a much higher rate was found[568] in tests at 10°C: nearly 14% in A_2 and 51% in A_2B. A_2 reacts more weakly than A_1 with anti-A. Opinion seems still to be divided whether the A_1 A_2 difference is qualitative or whether it is quantitative and merely reflects differences in number of antigen sites (Juel[45], 1959; Mäkelä, Ruoslahti and Ehnholm[595], 1969). A few samples cannot be classified either as A_1 or as A_2 and they are usually called 'intermediates': they are discussed on page 17.

The distinguishing between A_1 and A_2 was revolutionized by Bird's introduction[152,153] of anti-A_1 preparations from the seeds of *Dolichos biflorus*.

The subgroups of A increase the number of phenotypes from four to six: A_1 A_2, B, A_1B, A_2B and O.

In 1930 Thomsen, Friedenreich and Worsaae[5] put forward the four allele theory of inheritance to include the subgroups A_1 and A_2, which extended the theory of Bernstein. The four allele theory was supported by tests on 103 families (Friedenreich and Zacho[6], 1931).

A child receives from each parent one of the four genes A_1, A_2, B or O, which as shown in Table 3 combine to make ten genotypes.

Table 3. The A_1A_2BO groups as defined by anti-A, anti-A_1 and anti-B

Genotypes	Phenotypes
A_1A_1	
A_1A_2	A_1
A_1O	
A_2A_2	A_2
A_2O	
BB	B
BO	
A_1B	A_1B
A_2B	A_2B
OO	O

Using the antisera anti-A, anti-B and anti-A_1, all of which are readily available, six phenotypes can be distinguished. Without the information which may be given by family groupings, the genotypes A_1A_1, A_1A_2, A_1O are indistinguishable, as are the genotypes BB and BO, and A_2A_2 and A_2O.

The exact genotype of A_1B, A_2B and O people is apparent. Although it is impossible to distinguish the exact genotype of A_1, A_2 and B people with the use of anti-A, anti-B and anti-A_1 sera, the genotypes are often disclosed by blood grouping other members of the family. For example, in the first family in Figure 1 it is clear from the blood groups of the two elder children that each of the parents must possess an O gene. The father, therefore, is of the genotype BO and the mother A_1O. In the second family the father and the girl twin are of the phenotype A_1, and without the evidence provided by the genotypes of the mother and the

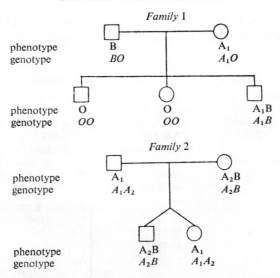

Fig. 1. The inheritance of the A_1A_2BO groups showing how genotypes may be disclosed by phenotypes of relatives.

boy twin their genotypes could not have been ascertained. The boy has received B from his mother and A_2 has come from his father, whose genotype must be A_1A_2. The girl of the phenotype A_1 has no B and must therefore have received A_2 from her mother; the genotype of the girl twin is consequently A_1A_2.

Finer points about the inheritance of the ABO groups are dealt with later in this chapter.

PHENOTYPE FREQUENCIES

During the 1914 war Hirszfeld and Hirszfeld[13] discovered that different peoples had different ABO group distributions. Since then hundreds of thousands of blood groups have been done for anthropological reasons from Tierra del Fuego to Lapland. A collection of the published results was made by Boyd[14] in 1939, by Mourant[15] in 1954, and, on a grand scale, by Mourant, Kopeć and Domaniewska-Sobczak[94] (1958) in *The ABO Blood Groups, Comprehensive Tables and Maps of World Distribution*. A record of the most detailed ABO blood analysis ever made of any country is *The Distribution of the Blood Groups in the United Kingdom* (1970) by Kopeć[580], compiled mainly from the records of the blood transfusion services. We hope that Dr Mourant's *magnum opus*, the second edition of *The Distribution of the Human Blood Groups and other Biochemical Polymorphisms*, will have appeared by the time this present book is published.

In Table 4 the results are shown of testing blood for the ABO groups at two levels of discrimination. The large numbers of Dobson and Ikin[18] may be taken as average for the whole of the United Kingdom. The samples were from airmen; it will be seen that the O and A ratios differ from those found in the wholly southern sample.

Table 4. ABO phenotype frequencies in Britain

Antisera Total	Dobson & Ikin[18] anti-A, -B 190,177 United Kingdom		Ikin et al.[19] anti-A, -A₁ & -B 3,459 S. England	
O	88,782 46·684%		O	1,503 43·45%
A	79,334 41·716%	A₁	1,204 34·81%	
		A₂	342 9·89%	
B	16,280 8·560%	B	297 8·59%	
AB	5,781 3·040%	A₁B	91 2·62%	
		A₂B	22 0·64%	

GENE FREQUENCIES

There are several reasons for finding out gene frequencies. They afford a more direct way of comparing the blood group content of different populations than do phenotype frequencies. They allow us to test the truth of theories concerning the manner of inheritance of the groups: knowing the gene frequencies we can calculate the expected frequency of children of different groups, from any type of mating. Most useful of all we can use the gene frequencies to show that a sample contains a reasonable distribution of the groups, and we can then take confidence in our technique.

Except in anthropological work, when computer methods are likely to be used, the calculation of ABO gene frequencies must be a very rare event nowadays. For this reason we are not repeating the various formulae given in previous editions. The references, however, are still in: (i) ABO: Bernstein[25], Taylor and Prior[26], Stevens[32], Fisher and Taylor[16], Dobson and Ikin[18], Fraser Roberts[22]; (ii) A₁A₂BO; Wellisch and Thomsen[31], Stevens[32], Hartmann, Hadland and Bjerkelund[27], Hartmann and Lundevall[28].

Gene frequencies in Britain

From the phenotype frequencies of Table 4 the following gene frequencies were calculated

$$O \quad 0\cdot6831$$
$$A \quad 0\cdot2569$$
$$B \quad 0\cdot0600$$

which may be taken as representative of the United Kingdom as a whole, and

$$O \quad 0\cdot6602$$
$$A_1 \quad 0\cdot2090$$
$$A_2 \quad 0\cdot0696$$
$$B \quad 0\cdot0612$$

which may be taken as representative of South England.

Phenotype and genotype frequencies based on these South English gene frequencies are in Table 5.

Table 5. Calculated frequencies of the A_1A_2BO phenotypes and genotypes in South England

Phenotypes		Genotypes			
O	0·4359	OO	0·4359		
A_1	0·3488	A_1A_1	0·0437	or 0·1253	
		A_1O	0·2760	or 0·7913	of all A_1
		A_1A_2	0·0291	or 0·0834	
A_2	0·0967	A_2A_2	0·0048	or 0·0496	of all A_2
		A_2O	0·0919	or 0·9504	
B	0·0845	BB	0·0037	or 0·0438	of all B
		BO	0·0808	or 0·9562	
A_1B	0·0256	A_1B	0·0256		
A_2B	0·0085	A_2B	0·0085		

ANALYSIS OF FAMILIES

Wiener[33] collected from the literature and critically analysed a vast body of data concerning the inheritance of the ABO groups. As a result it can be said that, however our ideas concerning the precise mechanism of inheritance may change, the triple allele theory of Bernstein is adequate for all practical purposes.

Wiener was able to collect from the literature over a thousand families tested for the A_1A_2BO groups and concluded 'that there could be no doubt regarding the accuracy of the theory of Thomsen, Friedenreich and Worsaae[5] in principle, despite the existence of one or two conflicting cases'. Wiener considered that most of the discrepancies were probably due to rare forms of the A antigen intermediate between A_1 and A_2—an opinion which has been confirmed by Wiener, Gordon and Cohen[34] (1954) who analysed 1,590 families tested in Dr Wiener's laboratory between 1929 and 1952.

We are not going to repeat the classical methods of analysing these families; they are admirably set out by Wiener[33]. Nor will we give here Fisher's method of analysis. The analysis of A_1A_2BO families must nowadays be rather a special event, in which the original and lucid account of Fisher's method, given by Taylor and Prior[35], should be consulted. (There are errors in the description of the treatment of the mating $A_1B \times B$, see Race, Ikin, Taylor and Prior[36].)

The various genetical and environmental modifications to be mentioned below must not be allowed to shake our confidence in the simple Mendelian inheritance of the groups. In the extremely rare cases where red cell antigens are inhibited the groups are abnormal and can be recognized as such; and the same applies to the *cis* AB condition, however it may alter our view of the fine structure of the *ABO* locus.

Linkage relations of the *ABO* locus

The *ABO* locus is within direct measurable distance of the locus for the nail-patella syndrome, *Np*, and the locus for the enzyme adenylate kinase, *AK*, but details are reserved for the chapter on blood groups and autosomal linkage.

THE PHENOTYPE A_3

This kind of blood was first recognized by Friedenreich[37] in 1936. The appearance of the agglutination caused by anti-A and by most group O (anti-A + B) sera is characteristic: very small clumps vastly outnumbered by unagglutinated cells. A_3 cells do not react with anti-A_1. Secretors of group A_3 have A substance in their saliva.

Friedenreich and later workers (notably Gammelgaard) considered the gene responsible for A_3 to be an allele at the A_1A_2BO locus. Gammelgaard's magnificent thesis[38] on the weak forms of A is now available in English[17]. He estimates that A_3 is found once in about a thousand Danish A people. Nevertheless he was able to test 26 families which included 170 A_3 members and 33 A_3B members in a total of 726 persons. (The incidence seems to be lower in Canada[20].)

Gammelgaard[38] wrote 'In the sera from 58 A_3 persons, no instance of an irregular α_1, active at room temperature, could be demonstrated.' And this has been the experience of Friedenreich[37]. Dunsford[108], on the other hand, found anti-A_1 in the serum of two out of 11 cases of A_3.

Cotterman[39] suggested that A_3 blood is a mosaic of A_2 and O, the result perhaps of gene controlled mutation. But this does not square with Gammelgaard's findings, that the cells which are not agglutinated by anti-A nevertheless combine with it; nor does it fit his observation[38], confirmed by Dunsford[108], that group O (anti-A + B) sera exist which can agglutinate all the cells of people of the genotype A_3O. The use of fluorescent anti-A has given somewhat contradictory results: Cohen and Zuelzer[21] found that the majority of cells of two A_3 samples did not fluoresce whereas Reed[20] found a marked cell to cell variability in fluorescence. It seems that A_3 truly is a weaker form belonging to the A_1A_2 series and that it is controlled by an allele properly called A_3.

The diagnosis of A_3B, unsupported by family evidence, should be taken with a grain of salt. Several families have been reported[40,41,109,23], showing that an apparent A_3B may be of the genotype A_2B.

An A_3 always presents a lively problem. It has to be distinguished from chimeras and other mixtures of blood and from a leukaemic change.

THE LAST FIFTY YEARS

We sometimes wonder whether since 1911, or say 1925 to take in Bernstein, the only contributions of the first magnitude to the system are to be found in the biochemical work on the ABH substances and in the work on the 'Bombay' phenotype; and in the recognition of the *cis* AB phenomenon and perhaps, on a more practical level, the finding of specific agglutinins in extracts of seeds and snails.

OTHER ABO VARIANTS

The subdivision between A_1 and A_2 is well established and most laboratories would probably classify them alike, and perhaps A_3 as well. But there are weaker forms of A (and of B) all of which are rare, and innumerable papers have been written about them, often with fine pedigrees showing how precisely the peculiarity is inherited.

Phenotypically there are two main groups of weak A which we may call A_x type and A_m type:

A_x type   Cells: negative or weak reaction with anti-A, good reaction with anti-A + B.
           Serum: no, or very weak, anti-A but usually anti-A_1.
           Saliva (if secretor): H but no A.
A_m type   Cells: negative or weak with anti-A and anti-A + B.
           Serum: no anti-A or anti-A_1.
           Saliva (if secretor): A and H.

The cells of both phenotypes react strongly with anti-H. Some rare weak forms of A, such as those called A_{end} and A_{el}, do not fit this phenotype classification but in spite of that we have found it useful. Rare types of B analogous to A_x and A_m are known.

The study of these phenotypes has been illuminated by work (to be described below) on the 'Bombay' phenotype, on the acquired B phenotype and on the phenotypes of certain patients with leukaemia. As a result three possible causes of variations of A or B have, so far, become clear:

1 Rare alleles of *ABO*.
2 Action of other genes on normal *ABO* genes.
3 Action of environment on normal *ABO* genes.

The A_m phenotype has been found with all three backgrounds, and A_x with the first and probably with the second also.

1. Variations due to rare alleles of *ABO*

The majority of weak As and weak Bs are dominant characters: they are, of course, masked by the presence of normal A or B antigen.

A_x (A_4, A_5, A_z, A_0)

This extremely rare type of blood was first clearly described by Fischer and Hahn[51] in 1935. The red cells distinguish themselves by the following agglutination reactions: negative or weak with anti-A sera, negative with anti-B, but positive with most group O sera (anti-A + B) and positive with anti-H. The agglutination by O sera is general and quite unlike that of A_3 cells which is remarkable for the vast number of cells left unagglutinated. Though A_x cells are not agglutinated by anti-A, eluates show that they must combine with it. The serum of A_x people usually contains anti-A_1[108,110]. A_x secretors have H but no A in their saliva, although traces of A have been detected on occasion[23,29,30,526]. According to Salmon[111] A_x occurs once in about 40,000 donors in France.

The phenotype is probably heterogeneous. In some of the reported families the inheritance appears straightforward, A_x apparently being an allele at the *ABO* locus (Gammelgaard[38]; Jonsson and Fast[50]; Dunsford and Aspinall[52]; Dunsford[53]; Estola and Elo[55]; Grove-Rasmussen, Soutter and Levine[54]; Ellis and Cawley[56]; Fine, Eyquem and Thébault[112]; Glover and Walford[113]; Salmon[29,111]; Vos[30]). In other families, however, the inheritance is not straightforward[57,58,59,29,62,526,527].

The subject was well reviewed in 1965 by Salmon, Salmon and Reviron[29].

Until A_x becomes clearer the original notation of Fischer and Hahn seems preferable to the later synonyms. The synonyms are the result, in our opinion, of too fine splitting of hairs. A_x can vary in its expression even within one family. For example, in the family reported by Dr Cahan and his colleagues it was noted that only two of the seven carriers of A_x gave identical A_x reactions. Dunsford[108], on the other hand, in testing ten families found that 'all members of the same family gave identical reactions, some through three generations, although there were variations from family to family'.

Wiener et al.[528] still hold to their earlier opinion[60] that cells of the type we are discussing have no A but are group C (page 49). But this opinion ignores the repeated demonstrations that these cells do indeed react in some way with anti-A from group B people (Dunsford[53], Cahan et al.[59], Alter and Rosenfield[23], Salmon et al.[29], Poskitt and Fortwengler[663]).

A_m

This phenotype is also very rare. Examples usually present themselves as group O with missing anti-A; the cells react strongly with anti-H. Then the cells are found to adsorb anti-A as shown by its subsequent elution and, if the person is a secretor, A as well as H is found in the saliva.

As we have said, the phenotype can have different causes and the subject is returned to later. That an allele of ABO can be responsible has been shown clearly by Salmon and his colleagues[114, 67], by Kindler[115], by Hrubiško and his colleagues[69, 70] and by Serim[529]. In a splendid investigation Hrubiško and his colleagues[70] tested six kindred and found two probable homozygotes, the product of a first cousin marriage.

'Intermediates', A_{int}

A kind of A intermediate in its reaction with anti-A_1 was first noted by Landsteiner and Levine[116] and further studied by Friedenreich and Zacho[6]. A_{int} is commoner in Negroes than in Whites: Wiener[117] found 5 in 59 Negro group A samples and 3 in 332 Caucasian group A samples. Bird[103] found 15 in 730 group A Maharastrian Indians. Using quantitative methods, Grundbacher and Summerlin[570] classified as A_{int} 31·6% of 114 group A Virginian Negroes and 2·5% of 199 Virginian Whites.

Instead of sandwiching intermediates between A_1 and A_2 we have put them in this section, for the following reason. We were given the opportunity to test two samples, one sent by Dr Hässig and one by Miss Sausais[118]. To our surprise we found that these cells react more strongly with anti-H than do A_2 cells. The observations on the first sample were very elegantly confirmed by Bird[119] by means of absorption curves. If A_{int} were intermediate between A_1 and A_2 the anti-H reactions should be intermediate too: it looks as if they are in a distinct class of their own. A_{int} is common in the Bantu, and Brain[93] further confirmed the strong reaction with anti-H.

A_{end} and A_{finn}

A weak A, apparently due to an allele of ABO, but which can be labelled neither A_x nor A_m, was described by W. Weiner, Sanger and Race[120], and was later named A_{end}[106]. It was found in two generations of a family and looked like an abnormally weak A_3 but the saliva of all three carriers contained H but no A.

Two similar examples were found in Canada[182,183]; the family of one propositus was available and showed the condition to be inherited. Another example was reported from Australia[135] and three families from France[530,531].

A very weak A which can only be distinguished with difficulty from A_{end} is reported by Mohn et al.[665] (1973). The distinction depends mainly on the weak reaction with anti-A being improved by enzymes in the case of A_{finn} but not in that of A_{end}. The antigen is commoner in Finland than anywhere else tested. Nevanlinna and Pirkola[671] (1973), in an admirable population study, investigated no less than 128 propositi and the families of many of them.

A_{el}

This A is even weaker than A_{end}: the A antigen can be demonstrated only by elution; the saliva of secretors contains H but no A. Reed and Moore[136] recognized the phenotype in an Italian Canadian donor apparently group O but lacking anti-A: her sister had the same phenotype. The inheritance of the condition was confirmed in three generations of an American family[137]. Further examples have been found in America, Sweden and West Germany[106], and in France[532]. An example in a Negro is also reported[533].

A_{bantu}

Brain[93] describes this interesting variant of A which he finds in 4% of Bantu A samples. The pattern of agglutination of the red cells is like that of A_3 but the saliva of secretors contains H but no A, and anti-A_1 is regularly present in the serum. As Brain points out, the phenotype appears to fall between A_3 and A_{end}. Jenkins[534] found the incidence of A_{bantu} to be 1 or 2% in 6000 South African Negroes of various tribes but up to 8% in the 'Bushman' and 'Hottentot' people.

Other A variants

Gold and Dunsford[158] described a curious form of A_1 the inheritance of which was not made clear by the groups of the family in which it occurred. Re-read 13 years later the puzzle remains.

A mixture of A and O cells was reported by Furuhata, Kitahama and Nozawa[162,184]. The condition was found in a Japanese man and in four of the six of his children who were tested. There are one or two misprints in the pedigree so that it appears that some of the members have mixtures of blood on other systems. The condition must not be confused with a chimera. We were kindly given the opportunity to test one of the members and found that some of his cells reacted like A_1, others like A_2 and the rest like weaker A.

The subject of A antigen strength is returned to under the heading 'quantitative measurements'.

Weak B

Variants of B are even rarer than variants of A, perhaps, as Boyd points out, because most of the work has gone on in countries where B is relatively infrequent. On the other hand, in Japan, where the incidence of group A is about twice that of group B, Yamaguchi, Okubo and Tanaka[535] in an immense survey found a much higher incidence of weak B than weak A.

During the course of the survey the same authors[535] encountered the first example of B_x, corresponding in its reactions to A_x. The propositus was A_1B_x, his father B_x and a sib B_x. The cells of the two B_x members were not agglutinated by anti-B but were agglutinated by most anti-A + B sera: fixation-elution tests with anti-B were, however, positive. Their saliva contained H but no B, and weak anti-B was present in their serum.

The cells of all other weak B examples we have read about or worked with reacted weakly or not at all with anti-B and with anti-A + B and strongly with anti-H. They may be placed in three categories. Those in category 1 have often been called B_v. By analogy with A_m, those in category 2 may be called B_m. Those in category 3 have been called B_3 and B_x but, by analogy with A_3 and A_x, neither name is appropriate.

1. *Anti-B in serum*; *B of some kind in saliva*

Mäkelä and Mäkelä[63]: A Finnish propositus with five group O sibs. Boorman and Zeitlin[185, 138]: apparently a dominant character found in two generations of an English family; the anti-B of the propositus reacted with all B cells tested except her own, her father's and those of the Mäkeläs' propositus. Bennett *et al.*[139]: three members of a Polish family. Battaglini *et al.*[471]: a donor with no living relatives. Ruoslahti *et al.*[486]; four members of a Finnish family (only one of whom secreted their special family B though all four secreted H). Hrubiško[572]: twelve members of a Czechoslovakian kindred.

Previously we headed this section boldly '*Anti-B in serum*; *B in saliva*' but a suggestion by Schneider[536] made us look again at the papers cited and climb down a little, for usually the salivary B had been demonstrated when the test system was anti-B with the person's own weak B cells as indicator: so perhaps the saliva contained only a fraction of the normal B antigen. The family investigated by Schneider[536] which turned his thoughts to this problem, and the father and son described by Mayr *et al.*[569], may belong to category 1, but Schneider thought a further category was probably needed.

2. *No anti-B in serum (or very weak cold anti-B)*; *B in saliva*

Levine, Celano and Griset[65]: a dominant character, called B_w, found in several members of a negro family. Yokoyama, Stacey and Dunsford[66, 176]: a dominant character, called B_x, in three members of a Japanese family. Yokoyama, Barber and Dunsford[186]: a dominant character in a Japanese family. Liotta, Russo and

Gandini[338]: in a Roman donor with no available relatives. Kout and Totin[143]: one member of a Prague family, considered B_x. Yamaguchi, Okubo, Hazama and Oyama[144]: three Japanese families, two of them showing the character to be dominant; the notation B_x was used. Furukawa and Iseki[145]: a dominant character in a Japanese family; notation B_m. Ikemoto, Kuniyuki and Furuhata[231]: a large Japanese family also illustrating dominance; notation B_m. Simmons and Kwa[489]: five members of two Chinese families. Sathe *et al.*[537]: seven members of a Bombay family also illustrating dominance; notation B_m. Garlick and Maldre[538]: two Canadian sisters; notation B_m. Moores[539]: eleven members of an Indian kindred. Ikemoto *et al.*[540, 541]: thirteen members of a Japanese kindred; notation B_m. Kogure and Iseki[542]: a three generation Japanese family with some disturbance of the normal inheritance; notation B_m.

3. *No anti-B in serum*; *H but no (or doubtful) B in saliva*

Moullec, Sutton and Burgada[64]: a dominant character, called B_3, in a French family. Vyas, Bhatia and Sanghvi[187]: a dominant character in three members of an Indian family. Sussman, Pretshold and Lacher[188]: a dominant character, called B_3, in an American mother of Italian extraction and her daughter. Bhatia, Undevia and Sanghvi[232]: an obviously important family, father O, mother A_1B, not consanguineous, one A_1 and two weak B offspring (called B_3); a modifying gene was considered a possible cause. Alter and Rosenfield[233]: one member of an American family; the condition is called B_x. Sathe *et al.*[537]: four members in four generations of an Indian family; notation B_x. Wiener and Cioffi[668]: two members of a negro family with only about a tenth of their cells giving the reaction of B, the rest that of O; as both were non-secretors our putting them in this category is questionable; the authors favoured the explanation suggested by Cotterman (page 14) for A_3; the condition was called B_3.

Something very like B_2 is described in a Greek mother and her two children by Jakobowicz, Simmons and Whittingham[339].

Other categories of weak B are dealt with later in this chapter under the headings B_h, acquired B, 'Is the *ABO* locus complex?' and 'quantitative measurements'.

2. Variations due to the action of other genes

Genes that are detected only by their effect on the expression of other genes are called modifying genes. The first precise knowledge of such genes in man is being gained from the study of the ABO groups. The secretor genes provided the first example but they are reserved for Chapter 8. None of the modifying genes so far recognized is linked to the *ABO* locus.

The 'Bombay' or O_h phenotype

The 'Bombay' phenotype is peculiar both in red cells and in serum: the cells are not agglutinated by anti-A, anti-B or anti-H and the serum contains anti-A, anti-B and anti-H. The cells are usually Le(a+). The condition is very rare but, as often happens, this observation of almost the least common variety in a system was to illuminate the whole. In the original description (Bhende, Deshpande, Bhatia, Sanger, Race, Morgan and Watkins[42], 1952) it was suggested that a 'new' allele at the *ABO* locus was the easiest explanation, but Ceppellini[43], on the contrary, suggested that an inhibitor gene was involved.

Later, but with no less foresight, Watkins and Morgan[192] wrote 'There remains the possibility that the H character is the result of the presence of a genetically independent blood group system *H-h*. The "Indian" type of bloods are completely devoid of H character and could therefore be homozygous for the rare allele of *H* i.e. *hh*.' With subsequent biochemical support this was to become the basis of the

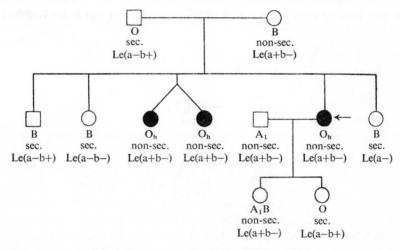

Fig. 2. Suppression of the blood group antigen B in a carrier of the gene *B*. O_h = 'Bombay' phenotype; arrow = propositus; the parents of the propositus are first cousins. (After Levine, Robinson, Celano, Briggs and Falkinburg[44], 1955.)

current way of looking at the genetical background of the ABO groups (see page 59).

Ceppellini's brilliant prediction of inhibition was shown to be right by Levine, Robinson, Celano, Briggs and Falkinburg[44] when they found, in an American family of Italian extraction, three more examples of the peculiar blood. The groups of the family (Figure 2) made it clear that the 'Bombay' propositus has no new kind of *ABO* allele but has an unexpressed but normal *B* allele which she has inherited from her mother and handed on to her elder daughter. It will be seen from the pedigree that the inheritance of secretion and of the Le^a antigen of the red cells is also disturbed. (This aspect of the problem is returned to on pages 312 and 342.)

Levine and his colleagues postulated the existence of 'a rare suppressor gene which in the homozygous state suppresses in the propositus the actions of gene *B* and secretor gene *Se*. The genes *B* and *Se* are fully expressed when transmitted to

2*

her offspring who are heterozygous for the suppression gene.' The rare gene was called x and its frequent allele X, and for the phenotype the symbol O_h was introduced. The gene symbols H and h have now generally replaced the original X and x. Figure 3 shows the important part of the family interpreted in terms of the Hh genes. We find it easier to think of the suppression as due to the absence of H rather than to the presence of two h, but this is merely a matter of choice.

Although in practice it makes no difference whether the symbols hh or xx are used to describe the genetic background of the Bombay condition they do represent two distinct outlooks. On the one hand, h is an allele at the H locus, on the other, x is an allele at an unknown locus X, perhaps unlinked to H, but which modifies or regulates the activity of H.

At first we preferred the hh interpretation as seeming the more economical, but now that we have come round to thinking that various lesser Bombay-like

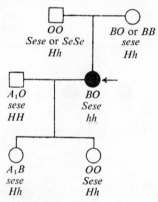

Fig. 3. Part of the previous pedigree (Figure 2) showing the ABO and secretor genotypes in the light of the Hh genes. (After Levine, Robinson, Celano, Briggs and Falkinburg[44], 1955.)

conditions (see below) are due to a modifying locus, Z, perhaps, for consistency, we ought to hold equally in mind the xx and hh interpretation of the Bombay phenotype. However, the difference is academic, for at present there seems no way of deciding between the two.

Other examples of O_h were soon found[46,47,48,194,195,240] but no further demonstration of inhibition was provided until 1961 when four families were reported: in one the inhibition again was of B and H and in another it was either of A and H or of B and H, the groups of the relatives did not show which (Hakim, Vyas, Sanghvi and Bhatia[196]).

That O_h could be the manifestation of inhibition of A_1 and A_2 as well as of B and H was ultimately demonstrated by two American families, one of English and the other of French extraction (Aloysia, Gelb, Fudenberg, Hamper, Tippett and Race[193], 1961). The inhibition of A_1, A_2 and B antigens, as well as H, was confirmed: A_1 in an American family[243], B in an American family[249], A_2 in a Dutch family[281], and A_1 and B in a French family[285].

At the suggestion of Dr Levine the symbol O_h was given a superscript, O_h^B, $O_h^{A_1}$, $O_h^{A_2}$, when family tests showed which antigen had been inhibited.

As with other rare recessive characters the parents of *hh* people have a high consanguinity rate[287,197].

The red cells of O_h people usually give the reaction Le(a+b−). An Le(a−b−) example is reported by Giles, Mourant and Atabuddin[294]. This is compatible with the 'genetical pathway' diagrams on page 61 and page 342: the saliva of the propositus contained no ABH, Le^a or Le^b substance. (An earlier example of O_h Le(a−) may have been found, but doubts were expressed about the condition of the sample[46].)

Further examples of O_h Le(a−b−) people have been found: the propositus in an Italian family (Gandini *et al.*[550], 1968); two sibs in a Canadian family (Pretty *et al.*[543], 1969); three sibs in a Natal Indian family (Moores[544], 1972). The last two families were particularly useful: that from Canada[543] strongly suggested that the *Hh* genes were not controlled from the *Le* locus and that from Natal[544] proved it. In the Natal family the father is *Hh lele* and the mother *Hh Lele*; three of the children are O_h, one of them *hh Lele* and two *hh lele*, at least one child must reflect recombination between the two loci.

This seems to clear the air of a further theory about the Bombay background: Yunis *et al.*[545] (1969) investigated a large inbred Orissa family in which O_h was present in two generations and the constellation of H and Lewis groups led them to postulate that the *H* and *Lewis* loci are adjacent, and to build an elaborate theory thereon involving unequal crossing-over. However, the Natal family seems to us rather to shake the foundations of this ingenious idea.

As Levine and his colleagues[44] pointed out, this apparent exception to the known manner of inheritance of the ABO groups does not in any way affect the use of these groups in medico-legal problems—the presence in a serum of anti-H, anti-A and anti-B shows that it cannot belong to a person of group O.

The antibodies in the serum of O_h people are referred to on page 51.

Independence of the Hh genes

The *Hh* genes are not sited at any of the following loci, *ABO, secretor, MNSs, P, Rh, Duffy* or *Kidd*, nor are they on the sex chromosomes[193]. To this list *Lewis*, referred to above [544], can now be added, and so can *Kell*[546]. The methods of reasoning behind such statements are given on page 411.

Eluates from O_h cells

Though Levine *et al.*[44] in their classical paper had adumbrated the possibility of elution tests as a key to the underlying Bombay ABO groups it was really Lanset, Ropartz, Rousseau, Guerbet and Salmon[285] (1966) who altered our way of thinking of the O_h phenotypes when they demonstrated that the suppressed A or B antigens could be identified, without recourse to family studies, by fixation-elution tests. They found this out when testing a fine family with four sibs, three of whom could be shown to be O_h^{AB} and one O_h^B.

The same observation was made, independently, by Mr A.G. Gelb when re-testing the $O_h^{A_1}$ family reported by Aloysia et al.[193]: at the earlier testing our attempts to make eluates were unsuccessful. The most extensive elution tests we know of were reported from Poland (Dzierzkowa-Borodej et al.[546], 1972).

So the A and B antigens of O_h red cells, though unfit for agglutination, must be present in some form.

The frequency of O_h

Four O_h people, all Indian, have been found as a result of the testing of random cell samples, and this allowed Bhatia and Sanghvi[197] to calculate that the phenotype has a frequency of one in about 13,000 Marathi-speaking people in and around Bombay. After applying some correction for inbreeding they estimated that the corresponding frequency of the gene h in these people is 0·0066. The phenotype must be very rare indeed in Europeans for many million blood donors must have been appropriately tested but without, as far as we know, the finding of a single O_h person. In Table 6, where an attempt is made to relate the serological reactions of Bombay and certain para-Bombay conditions, the number of O_h references gives an exaggerated idea of the frequency in Whites.

Since the last edition of this book many unreported examples of O_h must have been found, having selected themselves out of an unknown multitude by trouble arising from the anti-H in their serum. 'Bombay' cells and serum now have almost a routine place in the investigation of many blood group problems and the donors who give the samples and the transfusion services which distribute them are much to be thanked.

Glycosyltransferases in O_h sera

Recent work by Watkins and her colleagues[547-549] beautifully demonstrated that α-2-L-fucosyltransferase, the H gene product present in all normal sera, is absent from the serum of O_h persons. O_h^A sera have α-N-acetylgalactosaminyltransferase and O_h^B have α-D-galactosyltransferase and O_h^{AB} have both, but these enzymes cannot work in the absence of H from the red cells.

Para-Bombay phenotypes

In 1961, Levine, Uhlíř and White[334] reported the first example of a Bombay-like condition which they called A_h. The cells of a Czechoslovakian nurse, like O_h cells, did not react with anti-H but, unlike O_h, reacted weakly in straight agglutination tests with anti-A. Her serum contained anti-H and she was a non-secretor. The ABO groups of her family were unremarkable and a 'partial suppressor' was thought to be the most likely explanation.

In a fine investigation of a Catawba Indian family Solomon, Waggoner and Leyshon[313] (1965) found that the cells of three brothers, one of the phenotype O and two of A_x, failed to react with anti-H. Nevertheless, the saliva of all three contained H, and A was present in the saliva of the two A_x brothers. The sera of all three contained virtually no anti-H. The parents were consanguineous and the character was considered to be recessive. The phenotype notation O_m^h and A_m^h was proposed.

Since 1965 some fine families showing the effect of 'partial suppressors' have been reported and we have attempted to classify them in Table 6, which also shows, for comparison, the reactions of O_h cells. All the conditions are recessive and, as in O_h, the *A* or *B* alleles express themselves normally in parents and offspring. As expected, the consanguinity rate of the parents is high.

It may be seen in Table 6 that the essential phenotypic differences between O_h (row I) and A_h or B_h (row II) is that the A or B of the latter cells can be detected by

Table 6. Recessive Bombay and para-Bombay phenotypes

Row	Usual notation of phenotype	Reaction of red cells with anti- A B A+B H				Anti-H in serum	Antigens in saliva A B H			References
I	O_h O_h^A, O_h^B, O_h^{AB}	−	−	−	−	yes	−	−	−	Indians: 42,46,47,194,196,294, 544,545 Whites: 44,48,193,195,240,243, 249,281,285,543,546,550,573 Japanese: 551 Negroes: none
II	A_h B_h	± −	− ±	± ±	−* −	yes	−	−	−	Czech: Levine et al.[334]; Beranova et al.[552] French Canadian: Molthan[480] La Réunion: Liberge et al.[553]; Gerard et al.[554]
III	O_{Hm} or O_m^h O_{Hm}^A or A_m^h O_{Hm}^B or B_m^h	− ± −	− − ±	− ± ±	−* − −	probably no*	− + −	− − +	+ + +	American Indian: Solomon et al.[313] Japanese: Kitahama et al.[315]; Yamaguchi et al.[555]; Kogure et al.[556] French: Lewi[468] Sicilian: Fawcett et al.[557] Czech: Hrubiško et al.[558] Thai: Sringarm et al.[559] Singapore Chinese: Albrey[560] Persian: Rogers[561] Dutch: v.d. Hart[562]

±, When + always much weaker than A_2 or B controls.
* See text.

straight agglutination methods without the need of fixation-elution tests: the reactions with anti-A+B sera are stronger than with anti-A or anti-B.

The essential phenotypic difference between A_h and B_h (row II) and the variously termed samples of row III is that row II are non-secretors and row III are secretors (having normal amounts of A, B or H substances).

Hrubiško and his colleagues[558] in reporting the investigation of a large inbred Czechoslovak family with antigens suppressed in red cells but not in saliva (our row III) suggested that O_{Hm}, O_{Hm}^A, O_{Hm}^B, O_{Hm}^{AB} was a more appropriate notation than the O_m^h, A_m^h etc. which had previously been used. With this we agree and shall, with apologies, sometimes translate in quoting the work of others.

Bhatia[341,342,563] tested samples from three of the earlier families[334,313,315] of rows II and III and showed a small amount of H to be present on their red cells. Sringarm, Chupungart and Giles[559] noted that O_{Hm} (row III) cells although H negative as judged by *Ulex* did react with some anti-H from O_h people, and we also had noticed that some of these human anti-H sera reacted with A_h and O_{Hm}^A cells[480,561,562].

People in row I and row II have anti-H in their serum: those in row III are often reported as having anti-H, usually it is said to be rather weak and there is seldom mention of inhibition checks on the antibody. Sringarm and her colleagues[559] report that the apparent anti-H in their family was not inhibited by O secretor saliva and was therefore probably anti-HI; and we also found the apparent anti-H in three more row III propositi was not inhibited by secretor saliva. We guess that the row III antibody never is anti-H but is the sometime 'anti-O' now called anti-HI.

Several genetical theories have been suggested for the background of these near-Bombay phenotypes of rows II and III. For row II type a third allele at the Hh locus is proposed[334,342,552,553], one which produces only a limited amount of H substance which becomes completely converted into a small amount of A or B. For row III type, with their normal salivary antigens, a different locus, sometimes called Zz, is proposed[313,315,558,556,557] which controls the synthesis of red cell antigens only: row III people being zz.

Yamaguchi et al.[555] consider Z (which they call *Es*) to be a regulator gene controlling 'the expression of the H gene at sites of biosynthesis of the secreted glycoproteins'—a regulator opposite in its effects to the regulator secretor gene *Se*.

We would like to put forward a more economical suggestion that row II and row III have the same genetical background, say zz, which allows H etc. in saliva but no H in the red cells, and that row II people are zz, $sese$ and row III zz, Se. Incidentally this fits well the observation made by one of us[141] some years ago that anti-H is made by non-secretors and 'anti-O' (anti-HI) by secretors. We can find nothing in the published families to contradict this suggestion. If it is correct, and if the Zz locus is not very closely linked to the *secretor* locus, one could expect to find row II and row III people in the same sibship. Indeed, in the remarkable family of Hrubiško et al.[558], one sib secretes only traces of H and B (? row II) while the propositus and two other sibs secrete plenty (row III). Available details of row II families happen so far not to be informative about whether they may include row III members.

However, our idea would collapse if an A_h or B_h (row II) person with a non-secretor spouse produced a secretor child—that is, if the action of the Se gene were shown to be suppressed in this phenotype as it is in O_h (row I).

If homozygosity for a rare allele, zz, proves to be the correct background to rows II and III, then it could be argued that the notation A_h and B_h should be changed to O^A_{Hm} and O^B_{Hm} leaving their non-secretor, $sese$, symbols to show that they are in row II and not in row III. A precedent for this would be that in the symbols for the ABO groups of red cells no need is felt for indication of the secretor status. Presumably O^0_{Hm} non-secretors would be phenotypically indistinguishable from O^0_h except for a weak reaction of the cells of the former with some anti-H sera from O_h people.

The incidence of these para-Bombay phenotypes is unknown outside Thailand where Sringarm et al.[559] found 6 unrelated examples in 29,708 donors, a frequency of 0·02%. This was the fruit of including Ulex extract in their routine tests.

Schenkel-Brunner, Chester and Watkins[548] tested the serum of one B_h propositus[553] and found the B gene enzyme, α-galactosyltransferase, to be present in normal amounts but found no H enzyme, α-2-L-fucosyltransferase, an echo from a deeper level, of the serological message.

The evidence for the Yy genes

Evidence for the existence of a very common gene Y which is necessary for the development of the A antigen in red cells is given by W. Weiner, Lewis, Moores, Sanger and Race[49]. The Yy genes were invented to explain the following observations in two families.

The groups of the family of a healthy donor of the phenotype A_m proved that his genotype was A_1O. His cells were not agglutinated by anti-A but they could adsorb it; they were strongly agglutinated by anti-H. His serum contained anti-B but no anti-A and his saliva contained A and H substance.

The second example of what we presumed to be the same condition was found in a healthy person of the phenotype A_mB but whose genotype was shown, by the groups of her family, to be A_1B. Her cells were not agglutinated by anti-A nor did they adsorb detectable amounts of anti-A. (The A is known to be somewhat depressed in AB people and to this we attributed the difference in adsorptive behaviour of the two examples.) Her serum contained no antibody; her saliva contained A, B and H. Dr Weiner retested this perfectly healthy person five years after the first test: there was no change in the reactions of the red cells, serum or saliva.

We assumed that the absence of the gene Y, that is in the genotype yy, inhibits the development of the A antigen in the red cells but not in the saliva: Y is evidently not necessary for the development of B or H antigens. One of the families showed that the postulated Yy genes cannot be closely linked to the ABO locus.

Other examples of A_m and A_mB were reported[198,199], but the family groups did not disclose whether the phenotypes represented alleles of *ABO* or the effect of modifying genes. Environmental changes (e.g. leukaemia) can be excluded in the first case and are unlikely in the second for the propositus was a donor. The example of Darnborough *et al.*[564], on the other hand, was clearly the effect of modifying genes, for the family groups showed the A_m person to be of the genotype A_1O and, presumably, *yy*. The saliva, like that of the original case[49], contained less A and more H than the saliva of A_1 secretor controls.

Recessive inhibition of B

Though obviously not caused by the *yy* genes (which do not affect[49] the B antigen) this seems a convenient place to refer to analogous B phenotypes described by Gundolf and Andersen[565] and by Marsh *et al.*[664]. The cells of the first propositus[565] lack B but have H, her serum lacks anti-B, her saliva has H but only a little B. Though these reactions ape those of other weak B examples (page 19) the condition is recessive since her parents are both *BO* with normal B antigens. The second propositus[664] differed in that his saliva contained a lot of B; but he also must have a normal *B* gene for his father is O and his mother A_2B and his sibs A_2 and B.

Dominant inhibition of A and B

A good case for the existence of a dominant suppressor of both A and B (but not H) was made by Rubinstein *et al.*[672] (1973) from examination of a family in which two half-brothers were, at any rate superficially, group O, but one of them lacked anti-A and the other anti-B. A built in suppressor, rather than an unlinked suppressor, was favoured in this case.

Other possible genetic modifications

In this section are gathered some conditions that do not fit easily into our attempted classification though this may mean that they are all the more significant.

Though the phenotype A_x is apparently controlled in most families by an allele of ABO, other families strongly suggest that the phenotype can also be caused by modifying genes: van Loghem and van der Hart[57] and Beckers, van Loghem and Dunsford[58] reported two families in which A_x children occurred though both parents were group O, and McGuire *et al.*[527] report yet another A_x with both parents O.

Cahan *et al.*[59, 62] reported a family in which an A_2B man transmitted A_x to his daughter; A_x was present in three generations. Similar families are: father A_2B, mother O, six children A_x and one B (Salmon *et al.*[29]); father O, mother A_1, two children O, three A_x and three A_1 (Lanset *et al.*[526]); father A_x, mother B, three children A_x, three children A_2B, one of the A_2B children is married to an O and they have an A_x child. In this last family A_x was found in four generations (Ducos *et al.*[667]).

Prokop, Simon and Rackwitz[200] recorded an interesting family: father A_3 (weak), mother O, two children A_3 (weak), two O and one A_2. There is no reason to think that the A_2 child is extra-marital: his other groups fit and anatomical tests, measurements, finger-prints etc., are in favour of his being a full sib.

A Greek family in which an A_h-like condition is present was described by Jakobowicz, Simmons, Graydon, Constantoulakis and Ehrlich[314]. However, the serum of the propositus contained anti-Le^b and not anti-H: she was a non-secretor and her red cells gave the reactions Le(a–b–). There was a hint that the condition could only be expressed in females and a possible explanation involving an X-linked gene was put forward.

A peculiar form of A_h was described by Voak et al.[483]. Two English sisters react as A_2 but do not react with anti-H, their serum contains a 'cold' anti-H; one of the sisters has transmitted an A_1 allele to her child.

Hrubiško and his colleagues[343, 566] describe dominant depression of red cell H, A and A_1 in three Czechoslovak families whose salivary antigens were normal. How this ties up with the elaborate study by Voak et al.[567] of H, A and B strengths in Sheffield families is a question for more robust brains than remain to us.

3. Variations due to the action of the environment

Until 1957 blood group antigens were thought to be independent of the environment: it then emerged that they could on rare occasions be modified by disease.

Leukaemia and the antigen A

An extremely weak A antigen was found in a patient suffering from myeloblastic leukaemia who, a year before, had been grouped as A without difficulty or comment (van Loghem, Dorfmeier and van der Hart[61], 1957). It seemed possible that the change in the A antigen of his cells was associated in some way with his disease.

A similar change was observed by Stratton, Renton and Hancock[201] in a patient suffering from hypoplastic anaemia: he was proved to be A_1 by previous grouping and by family tests but his cells became inagglutinable by anti-A though they did not lose their power to adsorb anti-A. After the publication of the paper it was stated[202] that the patient had died of leukaemia.

An even more striking case was then reported by Gold, Tovey, Benney and Lewis[202, 203]. The cells of a patient, suffering from acute monoblastic leukaemia, gave a very feeble reaction with anti-A (2 per cent only were agglutinated) but the inagglutinable cells when separated were capable of adsorbing anti-A. During a remission of the disease the number of agglutinable cells rose to 35% only to fall again, just before death, to 8%. The 'inagglutinable' cells reacted more strongly with anti-H (Ulex) than did the cells which were agglutinable by anti-A. Family tests made it probable that the patient was A_1 rather than A_2.

Further cases were reported by Bhatia and Sanghvi[204], by Salmon and his colleagues[205–209], by Gandini and Ceppellini[324], by Hoogstraten, Rosenfield and

Wasserman[210]. Many papers followed and changes not only to A but also to H, B, I and D antigens were described[329,337,335,330,344–347,507] though the diminution of I is in question[508,509].

Salmon and Salmon[348] (1963) made the important observation that in the serum of a patient of the genotype A_1O, whose A antigen had been modified in the course of the disease, the anti-B was modified also: its affinity for B cells was reduced. In a later paper Salmon[345] considers that the anti-B change was a consequence of the change to the A antigen and not a primary effect of the disease on the manufacture of globulin.

That H as well as A can sometimes be modified suggests that the change can affect steps in the synthesis of the red cell antigens anterior to the time of action of the *ABO* genes, if the scheme in Figure 5, page 61, be correct (Salmon, Debray and Lemaire[349], 1964). A similar deficiency of H in the cells of certain patients of group O is reported by Salmon and Salmon[350], 1965.

Salmon[206,209] at first thought that somatic mutation afforded the best explanation of the antigenic change, but in a later paper [351]he points out the snag that the improbable event of mutation at both the AB and the H loci would have to be postulated, at any rate according to the current view that two independent loci are responsible for the A, B and the H antigens of the red cells.

Salmon, André and Philippon[352] injected A_1 cells into three patients with A antigen modified by the disease: the foreign cells kept their antigen intact. This seems an important observation, the meaning of which is not yet clear.

How lively was the interest taken in leukaemic changes in the antigens of red cells is well illustrated by the 'Confrontation Cytologique' at Hôpital St Louis, Paris, at which Dr Salmon had to face questions from a most talented range of experts with the common interest of leukaemia[353].

An attempt to assess the frequency with which leukaemia affects the antigens of red cells was made by Ayres, Salzano and Ludwig[354] (1966) in Brazil.

Salmon and his colleagues[487] discuss the possibility of chromosome inactivation as a background to the leukaemic changes of red cell antigens.

Since the last edition of this book many more cases have been reported but the nature of the change still remains unknown. A scholarly setting out of the problem will be found in Salmon[510].

Kassulke, Hallgren and Yunis[511] found that, during the course of leukaemia, leucocytes may lose their A and H antigens and, what is more surprising, may acquire appropriate M or N antigens not detectable in normal leucocytes.

Scott and Rassbridge[512] reported diminution of A and I antigens in a case of Hodgkin's disease. Kahn *et al.*[513] describe a patient with erythroleukaemia known to have been A_1 but who came to lose the A antigen from 50% of his cells. The abnormal cells when separated were found to show various enzyme changes but most notably a great fall in adenylate kinase (AK), suggesting a chromosome lesion, for *ABO* and *AK* are known to be fairly closely linked. Salmon *et al.*[522] had previously reported a persisting mixture of A_1 and weak A in an apparently healthy old lady whose two populations of red cells differed in their AK reactions.

Salmon et al.[514], using quantitative agglutination methods found modifications of A, B, H, I and i in ten of eleven cases of refractory anaemia, which suggested a relation between this disorder and leukaemia.

Possible age effects

A few lines above, an A: weak A mixture in a healthy old lady is quoted from Salmon et al.[522]. The case was republished[523] together with two other examples of A: weak A mixtures in healthy people, neither of whom showed AK mixtures.

The red cells of an old man investigated in the laboratory of Professor Sansone in Genoa (Rasore-Quartino and Galletti[524]) were normal group A in 1965 but in 1969 were mosaic, only about 30% being A_1 and the rest apparently O. Before his death in 1970, at the age of 79, the proportion of A_1 decreased further. The patient had shown no sign of haematological disease. We were kindly sent samples of this blood and have recorded a few details[525].

Acquired B

It dawned slowly to Cameron, Graham, Dunsford, Sickles, Macpherson, Cahan, Sanger and Race[211] (1959) that a certain kind of weak B antigen in seven samples of otherwise group A_1 blood which they had tested over the years was, contrary to all previous experience, an acquired and not an inherited antigen. The proof that the antigen was acquired rather than inherited depended mainly on the following observations. All seven patients were A_1 and four of them had group O children, thus their genotype must be A_1O with no room for a weak B allele. Their serum contained anti-B. Those who were secretors secreted A and H but not B. The character could be transient, and it was clearly associated either with age or disease (notably carcinoma of the rectum or colon) or both. Later we came to realize that age was merely secondary to disease. The absence of group O from the seven was highly significant.

Some anti-B are better than others at detecting this antigen: characteristically, many cells remain unagglutinated but the proportions may vary from time to time in the same patient.

An eighth example was very fully investigated by Marsh, Jenkins and Walther[212] who also described how they had been able to induce a similar change in vitro by treating A_1 cells with a bacterial filtrate. They concluded that the B-like antigen was probably acquired through the action of a bacterial enzyme. They referred to the antigen as pseudo-B.

It has been known for some years from the work of Springer and of Iseki that there was a close serological relationship between E. coli O_{86} and blood group B (see references in Williamson and Springer[213]) and a search was made for this organism in the faeces of some of his acquired B patients by Dr Cameron, but without success. Stratton and Renton[214] suggested that the change might be due to adsorption of a B-like bacterial polysaccharide on to the red cells. Later, Springer and Ansell[215] reported that purified lipopolysaccharides and protein-lipopolysaccharides from *E. coli.* O_{86} and from a number of other organisms[216] could be adsorbed on to A and O red cells giving them a B-like antigen which could be shown by exposure of these cells to anti-B and subsequent elution of that antibody. This roundabout method was necessary because the cells became polyagglutinable after adsorption of the polysaccharides.

If *E. coli.* O_{86} polysaccharide be responsible the question immediately arises, why does it stick on to O cells *in vitro* but not *in vivo*? To this question we have no answer. Pettenkofer, Maassen and Bickerich[217] found that *E. coli* O_{86} had A as well as B specificity. The same observation was made independently by Modiano, Gonano and De Andreis[218] and by Marsh (personal communication).

Marsh[219] reported that a bacterial filtrate, which was also a powerful T activator (supplied by Dr Friedenreich), could induce the B change in O cells as well as in A cells, and that the T changing factor could be separated from the B changing factor.

Once the condition was clearly recognized it could be seen that three puzzling cases previously reported were probably examples of the same thing. (Prokop and Schuberth[220], 1954, one case; Stratton and Renton[221], 1958, two cases.)

We now know of 42 examples of acquired B and some of them have been reported[222,223,227,335-338,515-521,660]. Of the 42 people 39 were A_1, 2 were A_2 and 1 was an inhibited A ('A_h^m'). The shortage of A_2 in the sample is significant at about the 1 in 100 level of probability. The statistical evidence is overwhelmingly against O cells acquiring B; and Marsh[516] cites experimental evidence in support: A_1 cells suitably marked for subsequent recovery were injected into an A_1 acquired B person and they too acquired the B, whereas O cells injected into an A_1 acquired B did not acquire the B.

A minor degree of polyagglutinability was noted in several of the acquired B cases.

The average age of the patients was well over 60: most of them had a carcinoma of the colon or rectum, a few had a carcinoma elsewhere (cervix, prostate and peritoneum) and the rest had infection of the intestine or gangrene of the legs, only one was thought to be healthy[521]. Ten of the 42 cases were found in Dundee, the fruits of a special search by Dr Cameron.

In 1960 Andersen published four papers[189,224-226] dealing with six cases of what we think is the same condition and with one case which, though serologically indistinguishable, was clearly shown to be an inherited group; this example is referred to on page 34. Andersen[226] found that anti-B sera from A_2 donors were more efficient than those from A_1 donors for detecting the B antigen he was describing. Andersen's thesis[359], 1963, which is in Danish but with summaries of each chapter in English, may also be consulted.

Mimic ABO variants

The effects of leukaemia, possibly of old age, and the acquisition of B by A_1 people might perhaps come under this heading but they have already been discussed. The purpose of this section is to recall that a mixture of blood may be the cause of an apparent ABO variant.

Transfused cells

Transfusion is of course the commonest cause of a transient mixture of blood. The blood of an A_2 person transfused with O cells could be difficult to distinguish from A_3.

Foetal bleeding

It is now well established that foetal red cells can get into the mother's circulation. A paternal antigen (*via* the foetus) in the maternal circulation might give the appearance of a weak A or B.

Polyagglutinability

Polyagglutinable O cells can be mistaken for a weak A variant or for a mixture of O+A cells. This is because polyagglutinable cells react rather more strongly with sera containing anti-A than with those lacking it (page 490).

Twin and dispermic chimeras

These chimeras (Chapter 26) might at first be mistaken for an ABO variant. Therapeutic chimeras, the consequence of marrow grafting, would not confuse the ABO groups because recipient and donor would presumably be of the same group.

OTHER ASPECTS OF ABO

Is the *ABO* locus complex?

For practical purposes the ABO groups are inherited through multiple alleles at one locus, as seen by Bernstein nearly 50 years ago. On the other hand evidence has been accumulating during the last 10 years that promises a deeper insight into the *ABO* locus.

It seems that we shall have to accept that some if not all blood group loci are like bacterial loci and include many sites where mutation can go on and between which, as an extreme rarity, crossing-over can happen. The Rh, MNSs and Kell systems have long pointed in this direction and now ABO is beginning to do so too.

Furuhata[360,361], in 1927, proposed a scheme for the inheritance of ABO involving two mutable sites, one for *A* or *not A* and one for *B* or *not B*. Pedigree evidence showed that the sites would have to be completely linked and so did the frequency of the alleles in the population.

The general opinion, clearly expressed by Lattes[362] and by Wiener[33] was that, if the two loci were absolutely linked, Furuhata's scheme merely reduced to that of Bernstein[11,12]. Lattes concluded that 'for practical purposes, Bernstein's theory and Furuhata's are identical'. And this is true, for practical purposes. But now that we know crossing-over can happen within a gene, though it be an extreme rarity, the two schemes no longer appear identical.

Before the days of cistrons, Komai[363] (1950) in a paper on 'Semi-allelic genes' considered the ABO groups and said:

This author [Bernstein[364]] has shown conclusively that, if crossing over occurs between A and B, however low its frequency might be, it will eventually bring about a situation very different from the actual state. This argument is undoubtedly convincing on the whole; still it does not seem to have thoroughly disproved the semi-allelic interrelation of A and B, and the possibility of very rare, rather exceptional, occurrence of recombination.

The family which first strongly suggested that A and B could be inherited together from one parent was described by Seyfried, Walewska and Werblińska[365] (1964). An A_2B daughter of an O mother was married to an O husband and had two A_2B children. The B antigen was weaker than normal and the serum contained some kind of anti-B. A antigen and weak B antigen were present in the saliva.

The next family was reported by Yamaguchi, Okubo and Hazama[366] (1965). Again A_2 and a weak B antigen were apparently being inherited together. The authors considered the condition to be the same as that described by Seyfried and her colleagues. Professor Komai added a note to the paper suggesting that the weak B reflected a position effect, the B gene giving a weaker effect in the *cis* arrangement with A (AB/O) than in the normal *trans* arrangement (A/B).

Another family with 'A_2B_3' children of 'A_2B_3' × O parents was reported by Yasuda, Amano, Matsunaga and Hayama later in 1965 at a meeting of the Japanese Society of Haematology at Kyoto and again early in 1966 at the Annual Meeting of the Japan Society of Blood Transfusion at Tokyo.

In the light of these families it could be seen that inheritance of A and B on one chromosome was the most entertaining explanation of the family reported by Moullec and Le Chevrel[190, 191] (1959): again A_2 and again a weak B were inherited together, this time through four generations of the family. A puzzling family reported by Andersen[189] (1960) might have been another example—the pedigree very nearly fits. Boettcher[367] (1966) proposed an ingenious scheme of crossing-over which could explain these families.

The condition must be less rare in Japan than in Europe: another family (father O, mother 'A_2B_3', three children 'A_2B_3') was reported by Yamaguchi, Okubo and Hazama[371] (1966). In their paper they introduced the notation '*cis*-AB'. In 1970 Yamaguchi, Okubo and Tanaka[368] gave pedigrees of the nine Japanese *cis* AB families then known, and in 1971 Kogure[369] added another and in 1973 Dr Hosoi, of Kyoto, found *cis* AB in three generations of a Japanese family (personal communication).

Miss Greta Madsen, of Dr Heistö's laboratory, when working in Korea, found a fine family[472]; mother O, one child O, three children A_2B with anti-B in their seru ; the father was dead.

An extension of the French family[190] and another white family are on record[666, 661].

The first example of *cis* A_1B (as opposed to *cis* A_2B) was reported from the Centre Départemental de Transfusion Sanguine in Paris[477,478]. From the excellent investigations it emerges that the B antigen resulting from the *cis* A_1B complex is part of the normal B antigen: the anti-B of such people is directed at the remaining part of the B antigen. The two A_1B/O members of the family were secretors and the B they secreted corresponded to the partial B of their red cells. Anti-B sera of A_2 donors reacted more strongly with the A_1B/O cells than did the anti-B of A_1 donors; indeed, one good A_1 anti-B did not react at all. Normal A_1B cells have less of the A_1B/O fraction of B antigen than do B or A_2B cells. Intragenic exchange was proposed as the most likely explanation of the condition, in conformity with the opinion of Yamaguchi *et al.*[371] (1966). Thermodynamic investigation of this *cis* A_1B by Bouguerra-Jacquet *et al.*[370] (1969) showed that the B was different from other B antigens.

It should be mentioned that this fascinating development in the ABO system does not invalidate its use in paternity tests: the weakness of the B antigen and the simultaneous presence of some kind of anti-B should prevent any conclusions being drawn from the ABO groups.

Although recombination within a complex locus is the most attractive and, by analogy with the MNSs, Rh and Kell systems, the most likely explanation of the families above, it can be argued that a rare allele is responsible, one which results in an antigen with some of the properties of A and of B. That the phenotype is evidently less rare in Japan may lean towards the duller, allelic, explanation. However, it may be that a relatively high *B* gene frequency, coupled with serological skill, is needed for recombination to be detected, and this would march with examples having been found in Japan and in Poland.

But, anyhow, a new ABO group has certainly emerged.

Quantitative measurements

Several facts have long been known, as, for example, that the A in A_2B is weaker than in A_2 and that A_1 is weaker in A_1B than in A_1, and that the descending order of strength of H is O, A_2, B, A_1. The balance sheet of the antigens is neatly demonstrated by Brain[93,372]: Bantus of groups O, A_2 and A_1 have more H antigen than do Europeans of these groups, but the amount of H is the same in group B people of both races. However, Bantus have a much stronger B antigen than do Europeans. Brain points out that his findings support the theory of Watkins and Morgan that H substance is competed for by the *A* and *B* genes and that 'the more A or B substance that is produced, the less should be the amount of H remaining'. Grundbacher and Summerlin[570], in Virginia, confirmed the stronger H of Negroes compared with Whites. In Durban, Milner and Calitz[571] confirmed the finding of Brain that Negroes had stronger B than Whites and, further, stronger B than Asiatics. The mean strength of B was similar in Whites and Asiatics but the Asiatics showed greater variation in strength: amongst them were found the strongest and the weakest Bs in all three populations.

Earlier in this chapter we attempted to classify weak As and weak Bs at the level at which they are usually investigated. However, more refined quantitative techniques can provide a more objective classification of differences in agglutinability. The methods mostly stem from the brilliant work of Filitti-Wurmser, Jacquot-Armand and Wurmser[296] and have been notably applied by Salmon and his colleagues. The strength of the antigen is expressed as the percentage of cells agglutinated by selected antisera at a certain dilution and temperature. By this method Salmon and Reviron[373] identified three weak Bs as B_{80}, B_{60} and B_0 compared with the normal, B_{100}. The wider applications of this work to the study of agglutination are to be found in an important paper by Salmon, Salmon and Reviron[374]. By the same method Salmon, de Grouchy and Liberge[375] identified a sample of blood, $A_{1(80)}$, only 80 % of the cells being agglutinated by anti-A_1: the reaction with anti-H was that expected of A_2. The saliva contained a normal amount of A substance. The character is clearly a new one and was shown to be inherited. In recent years many papers applying these thermodynamic methods to rare ABO phenotypes have been published in *Nouvelle Revue Française d'Hématologie*.

In America, quantitative agglutination and haemolytic techniques show that the amount of A in normal A_1 cells and in normal A_2 cells is variable, though different methods give different frequencies in the categories strong, medium and weak[376-378]; the pattern evidently depends on the antiserum used[379]. Gibbs, Akeroyd and Zapf[380] found marked differences in the antigen strength of normal group B people. The method used by Salmon and Reviron[373] did not show this but, as the latter authors point out, the differences may appear at only certain concentrations of antibody.

These quantitative aspects of haemagglutination have acquired a daunting literature, references to which may be found in very useful reviews by Solomon, Gibbs and Bowdler[381,382] and by Grundbacher[378].

Inagglutinable cells

Though the vast majority of red cells in a sample of, say, A blood are agglutinated by anti-A a small proportion are usually left unagglutinated. These free cells have been studied by Goudie and by Atwood and his colleagues who were seeking evidence of somatic segregation, on the one hand, and somatic mutation, on the other.

Somatic, or mitotic, crossing-over and subsequent segregation was discovered by Stern[238] (1936) in *Drosophila melanogaster*: it can only make an observable difference when it happens in a heterozygous cell. If it can occur in haemopoietic tissue in man its effect as far as the *ABO* genes are concerned would be that an *AB* cell could have *AA* or *BB* daughter cells, and *AO* could have *AA* and *OO* daughter cells and a *BO* cell could have *BB* and *OO* daughter cells. Somatic crossing-over could introduce no incompatible cells into the circulation.

Somatic mutation is quite different; it can affect homozygotes or heterozygotes. If it can occur in haemopoietic tissue in man its effect, as far as *ABO* genes are concerned, would be that, for example, an *AO* cell could have a *BO* daughter cell, an *OO* cell an *AO* daughter cell, etc. Somatic mutation would, of course, often introduce incompatible cells into the circulation.

If both events occur in man, then, as far as the ABO groups are concerned, somatic mutation has the more interesting theoretically possible consequences. (1) Occurring early in development it might result in a sector of blood forming tissue sufficiently large to cause, later in life, a detectable mixture of blood. A lesser dose of mutant cells if incompatible might induce the acquisition of toler-ance, of which, later on, the outward sign would be a 'missing agglutinin' (2) Incompatible mutant cells produced shortly after birth might provide one of the antigenic stimuli responsible for the presence of anti-A and anti-B. (3) After the establishment of anti-A and anti-B any incompatible mutant red cells would presumably have but a short life in the circulation.

According to Bessis[239] 250 thousand million new red cells enter the circulation each day. If somatic mutation does occur then we must suppose that B and O cells, for example, are being constantly launched into an A circulation. The *proportion* of mutant cells would of course be infinitely small.

The inagglutinable cells here being considered are those found in ordinary A_1, A_2, B, A_1B, and A_2B blood; they are not the inagglutinable cells present in gross amount in a range of conditions mentioned earlier in this chapter, A_3, A_m, A_x, etc., which cells, though not agglutinated by anti-A, can be shown to adsorb anti-A: nor are they true mosaics (page 519). Since mutant incompatible cells would presumably be quickly eliminated the only cells which we could hope to recognize resulting from either somatic segregation or mutation would be A, B or O in AB, A_2 in A_1 or in A_1B, O in A, O in B, all of which unfortunately would pre-sent themselves in a negative way as cells inagglutinable by anti-A, anti-A_1 or anti-B as the case may be.

A great deal of very intricate but inconclusive work has been devoted to the subject by Goudie[241], Bird[119], Atwood and colleagues[242,245,246,336] and by McKerns and Denstedt[244]. As far as B is concerned the very clear answer is that the inagglutinable cells do have B antigen (Winkelstein and Mollison[383]).

Perhaps the most striking thing about this problem is the lack of evidence for somatic mutation and mitotic crossing-over, and one begins to wonder whether there is some mechanism to prevent them happening in the haemopoietic system. If they do happen, that would be interesting: if they do not happen, that would be still more interesting.

Development of ABH antigens of the red cells

A and B

The antigens A and B are detectable long before birth: Kemp[68] holds the record, he detected A in a foetus aged 37 days. Constantoulakis and Kay[247] tested a number of foetuses. They find no increase of strength of A and B during foetal life; the antigens are weaker in absorptive power than adult cells and are qualitatively different in that they lack 'representation of some of the adult spectrum of antigenic groupings' including that for A_1. Constantoulakis, Kay, Giles and Parkin[384] found that the A_2 gene expressed itself in the foetus as a phenotype somewhat like A_x: the cells were agglutinated weakly by anti-A from B donors but strongly by anti-A from O donors.

It is well known (Wiener[33]) that at birth there may be difficulty in distinguishing between A_1 and A_2. In our experience *Dolichos biflorus* anti-A_1 is much better than human anti-A_1 at making this distinction.

After birth the strength of A and B rises (Bjorum and Kemp[248]). After about three years of age the antigen strength remains steady for life (Grundbacher[385]). Skov, Eriksen and Hagerup[574] found no difference in the A_1A_2BO groups of 802 Danes in their 50th year and 427 in their 70th year.

Ageing, in a different sense, was investigated by van Gastel and Dudok de Wit[575]. Group A_1 red cells were ultracentrifuged and the denser, older, portion separated from the lighter, younger portion. There was no definite difference in their agglutinability by anti-A though in some of the experiments there was a suggestion that the younger cells were the slightly less agglutinable.

H

Constantoulakis *et al.*[384] showed that the H antigen is expressed in foetal red cells of all ABO groups. Though not so strong as in the adult its relationship to the A and B antigens is the same.

In our experience H is pretty well developed at birth if it is measured by anti-H from O_h persons or from extracts of the seeds of *Ulex europaeus*, and this has also been the experience of Bhatia[386] with a variety of anti-H reagents. Pioneer work by Formaggio[71] and by Watkins[72] on the 'O' and H antigens of cord cells gave variable answers according to the antiserum used.

More recent work on the development of H has shown the subject to be extremely complicated owing to varying anti-H, anti-I, anti-HI etc. components in the reagents and different rates of development of the corresponding antigenic components. At least one of the components of H is developed after birth (Bhatia[386], Gold and Bhatia[576], Wiener *et al.*[446], Dzierzkowa-Borodej *et al.*[577], Kuśnierz and Leśkiewicz[578]).

Number of A and B antigen sites on a red cell

Filitti-Wurmser and her colleagues[107] estimated that the number of B antigen sites on one red cell of the genotype *BO* or A_1B was about 500,000. An estimate of A sites by Greenbury, Moore and Nunn[433] was of very much the same order: 830,000 for A_1, fewer for A_2.

Economidou, Hughes-Jones and Gardner[435] (1967) in an important paper give the following most interesting figures:
A antigen sites

A$_1$ adult	810,000–1,170,000
A$_1$ cord	250,000–370,000
A$_1$B adult	460,000–850,000
A$_1$B cord	220,000
A$_2$ adult	240,000–290,000
A$_2$ cord	140,000
A$_2$B adult	120,000

B antigen sites

B adult	610,000–830,000
A$_1$B adult	310,000–560,000

The range covers three, four or five samples of each kind: single samples were tested of A$_1$B cord, A$_2$ cord and A$_2$B adult.

Williams and Voak[579] concentrated on the difference between A$_1$ and A$_2$. They used ferritin labelled *Dolichos* lectin and an electron microscope: their estimate was about 800,000 A$_1$ sites and 150,000 A$_2$ sites.

Boyd and his colleagues[434] to their surprise reached a higher figure in calculations based on the reaction of Lima bean lectin: eight to ten million A sites. But this is not really worrying; for it is the comparisons between the groups that are interesting rather than the exact number: the imagination has collapsed anyhow, even before remembering all the other sites, MN, Rh and so on, for which room has to be found.

ABH antigens in other places

It has long been known that the blood group antigens are not confined to red cells and saliva but are to be found in most secretions and tissues of the human body[33]. The classical work on the subject is *Group Antigens in Human Organs* by Grethe Hartmann (Munksgaard, 1941), now reprinted[17]. The antigens in saliva are dealt with in Chapter 8.

In the words of Davidsohn and Stejskal[491] (1972) 'The isoantigens A, B and H of blood groups A, B and O are present in some epithelial cells and in all endothelial cells lining the blood vessels. They are absent in connective tissues, in the central nervous system and in some epithelial cells.'

Outside the human body substances like A, B and H are widely distributed in nature; they have been found in many animals, some plants[73] and many bacteria[73,213,217,250–252,323,387,388]. A jolt to our anthropocentric outlook is provided by Springer in a summary[387]:

The name 'blood group substances' for the ABO and MN substances is a 'misnomer' and can only be explained by the history of the discovery of these surface structures some of which are ubiquitously distributed throughout the animal and plant kingdoms and seem to represent a surface structure principle which Nature has preserved from microorganisms and plants up to man. As surface structures the substances have receptor properties. Antibodies, viruses, toxins and pharmacological agents specificially interact with them.

Returning to man, the biochemists have found rich veins of ABO substances in the most retired places: Morgan and van Heyningen[74] discovered them in the fluid of pseudomucinous ovarian cysts of secretors; Yosida[75], Sekimoto[76] and Buchanan and Rapoport[77] found them in large amounts in the meconium of secretor babies. The substances have also been found in pre-Columbian Peruvian mummies[253,78,254] in predynastic Egyptian mummies[78] and in the mummies of Governor-Generals of Provinces in the northern part of Japan[79].

Serum

The question often arises whether the serum of secretors contains more group substance than that of non-secretors. Early work on the subject by Hartmann[257] and by Halvorsen[258] did not give a clear answer. However, Høstrup[394,395] had a go at the problem and reached the following conclusions. In adults and in infants non-secretors have significantly less A than secretors, and A_2 people in each secretor category have less A than do A_1. No difference could be detected in the B of secretors and non-secretors. In tests on healthy people Fried et al.[493] found no relation between amount of A and B substance and the secretor state. By radio-immunoassay Holburn and Masters[675] found more A in the serum of A_1 than A_2 donors and more in the serum of secretors than non-secretors.

Thirteen interesting cases are reported[259–262,331,479,488,494] of people whose serum was so loaded with A or B substance that the reaction of their cells with anti-A or anti-B was inhibited if the cells were tested without the usual preliminary washing in saline. Eight of the cases were suffering from cancer, three from pseudomucinous ovarian cysts, one was an apparently healthy blood donor and one heterozygous for haemoglobin S. After removal of the ovarian cysts the serum of the three patients returned to normal[262], or nearly normal[331].

This may be as good a place as any to record a most interesting and surprising observation made by Renton and Hancock[396]. They took successive samples from A or B recipients of O transfusions. The separated donor cells were found to give a reaction with group O sera. The effect was transient and best demonstrated about two weeks after the transfusion. It seemed that the O cells had taken up some A or B substance: the effect could not be imitated in vitro.

However, Wherrett, Brown, Tilley and Crookston[581,582] confirming that transfused O cells could take up A or B antigen from a recipient's plasma, were successful in reproducing the effect in vitro. Again, only group O sera showed the effect, some better than others.

Mrs Crookston, in 1972, asked us whether we had noticed this effect in twin chimeras, whether O cells from a genetically A twin were known to have taken up

A antigen. Our records showed that the separated O cells of such chimeras had been tested only with anti-A and anti-B. Since that time we have tested several suitable chimera pairs and, as Mrs Crookston expected, the 'grafted' O cells in an A twin do take up some of the host's A antigen, as judged by agglutination by some group O sera.

Candela [255] first grouped dry bones. The technical difficulties are considerable. Toral and Salazar[256], unexpectedly finding the majority of a sample of bones from the Monte Alban tombs to give the reaction of A when Mexican Indians are mostly O, tested the surrounding dust to which they were returning and found that it too gave the reaction of A.

A and B antigens have been found in the human cornea (Nelken, Michaelson, Nelken and Gurevitch[177,178]), and it was suggested that ABO incompatibility might play a part in determining the success or failure of corneal grafting.

Many human tissues have now been tested for the antigen A using the mixed agglutination method[86,491] or the fluorescent antibody method[325,326,389,390,501] or both[263].

Antigens in tissue culture

Foetal tissue cells grown in culture have been successfully ABO grouped by the mixed cell method (Högman[264,265,332]) and so have HeLa cells[266]. After repeated subcultivation of foetal tissue the antigens could no longer be demonstrated[333]. Similar results were obtained by Chessin, Bramson, Kuhns and Hirschhorn who went on to try the effects of adding various blood group substances to the medium. (See also Kuhns et al.[392,393]). Friedhoff and Kuhns[492] using the mixed cell method were able to detect A, B, H, Tj[a], I and i on amnion cells, fresh and in culture. 'Decrease in the number of cells positive for Tj[a], and possibly for A and B, was observed in the course of cell passages. In cultures positive for H the percentage of positive cells, although small, generally continued as long as the culture was continued.' The maximum time of culture was 39 days. The antigens M, N, D and Yt[a] were not detected on the amnion cells or in their cultures.

The very surprising presence of P[k] on cultured fibroblasts[658,659] is dealt with in the chapter on P, and the potentially important detection of Xg[a] on fibroblasts on page 589.

Normoblasts

At what stage in its development does a red cell acquire blood group antigens is a question that is often asked. Some answer can be given: Yunis and Yunis[397-399] demonstrated the antigens A, B and H on normoblasts, and Mazumdar[400] the antigen D. Mazumdar concludes that D must be synthesized either by the earliest morphologically recognizable normoblasts or by 'a cell type that is not recognizable as a red cell precursor'.

Platelets

Platelets and white cells are now known to have a wonderful diversity of antigens but here our only concern is whether they have the red cell antigens with which we are familiar.

There is no longer any doubt that A and B antigens occur on platelets: Gurevitch and Nelken[80-83] first demonstrated them by direct agglutination; Moureau and André[84] confirmed their presence by inhibition tests using crushed platelets, and Dausset and Malinvaud[85] by a special agglutination technique, and Coombs and Bedford[86] by their mixed cell agglutination technique, and Janković and Arsenijevic[267] by the fluorescent method. Yunis and Yunis[399] find H to be present as well.

Attempts to demonstrate, by various techniques, other red cell antigens on platelets may be summarized thus: M and N, found[268], not found[87]; P_1, found[268], not found[87]; P (Tj^a) found[88,268]; Rh found[268-270], not found[87,88,271,272,401]; K found[268] and Fy^a found[268].

Lewis, Draude and Kuhns[273] coated O platelets with A and B substances and so wondered whether the A and B of platelets is intrinsic or is adsorbed from the surrounding plasma.

White cells

Thomsen[89], in 1930, showed by absorption tests that white cells had A and B antigens; agglutination tests he found gave inconsistent results, and this was confirmed by Dausset[90].

There now seems general agreement that A and B are present on white cells [274-276]: the agglutination results have been confirmed by absorption and elution tests and by mixed cell agglutination tests. The presence of A on leucocytes is independent of the secretor status[473,474]. If A is present on A_2 leucocytes it is weak[274,474]. Flory[474] could not detect the antigen H on O or A_2 leucocytes.

Attempts to demonstrate other red cell antigens on white cells, using various techniques, may be summarized thus: M and N, found[275], not found[276]; S, found[276]; P_1, not found[276], P(Tj^a) found[275,276]; Rh, found[269,277], not found[275,276,401]; Lu^a, equivocal[275]; Le^a, equivocal[275], not found[276].

Dausset[278] gives reason for believing that the A and B antigens are intrinsic in the white cells and not merely adsorbed from the plasma. Swisher[279] discusses some possible sources of error in the mixed cell agglutination technique.

Epidermal and epithelial cells

The elegant mixed agglutination technique of Coombs and Bedford[86] was applied by Coombs, Bedford and Rouillard[91] to show that skin cells also have A and B antigens—independent of whether the donor is a secretor or a non-secretor. The presence of the antigens was confirmed by Nelken, Gurevitch and Neuman[179], and by Yunis and Yunis[402] who also showed that H is present.

The question whether the antigens are secondarily adsorbed on to buccal epithelial cells is raised by the finding that the cells of A_2 non-secretors have very little A but that it can be augmented by immersing the cells in A secretor saliva; O cells will also take up A (Swinburne, Frank and Coombs[280]). Flory[403,485] has shown that buccal cells from secretors and non-secretors differ qualitatively in their content of H.

The mixed agglutination method has been applied by Fuchs, Freiesleben, Knudsen and Riis[92] to the grouping of desquamated epithelial cells in amniotic fluid. By taking a sample of the fluid the ABO group, as well as the sex, of the unborn baby could be determined. Ducos and his team in Toulouse[669,404] later simplified the grouping, for they found they could recover enough foetal red cells from an amniotic puncture for direct tests. They insisted, however, that radiological recognition of the position of the placenta should precede puncture, to avoid possible placental damage.

Cancer cells

Intensive work by Davidsohn and his colleagues at Chicago has given us a very clear picture of the state of the A, B and H antigens in cervical[495], pancreatic[496] and gastro-intestinal[497,498] carcinoma. A brilliant adaptation of the mixed-cell agglutination technique, called the specific red cell adherence test (SRCA), made possible the detection of the presence or the absence of the A, B and H antigens in old stained sections of tissue as well as in fresh material[491,495,496,498-500]. Briefly, the cancer cells progressively lose their A, B and H antigens, and this may become an important aid in prognosis. This subject is rather out of our field but we recommend Dr Davidsohn's Philip Levine Award Address[500] where are to be found references not only to the work of his own group but also to that of Szulman[501-503] and of others.

Spermatozoa

Whether or not spermatozoa possess intrinsic ABH substance, or whether when the substance is found it has been secondarily adsorbed from the seminal fluid, is an old problem. Edwards, Ferguson and Coombs[405] using the mixed cell technique found evidence of A or B on the spermatozoa of six secretors but not on those of four non-secretors. This suggested that the antigens were adsorbed rather than intrinsic. Boettcher[406,504] also considered the antigens to be adsorbed, and so did Parish, Carron-Brown and Richards[234] who further showed that spermatozoa from an A non-secretor and from an O person acquired A specificity when incubated with seminal fluid from an A secretor.

Edwards et al.[405] were 'inclined to accept the findings of Quinlivan and Masouredis[407] and Levine and Celano[340] that the rhesus antigen D is absent from spermatozoa.'

Edwards et al.[405] considered that they had established the presence of M and N and 'Tj^a' on spermatozoa but not of Xg^a. (Had Xg^a been present it might have afforded a way of separating X bearing from Y bearing sperm and thereby vastly complicating life.)

Alkaline phosphatase, ABO and secretor groups

Arfors, Beckman and their colleagues[408-411] (1963-6) found an association between a division of serum alkaline phosphatase and the ABO groups and secretor groups: all people[410] with the phosphatase group 2 were secretors and nearly all of them were B. Bamford, Harris, Luffman, Robson and Cleghorn[412] (1965) found that group 2 was a graded character and that sera giving the strongest group 2 reaction were from O or B secretors: possible backgrounds were discussed. Other references can be found in Hope and Mayo[505]. On the other hand, the amount of the serum enzyme acid phosphatase is higher in group A and AB persons (Beckman and Zoschke[506], 1968).

Animal red cells and the A and B antigens of man

Antigens with at least some of the serological properties of A and B are to be found in the red cells and tissues of a very wide range of animals. The subject was reviewed by Joysey[282].

Absorptions with animal blood have been used to prepare sera to demonstrate the existence of different components ('partial receptors') of the B antigen in human red cells. Friedenreich and With[95], in 1933, absorbed human anti-B with rabbit cells and with guinea-pig cells and conclude that the human B antigen has at least three components (B_1, B_2, B_3). At the same time it was shown that different samples of human anti-B were not all the same.

In another important paper Owen[96] reported the use of opossum cells to make similar distinctions. Owen, if we understand him correctly, prefers to think that the differences observed are not so concrete as symbols such as B_1 and B_2 suggest, but that they reflect cross-reactions of antibodies that are heterogeneous. Jacquot-Armand, Théoleyre and Filitti-Wurmser[97] brought their physico-chemical methods to bear on the opossum and anti-B.

By the use of pig red cells Winstanley, Konugres and Coombs[181] identified a component of the human A antigen complex, called A^p. Group A pig red cells absorb the haemolytic fraction of 'immune' anti-A but do not absorb the agglutinin of 'natural' anti-A: thus the two anti-A fractions are seen to have different specificities. In a second paper Konugres and Coombs[283] show that the anti-A^p fraction of 'immune' anti-A is that fraction which fails to be inhibited by A substance in Witebsky's[105] partial neutralization test for 'immune' anti-A. Yokoyama and Fudenberg[413] find evidence that the antigen A^p in pig red cells is heterogeneous.

The subject is clearly of fundamental serological importance but does not yet seem ready to be applied to immunogenetics, though pig A cells have been found useful[414] in the prediction of haemolytic disease of the newborn due to anti-A.

ABO ANTIBODIES

Anti-A and anti-B

In adults anti-A and anti-B are almost invariably present in blood when the corresponding antigen is absent. If an expected agglutinin is not found, the blood and saliva of the donor and of his family should be tested. Missing agglutinins are very rare and they usually have some interesting explanation: they may, for example, be the first indication of the phenotype A_m, of a chimera, of dispermy or of hypogammaglobulinaemia. In the last 20 years we can remember testing only two examples of missing agglutinins for which no cause could be found[286, 417], but a good case was reported recently[674].

It used to be thought that any anti-A or anti-B present in cord serum had been passively derived from the mother but this is now known not always to be the case. Toivanen and Hirvonen[589] (1969) found anti-A when the mother was A or anti-B when the mother was B in 8 out of 44 neonatal sera and they give references to two earlier accounts, in 1967 and 1968.

Between three and six months of age the child regularly begins to make its own agglutinins[99-101]. The strength of the agglutinin rapidly rises and is at its maximum at five to ten years of age, after this it gradually falls[102].

A seasonal variation in anti-A and anti-B titre observed by Shaw and Stone[104] in Wisconsin in 1957 could not be detected by Grundbacher in Virginia[583], but variation was found by Mayeda[584] in Salt Lake City, and in outdoor but not urban workers in Northern England by L.A.D. Tovey, Taverner and Longster[585]. In Oslo, with its great seasonal differences, Heistö and Uggerud[586] could find no variation in twelve urban donors tested monthly for two years. We do not know what to make of this, does it mean that pollen can do more than petrol can? Ssebabi[673] found fluctuations in Uganda, where the seasons vary but little.

Anti-A and anti-B are also to be found in milk and in ascitic fluid[33].

Putkonen[587], in 1930, gives priority to Yoshida (1928) for the recognition of isoagglutinins in the saliva. Later Japanese workers[327] found that anti-A or anti-B were present in the saliva of certain people and they postulated a pair of alleles, independent of the *ABO* genes, to account for it. Prokop[328], on the other hand, found that antibody is present much more frequently in group O salivas than in those of other groups and this makes the genetic theory untenable. Prokop's observations have been confirmed[418-420,482,588,655,657]. Hummel and Schöch[481] using a special technique were able to demonstrate the presence of the expected agglutinins in all saliva samples tested; O saliva was the most active. Schlesinger and Osińska[420] found the incidence of detectable agglutinins to be lower during pregnancy. Jakobowicz and her colleagues[421,656] found that in the saliva of postpartum mothers the presence or absence of anti-A or anti-B was related to the presence or absence of maternal 'immune' antibodies.

Anti-A and anti-B have been found in the cervical secretion of about 20% of

3

women, most of whom were group O, anti-A being commoner than anti-B (Gershowitz et al.[422], Solish et al.[423], Parish et al.[234]).

Putkonen[587] found that tears, induced by chopped onions, sometimes contained the appropriate anti-A or anti-B. Prokop, Bundschuh and Geserick[424] very simply demonstrated the presence of anti-A or anti-B in lacrymal fluid by dropping suspensions of red cells into the eyes of volunteers: the appropriate antibodies were found in 16 out of the 20 subjects. Our German is not good enough to say whether the volunteers also could observe the agglutination which took place.

Antibodies, closely related to anti-A and anti-B, of animal and plant origin will be described later in this chapter.

Origin of anti-A and anti-B

The origin of anti-A and anti-B has long been a matter for conjecture: the two extreme views were that these antibodies are wholly genetically determined or wholly the result of immunization by A and B substances of the environment.

An excellent and brief summary of the views of the protagonists is to be found in Springer, Horton and Forbes[288] in the paper in which they have, for the present at any rate, swayed opinion very much towards the 'acquired' view first expressed so clearly by Mlle Dupont[289] in 1934. White Leghorn chicks when a few weeks old have an agglutinin for human red cells which is mostly anti-B, but no antibody appears if the chicks have been hatched and kept in a germ-free environment[288,290-292]. Springer and his colleagues thus demonstrated that the anti-B in White Leghorn chicks is an acquired character. One cannot resist applying this to man, though Springer and his colleagues showed a more admirable restraint; they also remind us that their data are in agreement with the conclusions of earlier workers that the *capacity* to make antibodies is an inherited character.

The view we take involves the genetics of the red cells as well as the environment: it is based on the work of the Wurmsers[107] on the physicochemical differences between the anti-B produced by A_1A_1, A_1O and OO persons and on the observation by Salmon[345], noted earlier in this chapter, that people whose red cell antigen A had been changed by leukaemia (or by massive transfusion of washed O cells[425]) showed changes in the physical properties of their anti-B. This suggests that the finished antibody is not under complete and direct genetic control but rather that the antibody making apparatus is reflecting the state, which may be transient, of the antigens with which it is faced.

'Immune' anti-A and anti-B

If the 'naturally occurring' antibodies in man do arise like anti-B in the White Leghorn chick then the distinction between 'naturally occurring' and 'immune' antibodies loses a good deal of its meaning, and some phrase other than 'immune anti-A' or 'immune anti-B' is needed to describe the changes which take place following frank immunization. Unfortunately the only candidates so far seem to be 'boosted,' or 'hyper'-immunized.

Examples of such changes are: rise in titre of the agglutinin; increase of avidity; the antibody becomes more difficult to neutralize with A or B substance; haemolysins may appear or may increase; a zone may appear; the antibody may become more active at 37°C. than at 4°C.—the reverse of the usual behaviour.

There are several ways in which a person may become 'hyper'-immunized to A and B: by injection of A or B substance with the intention of producing powerful blood grouping serum; by pregnancy with an incompatible foetus; by transfusion of incompatible blood; by transfusion of incompatible plasma; by injection of horse serum, as in anti-tetanus inoculation; by injection of the non-dialysable part of influenza virus vaccine[426].

For an expert account of immune responses to A and B antigens the reader is referred to Mollison's *Blood Transfusion in Clinical Medicine*, now in its fifth edition.

Acquired tolerance to A

If an animal is exposed to a foreign antigen during foetal life its antibody forming apparatus then developing is somehow impressed so that, later in life, it may not respond in the usual way to the antigen concerned. Fully developed immune tolerance is seen in the chimeras when a twin is, for example, genetically O but lacks anti-A because it has been grafted with A cells from its fellow twin during embryonic life.

The establishment of a partial tolerance has been invoked to explain the following observations: Jakobowicz, Crawford, Graydon and Pinder[293] measured by various methods the strength of anti-A in the serum of 230 group O and B recruits before and after injections of tetanus toxoid (which contained A substance[101]); the mothers of the recruits were grouped. The average rise in antibody was significantly less if the mother had A than it was if she lacked it.

On the other hand no relation has been found between ABO group of mothers and antibody titre of their offspring[427-429].

Konugres[430] approached the problem in the way suggested by Professor Rogers Brambell and Mr N.A.Mitchison for Rh (page 238). The maternal grandmothers of children with haemolytic disease of the newborn due to anti-A or anti-B were grouped to see whether too many of them were group O. Group O women could not endow their daughters *in utero* with any hypothetical tolerance to A or B and these daughters might be the ones most likely to respond by making 'immune' anti-A or anti-B against their own children *in utero*. The results suggested 'that some degree of tolerance to A or B can be developed *in utero*'. Some one should test some more of these families. The evidence is much against any such tolerance to Rh (page 239).

Wiener, Nieberg and Wexler[431] failed to find any evidence that massive transfusion, shortly after birth, of ABO incompatible red cells affected the antibody titre of the infant later in life.

On the other hand, there has been clear warning that transfusion *before* birth may result in some complicated immunological problems. It may be a question of how early the intrauterine transfusion is given: Naiman, Punnett, Destiné and Lischner[432,590] proved that donor lymphocytic cells had taken root in a foetus first transfused at 27 weeks' gestation. Ten weeks after birth the grafting was detected in a most interesting way: the male child's lymphocytes were a mosaic of cells, some with a big Y chromosome and some with a small Y. Size of the Y chromosome is rigorously inherited: the father had a big Y and the donor a small Y. The child suffered severely from what was thought to be a graft *versus* host reaction.

Physico-chemical investigations of the B:anti-B reaction

Filitti-Wurmser, Jacquot-Armand, Aubel-Lesure and Wurmser summarized in English their work up to 1954[107] and to 1956[295] on the combination of anti-B and the antigen B of red cells. By calculations based on the number of cells agglutinated by a particular serum at different temperatures they were able to distinguish between anti-B from OO, A_1O and A_1A_1 donors. The work was criticized by Kabat[98] and the criticisms were answered by Filitti-Wurmser, Jacquot-Armand and Wurmser[296] in a paper which included references to their previous work.

There are two theses on this subject, Salmon[111] (Paris) and Eigel[297] (Bonn); both confirm the original distinctions. The methods have been successfully applied by Dr Salmon and his colleagues to a variety of problems already noted in this chapter.

Cross-reacting anti-A and anti-B in group O serum

The old and still puzzling observation that A cells can apparently combine with some anti-B, and likewise B cells with some anti-A, when mixed with anti-A,B (group O) serum goes on being studied and argued about.

Landsteiner and Witt[121], in 1926, confirmed the curious fact (first reported, we believe, by Hektoen in 1907) that A cells, mixed with anti-A,B serum then washed, would give up, on elution, not only the expected anti-A but also some agglutinin for B cells; after similar treatment B cells would give up not only anti-B but some agglutinin for A cells. Such unexpected elution results did not follow when the experiments were done with an artificial anti-A+anti-B serum made by mixing anti-A from a B person and anti-B from an A person (Dodd[124], Bird[125]).

Bird[125,126] focused attention on the curious and not infrequent phenomenon of asymmetry in the cross-reaction: from some cross-reacting O sera A cells adsorb and give up on elution agglutinin for B, though B cells will not give up agglutinin for A.

Rosenfield[129] made an important observation: when a mother and baby are both group O the isoagglutinins are detectable in the baby's serum more regularly than when they are both group A or both group B. Furthermore, Rosenfield[129,436] found that cross-reacting anti-A,B antibodies pass the placenta more easily than the more specific antibodies, and this was attributed to their small molecular size, for they were found to be of the '7Sγ^2 globulin' type[437]. Whatever their serological background, Rosenfield's term 'cross-reacting' seems to be the most convenient name for these antibodies.

There is no agreement yet about the serological explanation but there are four suggestions:

1 That there is a third antibody, besides anti-A and anti-B, called anti-C present in group O serum; and that A and B and AB people have the corresponding antigen C on their red cells. The first tabulation of this scheme that we have been able to find is in Koeckert[122], 1920; Koeckert attributes the scheme to Moss[123], 1910, though he seems to have varied it a little. This hypothesis has long been supported in Japan and references may be found in Matsunaga[128] (1950); Matsunaga writes in English, but many references to the work of his countrymen on the subject are in Japanese. The C:anti-C explanation was championed by Wiener[60] in a review on the subject, and by Wiener, Samwick, Morrison and Cohen[130] and by Unger and Wiener[131], and by Wiener, Socha and Gordon[528].

2 That certain single antibody molecules in group O serum have a double specificity, anti-A and anti-B, and consequently such antibody molecules can react with A cells and with B cells. This view has had the support of Dodd[124,298] and of Bird[125,126] who have both done a great deal of work on the problem. With a slight modification, Milgrom[127] also supported this view. Jones and Kaneb[299] add their support: they approached the problem from a different direction by means of their sensitive minor cell population technique[300,301]. They conclude that their blocking tests establish that the site of attachment of the cross-reacting antibody is at the A or B site and that the hypothetical C antigen either does not exist or is an integral part of the A and B antigens. Titration tests by the special technique confirmed that the cross-reacting antibody can react asymmetrically which, according to the authors, 'anti-C' should not do. (However, Bird[126] did not think the asymmetrical cross-reaction absolutely ruled out the anti-C hypothesis.)

3 The third possibility is most clearly stated by Kabat[98] who says that it 'would postulate, since such close similarities between the A, B and O substances exist, that the individual of group O may form part of his anti-A and anti-B of such specificity that it is directed not exclusively against A or against B specific groupings on the molecule but against some portion of the molecule involving structures which are similar in the A and B substances in addition to parts of the characteristic A or B structures. Thus, one might consider that the combining site of a 'linked' antibody molecule might be directed towards a larger area of the blood group A or B substance than the specific anti-A or anti-B groupings in such a manner that it involved a portion of the antigenic structure possessed by both.' Kabat thinks this the most attractive explanation; and so, it seems to us, do Schiffman and Howe[438]. Franks and Liske[490] agree with Kabat about there being a common part to the A and B antigenic determinants but diverge in holding that the combining site on the cross-reacting antibody is smaller than that of anti-A and anti-B.

4 Ogata, Matuhasi and Usui in a series of short and interesting papers[439-441] point out that a phenomenon, non-specific antibody adhesion to an antigen-antibody complex, should at least be remembered when theories about cross-reacting antibodies are being engendered. They find that A cells when exposed to a mixture of anti-A (from a B person) and anti-B (from an A person) will attach to themselves some anti-B and, conversely, B cells will attach some anti-A. The faculty of a specific antigen-antibody complex to attach non-specific antibody was found to apply not only to other blood group systems[439] but also to a syphilis antigen-antibody precipitate[441]. We can only suppose that differences in technique account for the discrepancy between these observations and those of Dodd[124] and Bird[125] who found no non-specific antibody in eluates from A or B cells exposed to mixtures of anti-A and anti-B.

The work of Bove, Holburn and Mollison[600] (see page 485) has altered our ideas about the nature of the Matuhasi–Ogata phenomenon, but has not invalidated its contribution to 'cross-reacting' thoughts.

Matuhasi[442] claims to confirm, in a different way, that anti-A,B (group O) serum does not contain an antibody component capable of reacting with both A and B cells. A mixture of ordinary B cells and fluorescent[443] A cells when exposed to anti-A,B (group O) serum gives agglutinates which are either fluorescent or not fluorescent; mixed agglutinates were not seen. Mixed agglutinates might have been expected if a third antibody capable of combining with A *and* B were present.

The problem of the specificity of the cross-reacting component remains a puzzle. As Dodd, Lincoln and Boorman[444] pointed out in their important paper, understanding may come when the chemistry of A and B of red cells is as well worked out as that of the secretions.

In another important paper Lincoln and Dodd[591] (1969) conclude that a cross-reacting antibody stimulated by A differs from one stimulated by B. Further, elution experiments led them to suggest that these antibodies 'may become denatured after combination with the corresponding antigen yet retain some combining capacity'.

Voak[592] (1968) deals with cross-reacting antibody in relation to ABO haemolytic disease of the newborn and gives an admirable short history of this teasing antibody.

Anti-H and 'anti-O'

These antibodies react much more strongly with red cells of group O and A_2 than with A_1 or A_1B; the reaction with B is usually intermediate between that with O and with A_1. They are found in the serum of certain humans, oxen, goats, chickens, eels, cats, dogs, pigs, sheep, rabbits and in extracts of some seeds. For years the relationship of such antibodies to the ABO group was obscure. (References to the earlier work may be found in reviews by Grubb[132,133] and by Watkins and Morgan[134].)

The first step towards clarification was made in 1948 when Morgan and

Watkins[140] divided what had been called anti-O sera into those which were inhibited by secretor saliva of any group, anti-H, and those which were not, 'anti-O.' Sanger[141] then noticed that the donors of anti-H were Le(a+) unlike the donors of 'anti-O' who appeared to have the normal distribution of Lewis groups. She assumed that the decisive factor was the non-secretor state rather than the Lewis phenotype.

Anti-H

By definition these antibodies are alike in being inhibited by secretor saliva but they are known to differ slightly in the specificity of their reactions, which is not surprising considering their different origins.

In the serum of O_h persons

This must be considered the veritable anti-H: it is regularly present, like anti-A and anti-B, when the corresponding antigen is absent from the red cells. Some examples react as strongly at 37°C. as at lower temperatures[42,47,48,195]; others react better at lower temperatures[44,46,193]. The anti-H can be removed from O_h sera leaving anti-A and anti-B, but so far it has not proved possible to absorb anti-A and anti-B and leave a good anti-H: this is not surprising since even A_1B cells have some H.

In the serum of not-O_h persons

These anti-H tend to be much weaker than those in the serum of O_h people and usually they act only at low temperatures. Since they are formed in people who presumably have some H they may ultimately prove to be analogous to anti-A_1.

An anti-H serum Toml.[142] is exceptional not only in being very powerful but also in coming from a person whose red cells were Le(a−) and who was a secretor and whose saliva inhibited her own antibody. The antibody is not anti-I: it reacts strongly with cord cells and with a sample of O i cells, it fails to react with Bombay cells and it is inhibited by secretor saliva.

In extracts of seeds

The discovery that extracts of certain seeds, notably those of *Ulex europaeus*, contain anti-H was of great importance in providing an easy source of the antibody. The subject is returned to on page 56.

The relationship between anti-H and anti-Le^b (page 339) is still puzzling: Bird[302] suggested that anti-H could be anti-HH$_1$ (as anti-A from a B person is anti-AA$_1$) and that H positive cells are H or HH$_1$, the former being Le(b−) and the latter Le(b+) and anti-Le^b, according to the theory, anti-H$_1$.

In the serum of animals

Bhatia[445] had great success in preparing anti-H in chickens by immunizing with
O cells and subsequently removing the species agglutinins by absorption with O_h
cells: O_h cells were also used to absorb species agglutinins from cattle, goat and
rabbit sera containing non-immune anti-H.

Bhatia[445] as the result of a comprehensive series of tests concluded that the
antibodies to the H antigen show striking similarity to the antibodies to the A
antigen, suggesting that H is divided in a way comparable to A_1 and A_2.

The subject of anti-H is returned to in the chapter on I (page 457).

'Anti-O'

The realization that neither anti-H nor 'anti-O' reacts with a product of the O gene
is no longer surprising, provided we are right in thinking of O as an amorph.

'Anti-O' sera strong enough to use with confidence are rare but they do seem
to exist as a separate entity and they do seem to be associated with the ABO groups
because they do not react with O_h cells. Most of those which we have tested do not
react with cord cells.

That some 'anti-O' are really anti-I was recorded, for the first time, in our
fourth edition. There are now a number of papers on the subject and they will
be faced in the chapter on I. Wiener, Moor-Jankowski and Gordon[446] (1965),
reasoning that the H antigen of red cells differs from the H of saliva, divide anti-H
into two components: anti-H^c, which is not inhibitable by secretor saliva (referred
to here as 'anti-O') and anti-H^s, which is inhibitable by secretor saliva (referred
to above as anti-H).

Voak, Lodge, Hopkins and Bowley[593] tested a large series of anti-H and 'anti-
O' sera against a range of cells of known H and I or B and I status and gained a
view of the great variation of the anti-H and anti-I components of such sera. The
notation H^c and H^s suggested by Wiener *et al.*[446] was adopted.

In this section on anti-H and 'anti-O' there has been no mention of anti-Le^b,
an antibody which will be described in the chapter on the Lewis groups, but it
should at least be referred to here. Anti-Le^b shares several of the properties of
anti-H: it works best with O and A_2 cells; saliva which inhibits anti-Le^b inhibits
anti-H, and the two antibodies are often found together in the same serum.

Cold agglutinins

The name 'cold agglutinins' can be used in a general way to distinguish agglutinins
more active at lower temperatures from 'warm agglutinins' which are more active
at higher temperatures. In practice 'cold agglutinin' is quite a useful way of
describing any cold agglutinin before its specificity is worked out. If the investigation be pursued the name usually gives way to anti-P_1, anti-A_1, anti-H, anti-Le^a,
anti-Le^b, anti-M, anti-N or anti-I.

A fairly common agglutinin sometime called 'non-specific complete cold auto-agglutinin' is now known to be anti-I (see page 456). The presence of anti-I should be suspected if a serum agglutinates all cells except cord cells. Anti-I is the commonest antibody in the serum of sufferers from acquired haemolytic anaemia of the 'cold antibody type.'

In normal fresh sera some cold agglutinin can usually be found. Incomplete cold anti-H was found by Crawford, Cutbush and Mollison[171] in all human sera tested.

'Suppressed' or 'latent' antibodies have been described by Bird[172-174]. Sera from four healthy A_1B people containing cold auto-antibodies were found to agglutinate O cells strongly and A and B cells weakly. Absorption with O cells removed the agglutinin for O cells but brought to light strong anti-A and anti-B, which antibodies could subsequently be separated by further absorption by B or A cells. Possible explanations of the phenomenon are discussed by Bird[174] who also describes the same behaviour of the cold agglutinins present in the extract of the seeds of Glycine soja.

Four other examples of cold ABO auto-antibodies perhaps fit in here. Kissmeyer-Nielsen, Nedergaard and Tippett[322] found anti-A and anti-A_1 in the serum of an A_2 secretor and anti-A_1, plus a trace of anti-A, in the serum of an A_1 secretor: neither antibody could be inhibited by A secretor saliva. The antibodies were referred to as 'pseudo anti-A', The Ii groups were shown not to be involved. An apparently normal healthy A_1B person but with anti-B in her serum is reported by Seyfried, Walewska and Giles[447]. Ehnholm and Mäkelä[594] described another healthy A_1B person with anti-B in her serum: the anti-B failed to agglutinate about 50% of B samples but these samples did absorb the antibody. For a subtle discussion of the possible background to such ABO specific autoagglutinins the paper should be read, and so should an earlier one by Mäkelä, Ruoslahti and Ehnholm[595].

Antibodies of other systems susceptible to the ABO groups

A fascinating antiserum was reported by Ikin, Mourant and Pugh[175]. The serum, from a group A Rh negative patient, gave the normal reactions expected of incomplete anti-D (the commonest Rh antibody) against red cells suspended in albumin, but tested against cells suspended in saline its reactions were extraordinary: it agglutinated only those cells with both D and A antigens. The agglutination was greater with A_1, D cells than with A_2, D cells. The antibody could be completely absorbed by O, D cells but not at all by A_1, dd cells. A mixture of A_1, dd and O, D cells was not agglutinated.

Tippett and her collaborators[448] first noted that the reactions of some examples of anti-I are influenced by the ABO groups (see page 452). For example, an antibody is described which behaved, when slightly diluted with saline, like a normal anti-A_1 but it was from an A_1 person; it was not inhibited by A secretor saliva and it did not agglutinate A_1 cells of the very rare phenotype i.

3*

An antibody called Luke (Tippett, Sanger, Race, Swanson and Busch[449]) without doubt owes its first allegiance to the P system but nevertheless is influenced in its reactions by the A_1A_2BO groups (see page 163).

Here mention may be made of a component of the lectin in the seeds of *Moluccella laevis* which has anti-(A+N) specificity (Bird and Wingham[601]).

Satisfactory explanations of such interactions between systems known to be genetically unrelated will probably have to await chemical enlightenment.

Plant agglutinins

This branch of blood group knowledge has blossomed so luxuriantly that we feel capable only of giving an outline of the subject. For those who need more information there is Mäkelä's excellent thesis[151] which is in English and which, fortunately, is published; Bird's thesis[119] (London) can hardly be considered accessible, and Krüpe's book[170], the first in the field, is, unfortunately for us, in German; and there are somewhat more recent reviews by Bird[302], by Saint-Paul[450] and by Boyd[451].

Since the last century certain seed extracts have been known to agglutinate human and animal red cells. According to Mäkelä[151] the first attempts to find blood group specific agglutinins in these extracts were made by Marcusson-Begun in 1926 and by Sievers in 1927 but they were unsuccessful. The discovery was reserved for Renkonen[146] (1948) and for Boyd and Reguera[147] (1949), working independently.

The results of extensive surveys have been reported by Renkonen[146] in Helsinki, Boyd and Reguera[147] in Boston, Boyd[149] in Egypt, Bird[150] in India, Mäkelä[151] (seeds from many parts of the world collected by Professor Renkonen), Krüpe[170], Cazal and Lalaurie[159], Boyd et al.[303], Martin and Bomchil[452] and many others, references to which will be found in Mäkelä[151] or in Boyd[451].

Two names have been suggested for plant agglutinins: phytagglutinins and lectins, the latter for the agglutinins which show specificity.

Inhibition tests of lectins with simple sugars have indicated that anti-A is inhibited by N-acetyl-D-galactosamine, anti-B by D-galactose and anti-H sometimes by L-fucose and sometimes by N-acetylglucosamine.

Anti-A

Anti-A was the first agglutinin with blood group specificity to disclose itself. Renkonen[146] found it in *Vicia cracca* and Koulumies[148] showed that it could be of practical use in making the $A_1 A_2$ distinction. Boyd and Reguera[147] found it in *Phaseolus limensis* (Lima Bean).

Probably the most useful anti-A was found by Bird[152,153] in *Dolichos biflorus*: the extract agglutinates A_1 and A_1B cells very avidly and to high dilution; it reacts relatively weakly with A_2 cells and is practically negative with A_2B cells. An excellent anti-A_1 can be prepared from these seeds and commercial preparations are available. The *Dolichos biflorus* extract has the advantage that it does not react with O or B cells suspended in albumin or treated with enzymes as other seed anti-A preparations tend to do. The extract can be purified and a very avid anti-A_1 results. We have found this preparation particularly useful in separating A_1 cells from mixtures of A_1 and O blood (see chimera sections in Chapter 26).

Boyd and Shapleigh[161] found that the *Dolichus biflorus* extract would precipitate with the saliva of secretors of group A_1, but not A_2. Bird[302] found that his purified extract would precipitate with both A_1 and A_2 secretor saliva, the precipitation being heavier with A_1 saliva.

Bird[304] has used the purified preparation to show, by the agar gel diffusion method, that *Dolichos* reacts with a common component of the A complex in A_1 (cyst preparation), A_2 (cyst preparation) and hog gastric mucin. He concludes that the lighter precipitate with A_2 saliva compared with that of A_1 is measuring a quantitative and not a qualitative difference.

The extract *Dolichos biflorus* does not react with the Forssman antigen[154] nor with the T antigen of 'changed' cells[155]: it does, however, react with O and B cells of the very rare Sd(a++) phenotype (see Chapter 17).

Anti-A has been found in several other plants belonging to the Leguminosae; so far it has been found in only two non-leguminous plants both of the order Labiatiae. The agglutinin in *Hyptis suaveolens* Poit is mainly anti-A_1 (Bird[305, 306]). The agglutinin extracted[601] from *Moluccella laevis* was surprising for although it agglutinated all A cells it behaved as anti-N with O and B cells: the unsplittable agglutinin evidently had the specificity anti-(A+N).

The oldest red cell agglutinin so far tested must surely be that extracted by Jones[307] from *Vicia cracca* seeds harvested in 1852.

Anti-B

Only a few extracts are specific for B cells. Mäkelä and Mäkelä[156] prepared one from 'old' samples of the seeds of *Bandeiraea simplicifolia* collected more than a year before (the age since harvesting was found to be important: fresh seeds had some anti-A agglutininating faculty as well).

Elo, Estola and Malmström[157] found something very like anti-B in the extract of a mushroom, *Marasmius oreades*; they had tested 139 species of fungi.

Specific anti-B was found[308] in an extract of the fungus *Fomes fomentarius*, L. (Polyporus). It was used[309] to demonstrate that the B antigen, as measured by the extract, is weaker in A_1B than in A_2B cells.

In 1968 anti-B in the seed cover of several varieties of *Evonymus* was recognized in Moscow by Potapov[596, 597] and, independently, by Ottensooser, Sato and Sato[598] working in São Paulo and Tokyo. It had been observed that the crude extract, which also reacted weakly with O and A cells, increased in its anti-B content on storage (perhaps echoing the behaviour of *Bandeiraea simplicifolia* noted above by the Mäkeläs) and Ottensooser, Sato, Sato and Kurata[599] discovered the very interesting reason why. The increased relative amount of anti-B is due to

infection with the fungus *Fusarium roseum* which greatly diminishes the agglutinin
for A and O cells.

Anti-A+B

Extracts which agglutinate A and B cells more strongly than O cells have been prepared from the following seeds: *Sophora japonica*[167], *Crotolaria striata*[168],
Bandeiraea simplicifolia, fresh seeds[156], *Calpurnia aurea*[180] and *Crotolaria mucro-
nata*[453], *Phlomis fructicosa* (Jerusalem sage)[602]. These extracts have lent themselves
to some fine serological and immuno-chemical investigations. The general conclusion seems to be that the anti-A and the anti-B are one agglutinin reacting with
some antigenic component common to A and to B cells, and thus closely resembling the cross-reacting antibody in group O serum (see page 48). However, with
some extracts changes of temperature have not had the same effect on the reaction
with A cells as with B cells[151,453]. Other important references to the study of this
group of agglutinins are: Morgan and Watkins[165] (*Sophora japonica*) and Furuhata and Nakajima[310] (*Sophora japonica*).

Anti-H

Agglutinins giving the reaction of anti-H were first found by Renkonen[146] (1948)
in extracts of the seeds of *Cytisus sessilifolius*, *Laburnum alpinum* and *Lotus tetragonolobus*. Five years later Cazal and Lalaurie[159] found anti-H in three species of
Ulex.

These are still the most widely used: anti-H has also been extracted from the
roots of *Ononis spinosa*[454] and from the fruit pulp of *Clerodendrum viscosum*[455].

The recognition of the usefulness of the anti-H in the seeds of *Ulex europaeus*
(common gorse) by Boyd and Shapleigh[160] reanimated the secretor system.
Group A, B or AB people had for long been easily divided into secretors or non-
secretors, but it was difficult to classify people of group O, because of the lack of
anti-H reagent: humans with good anti-H in their serum were too rare, eels too
difficult to handle and *Lotus tetragonolobus* too awkward to pronounce. Though
we find *Ulex* invaluable in classifying O saliva we do not think it reliable for A_1B
saliva. It was the use of *Lotus tetragonolobus* that led Bird to his theory about the
relation of anti-Le^b to anti-H (page 339).

Notable investigations of the variability of anti-H lectins are to be found in
Bird and Wingham[603], Voak and Lodge[604] and Matsumoto and Osawa[605].

Non-specific agglutinins

Bird[316] tested some of the seed extracts which had agglutinated cells of all ABO
groups with rare samples of cells lacking various very common antigens. All the
cells were agglutinated by all the extracts. In this way it was shown that these extracts did not contain, at any rate unmixed, anti-H, anti-Ss (-U), anti-P, anti-e,

anti-Lu[b], anti-k, anti-Yt[a], anti-I nor the theoretically possible anti-Fy. Bhatia and his colleagues[456,606] tested 'non-specific' agglutinins from seed extracts against a range of human red cells of rare phenotype. O_h cells alone gave any lead: five of the extracts reacted comparatively weakly, and were inhibitable by secretor saliva and this suggested anti-H, but they did not give the reactions of anti-H with the ordinary run of cell samples.

Bird[317,319,320] considered that the extract of *Ricinus communis* and that of *Abrus precatorius* react with the 'basic chemical substrate common to the ABH and Le[a] substances': agar gel diffusion tests had shown that the extract precipitated equally with secretor or non-secretor saliva and with saliva devoid of A, B, H and Le[a] substance. Drysdale *et al.*[607], on the other hand, decided that *Ricinus* reacts with a small part only of the galactose molecule and 'cannot be said to react specifically with the precursor of the blood group substance'.

Other observations on plant agglutinins

Bird[165] used a battery of plant agglutinins to distinguish the blood of various animals. Mäkelä[151] in his large summary of Leguminosae used, as well as human cells, those from cow, sheep, rabbit, guinea-pig and chick.

Reimann and Popwasileff[318] used an extract of *Sophora japonica* to distinguish between human blood stains and those from horse, cat, dog and cow.

From breeding experiments Schertz, Jurgelsky and Boyd[228] found that the strength of the anti-A_1 in *Phaseolous lunatus* was under genetic control.

Seed agglutinins have been useful in studying the chemistry of the red cell antigens by virtue of their property of being neutralized by simple sugars, a property not shared by human agglutinins (for references see[151,170,302,321,485] or almost any issue of *Vox Sanguinis* in recent years).

Plant agglutinins have contributed to biology in two further important ways: the rapid agglutination and sedimentation of red cells is used to obtain white cell suspensions, and the surprising power of certain agglutinins to stimulate mitosis has great use in cytogenetics.

The seed agglutinins themselves are believed to be globulins[170] and their structure to be less complex than that of the agglutinins of man. Bird[119] found the molecular weight of purified *Dolichos biflorus* agglutinin to be about one-third that of human anti-A and anti-B globulins.

Mäkelä[151] shares the opinion of Boyd and Shapleigh[169] that whatever the usefulness to the plant of the particular globulins their fit with the red cell antigens is accidental. Boyd[451] still holds this view: he does not consider that lectins are antibodies. In discussing the possible reasons for their presence he favours the suggestion of Krüpe that their function may be to 'combine with, transport and perhaps immobilize in the seed one or more of the carbohydrates with which they have the power to combine'. Jones[457] suggests, very tentatively, that one function of the lectin in *Vicia cracca*, though perhaps not the main one, may be to inhibit a soil bacterium which causes the seed coat of the plant to decay.

Lectins of specificities outside the ABO system are dealt with in the chapters on MNSs, Sid, En and T and polyagglutinability.

Though lectins have provided enormously useful reagents and have contributed to chemical knowledge about antigenic structure, they have not so far led to the recognition of any new blood group system.

Agglutinins in snails, fish roe etc.

The exciting discovery that the familiar snail contained powerful anti-A was reported in 1965 by Prokop and his colleagues[460-462] at Humboldt University in East Berlin, and later in the same year, independently by Boyd and Brown[463], in Boston.

In the first account Prokop, Rackwitz and Schlesinger[460] showed that an extract of *Helix hortensis*, agglutinated A_1, A_2, A_1B and A_2B red cells but not those of groups O or B. The strength of the reaction was the same with A_1 as with A_2, and they concluded that this anti-A agglutinin is demonstrating a 'new' blood group receptor in man, A_{hel}. Further, an extract of cooked snail gave the reactions of B substance. In an addendum is reported the finding of anti-A_{hel} and B substance, in *Helix pomatia* also (A_{hel} was later to be called A_{HP}, A_{HH} etc.).

In the first account in German, by the same authors[461], the extraordinary heat stability of the agglutinating factor in *Helix pomatia* is recorded: heating up to 80°C. for one hour actually increases the strength of the reaction. Dissection of the snail located the activity in the Eiweissdrüse (egg white gland).

In a third paper, Prokop and Rackwitz[462] record how anti-A_{hel} differs strikingly from human anti-A in its reaction with the cells of various farm animals.

The immunochemical properties of anti-A_{hel} soon began to be explored[464,465,470].

Boyd and his colleagues[463,466,465] used the fluid expressed from the land snail, *Otala lactea*: the anti-A was powerful and specific but here the reaction with A_1 cells was stronger than that with A_2.

In testing species of snails with terrestrial lungs, Krüpe and Pieper[467] found many with anti-A and three with anti-B: *Iphygena plicatula*, *Leciniaria biplicata* and *Balea perversa*. The anti-B reaction was observed using Löw's papain technique: without the enzyme there was no reaction. In 1964 Johnson[459] had found anti-A_1 in extracts of butter clams (*Saxidomus giganteus*) taken from Oyster Bay, Southern Puget Sound, Washington, and this may possibly have turned the thoughts of Prokop and his colleagues[475,476] to marine animals, for in tinned salmon caviar they found an incomplete anti-B-like reagent and, once again, set off a long train of work. (Here we cannot resist noting the not very practical finding by Tippett and Teesdale[670] of an anti-B-like agglutinin in the plasma of one of the two, untinned, coelacanths they tested.)

So much for the history of this discovery which was to contribute greatly to practical blood grouping and, like the discovery of lectins, to chemical knowledge of the antigens involved. Since our last edition the number of papers on anti-A and anti-B in many snails, in various fish roes and in mussels has grown over-whelmingly. We decided all we could do was to give references to papers we have seen (608–636), in the hope that their titles may help the reader to find what he wants. However, a few of more general interest will now be mentioned.

An outstanding review of the whole subject of agglutinins in snails and fish roes by Prokop, Uhlenbruck and Köhler[609] appeared in 1968; this paper also laid down a standard notation.

Many useful references are to be found in the review by Schnitlzer[631] (1971) in which are listed the specificities of extracts from 59 different kinds of Land-lungenschnecken (which, according to our dictionary, may be translated as land-loitering snails).

Many papers deal with the inhibition by sugars of the agglutinins in the snail extracts: comparisons are made with the inhibition of *Dolichos biflorus* and other anti-A lectins by Uhlenbruck *et al.*[622] (1970) and by Wiener[624] (1970).

Schnitzler, Uerlings and David[632] (1971) in an electronmicroscopic study of purified anti-A_{HP} found the molecules to be egg shaped and to represent 'the smallest antibody-like structure ever encountered'.

BIOCHEMICAL BASIS OF THE ABH ANTIGENS

We confessed in the preface to the first edition of this book that we were totally unfitted to write about the brilliant work on the chemistry of the blood group antigens that emerged from the schools of Witebsky, of Morgan and Kabat. But even without special knowledge one cannot fail to see how triumphant has been the chemical analysis that has brought to light the very complicated genetic back-ground to the ABO, Hh, secretor and Lewis phenotypes. The reader is referred to writings by Morgan and Watkins[284,415,416,648] where many of the earlier references can be found.

In this chapter we shall confine the brief summary to the A, B and H antigens, a detail from the larger canvas of ABH, secretor and Lewis (page 342).

The first stage was the working out of the chemical constitution of the water soluble A, B and H substances from a variety of sources, notably the fluid from ovarian cysts. Figure 4, taken from a paper by Professor Watkins in *Science*[416], tells this part of the story: the gene *H* adds L-fucose to precursor carbohydrate chains and to these H-activated chains the gene *A* further adds *N*-acetyl-D-galac-tosamine and the gene *B* adds D-galactose.

Another step was the visualization of the order in which the genes worked on the precursor substance, the genetical pathways. The map in Figure 5 summarized the beautiful solution. (The pathways leading to the presence of antigens in the saliva are more elaborate, see Figure 22, page 342, because of the bifurcations con-trolled by the secretor and Lewis genes.) This kind of map was originally suggested to us by Dr Eloise Giblett: it is a paraphrase of part of Table I in Watkins[235] and a slight variation on Figure 1 in Ceppellini[236].

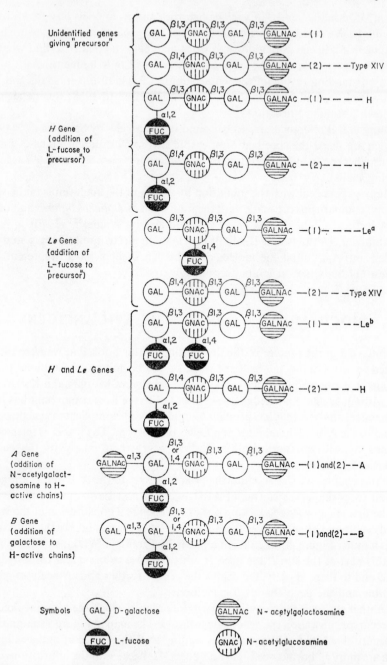

Fig. 4. Representation of the structures proposed for the carbohydrate chains in the precursor glycoprotein and the additions to these chains controlled by the *H*, *Le*, *A*, and *B* genes. (From Watkins[416]. Copyright 1966 by the American Association for the Advancement of Science.)

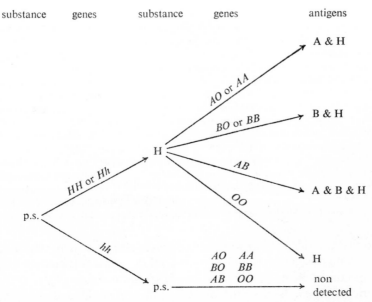

substance   genes   substance   genes   antigens

Fig. 5. The genetical pathways leading to the A, B and H antigens of the red cells. (From the work of Morgan and Watkins, and Ceppellini.) The genes *h* and *O* are considered amorphs.

Incidentally it should be remembered, as Watkins[638] points out, that as early as 1941 Witebsky and Klendshoj in a prophetic sentence wrote 'On the other hand, the possibility could be entertained that there is a basic substance constituting the bulk of the group specific substances, somewhat incorrectly referred to as O substance, on top of which the A and the B property might be present or absent.'

The sequence was based on a vast amount of work on the substances in body fluids: it begins with a precursor glycoprotein which is moulded by the gene *H* into H substance which, in its turn, is partly converted by the independent *A* or *B* genes into A or B antigen; the conversion by A_1 is more complete than that by A_2. *O* is an amorph which effects no conversion[192,237]. The gene *h* is an amorph too, and it fails to produce any H substance for the *A* or *B* genes to convert or for the *O* gene to let through unchanged. The red cells of a person homozygous for *h* are of the O_h phenotype having no A, B or H antigens; no antibody specific for the theoretical precursor substance which may be present on O_h red cells has yet been identified.

Not everyone supports this place of action of *H* in the pathway (Solomon *et al.*[313], Wiener *et al.*[446,639], Voak and Lodge[640]): the objections are serologically based and seem to us rather light against the weight of biochemical evidence. We guess the last word will be with the biochemists.

The gene-enzyme relationships in the pathways were beautifully adumbrated by Watkins[484] in the abstract of her paper to the American Association of Blood Banks, 1967:

The uncomplicated manner of inheritance of most of the blood-group characters indicates a close relationship between the genes and the antigens on the red cells. Detailed chemical investigations on the substances in secretions that have the same serological specificity as the A, B, H, and Lewis antigens on red cells, however, reveal that the blood group specificity is associated with carbohydrate structures. Since the genetic material in the chromosomes (DNA) carries information for the synthesis of proteins, the question that has to be answered is how the information in the blood group genes is translated into carbohydrate structures of defined sequence and pattern. The most plausible explanation is that the genes control the formation or functioning of proteins that are specific enzymes responsible for the assembly of the carbohydrate subunits. These enzymes catalyze the transfer of sugars from an activated donor substrate to carbohydrate chains in a precursor molecule. It is proposed that the protein specified by the *H* gene is an α-L-fucosyltransferase that conveys fucose to a precursor substance to give H specific structures which then constitute acceptors for sugars added by the α-N-acetyl-D-galactosaminyl and D-galactosyltransferases specified by the allelic *A* and *B* genes, respectively. The enzymic product of the *Le* gene, also an α-L-fucosyltransferase, adds fucose to the same precursor as the *H* gene transferase, but to a different sugar in the carbohydrate chain and in different linkage.

To give some idea of how this forecast proved correct we may, this time, quote two separate paragraphs from Professor Watkins' admirable account of the unfolding of the whole story, taken from the *Lister Institute Report*[638] in 1972, which also bridges the gap between the antigens of the body fluids and of the red cells; we have added our reference numbers.

So far mention has been made only of the glycoprotein blood group substances found in tissue fluids and secretions. Since the earliest attempts to identify the blood group A and B factors it appeared probable that, according to the source of the specific material, the characteristic serological properties could be associated with more than one kind of macromolecule. The work of Yamakawa and Suzuki[641] (1952), Koscielak[642] (1963), and Hakomori and Strycharz[643] (1968) established that A and B specificity on the erythrocyte surface is associated, at least in part, with glycolipid molecules. The materials contain sphingosine, fatty acids and the sugars L-fucose, D-galactose, D-glucose and N-acetylglucosamine. The A-active glycolipid has in addition N-acetylgalactosamine. The order, glycosidic linkages and anomeric forms of the individual sugars are not established but on the basis of the molar ratios of the component sugars in the preparations isolated by Hakomori and Strycharz structures for the A and B glycolipids can be proposed that are identical with the serologically active units isolated from A- and B-active glycoproteins. Indirect evidence from haemagglutination and enzymic inhibition experiments established that the same immunodominant sugars are involved in the A and B determinants on the red cell as in the secreted substances (Watkins *et al.* [644]1964). Therefore, although strict proof is not yet available, these results on the glycolipid substances support the belief that the serologically active structures are the same in the glycoprotein and glycolipid substances despite the overall disimilarity of the macromolecules. The same blood group gene specified glycosyltransferases are considered to control the formation of the active structures in the glycolipids and the only difference in the biosynthetic pathway for the formation of the ABH erythrocyte substances is that the secretor gene *Se* does not control the expression of the *H* gene; consequently, H, A and B substances, are formed on the red cell whenever the *H*, *A* and *B* genes are part of the genotype.

Experimental verification of the biosynthetic pathways proposed for the formation of the A, B, H, Le^a and Le^b specific structures has been obtained by examination of tissues from donors of known blood group and secretor status, for glycosyltransferases of the required specificity. An α-N-acetylgalactosaminyl transferase found only in tissues from group A and AB subjects occurs in human submaxillary glands and stomach mucosal linings (Hearn *et al.*[645], 1968; Tuppy and Schenkel-Brunner[646], 1969), milk (Kobata *et al.*[647], 1968), plasma (Sawicka,[648] 1971) and ovarian cyst linings and fluids (Hearn et al.[649], 1972). An α-galactosyltransferase occurring only in group B and AB subjects is demonstrable in the same types of tissue (C. Race et al.[650], 1968; Kobata et al.[651], 1968; Sawicka[648], 1971; Hearn et al.[649], 1972; Poretz and Watkins[652], 1972). These enzymes have an absolute requirement for H-active structures in low-molecular weight acceptors.

The enzyme for H, α-2-fucosyltransferase, was found in milk (Shen et al.[653], 1968) and other sites. In 1972 Schenkel-Brunner et al.[548] report 'In contrast to the α-2-L-fucosyltransferases in human milk, submaxillary glands and stomach mucosa that occur only in ABH secretors, an enzyme that transfers L-fucose to the C-2 position of non-reducing β-galactosyl residues was found in the serum of all normal ABO donors irrespective of their ABH secretor-nonsecretor status.'

Work on the N-acetyl-D-galactosaminyltransferases produced by A_1 and A_2 was interpreted as evidence of a qualitative rather than a quantitative difference between the two enzymes (Schachter et al.[654], 1973).

Even non-biochemists can scarce forbear to cheer on reading (Schenkel-Brunner et al.[548] and C. Race and Watkins[549]) that O_h people, unlike people of ordinary ABO groups, lack in their serum the α-2-L-fucosyltransferase needed for H formation yet have the A and B enzymes, α-N-acetyl-D-galactosaminyl and α-D-galactosyltransferases, appropriate to their true ABO genotype.

REFERENCES

1 LANDSTEINER K. (1900) Zur Kenntnis der antifermentativen, lytischen und agglutinierenden Wirkungen des Blutserums und der Lymphe. Zbl. Bakt., 27, 357–362. (See ref. 17.)
2 LANDSTEINER K. (1901) Über Agglutinationserscheinungen normalen menschlichen Blutes, Wien. klin. Wschr., 14, 1132–1134. (See ref. 17.)
3 DECASTELLO A. v. and STURLI A. (1902) Über die Isoagglutinine im Serum gesunder und kranker Menschen. Munchen. med. Wchnschr., 1090–1095. (See ref. 17.)
4 DUNGERN E. v. and HIRSZFELD L. (1911) Über gruppenspezifische Strukturen des Blutes III. Z. Immun. Forsch., 8, 526–562. (See ref. 17.)
5 THOMSEN O., FRIEDENREICH V. and WORSAAE E. (1930) Über die Möglichkeit der Existenz zweier neuer Blutgruppen; auch ein Beitrag zur Beleuchtung sogennanter Untergruppen. Acta path. microbiol. scand., 7, 157–190.
6 FRIEDENREICH V. and ZACHO A. (1931) Die Differentialdiagnose zwischen den 'Unter'-gruppen A_1 und A_2. Z. Rassenphysiol, 4, 164–191.
7 FRIEDENREICH V. (1931) Ueber die Serologie der Untergruppen A_1 and A_2. Z. ImmunForsch. 71, 283–313.
8 TAYLOR G.L., RACE R.R., PRIOR AILEEN M. and IKIN ELIZABETH W. (1942) Frequency of the iso-agglutinin α_1 in the serum of the subgroups A_2 and A_2B. J. Path. Bact., 54, 514–516.
9 EPSTEIN A.A. and OTTENBERG R. (1908) Simple method of performing serum reactions. Proc. N.Y. path. Soc., 8, 117–123.
10 DUNGERN E. v. and HIRSZFELD L. (1910) Ueber Vererbung gruppenspezifischer Strukturen des Blutes. Strukturen des Blutes. Z. ImmunForsch., 6, 284–292. (A translation by G.P. Pohlmann: Transfusion, Philad. 1962, 2, 70–74.)
11 BERNSTEIN F. (1924) Ergebnisse einer biostatischen zusammenfassenden Betrachtung uber die erblichen Blutstrukturen des Menschen. Klin. Wschr., 3, 1495–1497. (See ref. 17.)
12 BERNSTEIN F. (1925) Zusammenfassende Betrachtungen über die erblichen Blutstrukturen des Menschen. Z. indukt. Abstamm. u. VererbLehre., 37, 237–270. (See ref. 17.)

[13] HIRSZFELD L. and HIRSZFELD H. (1919) Serological differences between the blood of different races. The result of researches on the Macedonian front. *Lancet*, **ii**, 675–679.

[14] BOYD W.C. (1939) Blood Groups. *Tabulae Biologicae*, **17**, 113–240.

[15] MOURANT A.E. (1954) *The Distribution of the Human Blood Groups*, Blackwell Scientific Publications, Oxford.

[16] FISHER R.A. and TAYLOR G.L. (1940) Scandinavian influence in Scottish ethnology. *Nature, Lond.*, **145**, 590.

[17] Translations of these papers have been published by the Blood Transfusion Division, U.S. Army Medical Research Laboratory, Fort Knox, Kentucky, 40121.

[18] DOBSON AILEEN M. and IKIN ELIZABETH W. (1946) The ABO blood groups in the United Kingdom; frequencies based on a very large sample. *J. Path. Bact.*, **48**, 221–277.

[19] IKIN ELIZABETH W., PRIOR AILEEN M., RACE R.R. and TAYLOR G.L. (1939) The distribution of the A_1A_2BO blood groups in England. *Ann. Eugen., Lond.*, **9**, 409–411.

[20] REED, T.E. (1964) The frequency and nature of blood group A_3. *Transfusion, Philad.*, **4**, 457–460.

[21] COHEN FLOSSIE and ZUELZER W.W. (1965) Interrelationship of the various subgroups of the blood group A: study with immunofluorescence. *Transfusion, Philad.*, **5**, 223–229.

[22] ROBERTS J.A.F. (1948) The frequencies of the ABO blood groups in South-Western England. *Ann. Eugen., Lond.*, **14**, 109–116.

[23] ALTER A.A. and ROSENFIELD R.E. (1964) The nature of some subtypes of A. *Blood*, **23**, 605–620.

[24] JUEL E. (1959) Anti-A agglutinins in sera from A_2B individuals. *Acta path. microbiol scand.*, **46**, 91–95.

[25] BERNSTEIN F. (1930) Fortgesetzte Untersuchungen aus der Theorie der Blutgruppen. *Z. indukt. Abstamm. u. VererbLehre*, **56**, 233–273 (See ref. 17.)

[26] TAYLOR G.L. and PRIOR AILEEN M. (1938) Blood groups in England. II. Distribution in the population. *Ann. Eugen., Lond.*, **8**, 356–361.

[27] HARTMANN O., HADLAND K. and BJERKELUND C.J. (1941) *Blood Group Distribution in Norway*, 1 Kommisjon Hos Jacob Dybwad, Oslo.

[28] HARTMANN O. and LUNDEVALL J.U. (1944) *Blood Group Distribution in Norway with Special Regard to the MN and OA_1A_2B System*, 1 Kommisjon Hos Jacob Dybwad, Oslo.

[29] SALMON C., SALMON DENISE and REVIRON J. (1965) Étude immunologique et génétique de la variabilité du phénotype A_x. *Nouv. Revue fr. Hémat.*, **5**, 275–290.

[30] VOS G.H. (1964) Five examples of red cells with the A_x subgroup of blood group A. *Vox Sang.*, **9**, 160–167.

[31] WELLISCH S. and THOMSEN O. (1930) Uber die vier-gen-hypothese Thomsens. *Hereditas, Lund*, **14**, 50–52.

[32] STEVENS W.L. (1938) Estimation of blood group gene frequencies. *Ann. Eugen., Lond.*, **8**, 362–375.

[33] WIENER A.S. (1943) *Blood Groups and Transfusion*, 3rd edition, Thomas, Springfield.

[34] WIENER A.S., GORDON EVE B. and COHEN L. (1954) Studies on the heredity of the human blood groups II. The A-B-O groups. *Acta Genet. Med. Gemell.*, **3**, 29–33.

[35] TAYLOR G.L. and PRIOR AILEEN M. (1939) Blood Groups in England. III. Discussion of the family material. *Ann. Eugen., Lond.*, **9**, 18–44.

[36] RACE R.R., IKIN ELIZABETH W., TAYLOR G.L. and PRIOR AILEEN M. (1942) A second series of families examined in England for the A_1A_2BO and MN blood group factors. *Ann. Eugen., Lond.*, **11**, 385–394.

[37] FRIEDENREICH V. (1936) Eine bisher unbekannte Blutgruppeneigenschaft (A_3). *Z. Immun-Forsch.*, **89**, 409–422. (See ref. 17.)

[38] GAMMELGAARD A. (1942) Om Sjaeldne, Svage A-receptorer (A_3, A_4, A_5, og A_x). *Hos Mennesket*. Published by Nyt Nordisk Forlag. Arnold Busck. (See ref. 17.)

[39] COTTERMAN C.W. (1956) Somatic mosaicism for antigen A_2. *Abstracts, 1st int. Congr. hum. Genet.*, p. 94.

[40] YOUNG L.E. and WITEBSKY E. (1945) Studies on the sub-groups of blood groups A and AB. II. The agglutinogen A_3: its detection with potent B serum and an investigation of its inheritance. J. Immunol., 51, 111–116.

[41] SCHMID A. (1956) Ueber Intermediarformen der A-Untergruppen. Inaugural dissertation, Univ. of Bern.

[42] BHENDE Y.M., DESHPANDE C.K., BHATIA H. M., SANGER RUTH, RACE R.R., MORGAN W.T.J. and WATKINS WINIFRED M. (1952) A 'new' blood-group character related to the ABO system. Lancet, i, 903–904.

[43] CEPPELLINI R., NASSO S. and TECILAZICH F. (1952) La Malattia Emolitica del Neonato, Istituto Sieroterapico Milanese Serafino Belfanti Milano (p. 204.)

[44] LEVINE P., ROBINSON ELIZABETH, CELANO M., BRIGGS OLIVE and FALKINBURG L. (1955) Gene interaction resulting in suppression of blood group substance B. Blood, 10, 1100–1108.

[45] JUEL E. (1959) Studies in the subgroups of the blood group A. Absorption experiments indicating qualitative differences between subgroups A_1 and A_2. Acta path. microbiol. scand., 46, 251–265.

[46] SIMMONS R.T. and D'SENA G.W.L. (1955) Anti-H in group O blood. J. Ind. med. Ass., 24, 325–327.

[47] BHATIA H.M., SANGHVI L.D., BHIDE Y.G. and JHALA H.I. (1955) Anti-H in two siblings in an Indian family. J. Ind. med. Ass., 25, 545–548.

[48] PARKIN DOROTHY M. (1956) Study of a family with unusual ABO phenotypes. Brit. J. Haemat., 2, 106–110.

[49] WEINER W., LEWIS, H.B.M., MOORES PHYLLIS, SANGER RUTH and RACE R.R. (1957) A gene, y, modifying the blood group antigen A. Vox Sang,, 2, 25–37.

[50] JONSSON B. and FAST K. (1948) Ein eigenartiger, familiärer typus von extrem schwachem A-faktor, 'A_6'. Acta. path. microbiol. scand., 25, 649–655.

[51] FISCHER W. and HAHN F. (1935) Ueber auffallende Schwache der gruppenspezifischen Reaktionsfahigkeit bei eniem Erwachsenen. Z. ImmunForsch., 84, 177–188. (See ref. 17.)

[52] DUNSFORD I. and ASPINALL P. (1952) An A_4 $cD^u e/cde$ blood in an English family. Ann. Eugen., Lond., 17, 30–34.

[53] DUNSFORD I. (1952) Group A blood weaker in reaction than A_3. Bulletin of the Central Laboratory of the Netherlands Red Cross Blood Transfusion Service, 2, 209–219.

[54] GROVE-RASMUSSEN M., SOUTTER L. and LEVINE P. (1952) A new blood subgroup (A_0) identifiable with group O serums. Amer. J. clin. Path., 22, 1157–1163.

[55] ESTOLA E. and ELO J. (1952) Occurrence of an exceedingly weak 'A' blood group property in a family. Ann. Med. exp. Fenn., 30, 79–87.

[56] ELLIS F.R. and CAWLEY L.P. (1958) The third instance of agglutinogen A_0. Report of a family study. Proc. 6th Congr. Int. Soc. Blood Transf., 135.

[57] LOGHEM J.J. VAN and HART MIA V.D. (1954) The weak antigen A_4 occurring in the offspring of group O parents. Vox Sang. (O.S.), 4, 69–75.

[58] BECKERS THEODORA, LOGHEM J.J. VAN and DUNSFORD I. (1955) A second example of the weak antigen A_4 occurring in the offspring of group O parents. Vox Sang. (O.S.), 5, 145–147.

[59] CAHAN A., JACK J.A., SCUDDER J., SARGENT MARY, SANGER RUTH and RACE R.R. (1957) A family in which A_x is transmitted through a person of the blood group A_2B. Vox Sang., 2, 8–15.

[60] WIENER A.S. (1953) The blood factor C of the A-B-O system, with special reference to the rare blood group C. Ann. Eugen., Lond., 18, 1–8.

[61] LOGHEM J.J. VAN, DORFMEIER HANNY and HART MIA V.D. (1957) Two A antigens with abnormal serologic properties. Vox Sang., 2, 16–24.

[62] FISHER NATHALIE and CAHAN A. (1962) An addition to the family in which A_x is transmitted through a person of the blood group A_2B. Vox Sang., 7, 484.

63 MÄKELÄ O. and MÄKELÄ PIRJO (1955) A weak B containing anti-B. *Ann. Med. exp. Fenn.*, **33**, 33–40.

64 MOULLEC J., SUTTON ELLAINE and BURGADA M. (1955) Une variante faible de l'agglutinogène de groupe B. *Rev. Hémat.*, **10**, 574–582.

65 LEVINE P., CELANO M.J. and GRISET T. (1958) B_w: a new allele of the ABO locus. *Proc. 6th Congr. int. Soc. Blood Transf.*, 132–135.

66 DUNSFORD I., STACEY S.M. and YOKOYAMA M. (1956) A rare variety of the human blood group B. *Nature, Lond.*, **178**, 1167–1168.

67 SALMON C., REVIRON J. and LIBERGE GENEVIÈVE (1964) Nouvel exemple d'une famille ou le phénotype A_m est observé dans 2 générations. *Nouv. Revue fr. Hémat.*, **4**, 359–364.

68 KEMP T. (1930) Uber den Empfindlichkeitsgrad der Blutkörperchen gegenüber Isohämagglutininen im Fötatteben und im Kindersalter beim Menschen. *Acta path. microbiol. scand.*, **7**, 146–156.

69 HRUBIŠKO M., ČALKOVSKÁ ZDENKA, MERGANCOVÁ OLGA and GALLOVÁ KATARÍNA (1966) Beobachtungen über Varianten des Blutgruppensystems ABO. I. Studies der Variante A_m. *Blut*, **13**, 137–142.

70 HRUBIŠKO M., ČALKOVSKÁ ZDENKA, MERGANCOVÁ OLGA and GALLOVÁ KATARÍNA (1966) Beobachtungen über Varianten des Blutgruppensystems ABO. II. Beitrag zur Erblichkeit der A_m-Variante. *Blut*, **13**, 232–239.

71 FORMAGGIO T.G. (1951) Development and secretion of the blood group factor O in the newborn. *Proc. Soc. exp. Biol. N.Y.*, **76**, 554–556.

72 WATKINS WINIFRED M. (1952) The O and H blood group characters in the newborn. *Brit. J. exp. Path.*, **33**, 244–257.

73 SPRINGER G.F. (1956) Inhibition of blood-group agglutinins by substances occurring in plants. *J. Immunol.* **76**, 399–407.

74 MORGAN W.T.J. and VAN HEYNINGEN RUTH (1944) The occurrence of A, B and O blood group substances in pseudo-mucinous ovarian cyst fluids. *Brit. J. exp. Path.*, **25**, 5–15.

75 YOSIDA K.L. (1928) Cited by Buchanan and Rapoport.[77]

76 SEKIMOTO H. (1940) Cited by Buchanan and Rapoport.[77]

77 BUCHANAN DOROTHY J. and RAPOPORT S. (1951) Composition of meconium. Serological study of blood-group-specific substances found in individual meconiums. *Proc. Soc. exp. Biol. N.Y.*, **77**, 114–117.

78 BOYD W.C. and BOYD LYLE G. (1937) Blood grouping tests on 300 mummies. *J. Immunol.*, **32**, 307–319.

79 FURUHATA T., OKAJIMA M. and SHIMIZU S. (1950) Blood group determinations of eight hundred years old mummies of Governor-Generals in four generations at Chusonji. *Proc. imp. Acad. Japan*, **26**, 78–80.

80 GUREVITCH J. and NELKEN D. (1954) ABO blood groups in blood platelets. *Nature, Lond.*, **173**, 356.

81 GUREVITCH J. and NELKEN D. (1954) ABO groups in blood platelets. *J. Lab. clin. Med.*, **44**, 562–570.

82 GUREVITCH J. and NELKEN D. (1955) Elution of isoagglutinins adsorbed by platelets. *Nature, Lond.*, **175**, 822.

83 GUREVITCH J. and NELKEN D. (1955) Studies on platelet antigens. II. A_1 and A_2 subgroups in blood platelets. *J. Lab. clin. Med.*, **46**, 530–533.

84 MOUREAU P. and ANDRÉ A. (1954) Présence des antigènes A et B dans les plaquettes. *Vox Sang.* (O.S.), **4**, 46–51.

85 DAUSSET J. and MALINVAUD G. (1954) Normal and pathological platelet agglutinins investigated by means of the shaking method. *Vox Sang.* (O.S.), **4**, 204–213.

86 COOMBS R.R.A. and BEDFORD D. (1955) The A and B antigens on human platelets demonstrated by means of mixed erythrocyte-platelet agglutination. *Vox Sang.* (O.S.), **5**, 111–115.

87 MEYER W., WUILLERET B. and HÄSSIG A. (1955) Uber den Nachweis von Blutgruppen-antigenen in Thrombozyten. *Z. ImmunForsch.*, **112**, 369–372.

88 ASHHURST DOREEN E., BEDFORD D. and COOMBS R.R.A. (1956) Examination of human platelets for the ABO, MN, Rh, Tj^a, Lutheran and Lewis system of antigens by means of mixed erythrocyte-platelet agglutination. *Vox Sang.*, **1**, 235–240.

89 THOMSEN O. (1930) Untersuchungen über die serologische Gruppendifferenzierung des Organismus. *Acta path. microbiol. scand.*, **7**, 250. Cited by Dausset.[90]

90 DAUSSET J. (1954) Présence des antigènes A et B dans les leucocytes décelée par des épreuves d'agglutination. *C. r. Soc. Biol., Paris*, **148**, 1607.

91 COOMBS R.R.A., BEDFORD D. and ROUILLARD L.M. (1956) A and B blood-group antigens on human epidermal cells demonstrated by mixed agglutination. *Lancet*, **i**, 461–463.

92 FUCHS F., FREIESLEBEN E., KNUDSEN ELSE E. and RIIS P. (1956) Determination of foetal blood-group. *Lancet*, **i**, 996.

93 BRAIN P. (1966) Subgroups of A in the South African Bantu. *Vox Sang.*, **11**, 686–698.

94 MOURANT A.E., KOPEĆ ADA C. and DOMANIEWSKA-SOBCZAK KAZIMIERA (1958) *The ABO Blood Groups. Comprehensive Tables and Maps of World Distribution*, pp. 276, Blackwell Scientific Publications, Oxford.

95 FRIEDENREICH V. and WITH S. (1933) Ueber B-Antigen und B-Antikörper bei Menschen und Tieren. *Z. ImmunForsch.*, **78**, 152–172.

96 OWEN R.D. (1954) Heterogeneity of antibodies to the human blood groups in normal and immune sera. *J. Immunol.*, **73**, 29–39.

97 JACQUOT-ARMAND YVETTE, THÉOLEYRE MADELEINE and FILITTI-WURMSER SABINE (1956) Sur l'absorption des isohémagglutinines humaines anti-B par les hématies de lapin et d'opossum. *Rev. Hémat.*, **11**, 63–78.

98 KABAT E.A. (1956) *The Blood Group Substances*, p. 267, Academic Press Inc. Publishers, New York.

99 MORVILLE, P. (1929) Investigation on iso-haemagglutination in mothers and newborn children. *Acta path. microbiol. scand.*, **6**, 39. Cited by Mollison.[101]

100 YLIRUOKANEN A. (1948) Blood transfusion in premature infants. *Ann. Med. exp. Biol. Fenn.*, **26**, supp. 6. Cited by Mollison.[101]

101 MOLLISON P.L. (1956) *Blood Transfusion in Clinical Medicine*, 2nd edition, Blackwell Scientific Publications, Oxford.

102 THOMSEN O. and KETTEL K. (1929) Die Stärke der menschlichen Isoagglutinine und entsprechender Blutkörperchenrezeptoren in verschiedenen Lebensaltern. *Z. Immun-Forsch.*, **63**, 67–93.

103 BIRD, G.W.G. (1964) A— intermediates in Maharastrian blood donors. *Vox Sang.*, **9**, 629–630.

104 SHAW D.H. and STONE W.H. (1957) Seasonal variation of natural occurring isoantibodies of man. *Trans 6th Congr. europ. Soc. Hemat.*, 724–732.

105 WITEBSKY E. (1948) Interrelationship between the Rh system and the ABO system. *Blood 3*, suppl., **2**, 66–78.

106 STURGEON P., MOORE B.P.L. and WEINER W. (1964) Notations for two weak A variants: A_{end} and A_{el}. *Vox Sang.*, **9**, 214–215.

107 FILITTI-WURMSER SABINE, JACQUOT-ARMAND YVETTE, AUBEL-LESURE G. and WURMSER R. (1954) Physico-chemical study of human isohaemagglutination. *Ann. Eugen., Lond.*, **18**, 183–302.

108 DUNSFORD I. (1959) A critical review of the ABO sub-groups. *Proc. 7th Congr. int. Soc Blood Transf.*, 685–691.

109 DUNSFORD I. (1959) Interaction between the A and B blood group genes. *Proc. 7th Congr. int. Soc. Blood Transf.*, 707–709.

110 ANDRÉ R. and SALMON C. (1957) Étude sérologique comparée de neuf exemples non apparentés de groupe sanguin 'A faible'. *Rev. Hémat.*, **12**, 668–678.

[111] SALMON C. (1960) *Étude thermodynamique de l'anticorps anti-B des sujets de phenotype A_x.* D.Sc. thesis, University of Paris.

[112] FINE M., EYQUEM A. and THÉBAULT J. (1956) Contribution a l'étude de l'antigène érythrocytaire humain A_4. *Ann. Inst. Pasteur*, **91**, 892–897.

[113] GLOVER S.M. and WALFORD R.L. (1958) A serologic and family study of the rare blood group A_x. *Amer. J. clin. Path.*, **30**, 539–546.

[114] SALMON C., BORIN P. and ANDRÉ R. (1958) Le groupe sanguin A_m dans deux générations d'une même famille. *Rev. Hémat.*, **13**, 529–537 and (1959), *Proc. 7th Congr. int. Soc. Blood Transf.*, 709–715.

[115] KINDLER M. (1958) Ein weiteres Beispiel einer schwachen A-Eigenschaft (A_m). *Blut.* **4**, 373–377.

[116] LANDSTEINER K. and LEVINE P. (1930) Differentiation of a type of human blood by means of normal animal serum. *J. Immunol.*, **18**, 87–94.

[117] WEINER A.S. (1950) Heredity of the Rh blood types. IX. Observations in a series of 526 cases of disputed parentage. *Amer. J. hum. Genet.*, **2**, 177–197.

[118] TIPPETT PATRICIA, NOADES JEAN, SANGER RUTH, RACE R.R., SAUSAIS LAIMA, HOLMAN C.A. and BUTTIMER R.J. (1960) Further studies of the I antigen and antibody. *Vox Sang.*, **5**, 107–121.

[119] BIRD G.W.G. (1958) Erythrocyte agglutinins from plants. Ph.D. thesis, London.

[120] WEINER W., SANGER RUTH, and RACE R.R. (1959) A weak form of the blood group antigen A: an inherited character. *Proc. 7th Congr. int. Soc. Blood Transf.*, 720–725.

[121] LANDSTEINER K. and WITT D. (1926) Observation on the human blood groups. *J. Immunol.*, **11**, 221–247.

[122] KOECKERT H.L. (1920) A study of the mechanism of human isohemagglutination. *J. Immunol.*, **5**, 529–537.

[123] MOSS W.L. (1910) Studies on isoagglutinins and isohemolysins. *Bull. Johns Hopkins Hosp.*, **21**, 63–70.

[124] DODD BARBARA E. (1952) Linked anti-A and anti-B antibodies from group O sera. *Brit. J. exp. Path.*, **33**, 1–18.

[125] BIRD G.W.G. (1953) Observations on haemagglutinin 'linkage' in relation to isoagglutinins and auto-agglutinins. *Brit. J. exp. Path.*, **34**, 131–137.

[126] BIRD G.W.G. (1954) The hypothetical factor C of the ABO system of blood groups. *Vox Sang.* (O.S.), **4**, 66–68.

[127] MILGROM F. (1952) Recherches sur la structure des isoanticorps groupaux. *Rev. Immunol.*, **16**, 86–109.

[128] MATSUNAGA E. (1950) Heredity of the agglutinogen C and the anti-C agglutinin in human blood. *Proc. imp. Acad. Japan*, **26**, 59–64.

[129] ROSENFIELD R.E. (1953) AB hemolytic disease of the newborn. *Prog. Amer. Ass. of Blood Banks*. Also (1955) AB hemolytic disease of the newborn: analysis of 1,480 cord blood specimens, with special reference to the direct antiglobulin test and to the role of the group O mother. *Blood*, **10**, 17–28.

[130] WIENER A.S., SAMWICK A.A., MORRISON H. and COHEN L. (1953) Studies on immunization in man II. The blood factor C. *Exp. Med. Surg.*, **11**, 276–285.

[131] UNGER L.J. and WIENER A.S. (1954) Studies on the C antibody of group O serum with special reference to its role in hemolytic disease of the newborn. *J. Lab. clin. Med.*, **44**, 387–399.

[132] GRUBB R. (1949) Some aspects of the complexity of the human ABO blood groups. *Acta path. microbiol., scand.*, suppl. **84**, 1–72.

[133] GRUBB R. (1950) Quelques aspects de la complexité des groupes ABO. *Rev. Hémat.*, **5**, 268–275.

[134] WATKINS WINIFRED M. and MORGAN W.T.J. (1955) Some observations on the O and H characters of human blood and secretions. *Vox Sang.* (O.S.), **5**, 1–14.

[135] JAKOBOWICZ RACHEL, NOADES JEAN E. and SIMMONS R.T. (1963) A further example of an unnamed variant of blood group A. *Med. J. Aust.*, **i**, 657–658.

136 REED T.E. and MOORE B.P.L. (1964) A new variant of blood group A. *Vox Sang.*, **9**, 363–366.

137 SOLOMON J.M. and STURGEON P. (1964) Quantitative studies of the phenotype A_{el}. *Vox Sang.*, **9**, 476–486.

138 BOORMAN KATHLEEN E. and ZEITLIN R.A. (1964) B_v—a sub-group of B which lacks part of the normal human B antigen. *Vox Sang.*, **9**, 278–288.

139 BENNETT M.H., BROMLEY ANNE, GILES CAROLYN M., JAMES J.D., MOURANT A.E. and PLAUT GERTRUDE (1962) A blood group B gene with variable expression. *Vox Sang.*, **7**, 579–584.

140 MORGAN W.T.J. and WATKINS WINIFRED M. (1948) The detection of a product of the blood group O gene and the relationship of the so-called O substance to the agglutinogens A and B. *Brit. J. exp. Path.*, **29**, 159–173.

141 SANGER RUTH (1952) A relationship between the secretion of the blood group antigens and the presence of anti-O or anti-H in human serum. *Nature, Lond.*, **170**, 78.

142 WATKINS WINIFRED M. and MORGAN W.T.J. (1954) A potent group—O cell—agglutinin of human origin with H-specific character. *Lancet*, **i**, 959–961.

143 KOUT M. and TOTÍN P. (1963) A case of very weak B agglutinogen. *Vox Sang.*, **8**, 741–746.

144 YAMAGUCHI H., OKUBO Y., HAZAMA F. and OYAMA S. (1964) B_x, another allele of the ABO locus and its heredity. *Proc. imp. Acad. Japan*, **40**, 357–361.

145 FURUKAWA K. and ISEKI S. (1963) An example of a family with blood group B_m. *Proc. 1st Asian Congr. Blood Transf.*, 183–188.

146 RENKONEN K.O. (1948) Studies on hemagglutinins present in seeds of some representatives of the family of Leguminoseae. *Ann. Med. exp., Fenn.*, **26**, 66–72.

147 BOYD W.C. and REGUERA ROSE M. (1949) Hemagglutinating substances for human cells in various plants. *J. Immunol.*, **62**, 333–339.

148 KOULUMIES R. (1949) The subgroups A_1, A_2 and A_1B, A_2B and their relation to some hemagglutinins present in seeds of *Vicia Cracca*. *Ann. Med. exp. Fenn.*, **27**, 20–24.

149 BOYD W.C. (1950) Hemagglutinating substances for human cells in various Egyptian plants. *J. Immunol.*, **65**, 281–284.

150 BIRD G.W.G. (1955) Haemagglutinins in Indian plants. *Army Medical Corps Journal*, **11**, 17–25.

151 MÄKELÄ O. (1957) Studies in hemagglutinins of Leguminosae seeds. Thesis, Supplement No. 11, *Ann. Med. exp. Fenn.*, **35**, 1–133.

152 BIRD G.W.G. (1951) Specific agglutinating activity for human red blood corpuscles in extracts of *Dolichos biflorus*. *Curr. Sci.*, **20**, 298–299.

153 BIRD G.W.G. (1952) Relationship of the blood sub-groups A_1, A_2 and A_1B, A_2B to haemagglutinins present in the seeds of *Dolichos biflorus*. *Nature, Lond.* **170**, 674.

154 BIRD G.W.G. (1952) Anti-A haemagglutinins in seeds. *J. Immunol.*, **69**, 319–320.

155 BIRD G.W.G. (1954) Seed agglutinins and the T receptor. *J. Path. Bact.*, **68**, 289–291.

156 MÄKELÄ O. and MÄKELÄ PIRJO (1956) Some new blood group specific phytagglutinins. *Ann. Med. exp. Fenn.*, **34**, 402–404.

157 ELO J., ESTOLA E. and MALMSTRÖM N. (1951) On phytagglutinins present in mushrooms. *Ann. Med. exp. Fenn.*, **29**, 297–308.

158 GOLD E. and DUNSFORD I. (1960) An A_1 antigen with abnormal serological properties. *Vox Sang.*, **5**, 574–578.

159 CAZAL P. and LALAURIE M. (1952) Recherches sur quelques phyto-agglutinines spécifiques des groups sanguins ABO. *Acta haemat.*, **8**, 73–80.

160 BOYD W.C. and SHAPLEIGH ELIZABETH (1954) Separation of individuals of any blood group into secretors and non-secretors by use of a plant agglutinin (lectin). *Blood*, **9**, 1195–1198.

161 BOYD W.C. and SHAPLEIGH ELIZABETH (1954) Specific precipitating activity of plant agglutinins (lectins). *Science*, **119**, 419.

[162] FURUHATA T., KITAHAMA M. and NOZAWA T. (1959) A family study of the so-called blood group chimera. *Proc. imp. Acad. Japan*, **35**, 55–57.

[163] OTTENSOOSER F. and SILBERSCHMIDT K. (1953) Haemagglutinin anti-N in plant seeds. *Nature, Lond.*, **172**, 914.

[164] LEVINE P., OTTENSOOSER F., CELANO M.J. and POLLITZER W. (1955) On reactions of plant anti-N with red cells of chimpanzees and other animals. *Amer. J. phys. Anthrop.*, **13**, 29–36.

[165] BIRD G.W.G. (1954) Observations on the interactions of the erythrocytes of various species with certain seed agglutinins. *Brit. J. exp. Path.*, **35**, 252–254.

[166] MORGAN W.T.J. and WATKINS WINIFRED M. (1953) The inhibition of the haemagglutinins in plant seeds by human blood group substances and simple sugars. *Brit. J. exp. Path.*, **34**, 94–103.

[167] KRÜPE M. and BRAUN CHRISTA (1952) Über ein pflanzliches Hämagglutinin gegen menschliche B-Blutzellen. *Naturwissenschaften*, **39**, 284–285.

[168] BIRD G.W.G. (1956) The haemagglutinins of *Crotalaria striata*. Further evidence of similarity of the A and B agglutinogens. *Vox Sang.*, **1**, 167–171.

[169] BOYD W.C. and SHAPLEIGH ELIZABETH (1954) Antigenic relations of blood group antigens as suggested by tests with lectins. *J. Immunol.*, **73**, 226–231.

[170] KRÜPE M. (1956) *Blutgruppenspezifische Pflanzliche Eiweisskörper* (*Phytagglutinine*), Ferdinand Enke Verlag, Stuttgart. Cited by Mäkelä and Mäkelä.[156]

[171] CRAWFORD HAL, CUTBUSH MARIE and MOLLISON P.L. (1953) Specificity of incomplete 'cold' antibody in human serum. *Lancet*, i, 566–567.

[172] BIRD G.W.G. (1951) The nature of auto-agglutinins. *Lancet*, i, 997.

[173] BIRD G.W.G. (1951) Auto-agglutinin components. *Lancet*, ii, 128.

[174] BIRD G.W.G. (1955) Observations on 'suppressed' or 'latent' haemagglutinins. *Brit. J. Haemat.*, **1**, 375–377.

[175] IKIN ELIZABETH W., MOURANT A.E. and PUGH V.W. (1953) An anti-Rh serum reacting differently with O and A red cells. *Vox Sang.* (O.S.), **3**, 74–78.

[176] YOKOYAMA M., STACEY S.M. and DUNSFORD I. (1957) B$_x$—a new sub-group of the blood group B. *Vox Sang.*, **2**, 348–356.

[177] NELKEN E., MICHAELSON I.C., NELKEN D. and GUREVITCH J. (1956) ABO antigens in the human cornea. *Nature, Lond.*, **177**, 840.

[178] NELKEN E., MICHAELSON I.C., NELKEN D. and GUREVITCH J. (1957) Studies on antigens in the human cornea and their relationship to corneal grafting in man. *J. Lab. clin. Med.*, **49**, 745–752.

[179] NELKEN D., GUREVITCH J. and NEUMAN Z. (1957) A and B antigens in the human epidermis, *J. clin. Investig.*, **36**, 749–751.

[180] BIRD G.W.G. (1957) Haemagglutinins in *Calpurnia aurea*. *Nature, Lond.*, **180**, 657.

[181] WINSTANLEY D.P., KONUGRES ANGELYN and COOMBS R.R.A. (1957) Studies on human anti-A sera with special reference to so-called 'immune' anti-A. 1. The A^P antigen and the specificity of the haemolysin in anti-A sera. *Brit. J. Haemat.*, **3**, 341–347.

[182] MOORE B.P.L., NEWSTEAD P.H. and JOHNSON JOANNE (1961) A weak example of the blood group antigen A, *Vox Sang.*, **6**, 151–156.

[183] MOORE B.P.L., NEWSTEAD P.H. and MARSON ANNE (1961) A weak inherited, group A phenotype. *Vox Sang.*, **6**, 624–626.

[184] KITAHAMA M. (1959) Chimera and mosaic in blood group. *J. Japan Soc. Blood Transf.*, **5**, 210–212.

[185] BOORMAN KATHLEEN E. and ZEITLIN R.A. (1959) A sub-group of B. *Proc. 7th Congr. int. Soc. Blood Transf.*, 716–720.

[186] YOKOYAMA M., BARBER MARGARET and DUNSFORD I. (1959) The sub-groups of blood group B in man. *Juntendo Med. J.*, **5**, 273–277.

[187] VYAS G.N., BHATIA H.M. and SANGHVI L.D. (1960) Three cases of weak B in an Indian family. *Vox Sang.*, **5**, 509–516.

188 SUSSMAN L.N., PRETSHOLD HANNAH and LACHER M.J. (1960) A second example of blood group B_3. *Blood*, 16, 1788–1794.

189 ANDERSEN J. (1960) An inheritable B-like character in persons of blood group A. *Blood*, 16, 1163–1172.

190 MOULLEC J. and LE CHEVREL P. (1959) A rare variant of B in a human blood sample belonging to group AB. *Nature, Lond.*, 183, 1733.

191 MOULLEC J. and LE CHEVREL B. (1959) Un facteur B faible dans un sang du groupe AB. *Transfusion, Paris*, 2, 47–56.

192 WATKINS WINIFRED M. and MORGAN W.T.J. (1955) Some observations on the O and H characters of human blood and secretions. *Vox Sang.* (O.S.), 5, 1–14.

193 ALOYSIA MARY, GELB A.G., FUDENBERG H., HAMPER JEAN, TIPPETT PATRICIA and RACE R.R. (1961) The expected 'Bombay' groups O_h^{A1} and O_h^{A2}. *Transfusion, Philad.*, 1, 212–217.

194 ROY M.N., DUTTA S., MITRA P.C. and GHOSH S. (1957) Occurrence of natural anti-H in a group of individuals. *J. Indian med. Ass.*, 29, 224–226.

195 PETTENKOFER H.J., LUBOLDT W., LAWONN H. and NIEBUHR R. (1960) Über genetische Suppression der Blutgruppen ABO Untersuchungen an einer Familie, bei der die Unterdrückung nicht das Blutgruppenmerkmal B betrifft. *Z. ImmunForsch.*, 120, 288–294.

196 HAKIM S.A., VYAS G.N., SANGHVI L.D. and BHATIA H.M. (1961) Eleven cases of 'Bombay' phenotype in six families: suppression of ABO antigen demonstrated in two families. *Transfusion, Philad.*, 1, 218–222.

197 BHATIA H.M. and SANGHVI L.D. (1962) Rare blood groups and consanguinity: 'Bombay' phenotype. *Vox Sang.*, 7, 245–248.

198 DODD BARBARA E. and GILBEY B.E. (1957) An unusual variant of group A. *Vox Sang.*, 2 390–398.

199 JUNQUEIRA P.C., GARANGAU F.M. and WISHART P.J. (1957) An example of A_x or A_m reactions in group AB. *Vox Sang.*, 2, 386–389.

200 PROKOP O., SIMON A. and RACKWITZ A. (1960) Ein seltener schwacher A_3-Rezeptor 'A_3^w,' seine Analyse und Vererbung. Zugleich ein Beispiel für die mögliche Wirkung von modifizierenden Genen. *Dtsch. Z. ges. gerichtl. Med.*, 50, 448–456.

201 STRATTON F., RENTON P.H. and HANCOCK JEANNE A. (1958) Red cell agglutinability affected by disease. *Nature, Lond.*, 181, 62–63.

202 GOLD E.R., TOVEY G.H., BENNEY W.E. and LEWIS F.J.W. (1959) Changes in the group A antigen in a case of leukaemia. *Nature, Lond.*, 183, 892–893.

203 TOVEY G.H. (1960) Changes in the group A antigen in leukaemia. *Proc. 7th Congr. europ. Soc. Hemat.*, London 1959, 1167–1170.

204 BHATIA H.M. and SANGHVI L.D. (1960) A variant of blood group A in a leukaemia patient. *Indian J. med. Sci.*, 14, 534–535.

205 SALMON C., DREYFUS B. and ANDRÉ R. (1958) Double population de globules, différant seulement par l'antigène de groupe ABO, observée chez un malade leucémique. *Rev. Hémat.*, 13, 148–153.

206 SALMON C., ANDRÉ R, and DREYFUS B. (1960) Arguments en faveur de mutations somatiques du gène de groupe sanguin A au cours de certanes leucémies aiguës. *Proc. 7th Congr. europ. Soc. Hemat.*, 1171–1177.

207 SALMON C., ANDRÉ R. and DREYFUS B. (1959) Existe-t-il des mutations somatiques du gène de groupe sanguin A au cours de certaines leucémies aiguës? *Rev. franc. Étud. clin. biol.*, 4, 468–471.

208 SALMON C. and BERNARD J. (1960) Nouvelle observation d'antigène A 'faible' chez un malade atteint de leucémie aiguë. *Rev. franc. Étud. clin. biol.*, 5, 912–916.

209 SALMON C. (1959) Leucémie aiguë et mutations somatiques des substances de groupe sanguin. *Rev. Hémat.*, 14, 205–208.

210 HOOGSTRATEN B., ROSENFIELD R.E. and WASSERMAN L.R. (1961) Change of ABO blood type in patients with leukemia. *Transfusion, Philad.*, 1, 32–35.

[211] CAMERON C., GRAHAM FRANCES, DUNSFORD I., SICKLES GRETCHEN, MACPHERSON C.R., CAHAN A., SANGER RUTH and RACE R.R. (1959) Acquisition of a B-like antigen by red blood cells. *Brit. med. J.*, **ii**, 29–32.

[212] MARSH W.L., JENKINS W.J. and WALTHER W.W. (1959) Pseudo B: an acquired group antigen. *Brit. med. J.* **ii**, 63–66.

[213] WILLIAMSON P. and SPRINGER G.F. (1959) Blood-group B active somatic antigen of *E. coli* O_{86}:B7. *Fed. Proc.*, **18**, 604.

[214] STRATTON F. and RENTON P.H. (1959) Acquisition of B-like antigen. *Brit. med. J.*, **ii**, 244.

[215] SPRINGER G.F. and ANSELL NORMA J. (1960) Acquisition of blood-group B-like bacterial antigens by human A and O erythrocytes. *Fed. Proc.*, **19**, 70.

[216] SPRINGER G.F. and ANSELL HAHN NORMA J. (1960) Acquisition of blood-group B-like bacterial antigens by human A and O erythrocytes. *Prog. 8th int. Soc. Blood. Transf.*, II-b-5.

[217] PETTENKOFER H.J., MAASSEN W. and BICKERICH R. (1960) Antigen-gemeinschaften zwischen menschlichen Blutgruppen und Enterobacteriaceen. *Z. ImmunForsch.*, **119**, 415–429.

[218] MODIANO G., GONANO F. and DE ANDREIS M. (1961) Relationships between the somatic antigens of *E. coli* O_{86} B:7 and blood group A and B substance. *Vox Sang.*, **6**, 683–691.

[219] MARSH W.L. (1960) The pseudo B antigen. A study of its development. *Vox Sang.*, **5**, 387–397.

[220] PROKOP O and SCHUBERTH G. (1954) Blutgruppen-autoantikörper im ABO-system. *Klin. Wschr.*, **32**, 183–185.

[221] STRATTON F. and RENTON P.H. (1958) *Practical Blood Grouping*, p. 112. Blackwell Scientific Publications, Oxford.

[222] GILES CAROLYN M., MOURANT A.E., PARKIN DOROTHY M., HORLEY J.F. and TAPSON K.J. (1959) A weak B antigen, probably acquired. *Brit. med. J.*, **ii**, 32–34.

[223] STRATTON F. and RENTON P.H. (1959) Acquisition of B-like antigen. *Brit. med. J.*, **ii**, 244.

[224] ANDERSEN J. (1960) B-like character in certain individuals of group A. *Proc. 7th Congr. europ. Soc. Hemat.*, 1183–1185.

[225] ANDERSEN J. (1960) Weak atypical B-like character in the blood cells of a group A person. *Acta path. microbiol. scand.*, **48**, 280–288.

[226] ANDERSEN J. (1960) A weak atypical B-like character in the blood cells of 7 group A persons. *Acta path. microbiol. scand.*, **48**, 289–304.

[227] CAMERON C. (1960) An acquired B-like antigen in human red blood cells, *Proc. 7th Congr. europ. Soc. Hemat.*, 1178–1182.

[228] SCHERTZ K.F., JURGELSKY W. and BOYD W.C. (1960) Inheritance of anti-A_1 haemagglutinating activity in lima beans, *Phaseolus lunatus. Proc. nat. Acad. Sci. Wash.*, **46**, 529–532.

[229] KRÜPE M. and DÖTZER W. (1957) Blood group A_1. A possible subdivision into two types probably heritable. *Ann. Med. exp. Fenn.*, **35**, 1–9.

[230] BOYD W.C., GREEN DOROTHY M., FUJINAGA DOROTHY M., DRABIK J.S. and WASZCZENKO-ZACHARCZENKO EUGENIA (1959) A blood factor, possibly new, detected by extracts of *Arachis hypogaea*. *Vox Sang.*, **4**, 456–467.

[231] IKEMOTO S., KUNIYUKI M. and FURUHATA T. (1964) A finding of rare B_m blood-type in Japanese. *Proc. Jap. Acad.*, **40**, 362–363.

[232] BHATIA H.M., UNDEVIA J.V. and SANGHVI L.D. (1965) Second Indian family of weak B(B_3). *Vox Sang.*, **10**, 506–510.

[233] ALTER A.A. and ROSENFIELD R.E. (1964) B_x a subtype of B. *Blood*, **23**, 600–604.

[234] PARISH W.E., CARRON-BROWN J.A. and RICHARDS C.B. (1967) The detection of antibodies to spermatozoa and to blood group antigens in cervical mucus. *J. Reprod. Fertil.*, **13**, 469–483.

[235] WATKINS WINIFRED M. (1959) Some genetical aspects of the biosynthesis of human blood group substances. Ciba Found. Symp. on *Biochemistry of Human Genetics*, 217–238. Churchill, London.

236 CEPPELLINI R. (1959) Physiological genetics of human factors. Ciba Found. Symp. on *Biochemistry of Human Genetics*, 242–261. Churchill, London.

237 WATKINS WINIFRED M. and MORGAN W.T.J. (1959) Possible genetical pathways for the biosynthesis of blood group mucopolysaccharides. *Vox Sang.*, 4, 97–119.

238 STERN C. (1936) Somatic crossing over and segregation in *Drosophila melanogaster*. *Genetics*, 21, 625–730.

239 BESSIS M. (1957) *Le Sang et la Transfusion Sanguine*, pp. 139, Dunod, Paris.

240 JAKOBOWICZ RACHEL, WHITTINGHAM SENGA and SIMMONS R.T. (1961) Investigations on two examples of the 'Bombay' type O_h blood, possibly O_h^A of the ABO system, found in two women siblings of Greek origin. *Med. J. Aust.*, ii, 868–871.

241 GOUDIE R.B. (1957) Somatic segregation of 'inagglutinable' erythrocytes. *Lancet*, i, 1333.

242 ATWOOD K.C. (1958) The presence of A_2 erythrocytes in A_1 blood. *Proc. nat. Acad. Sci. Wash.*, 44, 1054–1057.

243 AUST C.H., HOCKER NARCISSA D., KELLER ZOETTA G. and ARBOGAST J.L. (1962) A family of 'Bombay' blood type with suppression of blood group substance A_1. *Amer. J. clin. Path.*, 37, 579–583.

244 McKERNS K.W. and DENSTEDT O.F. (1950) The free-cell phenomenon in isohaemagglutination. *Canad. J. Res.*, E, 28, 152–168.

245 ATWOOD K.C. and SCHEINBERG, S.L. (1958) Somatic variation in human erythrocyte antigens. *J. cellular comp. Physiol.*, 52, supp. 1, 97–123.

246 ATWOOD K.C. and SCHEINBERG S.L. (1959) Isotope dilution method for assay of inagglutinable erythrocytes. *Science*, 129, 963–964.

47 CONSTANDOULAKIS M. and KAY H.E.M. (1962) A and B antigens of the human foetal erythrocyte. *Brit. J. Haemat.*, 8, 57–63.

248 BJØRUM A. and KEMP T. (1929) Untersuchungen über den Empfindlichkeitsgrad der Blutkörperchen gegenüber Isoagglutininen im Kindersalter. *Acta path. microbiol. scand.*, 6, 218–234.

249 BUSCH SHIRLEY (1965) Personal communication.

250 SPRINGER G.F. (1958) Relation of blood group active plant substances to human blood groups. *Acta haemat.*, 20, 147–155.

251 ISEKI S., ONUKI E. and KASHIWAGI K. (1958) Relationship between somatic antigen and blood group substance, especially B substance, of bacterium. *Gunma J. med. Sci.*, 7, 7–12.

252 MUSCHEL L.H. and OSAWA E. (1959) Human blood group substance B in *Escherichia coli* O_{86}. *Proc. Soc. exp. Biol.*, N.Y., 101, 614–617.

253 YAMAMOTO T. and AMAGASA S. (1934) Rinshobijorigaku Ketsuekigaku Zasshi, 3, 893–896. Cited by Furuhata *et al.*[254]

254 FURUHATA T., NAKAJIMA H., ISHIDA E., IZUMI S., TERADA K. and AMANO Y. (1959) Blood group determinations of Peruvian Mummies. *Proc. imp. Acad. Japan*, 35, 305–306.

255 CANDELA P.B. (1936) Blood group reactions in ancient human skeletons. *Amer. J. phys. Anthrop.*, 21, 429–432.

256 TORAL ROSA E. and SALAZAR M.M., cited by SALAZAR M.M. (1951) Estudio immunologico de restos oseos antiguos. *Gac. méd. Méx.*, 81, 122–128.

257 HARTMANN GRETHE (1941) *Group Antigens in Human Organs*, Munksgaard, Copenhagen.

258 HALVORSEN K. (1944) The significance of blood group characteristics in serum and plasma transfusions. *Acta chir. scand.*, 90, 80–88.

259 BARBER M. and DUNSFORD I. (1959) Excess blood-group substance A in serum of patient dying with carcinoma of stomach. *Brit. med. J.*, i, 607–609.

260 MOULLEC J., BORIN P. and FINE J.M. (1960) Forte concentration de substance de groupe A dans le sérum d'une malade porteuse d'une tumeur de l'ovaire. *Transfusion*, Paris, 3, 81–89.

261 SALMON C. and MALASSENET R. (1960) A propos des substances de groupes ABO présentes en grande quantité dans le sérum humain: deux observations nouvelles. *Transfusion*, Paris, 3, 91–94.

262 FREIESLEBEN E., KISSMEYER-NIELSEN F., CHRISTENSEN J., JENSEN K.G. and KNUDSEN, E.E. (1961) Excessive content of blood-group substance in serum from patients with ovarian cysts. *Vox Sang.*, 6, 304–311.

263 HOLBOROW E.J., BROWN PATRICIA C., GLYNN L.E., HAWES MARY D., GRESHAM G.A., O'BRIEN T.F. and COOMBS R.R.A. (1960) The distribution of the blood group A antigen in human tissues. *Brit. J. exp. Path.*, 41, 430–437.

264 HÖGMAN C. (1959) The principle of mixed agglutination applied to tissue culture systems. *Vox Sang.*, 4, 12–20.

265 HÖGMAN C.F. (1959) Blood group antigens A and B determined by means of mixed agglutination on cultured cells of human fetal kidney, liver, spleen, lung, heart and skin. *Vox Sang.*, 4, 319–332.

266 KELUS A., GURNER B.W. and COOMBS R.R.A. (1959) Blood group antigens on HeLa cells shown by mixed agglutination. *Immunology*, 2, 262–267.

267 JANKOVIĆ B.D. and ARSENIJEVIĆ K. (1959) Histochemical demonstration of A and B antigens in platelets. *Nature, Lond.*, 183, 695–696.

268 DUCOS J., BROUSSY J. and RUFFIÉ J. (1959) Peut-on affirmer que les antigènes de groupes sanguins érythrocytaires existent dans les thrombocytes? *Sang.*, 30, 548–559.

269 DAUSSET J., COLOMBANI J. and EVELIN J. (1958) Présence de l'antigène Rh(D) dans les leuco-cytes et les plaquettes humaines. *Vox Sang.*, 3, 266–276.

270 MOULINIER J. and SERVANTIE X. (1958) Détection par le test de consommation d'anti-globuline de l'antigène D sur les plaquettes des individus Rh-positif (D+). *Vox Sang.*, 3, 277–283.

271 LUNDEVALL J. (1958) *Serological Studies of Human Blood Platelets*, pp. 122, Oslo University Press.

272 GUREVITCH J. and NELKEN D. (1957) Studies on platelet antigens. III. Rh-Hr antigens in platelets. *Vox Sang.*, 2, 342–347.

273 LEWIS J.H., DRAUDE J. and KUHNS W.J. (1960) Coating of 'O' platelets with A and B group substances. *Vox Sang.*, 5, 434–441.

274 BERROCHE L., MAUPIN B., HERVIER P. and DAUSSET J. (1955) Mise en évidence des anti-gènes A et B dans les leucocytes humains par des épreuves d'absorption et d'élution. *Vox Sang.* (O.S.), 5, 82–93.

275 GURNER B.W. and COOMBS R.R.A. (1958) Examination of human leucocytes for the ABO, MN, Rh, Tjᵃ, Lutheran and Lewis systems of antigens by means of mixed erythrocyte-leucocyte agglutination. *Vox Sang.*, 3, 13–22.

276 ARCHER G.T. and KOOPTZOFF OLGA (1958) Blood group antigens in white cells. *Aust. J. exp. Biol. med. Sci.*, 36, 373–382.

277 JANKOVIĆ B.D. and LINCOLN T.L. (1959) The presence of D (Rh) antigen in human leuko-cytes as demonstrated by the fluorescent antibody technique. *Vox Sang.*, 4, 119–126.

278 DAUSSET J. (1958) Iso-leuco-anticorps. *Acta haemat.*, 20, 156–166.

279 SWISHER S.N. (1958) Comments on mixed agglutination reactions as a source of false positive tests in studies of leucocyte and platelet antigens and antibodies. *Vox Sang.*, 3, 43–44.

280 SWINBURNE LAYINKA M., FRANK BARBARA B. and COOMBS R.R.A. (1961) The A antigen on the buccal epithelial cells of man. *Vox Sang.*, 6, 274–286.

281 HART MIA V. D. and VAN LOGHEM J.J. (1963) Personal communication.

282 JOYSEY VALERIE C. (1959) The relation between animal and human blood groups. *Brit. med. Bull.*, 15, 158–164.

283 KONUGRES ANGELYN and COOMBS R.R.A. (1958) Studies on human anti-A sera with special reference to so-called 'immune' anti-A. II. Identification of the antibody detected by Witebsky's 'partial neutralization' tests as anti-Aᵖ and the occurrence of the Aᵖ antigen on human and animal red cells. *Brit. J. Haemat.*, 4, 261–269.

284 MORGAN W.T.J. (1960) A contribution to human biochemical genetics; the chemical basis of blood-group specificity. *Proc. roy. Soc., B*, 151, 308–347. (The Croonian Lecture.)

285 LANSET SUZAENNE, ROPARTZ C., ROUSSEAU P.-Y., GUERBET Y. and SALMON C. (1966) Une famille comportant les phénotypes Bombay: O_h^{AB} et O_h^B. *Transfusion, Paris*, **9**, 255–263.

286 WEISERT O. and HEIER ANNE-MARGRETHE (1961) A case of defective ABO groups. *Vox Sang.*, **6**, 692–697.

287 RACE R.R. and SANGER RUTH (1960) Consanguinity and certain rare blood groups. *Vox Sang.*, **5**, 383–384.

288 SPRINGER G.F., HORTON R.E. and FORBES M. (1959) Origin of anti-human blood group B agglutinins in White Leghorn chicks. *J. exp. Med.*, **110**, 221–244.

289 DUPONT MADELEINE (1934) Contribution á l'étude des antigènes des globules rouges. *Arch. int. Med. exp.*, **9**, 133–167.

290 SPRINGER G.F., HORTON R.E. and FORBES M. (1958) Immunogenic origin of anti-human blood-group agglutinins in 'germfree' chicks. *Fed. Proc.*, **17**, 535.

291 SPRINGER G.F., HORTON R.E. and FORBES M. (1959) Origin of anti-human blood group B agglutinins in White Leghorn chicks. *Proc. 7th Congr. int. Soc. Blood Transf.*, 529–535.

292 SPRINGER G.F., HORTON R.E. and FORBES M. (1959) Origin of antihuman blood group B agglutinins in germfree chicks. *Ann. N.Y. Acad. Sci.*, **78**, 272–275.

293 JAKOBOWICZ RACHEL, CRAWFORD HAL, GRAYDON J.J. and PINDER MARJORIE (1959) Immunological tolerance within the ABO blood group system. *Brit. J. Haemat.*, **5**, 232–244.

294 GILES CAROLYN M. MOURANT A.E. and ATABUDDIN A.-H. (1963) A Lewis-negative 'Bombay' blood. *Vox Sang.*, **8**, 269–272.

295 WURMSER R. and FILITTI-WURMSER SABINE (1957) Thermodynamic study of the isohaemagglutinins. *Progr. Biophys.*, **7**, 88–113.

296 FILITTI-WURMSER SABINE, JACQUOT-ARMAND Y. and WURMSER R. (1960) Sur les isohémagglutinines naturelles du système A, B, O. *Rev. Hémat.*, **15**, 201–216.

297 EIGEL M. (1960) *Untersuchungen über die Unterscheidungsmöglickeit der Génotypen der Blutgruppe A durch bestimmung des N_4/N_{37} Quotienten*. Inaugural Doctorate Thesis, pp. 32, Bonn University.

298 DODD BARBARA E. (1958) Further studies of antibody molecules having both A and B specificity. *Trans. 6th Congr. europ. Soc. Haemat.*, 733–739.

299 JONES A.R. and KANEB LORRAINE (1960) Some properties of cross reacting antibody of the ABO blood group system. *Blood*, **15**, 395–403.

300 JONES A.R. and KANEB LORRAINE (1959) A new property of iso-agglutinins of the ABO blood group system. *Blood*, **14**, 1094–1102.

301 JONES A.R., KANEB LORRAINE and ABRAHAMOV A. (1959) A technique for the titration of 'cross-reacting antibody' in group O serum. *J. Lab. clin. Med.*, **54**, 779–783

302 BIRD G.W.G. (1959) Haemagglutinins in seeds. *Brit. med. Bull.*, **15**, 165–168.

303 BOYD W.C., WASZCZENKO-ZACHARCZENKO EUGENIA and GOLDWASSER SANDRA M. (1961). List of plants tested for haemagglutinating activity. *Transfusion, Philad.*, **1**, 374–382.

304 BIRD G.W.G. (1959) Agar gel studies of blood group specific substances in precipitins of plant origin. I. The precipitins of *Dolichos biflorus*. *Vos Sang.*, **4**, 307–313.

305 BIRD G.W.G. (1959) Anti-A haemagglutinins from a non-Leguminous plant—*Hyptis suaveolens* Poit. *Nature, Lond.*, **184**, 109.

306 BIRD G.W.G. (1960) Anti-A agglutinins from the seeds of *Hyptis suaveolens* Poit. *Brit. J. Haemat.*, **6**, 151–153.

307 JONES D.A. (1961) Lectins in old seeds. *Vox Sang.*, **6**, 502–505.

308 MÄKELÄ O., MÄKELÄ PIRJO and KRÜPE M. (1959) Zur Spezifität der anti-B Phythämagglutinine. *Z. ImmunForsch.*, **117**, 220–229.

309 GILLESPIE E.M. and GOLD E.R. (1960) Weakening of the B-antigen by the presence of A_1 as shown by reactions with *Fomes fomentarius* (anti-B) extract. *Vox Sang.*, **5**, 497–502.

310 FURUHATA T. and NAKAJIMA H. (1959) On the anti-B and anti-C agglutinins contained in seeds of *Sophora japonica* L. *Proc. imp. Acad. Japan*, **35**, 53–54.

311   LEVINE P., CELANO M.J., LANGE S. and BERLINER V. (1957) On anti-M in horse sera. *Vox Sang.*, **2**, 433–439.

312   MÄKELÄ O. and HAUTALA TUULA (1958) Reactions of plant anti-N agglutinins with red cells treated with proteolytic enzymes. *Ann. Med. exp. Fenn.*, **36**, 323–327.

313   SOLOMON J.M., WAGGONER R. and LEYSHON W.C. (1965) A quantitative immunogenetic study of gene suppression involving A_1 and H antigens of the erythrocyte without affecting secreted blood group substances. The ABH phenotypes A_m^h and O_m^h. *Blood*, **25**, 470–485.

314   JAKOBOWICZ RACHEL, SIMMONS R.T., GRAYDON J.J., CONSTANTOULAKIS M. and EHRLICH MIRA (1965) Partial expression of A in group AB and group A members of a Greek family, not conforming with previously reported examples. *Vox Sang.*, **10**, 552–559.

315   KITAHAMA M., YAMAGUCHI H., OKUBO Y. and HAZAMA F. (1967) An apparently new B_h-like human blood-type. *Vox Sang.*, **12**, 354–360.

316   BIRD G.W.G. (1959) Observations on some non-specific plant haemagglutinins. *Vox Sang.*, **4**, 318–319.

317   BIRD G.W.G. (1959) Agar gel studies of blood group specific substances and precipitins of plant origin. II. The precipitins of *Ricinus communis*. *Vox Sang.*, **4**, 313–317.

318   REIMANN W. and POPWASILEFF I. (1960) Fleckentest zur Unterscheidung von Tierund Menschblut mittels Extrakten aus *Sophora japonica*. *Ztschr. f. d. ges. Hyg. i. Grenzgeb.*, **6**, 825–829.

319   BIRD G.W.G. (1960) Anti-pneumococcus Type XIV activity of precipitins from *Ricinus communis* seeds. *Nature Lond.*, **187**, 415–416.

320   BIRD G.W.G. (1961) Specific precipitins for Type XIV pneumococcus polysaccharide from *Abrus precatorius* seeds. *Experientia*, **17**, 71–72.

321   BOYD W.C. and WASZCZENKO-ZACHARCZENKO EUGENIA (1961) Erythrocyte receptors for two 'non-specific' lectins. *Transfusion, Philad.*, **1**, 223–227.

322   KISSMEYER-NIELSEN F., NEDERGAARD J. and TIPPETT P. (1964) Pseudo anti-A as a cold autoagglutinin. *Proc. 9th Congr. int. Soc. Blood Transf.*, Mexico 1962, 524–527.

323   SPRINGER G.F., WILLIAMSON P. and BRANDES W.C. (1961) Blood group activity of gram-negative bacteria. *J. exp. Med.*, **113**, 1077–1093.

324   GANDINI E. and CEPPELLINI R. (1960) Eterogeneita 'per il gruppo ABO per l'emoglobina F e per il numero cromosomico, in corso di leucemia. *Atti A.G.I.*, **5**, 283–292.

325   GLYNN L.E., HOLBOROW E.J. and JOHNSON G.D. (1957) The distribution of blood group substances in human gastric and duodenal mucosa. *Lancet*, **ii**, 1083–1088.

326   GLYNN L.E. and HOLBOROW E.J. (1959) Distribution of blood-group substances in human tissues. *Brit. med. Bull.*, **15**, 150–153.

327   FURUHATA T., NAKAMURA K., NAKAJIMA H. and SUZUKI M. (1959) Studies on the secretor (type v) and non-secretor (type V) of group specific agglutinin and their inheritance. *Proc. imp. Jap. Acad.*, **35**, 105–107.

328   PROKOP O. (1961) Studies on the excretion of antibodies in saliva. *Cong. Leg. Med., Vienna* 1961.

329   LEY A.B., HARRIS JEAN P. and BRINKLEY MARY (1961) Alteration of erythrocyte antigen B in acute leukemia. *Prog. Amer. Ass. Blood Banks*, page 72.

330   TOVEY G.H., LOCKYER J.W. and TIERNEY R.B.H. (1961) Changes in Rh grouping reactions in a case of leukaemia. *Vox Sang.*, **6**, 628–631.

331   HATTON JOAN and WALSH R.J. (1961) An unusual difficulty in blood grouping. Interference by soluble antigen in a patient's serum. *Vox Sang.*, **6**, 568–573.

332   HÖGMAN C.F. (1961) Interaction between human serum and human fetal cells grown in vitro studied with the aid of the mixed agglutination technique. *Acta path. microbiol. scand.*, **51**, 141–156.

333   HÖGMAN C.F. (1960) Blood group antigens on human cells in tissue culture. The effect of prolonged cultivation. *Exp. Cell Research*, **21**, 137–143.

334   LEVINE P., UHLÍŘ M. and WHITE JANE (1961) A_h, an incomplete suppression of A resembling O_h. *Vox Sang.*, **6**, 561–567.

335 JENKINS W.J. and MARSH W.L. (1961) Unpublished observations.

336 ATWOOD K.C. and PEPPER F.J. (1961) Erythrocyte automosaicism in some persons of known genotype. *Science*, **134**, 2100–2102.

337 RENTON P.H., STRATTON F., GUNSON H.H. and HANCOCK JEANNE A. (1962) Red cells of all four ABO groups in a case of leukaemia. *Brit. med. J.*, **i**, 294–297.

338 LIOTTA I., RUSSO G. and GANDINI E. (1961). A sample of B_m blood. *Vox Sang.*, **6**, 698–705.

339 JAKOBOWICZ RACHEL, SIMMONS R.T. and WHITTINGHAM SENGA (1961) A sub-group of group B blood. *Vox Sang.*, **6**, 706–709.

340 LEVINE P. and CELANO M.J. (1961) The question of D (Rh_0), antigenic sites on human spermatozoa. *Vox Sang.*, **6**, 720–723.

341 BHATIA H.M. (1962) A_h phenotype (further observations). *Vox Sang.*, **7**, 485–487.

342 BHATIA H.M. (1966) Serology and genetics of the variants of H antigen. *Indian Jour. Med. Res.*, **54**, 345–353.

343 HRUBIŠKO M. and MERGANCOVÁ OLGA (1966) Beobachtungen über Varianten des Blutgruppensystems ABO. III. Die neuen Variation O_{Hm} und A_{Hm}. Ein Beitrag zur Frage der Biosynthese der Blutgruppen-Antigene. *Blut.*, **13**, 278–285.

344 MCGINNISS MARY H., KIRKHAM W.R. and SCHMIDT P.J. (1964) Modified expression of the ABO, I and H antigens in acute myelogenous leukemia. (Abstract) *Transfusion, Philad.*, **4**, 310.

345 SALMON C. (1965) Données quantitatives et thermodynamiques sur les modifications leucémiques de groupes sanguins ABO. *Proc. 10th Congr. int. Soc. Blood Transf.*, Stockholm 1964, 337–342.

346 GOLD R. (1964) Modified A antigen in three cases of acute leukaemia and one case of pre-leukaemia. *Sangre*, **9**, 131–134.

347 UNDEVIA J.V., BHATIA H.M., SHARMA R.S. and PAREKH J.G. (1966) Modification of group B in acute myeloid leukaemia. *Indian J. med. Res.*, **54**, 1145–1149.

348 SALMON C. and SALMON DENISE (1963) Anomalies thermodynamiques de l'anti-corps anti-B chez un leucémique avec antigène A modifié. *Nouv. Revue fr. Hémat.*, **3**, 653–662.

349 SALMON C., DEBRAY J. and LEMAIRE A. (1964) Déficit de l'antigène H érythrocytaire chez une malade leucémique de phénotype A faible. *Nouv. Revue fr. Hémat.*, **4**, 245–252.

350 SALMON C. and SALMON DENISE (1965) Déficit en antigène H chez certains sujets de groupe O atteints de leucémie aiguë. *Revue fr. Étud. clin. biol.*, **10**, 212–214.

351 SALMON C. (1964) Sur le mécanisme des modifications de groupes sanguins au cours des leucémies aiguës. *Annls Génét.*, **7**, 3–6.

352 SALMON C., ANDRÉ R. and PHILIPPON J. (1961) Agglutinabilité normale des hématies A_1 transfusées à 3 malades leucémiques de phénotype A modifié. *Revue fr. Étud. clin. biol.*, **8**, 792–795.

353 BERNARD J., BESSIS M., BUSSARD A., DUCOS J., DE GROUCHY J., LEJEUNE J., SALMON C., SELIGMANN M. and FILITTI-WURMSER SABINE (1965) Confrontations cytologiques. IV. Changements de groups sanguins dans les leucémies. *Nouv. Revue fr. Hémat.*, **5**, 291–308.

354 AYERS M., SALZANO F.M. and LUDWIG O.K. (1966) Blood group changes in leukaemia. *J. med. Genet.*, **3**, 180–185.

355 CLAFLIN ALICE J. and ZINNEMAN H.H. (1963) Anti-B isohemagglutinins in the serum of a patient with a weak red cell B antigen. *Amer. J. clin. Path.*, **39**, 355–359.

356 JOUVENCEAUX A., BÉTUEL H., PAILLET H. and REVOL L. (1964) Un cas d'antigène pseudo-B permettant de découvrir un cancer du colon. *Transfusion, Paris*, **7**, 313–317.

357 BURNS W., FRIEND W. and SCUDDER J. (1965) Development of an acquired blood group antigen in surgical patients with peritonitis due to *Escherichia coli*. *Surg. Gynec. Obstet.*, **120**, 757–760.

358 MÁJSKÝ A. (1965) A weak transient B-like antigen in the red cells of a patient with chronic leukemia belonging to blood group A. *Neoplasma*, **12**, 617–623. (Abstract only seen).

359 ANDERSEN J. (1963) *Erhvervet blodtype B-egenskab hos mennesket*. M.D. Thesis, Copenhagen.

4

[360] FURUHATA T. (1927) On the heredity of the blood groups. *Japan med. World*, 7, 197–209.

[361] FURUHATA T. (1929) A summarized review of the gene-hypothesis of the blood groups. *Amer. J. phys. Anthrop.*, 13, 109–130.

[362] LATTES L. (1932) *The Individuality of the Blood* (translated by Bertie, L.H.W.), Oxford University Press.

[363] KOMAI T. (1950) Semi-allelic genes. *Amer. Nat.*, 84, 381–392.

[364] BERNSTEIN F. (1930) Uber die Erblichkeit der Blutgruppen. *Z. indukt. Abstamm. u. Vererb.*, 54, 400–426. (See ref. 17.)

[365] SEYFRIED HALINA, WALEWSKA IRENA and WERBLIŃSKA BOGUSLAWA (1964) Unusual inheritance of ABO group in a family with weak B antigens. *Vox Sang.*, 9, 268–277.

[366] YAMAGUCHI H., OKUBO Y. and HAZAMA F. (1965) An A_2B_3 phenotype blood showing atypical mode of inheritance. *Proc. imp Acad. Japan*, 41, 316–320.

[367] BOETTCHER B. (1966) Modification of Bernstein's multiple allele theory for the inheritance of the ABO blood groups in the light of modern genetical concepts. *Vox Sang.*, 11, 129–136.

[368] YAMAGUCHI H., OKUBO Y. and TANAKA M. (1970) '*Cis* AB' bloods found in Japanese families. *Jap. Jnl. Hum. Genet.*, 15, 198–215.

[369] KOGURE T. (1971) A family with unusual inheritance of ABO blood groups. *Jap. Jnl. Hum. Genet.*, 16, 69–87.

[370] BOUGUERRA-JACQUET ANNIE, REVIRON J., SALMON DENISE and SALMON C. (1969) Un exemple de chromosome *cis* A_1B. Étude thermodynamique de l'antigène B induit. *Nouv. Ref. franc. Hémat.*, 9, 329–338.

[371] YAMAGUCHI H., OKUBO Y. and HAZAMA F. (1966) Another Japanese A_2B_3 blood-group family with the propositus having O-group father. *Proc. imp. Acad. Japan*, 42, 517–520.

[372] BRAIN P. (1968) H, A and B titres in South African blood donors. *Vox Sang.*, 14, 119–123.

[373] SALMON C. and REVIRON J. (1964) Trois phénotypes 'B faible': B_{80}, B_{60}, B_0 définis par leur agglutinabilité, comparée a celle du phénotype normal. *Nouv. Revue fr. Hémat.*, 4, 655–668.

[374] SALMON C., SALMON DENISE and REVIRON J (1964) Données quantitatives et thermodynamiques comparées, concernant les antigènes B_{100}, B_{80}, B_{60} et B_0. Applications a l'étude de l'agglutination. *Nouv. Revue fr. Hémat.*, 4, 739–754.

[375] SALMON C., DE GROUCHY J. and LIBERGE GENEVIÈVE (1965) Un nouvel antigène du système ABO: $A_{1(80)}$. *Nouv. Revue fr. Hémat.*, 5, 631–637.

[376] COHEN FLOSSIE and ZUELZER W.W. (1965) Interrelationship of the various subgroups of the blood group A: study with immunofluorescence. *Transfusion, Philad.*, 5, 223–229.

[377] GIBBS MARY B. and AKEROYD J.H. (1959) Quantitative immunohematologic studies of hemagglutination. II-Assay of the agglutinogen A. *J. Immunol.*, 82, 577–584.

[378] GRUNDBACHER F.J. (1965) Sources of quantitative variation of the human A erythrocytes. *Amer. J. hum. Genet.*, 17, 399–409.

[379] TUGGLE J.M., GIBBS MARY B. and CAMP F.R. (1964) Quantitative hemagglutination studies of the reactivities of isohemagglutinins with A_1 and B antigens of human erythrocytes. (Abstract). *Transfusion, Philad.*, 4, 310.

[380] GIBBS MARY B., AKEROYD J.H. and ZAPF JULIA J. (1961) Quantitative sub-groups of the B antigen in man and their occurrence in three racial groups. *Nature, Lond.*, 192, 1196–1197.

[381] SOLOMON J.M., GIBBS MARY B. and BOWDLER A.J. (1965) Methods in quantitative hemagglutination. Part I. *Vox Sang.*, 10, 54–72.

[382] SOLOMON J.M., GIBBS MARY B. and BOWDLER A.J. (1965) Methods in quantitative hemagglutination. Part II. *Vox Sang.*, 10, 133–148.

[383] WINKELSTEIN J.A. and MOLLISON P.L. (1965) The antigen content of 'inagglutinable' group B erythrocytes. *Vox Sang.*, 10, 614–626.

[384] CONSTANTOULAKIS M., KAY H.E.M., GILES CAROLYN M. and PARKIN DOROTHY M. (1963). Observations on the A_2 gene and H antigen in foetal life. *Brit. J. Haemat.*, 9, 63–67.

385 GRUNDBACHER F.J. (1964) Changes in the human A antigen of erythrocytes with the individual's age. *Nature, Lond.*, **204**, 192–194.

386 BHATIA H.M. (1964) Serological specificity of anti-H blood group antibodies. *Indian J. med. Res.*, **52**, 5–14.

387 SPRINGER G.F. (1965) Microbes and higher plants. Their relation to blood group substances. *Proc. 10th Congr. int. Soc. Blood Transf.*, Stockholm 1964, 465–475.

388 SPRINGER G.F. (1966) Relation of microbes to blood-group active substances. *Angew Chem. internat. Edit.*, **5**, 909–920.

389 SZULMAN A.E. (1960) The histological distribution of blood group substances A and B in man. *J. exp. Med.*, **111**, 785–800.

390 SZULMAN A.E. (1962) The histological distribution of the blood group substances in man as disclosed by immunofluorescence. II. The H antigen and its relation to A and B antigens. *J. exp. Med.*, **115**, 977–996.

391 CHESSIN L.N., BRAMSON S., KUHNS W.J. and HIRSCHHORN K. (1965) Studies on the A,B,O(H) blood groups on human cells in culture. *Blood*, **25**, 944–953.

392 KUHNS W., FRIEDHOFF F., FAUR Y. and BRAMSON S. (1966) Blood groups on human cells growing in culture. *Bull. N.Y. Acad. Med.*, **42**, 412.

393 KUHNS W.J., FAUR Y. and BRAMSON S. (1966) Studies of blood groups on human cells grown in culture. *Abstracts, 11th int. Congr. Blood Transf.*, Sydney, 118.

394 HØSTRUP H. (1962) A and B blood group substances in the serum of normal subjects. *Vox Sang.*, **7**, 704–721.

395 HØSTRUP H. (1963) A and B blood group substances in the serum of the newborn infant and the foetus. *Vox Sang.*, **8**, 557–566.

396 RENTON P.H. and HANCOCK JEANNE A. (1962) Uptake of A and B antigens by transfused group O erythrocytes. *Vox Sang.*, **7**, 33–38.

397 YUNIS J.J. and YUNIS E. (1964) A study of blood group antigens on normoblasts. *Proc. 9th Congr. int. Soc. Blood Transf.*, Mexico 1962, 238–243.

398 YUNIS J.J. and YUNIS E. (1963) Cell antigens and cell specialization. I. A study of blood group antigens on normoblasts. *Blood*, **22**, 53–65.

399 YUNIS J.J. and YUNIS E. (1964) Cell antigens and cell specialization. IV. On the H blood group antigen of human platelets and nucleated cells of the human bone marrow. *Blood*, **24**, 531–541.

400 MAZUMDAR PAULINE M.H. (1966) Agglutination of normoblasts with anti-D. *Vox Sang.*, **11**, 90–98.

401 LAWLER SYLVIA D. and SHATWELL HELEN S. (1962) Are Rh antigens restricted to the red cells? *Vox Sang.*, **7**, 488–491.

402 YUNIS E. and YUNIS J.J. (1963) Cell antigens and cell specialization. III. On the H antigen receptors of human epidermal cells. *Blood*, **22**, 750–756.

403 FLORY L.L. (1966) Differences in the H antigen on human buccal cells from secretor and non-secretor individuals. *Vox Sang.*, **11**, 137–156.

404 DUCOS J. and MARTY Y. (1964) Nouvelle contribution à l'étude de la détermination du groupe sanguin du foetus in utero. *Proc. 9th Congr. int. Soc. Blood Transf.*, Mexico 1962, 244–250.

405 EDWARDS R.G., FERGUSON L.C. and COOMBS R.R.A. (1964) Blood group antigens on human spermatozoa. *J. Reprod. Fertil.*, **7**, 153–161.

406 BOETTCHER B. (1965) Human ABO blood group antigens on spermatozoa from secretors and non-secretors. *J. Reprod. Fertil.*, **9**, 267–268.

407 QUINLIVAN W.L.G. and MASOUREDIS S.P. (1963) Rh_0 (D) antigen content of human spermatozoa. *J. Immunol.*, **5**, 267–277.

408 ARFORS K.-E., BECKMAN L. and LUNDIN L.-G. (1963) Genetic variations of human serum phosphatases. *Acta genet., Basel*, **13**, 89–94.

409 ARFORS K.-E., BECKMAN L. and LUNDIN L.-G. (1963) Further studies on the association between human serum phosphatases and blood groups. *Acta genet., Basel*, **13**, 366–368.

[410] BECKMAN L. (1964) Associations between human serum alkaline phosphatases and blood groups. *Acta genet.*, *Basel*, 14, 286–297.

[411] BECKMAN L., BJÖRLING G. and HEIKEN A. (1966) Human alkaline phosphatases and the factors controlling their appearance in serum. *Acta. Genet.*, *Basel*, 16, 305–312.

[412] BAMFORD K.F., HARRIS H., LUFFMAN J.E., ROBSON E.B. and CLEGHORN T.E. (1965) Serum-alkaline-phosphatase and the ABO blood-groups. *Lancet*, i, 530–531.

[413] YOKOYAMA M. and FUDENBERG H.H. (1964) Heterogeneity of A^P antigen in pig red blood cells: significance for detection of human 'immune' anti-A_1. *J. Immunol.*, 92, 413–424.

[414] TOVEY G.H., LOCKYER J.W., BLADES A.N. and FLAVELL H.C.G. (1962) Antenatal prediction of ABO haemolytic disease. *Brit. J. Haemat.*, 8, 251–257.

[415] WATKINS WINIFRED M. (1965) Relationship between structure, specificity and genes within the ABO and Lewis blood-group systems. *Proc. 10th Congr. int. Soc. Blood Transf.*, Stockholm 1964, 443–452.

[416] WATKINS WINIFRED M. (1966) Blood-group substances. *Science*, 152, 172–181.

[417] CAMPBELL J.S. (1958) Unpublished observation.

[418] JAKOBOWICZ RACHEL, GRAYDON J.J. and SIMMONS R.T. (1966) Observations on saliva agglutinins. *Med. J. Aust.*, i, 399–401.

[419] BOETTCHER B. (1966) *Genetical Control of Blood Group Substances in Body Secretions.* Ph.D. thesis, University of Adelaide.

[420] SCHLESINGER DANUTA and OSIŃSKA MARIA (1964) The influence of pregnancy on salivary secretion of group isoantibodies. *Archwm. Immun. Terap. doswiad.*, 12, 297–307.

[421] JAKOBOWICZ RACHEL, EHRLICH MIRA and GRAYDON J.J. (1967) Crossreacting antibody and saliva agglutinins. *Vox Sang.*, 12, 340–353.

[422] GERSHOWITZ H., BEHRMAN S.J. and NEEL J.V. (1958) Hemagglutinins in uterine secretions. *Science*, 128, 719–720.

[423] SOLISH G.I., GERSHOWITZ H. and BEHRMAN S.J. (1961) Occurrence and titer of isohemag-glutinins in secretions of the human uterine cervix. *Proc. Soc. exp. Biol.*, *N.Y.*, 108, 645–649.

[424] PROKOP O., BUNDSCHUH G. and GESERICK G. (1963) Über blutgruppenreaktionen in der Tränenflüssigkeit. *Dtsch. Ges. wesen.*, 27, 1162–1165.

[425] SALMON C., SALMON DENISE and SAINT-PAUL B. (1965) Relation entre l'antigène ABH des hématies et al structure de l'isohémagglutinine révélée par des modifications réversibles d'affinité. *Nouv. Revue fr. Hémat.*, 5, 95–108.

[426] SPRINGER G.F. (1963) Influenza virus vaccine and blood group A-like substances. *Transfusion, Philad.*, 3, 233–236.

[427] TIILIKAINEN A., LEHTOVAARA R. and ERIKSSON A.W. (1959) Failure to demonstrate an acquired immunological tolerance of children to the ABO agglutinogens of their mother. *Ann. Med. exp. Fenn.*, 37, 414–418. (Not seen.)

[428] WICHER K. and WOZNICZKO-ORLOWSKA G. (1960) Próba wykazania róznic miana izoprezeciwciat grupowych u dzieci w zależnośki od grupy krwi matki. *Pol. Tyg. lek.*, 15., 481–482. (Not seen.)

[429] MAYEDA K. (1966) Study of tolerance to the ABO blood group antigens. *Vox Sang.*, 11, 33–37.

[430] KONUGRES ANGELYN A. (1964) Immunological tolerance of the A and B antigens. *Proc. 9th Congr. int. Soc. Blood Transf.*, Mexico 1962, 746–750.

[431] WIENER A.S., NIEBERG K.C. and WEXLER I.B. (1963) Observations on the effect of exchange transfusions in erythroblastotic babies on immunologic tolerance for the A-B-O agglutinogens. *Transfusion, Philad.*, 3, 269–273.

[432] NAIMAN J.L., PUNNETT HOPE H., DESTINÉ MARIE L. and LISCHNER H.W. (1966) Yy chromosomal chimaerism. *Lancet*, ii, 590.

[433] GREENBURY C.L., MOORE D.H. and NUNN L.A.C. (1963) Reaction of 7S and 19S components of immune rabbit antisera with human group A and AB red cells. *Immunol.*, 6, 421–433.

434 BOYD W.C., BHATIA H.M., DIAMOND M.A. and MATSUBARA S. (1962) Quantitative study of the combination of Lima bean lectin with human erythrocytes. *J. Immunol.*, **89**, 463–470.
435 ECONOMIDOU JOANNA, HUGHES-JONES N.C. and GARDNER B. (1967) Quantitative measurements concerning A and B antigen sites. *Vox Sang.*, **12**, 321–328.
436 ROSENFIELD R.E. and OHNO GRACE (1955) A-B hemolytic disease of the new-born. *Rev. Hémat.*, **10**, 231–235.
437 KOCHWA S., ROSENFIELD R.E., TALLAL L. and WASSERMAN L.R. (1961) Isoagglutinins associated with ABO erythroblastosis. *J. clin. Invest.*, **40**, 874–883.
438 SCHIFFMAN G. and HOWE C. (1965) The specificity of blood group A-B cross-reacting antibody. *J. Immunol.*, **94**, 197–204.
439 OGATA T. and MATUHASI T. (1962) Problems of specific and cross reactivity of blood group antibodies. *Proc. 8th Congr. int. Soc. Blood Transf.*, Tokyo 1960, 208–211.
440 MATUHASI T. and USUI M. (1963) Further studies on nonspecific antibody adhesion onto the antigen-antibody complex. *Proc. 1st Asian Congr. Blood Transf.*, Hakone, Japan 1963, 209–213.
441 OGATA T. and MATUHASI T. (1964) Further observations on the problems of specific and cross reactivity of blood group antibodies. *Proc. 9th Congr. int. Soc. Blood Transf.*, Mexico 1962, 528–531.
442 MATUHASI T. (1966) Evidence of monospecificity of anti-A and anti-B in group O serum. *Abstracts, 11th int. Congr. Blood Transf.*, Sydney, 142.
443 MATUHASI T. (1964) Fluorescent blood cells and anti-fluorescein antibodies. *Proc. 9th Congr. int. Soc. Blood Transf.*, Mexico 1962, 578–581.
444 DODD BARBARA E., LINCOLN P. J. and BOORMAN KATHLEEN E. (1967) The cross-reacting antibodies of group O sera: immunological studies and possible explanation of the observed facts. *Immunology*, **12**, 39–52.
445 BHATIA H.M. (1964) Serological specificity of anti-H blood group antibodies. *Indian J. med. Res.*, **52**, 5–14.
446 WIENER A.S., MOOR-JANKOWSKI J. and GORDON E.B. (1966) The relationship of the H substance to the A-B-O blood groups. *Int. Arch. Allergy*, **29**, 82–100.
447 SEYFRIED H., WALEWSKA I. and GILES CAROLYN M. (1963) A patient with apparently normal A₁B red cells whose serum contains anti-B. *Vox Sang.*, **8**, 273–280.
448 TIPPETT PATRICIA, NOADES JEAN, SANGER RUTH, RACE R.R., SAUSAIS LAIMA, HOLMAN C.A. and BUTTIMER R.J. (1960) Further studies of the I antigen and antibody. *Vox Sang.*, **5**, 107–121.
449 TIPPETT PATRICIA, SANGER RUTH, RACE R.R., SWANSON JANE and BUSCH SHIRLEY (1965) An agglutinin associated with the P and the ABO blood group systems. *Vox Sang.*, **10**, 269–280.
450 SAINT-PAUL M. (1961) Les hémagglutinines végétales. *Transfusion, Paris*, **4**, 3–37.
451 BOYD W.C. (1963) The lectins: their present status. *Vox Sang.*, **8**, 1–32.
452 MARTIN T. and BOMCHIL G. (1966) Haemagglutinins in Argentinean leguminosae seeds. *Vox Sang.*, **11**, 54–58.
453 OTTENSOOSER F. and SATO M. (1963) Cold lectins. *Vox Sang.*, **8**, 733–740.
454 HERZOG P. (1959) Spezifische Phytagglutinine aus Ononis spinosa—Wurzeln. *Z. Immun-Forsch*, **117**, 53–59.
455 BIRD G.W.G. (1961) Haemagglutinins from *Clerodendrum viscosum* Vent. *Nature, Lond.*, **191**, 292.
456 BHATIA H.M. and ALLEN F.H. (1962) 'Non-specific' seed agglutinins and blood group specificity. Study of fifteen lectins. *Vox Sang.*, **7**, 83–85.
457 JONES D.A. (1964) The lectin in the seeds of Vicia Cracca L. II. A population study and a possible function for the lectin. *Heredity*, **19**, 459–469.
458 BIRD G.W.G. (1964) Anti-T in peanuts. *Vox Sang.*, **9**, 748–749.
459 JOHNSON H.M. (1964) Human blood group A₁ specific agglutinin of the butter clam *Saxidomus giganteus*. *Science*, **146**, 548–549.

460 PROKOP O., RACKWITZ A. and SCHLESINGER D. (1965) A 'new' human blood group receptor A$_{hel}$. Tested with saline extracts from *Helix hortensis* (garden snail). *J. forens. Med.*, *S. Africa*, **12**, 108–110.

461 PROKOP O., SCHLESINGER D. and RACKWITZ A. (1965) Über eine thermostabile 'antibody like substance' (Anti-A$_{hel}$) bei *Helix pomatia* und deren Herkunft. *Z. ImmunForsch.*, **129**, 402–412.

462 PROKOP O. and RACKWITZ A. (1965) Weitere Untersuchungen mit Anti-A$_{hel}$ an Tierblutkörperchen. *Acta biol. med. germ.*, **15**, 191–192.

463 BOYD W.C. and BROWN REBECCA (1965) A specific agglutinin in the snail *Otala* (*Helix*) *lactea*. *Nature, Lond.*, **208**, 593–594.

464 UHLENBRUCK G. and PROKOP O. (1966) An agglutinin from *Helix pomatia*, which reacts with terminal N-acetyl-D-galactosamine. *Vox Sang.*, **11**, 519–520.

465 BHATIA H.M., BOYD W.C. and BROWN REBECCA (1967) Serological and immunochemical studies of snail (*Otala lactea*) anti-A: a simple purification method. *Transfusion, Philad.*, **7**, 53–59.

466 BOYD W.C., BROWN REBECCA and BOYD LYLE G. (1966) Agglutinins for human erythrocytes in mollusks. *J. Immunol.*, **96**, 301–303.

467 KRÜPE M. and PIEPER H. (1966) Hämagglutinine von Anti-A- und Anti-B-Charakter bei einigen Landlungenschnecken. *Z. ImmunForsch.*, **130**, 296–300.

468 LEWI S. (1967) Une variante rare du groupe A. Le phénotype A$_{2mh}$ (suppression partielle de A et totale de H sur les érythrocytes avec sécrétions salivaires normales). *Transfusion* (Paris), **10**, 335–350.

469 GOLD E.R., CANN G.B. and THOMPSON T.E. (1967) Studies on a mollusc extract using inhibiting and non-inhibiting salivas. *Vox Sang.*, **12**, 461–464.

470 KIM Z., UHLENBRUCK G., PROKOP O. and SCHLESINGER D. (1966) Über die B-Substanz und das Anti-A von *Helix pomatia Z. ImmunForsch.*, **130**, 290–295.

471 BATTAGLINI P., MELIS C. and BRIDONNEAU C. (1967) Un antigène B faible. *Transfusion, Paris*, **10**, 121–125.

472 MADSEN GRETHE and HEISTÖ H. (1968) A Korean family showing inheritance of *A* and *B* on the same chromosome. *Vox Sang.*, **14**, 211–217.

473 ANDERSEN R.E. and WALFORD R.L. (1963) Direct demonstration of A, B and Rh$_0$(D) blood group antigens on human leucocytes. *Amer. J. clin. Path.*, **40**, 239 (not seen, cited by Flory[474]).

474 FLORY L.L. (1967) A and H antigens on leucocytes. *Vox Sang.*, **13**, 362–365.

475 PROKOP O., SCHLESINGER D. and GESERICK G. (1967) Thermostabiles B-Agglutinin aus Konserven von Lachskaviar. *Z. ImmunForsch.*, **132**, 491–494.

476 UHLENBRUCK G. and PROKOP O. (1967) An incomplete antibody for red cells in salmon caviar. *Vox Sang.*, **12**, 465–466.

477 REVIRON J., JACQUET A., DELARUE F., LIBERGE G., SALMON DENISE and SALMON C. (1967) Interactions alléliques des gènes de groupes sanguins ABO. Résultats préliminaires avec l'anti-B d'un sujet 'cis AB' et étude quantitative avec l'anti-B d'un sujet A$_1$O. *Nouv. Revue fr. Hémat.*, **7**, 425–433.

478 REVIRON J., JACQUET ANNIE and SALMON C. (1968) Un exemple de chromosome 'cis A$_1$B'. Étude immunologique et gènetique du phenotype induit. *Nouv. Revue fr. Hémat.*, **8**, 323–338.

479 SAEED S.M. and FINE G. (1967) A-substance secretion by gastric carcinoma. *Transfusion, Philad.*, **7**, 384–5. (Abstract.)

480 MOLTHAN LYNDALL (1967) Second example of A$_h$ (Bombay with incomplete suppression of A$_1$.) *Transfusion, Philad.*, **7**, 384. (Abstract.)

481 HUMMEL K. and SCHÖCH J. (1967) Untersuchungen über die Ausscheidung von Anti-A- und Anti-B- Hämagglutininen im menschlichen Mundspeichel. *Z. ImmunForsch.* **133**, 80–100.

482 PHANSOMBOON S. (1968) The incidence of anti-A and anti-B agglutinins in the saliva of the Thai. *Vox Sang.*, **14**, 396–399.

483 VOAK D., STAPLETON R.R. and BOWLEY C.C. (1968) A_{2h}^{A1} A new variant of A_h, in two group A members of an English family. *Vox Sang.*, **14**, 18–30.

484 WATKINS WINIFRED M. (1967) Gene-enzyme relationships of the A, B, H and Le blood group genes. *Transfusion, Philad.*, **7**, 367. (Abstract.)

485 FLORY L.L. (1967) Comparison of lectin anti-H reagents. *Vox Sang.*, **13**, 357–361.

486 RUOSLAHTI E., EHNHOLM C. and MÄKELÄ O. (1967) A weak B blood group (B_v) in a Finnish family. *Vox Sang.*, **13**, 511–515.

487 SALMON C., JACQUET ANNIE, KLING C. and SALMON DENISE (1967) Analogie d'affinité entre un antigène B, modifié par la leucémie chez un sujet A_1B, et un antigène B partiel induit par un chromosome cis A_1B. *Nouv. Revue fr. Hémat.*, **7**, 755–764.

488 TREACY M., GEIGER J. and GOSS M.F. (1967) Substances in serum causing interference with blood group determination. *Transfusion, Philad.*, **7**, 443–446.

489 SIMMONS R.T. and KWA S.B. (1967) The first examples of subgroup B blood found in two unrelated Chinese families. *Med. J. Aust.*, **i**, 433–435.

490 FRANKS D. and LISKE ROSEMARY (1968) The specificity of the cross-reacting antibodies in blood group O sera which produce mixed agglutination. *Immunology*, **14**, 433–444.

491 DAVIDSOHN I. and STEJSKAL R. (1972) Tissue antigens A, B and H in health and disease. *Haematologia*, **6**, 177–184.

492 FRIEDHOFF F. and KUHNS W.J. (1968) Detection and characterization of blood group antigens on untransformed human amnion cells. *Transfusion*, Philad., **8**, 244–249.

493 FRIED D., SHILO R., STANECKI J. and GOTLIEB A. (1968) The antigenic substances 'A' and 'B' in the sera of healthy subjects. *Vox Sang.*, **15**, 427–434.

494 OTTENSOOSER F., ARAUJO J.T. DE and ROSALES T. (1970) Familial occurrence of increased activity of blood-group A in serum. *Transfusion, Philad.*, **10**, 6–9.

495 DAVIDSOHN I., KOVARIK S. and NI LOUISA Y. (1969) Isoantigens A, B and H in benign and malignant lesions of the cervix. *Arch. Path.*, **87**, 306–314.

496 DAVIDSOHN I., NI LOUISA Y. and STEJSKAL R. (1971) Tissue isoantigens A, B and H in carcinoma of the pancreas. *Cancer Res.*, **31**, 1244–1250.

497 DAVIDSOHN I., KOVARIK S. and LEE C.L. (1966) A, B and O substances in gastrointestinal carcinoma. *Arch. Path.*, **81**, 381–390.

498 DAVIDSOHN I., NI LOUISA Y. and STEJSKAL R. (1971) Tissue isoantigens A, B and H in carcinoma of the stomach. *Arch. Path.*, **92**, 456–464.

499 KOVARIK S., DAVIDSOHN I. and STEJSKAL R. (1968) ABO antigens in cancer. Detection with the mixed cell agglutination reaction. *Arch. Path.*, **86**, 12–21.

500 DAVIDSOHN I. (1972) Early immunologic diagnosis and prognosis of carcinoma. *Am. J. Clin. Path.*, **57**, 715–730.

501 SZULMAN A.E. (1965) The ABH antigens in human tissues and secretions during embryonal development. *J. Histochem. Cytochem.*, **13**, 752–754.

502 SZULMAN A.E. (1966) Chemistry, distribution, and function of blood group substances. *A. Rev. Med.*, **17**, 307–322.

503 SZULMAN A.E. (1971) The histological distribution of the blood group substances in man as disclosed by immunofluorescence. *Human Pathol.*, **2**, 575–585.

504 BOETTCHER B. (1968) Correlation between human ABO blood group antigens in seminal plasma and on seminal spermatozoa. *J. Reprod. Fert.*, **16**, 49–54.

505 HOPE R.M. and MAYO O. (1969) Relationship of human salivary alkaline phosphatase with ABO blood group and secretor status. *Aust. J. exp. Biol. med. Sci.*, **47**, 235–242.

506 BECKMAN L. and ZOSCHKE D.C. (1968) Serum acid phosphatase and ABO blood groups: a new blood group associated enzyme variation. *Acta genet.*, Basel, **18**, 289–299.

507 MÁJSKÝ A. (1967) Some cases of leukaemia with modifications of the $D(Rh_0)$-receptor. *Neoplasma*, **14**, 335–344.

508 SALMON C., SALMON DENISE, MICOUIN C. and BERTHIER JEANNE (1966) Étude quantitative

de l'antigène 'I' dans les érythrocytes des sujets atteints de leucémie aiguë. *Nouv. Rev. fr. Hémat.*, **6**, 563–567

509 FEIZI T. and HARDISTY R.M. (1966) I antigen in leukaemic patients. *Nature, Lond.*, **210**, 1066–1067.

510 SALMON C. (1969) A tentative approach to variations in ABH and associated erythrocyte antigens. *Ser. Haemat.*, **II**, 3–33.

511 KASSULKE J.T., HALLGREN H.M. and YUNIS E.J. (1969) Studies of red cell isoantigens on peripheral leukocytes from normal and leukemic individuals. *Am. J. Path.*, **56**, 333–349.

512 SCOTT G.L. and RASBRIDGE M.R. (1972) Loss of blood group antigenicity in a patient with Hodgkin's disease. *Vox Sang.*, **23**, 458–460.

513 KAHN A., VROCLANS M., HAKIM J. and BOIVIN P. (1971) Differences in the two red-cell populations in erythroleukaemia. *Lancet*, **ii**, 933.

514 SALMON C., ROCHANT H., MANNONI P., CARTRON J.-P., JACQUET A., LIBERGE G. and DREYFUS B. (1969) Étude des modifications des antigènes de groups sanguins dan 11 cas 'd'anémies réfractaires'. *Nouv. Rev. fr. Hémat.*, **9**, 113–124.

515 MARANTZ C. and DIMMETTE R.M. (1969) More about an acquired group B antigen. *Transfusion, Philad.*, **9**, 160–161.

516 MARSH W.L. (1970) Letter to Editor. *Transfusion, Philad.*, **10**, 41.

517 GERBAL A., LIBERGE G., LOPEZ M. and SALMON C. (1970) Un antigène B acquis chez un sujet de phénotype érythrocytaire A_h^m. *Rev. fr. Transf.*, **13**, 61–70.

518 SATHE M.S. and BHATIA H.M. (1970) Two cases of intestinal obstruction with acquired group B antigen. *Indian J. Med. Res.*, **58**, 863–865.

519 GARRATTY G., WILLBANKS ELEANOR and PETZ L.D. (1971) An acquired B antigen associated with *Proteus vulgaris* infection. *Vox Sang.*, **21**, 45–56.

520 BECK M.L., WALKER R.H. and OBERMAN H.A. (1971) Atypical polyagglutination associated with an acquired B antigen. *Transfusion, Philad.*, **11**, 296–301.

521 LANSET SUZANNE and ROPARTZ C. (1971) A second example of acquired B-like antigen in a healthy person. *Vox Sang.*, **20**, 82–84.

522 SALMON C., SÉGER JEANINE, MANNONI P., BAHNO-DUCHERY JEANINE and LIBERGE GENE-VIÈVE (1968) Une population d'érythrocytes avec anomalie simultanée des phénotypes induits par les gènes des locus ABO et adenylate kinase. *Revue fr. Étud. clin. biol.*, **13**, 296–298.

523 SALMON C., MANNONI P., SÉGER JEANINE, CARTRON, J.P., VROCLANS MILIA and LIBERGE GENEVIÈVE (1970) Double population de globules rouges pour les antigènes ABH chez trois sujets âgés. *Nouv. Rev. fr. Hémat.*, **10**, 303–312.

524 RASORE-QUARTINO A. and GALLETTI A. (1971) Mosaicismo gruppale (ABO) e cromosomico in un soggetto anziano con neoplasia vescicale. *Pathologica*, **63**, 37–41.

525 RACE R.R. and SANGER RUTH (1972) Blood group mosaics. *Haematologia*, **6**, 63–71.

526 LANSET S., LIBERGE G., GERBAL A., ROPARTZ C. and SALMON C. (1970) Lettre a la rédaction. Mise en évidence, dans une famille, d'une modification de l'expression des produits des locus *A.B.O. Rev. fr. Transf.*, **13**, 431–434.

527 McGUIRE D., WEBSTER G., MOUGEY R. and HOEVEN L. VAN DER (1972) A weak A antigen in children of group O patients. Abstracts AABB and ISH Meeting, Washington, p. 45.

528 WIENER A.S., SOCHA W.W. and GORDON EVE B. (1973) Further observations on the serological specificity C of the A-B-O blood group system. *Brit. J. Haemat.*, **24**, 195–203.

529 SERIM N. (1969) Lettres a la rédaction. Phénotype Am avec expression secondaire de l'antigène A dans les hématies. *Rev. fr. Transf.*, **12**, 277–280.

530 GERBAL A., LIBERGE G., CARTRON J.-.P. and SALMON C. (1970) Les phénotypes Aend: Étude immunologique et génétique. *Rev. fr. Transf.*, **13**, 243–250.

531 POIRIER R., POIRIER E. and GUIMBRETIÈRE J. (1970) Étude d'une famille comportant un gène 'A$_{end}$'. *Rev. fr. Transf.*, **13**, 365–371.

532 LANSET SUZANNE, LIBERGE GENEVIÈVE, GERBAL A., ROPARTZ C. and SALMON C. (1970) Le phénotype A$_{el}$: Étude immunologique et génétique. *Nouv. Rev. fr. Hémat.*, **10**, 389–400.

533 BEATTIE KATHRYN M., ROCCA F., PINES D.O. and ZUELZER W.W. (1971) A further example of A_{el}. AABB program, Chicago, p. 106.

534 JENKINS T. (1972) Blood group A_{bantu} population and family studies. Abstracts AABB and ISH Meeting, Washington, p. 11. See also (1974) *Vox Sang*, **26**, 537–550.

535 YAMAGUCHI H., OKUBO Y. and TANAKA M. (1970) A rare blood B_x analogous to A_x in a Japanese family. *Proc. Jap. Acad.*, **46**, 446–449.

536 SCHNEIDER W. (1969) Seltene Varianten der B-blutgruppe (Bv in einer deutschen Familie). *Blut.*, **19**, 3–7.

537 SATHE MALTI, SHARMA R.S., BHATIA H.M. and SAHIAR K.H. (1966) Pattern of weak B variants in India. *Ind. J. med. Res.*, **54**, 448–454.

538 GARLICK MARY and MALDRE LEIDA (1967) A weak subgroup of B, B_m, in a Canadian family. *J. med. Lab. Tech.*, **24**, 191–195.

539 MOORES PHYLLIS (1970) Weak B variant in an Indian family. Paper read at Blood Transfusion Congress, East London, South Africa.

540 IKEMOTO S., TERAMOTO T., MUKOYAMA H. and FURUHATA T. (1968) Genetical studies of B_m blood type on the twins. I. Heredity of Bm blood groups. *Proc. Jap. Acad.*, **44**, 727–729.

541 IKEMOTO S. and FURUHATA T. (1971) Serology and genetics of a new blood type Bm. *Nature New Biology*, **231**, 184–185.

542 KOGURE T. and ISEKI S. (1970) A family of B_m, due to a modifying gene. *Proc. Jap. Acad.*, **46**, 728–732.

543 PRETTY H.M., TALIANO V., FISET DENISE, BARIBEAU G. and GUÉVIN R. (1969) Another example of Lewis negative Bombay bloods. *Vox Sang.*, **16**, 179–182.

544 MOORES P.P. (1972) The 'Bombay' blood-type in Natal. Abstracts AABB and ISH Meeting, Washington, p. 11.

545 YUNIS E.J., SVARDAL JANET M. and BRIDGES R.A. (1969) Genetics of the Bombay phenotype. *Blood*, **33**, 124–132.

546 DZIERZKOWA-BORODEJ WANDA, MEINHARD WERONIKA, NESTOROWICZ STANISLAWA and PIROG JADWIGA (1972) Successful elution of anti-A and certain anti-H reagents from two 'Bombay' (O_h^A) blood samples and investigation of isoagglutinins in their sera. *Arch. Immunol. and Ther. Exp.*, **20**, 841–849.

547 WATKINS W.M., CHESTER M.A., RACE C. and SCHENKEL-BRUNNER H. (1972) Glycosyltransferases in serum from donors of the Bombay O_h phenotype. Abstracts AABB and ISH Meeting, Washington, p. 26.

548 SCHENKEL-BRUNNER H., CHESTER M.A. and WATKINS WINIFRED M. (1972) α-L-fucosyltransferases in human serum from donors of different ABO, secretor and Lewis bloodgroup phenotypes. *Eur. J. Biochem.*, **30**, 269–277.

549 RACE CAROLINE and WATKINS WINIFRED M. (1972) The enzymic products of the human *A* and *B* blood group genes in the serum of 'Bombay' O_h donors. *FEBS. Lett.*, **27**, 125–130.

550 GANDINI E., SACCHI R., REALI G., VERATTI M.A. and MENINI C. (1968) A case of Lewis negative 'Bombay' blood type. *Vox Sang.*, **15**, 142–146.

551 ISEKI S., TAKIZAWA H. and TAKIZAWA H. (1970) Immunological properties of 'Bombay' phenotype. *Proc. Jap. Acad.*, **46**, 803–807.

552 BERANOVÁ GERDA, PRODANOV P., HRUBIŠKO M. and ŠMÁLIK S. (1969) A new variant in the ABO blood group system: B_h. *Vox Sang.*, **16**, 449–456.

553 LIBERGE G., SALMON C., GERBAL A. and LOPEZ M. (1970) Le phénotype B_h: Étude immunologique et génétique d'un cas. *Rev. fr. Transf.*, **13**, 357–363.

554 GÉRARD G., GUIMBRETIÈRE J. and GUIMBRETIÈRE L. (1970) Difficultés de groupage chez un sujet vraisemblablement A_h. *Rev. fr. Transf.*, **13**, 267–274.

555 YAMAGUCHI H., OKUBO Y. and TANAKA M. (1972) Co-occurrence of A_m^h and B_m^h blood in a Japanese family. *Proc. Jap. Acad.*, **48**, 629–632.

556 KOGURE T., TOHYAMA H. and ISEKI S. (1968) An A_{2h}-like blood group with very weak H antigen. *J. Jap. Soc. Bld. Transf.*, **15**, 161.

4*

[557] FAWCETT K.J., ECKSTEIN EDITH G., INNELLA FILOMENA and YOKOYAMA M. (1970) Four examples of B_m^h blood in one family. *Vox Sang.*, **19**, 457–467.

[558] HRUBIŠKO M., LALUHA J., MERGANCOVÁ OLGA and ŽÁKOVICOVÁ SOŇA (1970) New variants in the ABOH blood group system due to interaction of recessive genes controlling the formation of H antigen in erythrocytes: the 'Bombay'-like phenotypes O_{Hm}, O_{Hm}^B and O_{Hm}^{AB}. *Vox Sang.*, **19**, 113–122.

[559] SRINGARM SOMMAI, CHUPUNGART CHUTAMARD and GILES CAROLYN M. (1972) The use of *Ulex europaeus* and *Dolichos biflorus* extracts in routine ABO grouping of blood donors in Thailand. *Vox. Sang.*, **23**, 537–545.

[560] ALBREY J.A. (1971) Personal communication.

[561] ROGERS K.L. (1969) Personal communication.

[562] HART MIA VAN DER (1971) Personal communication.

[563] BHATIA H.M. and SOLOMON J.M. (1967) Further observations on A_m^h and O_m^h phenotypes. *Vox Sang.*, **12**, 457–460.

[564] DARNBOROUGH J., VOAK D. and PEPPER R.M. (1973) Observations on a new example of the A_m phenotype which demonstrates reduced A secretion. *Vox Sang.*, **24**, 216–227.

[565] GUNDOLF F. and ANDERSEN J. (1970) Variant of group B lacking the B antigen on the red cells. *Vox Sang.*, **18**, 216–221.

[566] HRUBIŠKO M., PRODANOV P., ČALKOVSKÁ Z. and MERGANCOVÁ O. (1970) Beobachtungen uber Varianten des Blutgruppensystems ABO. IV. Weitere Beobachtungen der Variante A_{Hm}. *Blut*, **20**, 168–176.

[567] VOAK D., LODGE T.W., STAPLETON R.R., FOGG H. and ROBERTS H.E. (1970) The incidence of H deficient A_2 and A_2B bloods and family studies on the AH/ABH status of an A_{int} and some new variant blood types. *Vox Sang.*, **19**, 73–84.

[568] LENKIEWICZ BOGUSLAWA and SARUL BARBARA (1971) Anti-A_1 antibodies in blood donors in the Warsaw region. *Arch. Immunol.* and *Ther. Exp.*, **19**, 643–647.

[569] MAYR W.R., MICKERTS D. and PAUSCH V. (1969) Schwaches Isoagglutinogen der Blutgruppe B in einer österreichischen Familie. *Haematologia* 3, 17–22.

[570] GRUNDBACHER F.J. and SUMMERLIN D.C. (1971) Inherited differences in blood group A subtypes in Caucasians and Negroes. *Hum. Hered.*, **21**, 88–96.

[571] MILNER L.V. and CALITZ F. (1968) Quantitative studies of the erythrocytic B antigen in South African Caucasian, Bantu and Asiatic blood donors. *Transfusion, Philad.*, **8**, 277–282.

[572] HRUBIŠKO M. (1968) Exemple d'une interacton allélique chez l'homme: interaction entre une variante du gène B (Bx ou B_{20}) et A_2. *Nouv. Rev. fr. Hémat.*, **8**, 278 287.

[573] PRODANOV P., HRUBIŠKO M., BERANOVA GERDA, CALKOVSKA ZDENKA, VELVARTOVA MAGDA and DANKOVA ANA (1970) Étude quantitative du système de groups sanguins ABO. II. Paramètres quantitatifs de certaines catégories faibles des complexes agglutinogènes A et B et des phénotypes 'Bombay' $O_{,h}^{A1} A_h$ et B_h rares. Étude quantitative des phénotypes $O_{Hm} A_{Hm}$ et $A_{Hm}B$. *Nouv. Rev. fr. Hémat.*, **10**, 31–40.

[574] SKOV F., ERIKSEN MARIE and HAGERUP L. (1970) Distribution of the ABO, MNS, P, Rhesus, Lutheran, Kell, Lewis and Duffy blood groups and frequency of irregular red cell antibodies in a population of Danes aged fifty years and a population of Danes aged seventy years. *Acta path. microbiol. scand.*, **78**, 553–559.

[575] GASTEL C. VAN and DUDOK DE WIT C. (1970) The effect of red cell age on its agglutinablity by anti-A serum. *Vox Sang.*, **19**, 105–112.

[576] GOLD E.R. and BHATIA H.M. (1964) Observations on the H antigen. *Vox Sang.*, **9**, 625–628.

[577] DZIERZKOWA-BORODEJ WANDA, MEINHARD WERONIKA and NESTOROWICZ STANISLAWA (1971) Differences of H specificity of human group O erythrocytes. *Arch. Immunol.* and *Ther. Exp.*, **19**, 599–608.

[578] KUŚNIERZ GRAŻYNA and LEŚKIEWICZ ALDONA (1971) Studies on the ABH component of human newborn erythrocytes. *Arch. Immunol.* and *Ther. Exp.*, **19**, 635–641.

[579] WILLIAMS M.A. and VOAK D. (1972) Studies with ferritin-labelled *Dolichos biflorus* lectin

on the numbers and distribution of A sites on A_1 and A_2 erythrocytes, and on the nature of its specificity and enhancement by enzymes. *Brit. J. Haemat.*, **23**, 427–441.

580 KOPEĆ ADA C. (1970) *The Distribution of the Blood Groups in the United Kingdom.* Oxford University Press.

581 WHERRETT J.R., BROWN BARBARA L., TILLEY CHRISTINE A. and CROOKSTON MARIE C. (1971) A and B blood group substances in a glycosphingolipid fraction of human plasma. *Clin. Res.*, **29**, 784.

582 TILLEY C.A., CROOKSTON M.C., BROWN B.L. and WHERRETT J.R. (1975) A and B and A_1Le^b substances in glycosphingolipid fractions of human serum. *Vox Sang.*, **28**, 25–33.

583 GRUNDBACHER F.J. (1967) Quantity of hemolytic anti-A and anti-B in individuals of a human population: correlations with iso-agglutinins and effects of the individual's age and sex. *Z. Immun-forsch.*, **134**, 317–349.

584 MAYEDA K. (1966) Study of the seasonal variation of naturally occurring anti-A and anti-B antibodies of man. *Amer. J. Med. Tech.*, **32**, 187–190.

585 TOVEY L.A.D., TAVERNER J.M. and LONGSTER G.H. (1970) The effect of environment on ABO antibodies. *Vox Sang.*, **19**, 64–72.

586 HEISTO H. and UGGERUD B. (1972) Seasonal fluctuations in blood group antibodies hemo-globin concentration and sedimentation rate in Man: negative findings. *J. Oslo City Hosp.*, **22**, 17–25.

587 PUTKONEN T. (1930) Uber die gruppenspezifischen Eigenschaften verschiedener Korper-flussigkeiten. *Acta Soc. Med. fenn.*, 'Duodecim', A, **14**, No. 12, 113 pages (see ref. 17).

588 BADAKERE S.S. and BHATIA H.M. (1971) ABO agglutinins in the saliva of Indians from Bombay. *Proc. Indian Soc. Haemat. Blood Transf.*, Hyderabad, Jan. 1971, 13–17.

589 TOIVANEN P. and HIRVONEN T. (1969) Iso- and heteroagglutinins in human fetal and neo-natal sera. *Scand. J. Haemat.*, **6**, 42–48.

590 NAIMAN J.L., PUNNETT HOPE H., LISCHNER H.W., DESTINÉ MARIE L. and AREY J.B. (1969) Possible graft-versus-host reaction after intrauterine transfusion for Rh erythroblastosis fetalis. *New Engl. J. Med.*, **281**, 697–701.

591 LINCOLN P.J. and DODD BARBARA E. (1969) Antigen-antibody studies in the ABO blood group system with particular reference to cross-reacting antibodies in group O sera. *Immunology*, **16**, 301–310.

592 VOAK D. (1968) The serological specificity of the sensitising antibodies in ABO hetero-specific pregnancy of the group O mother. *Vox Sang.*, **14**, 271–281.

593 VOAK D., LODGE T.W., HOPKINS JEAN and BOWLEY C.C. (1968) A study of the antibodies of the H'OT-B complex with special reference to their occurrence and notation. *Vox Sang.*, **15**, 353–366.

594 EHNHOLM C. and MÄKELÄ O. (1970) ABO-specific autoagglutinins. *Vox Sang.*, **18**, 414–420.

595 MÄKELÄ O., RUOSLAHTI E. and EHNHOLM C. (1969) Subtypes of human ABO blood groups and subtype-specific antibodies. *J. Immunol.*, **102**, 763–771.

596 POTAPOV M.I. (1968) New anti-B lectins (phytohemagglutinins) including high-grade anti-B_1. *Izv. Akad. Nauk SSSR Ser. Biol.*, **5**, 712–720. (In Russian, with English summary.)

597 POTAPOV M.I. (1970) Untersuchung von Blutflecken und menschlichen Ausscheidungs-produkten mit dem Gruppenlektin Anti-B_1 (Evonymus alata). *Folia Haemat.*, **93**, 458–464.

598 OTTENSOOSER F., SATO R. and SATO M. (1968) A new anti-B lectin. *Transfusion, Philad.*, **8**, 44–46.

599 OTTENSOOSER F., SATO M., SATO R. and KURATA H. (1972) Lectin specificity induced by a fungus, *Vox. Sang.*, **22**, 354–358.

600 BOVE J.R., HOLBURN A.M. and MOLLISON P.L. (1973) Non-specific binding of IgG to anti-body-coated red cells. (The 'Matuhasi-Ogata phenomenon'). *Immunology*, **25**, 793–801.

601 BIRD G.W.G. and WINGHAM JUNE (1970) Agglutinins for antigens of two different human blood group systems in the seeds of *Moluccella laevis*. *Vox Sang.*, **18**, 235–239.

[602] BIRD G.W.G. and WINGHAM J. (1970) Agglutinins from Jerusalem sage (*Phlomis fruticosa*). *Experientia*, **26**, 1257–1258.

[603] BIRD G.W.G. and WINGHAM JUNE (1970) Anti-H from *Cerastium tomentosum* seeds. A comparison with other seed anti-H agglutinins. *Vox Sang.*, **19**, 132–139.

[604] VOAK D. and LODGE T.W. (1971) The demonstration of anti-HI/HI-H activity in seed anti-H reagents. *Vox Sang.*, **20**, 36–45.

[605] MATSUMOTO I. and OSAWA T. (1971) On the specificity of various heterologous anti-H hemagglutinins. *Vox Sang.*, **21**, 548–557.

[606] RANDERIA K.J. and BHATIA H.M. (1967) Further studies on the lectins from *Psofocarpus tetragonolobus*, *Erythrina subrosa* and *Galactia filiformis* showing anti-H specificity. *Indian J. Med. Res.*, **55**, 369–373.

[607] DRYSDALE R.G., HERRICK P.R. and FRANKS D. (1968) The specificity of the haemagglutinin of the castor bean, *Ricinus communis*. *Vox Sang.*, **15**, 194–202.

[608] BHATIA H.M., KIM Y.C. and BOYD W.C. (1968) Serological and immunochemical studies on the snail (*Otala lactea*). *Vox Sang.*, **14**, 170–178.

[609] PROKOP O., UHLENBRUCK G. and KÖHLER W. (1968) A new source of antibody-like substances having anti-blood group specificity. A discussion on the specificity of Helix agglutinins. *Vox Sang.*, **14**, 321–333.

[610] BRAIN P. and GRACE H.J. (1968) On the haemagglutinin of the snail *Achatina granulata*. *Vox Sang.*, **15**, 297–299.

[611] GOLD E.R. and THOMPSON T.E. (1969) Serological differences between related species of snails. I. Revealed by reverse passive agglutination tests. *Vox Sang.*, **16**, 63–66.

[612] GOLD E.R. and THOMPSON T.E. (1969) Serological differences between related species of snails. II. Revealed by haemolysis tests, agglutination tests with tumour cells and content of B-like substance. *Vox Sang.*, **16**, 119–123.

[613] LEE-POTTER J.P. (1969) Haemagglutinins in water snails. *Vox Sang.*, **16**, 500–502.

[614] PEMBERTON R.T. (1969) Studies on the human red cell agglutinins of the swan mussel (*Anodonta cygnea*). *Vox Sang.*, **16**, 457–464.

[615] PEMBERTON R.T. (1969) Incomplete antibodies for A₁ red cells in extracts of the molluscs *Bithynia tentaculata* and *Pomatias elegans*. *Vox Sang.*, **16**, 503–504.

[616] TOVEY G.H. and LOCKYER J.W. (1969) Valuable new sources of anti-A and anti-B. *J. med. Lab. Technol.*, **26**, 264–267.

[617] UHLENBRUCK G. (1969) Some remarks on the specificity of an agglutinin present in the snail Achatina. *J. forens. Med.*, **16**, 35–36.

[618] GRACE H.J. and UHLENBRUCK G. (1969) The agglutination of A_bantu and other human erythrocytes by reagents from snails. *J. forens. Med.*, **16**, 139–142.

[619] PEMBERTON R.T. (1970) Blood group A reactive substance in the common limpet (*Patella vulgata*). *Vox Sang.*, **18**, 71–73.

[620] PEMBERTON R.T. (1970) Haemagglutinins from the slug *Limax flavus*. *Vox Sang.*, **18**, 74–76.

[621] KHALAP S., THOMPSON T.E. and GOLD E.R. (1970) Haemagglutination and haemagglutination-inhibition reactions of extracts from snails and sponges. I. Agglutination of human and various animal red cells: its inhibition by sugars and aminosugars. *Vox Sang.*, **18**, 501–526.

[622] UHLENBRUCK G., SPRENGER I., LESENEY A.M., FONT J. and BOURRILLON R. (1970) Comparative studies of the anti-A agglutinins from *Dolichos biflorus* and certain snails. *Vox Sang.*, **19**, 488–495.

[623] ISHIYAMA I. and TAKATSU A. (1970) Anti-A hemagglutinin from the garden snail *Euphadra periomphala*: inhibition by *N*-acetyl-D-galactosamine and *N*-acetyl-D-glucosamine. *Vox Sang.*, **19**, 522–526.

[624] WIENER A.S. (1970) Immunochemical studies on group-specific agglutinins of diverse origin. *Haematologia*, **4**, 157–166.

[625] KHALAP S., THOMPSON T.E. and GOLD E.R. (1971) Haemagglutination and haemagglutination-inhibition reactions of extracts from snails and sponges. II. Haemagglutination-

inhibition tests with biological materials and some substances contained in them. *Vox Sang.*, **20**, 150–173.

626 PEMBERTON R.T. (1971) Observations on a haemagglutinin from the freshwater mussel *Anodonta anatina*. *Vox Sang.*, **21**, 159–174.

627 TODD G.M. (1971) Blood group antibodies in salmonidae roe. *Vox Sang.*, **21**, 451–454.

628 PEMBERTON R.T. (1971) Haemagglutinins from some British non-marine *Mollusca*. *Vox Sang.*, **21**, 509–521.

629 BIZOT M. (1971) Hemagglutinin from the snail *Eobania vermiculata*. *Vox Sang.*, **21**, 465–468.

630 BIZOT M. (1971) Activité hémagglutinante des extraits de glande d'albumine de *Helix* (*Cryptomphalus*) *Aspersa* et de *Helix* (*Helix*) *Pomatia*. *Rev. franc. Transf.*, **14**, 445–453.

631 SCHNITZLER S. (1971) Zu Eigenschaften und Anwendungsmöglichkeiten der Schnecken-agglutinine. *Kriminalistik und forensische Wissenschaften*, **4**, 135–141.

632 SCHNITZLER S., UERLINGS I. and DAVID H. (1971) Elektronenmikroskopische Darstellung der Antikörper aus Helix pomatia L. *Acta biol. med. germ.*, **26**, 193–203.

633 ISHIYAMA I., TAKATSU A., UHLENBRUCK G., REIFENBERG U., SCHNITZLER S. and PROKOP O. (1971) Serological behaviour of an 'incomplete' and 'superagglutinating' anti-A from the snail *Helix pomatia*. *Z. Naturf.*, **26b**, 171.

634 KHALAP S., PHELPS C.F., FUDENBERG H.H. and GOLD E.R. (1972) Separation of haemagglutinins from haemolysins in extracts of the albumin gland of *Helix aspersa*. *Vox Sang.*, **23**, 218–221.

635 ANSTEE D.J., HOLT P.D.J. and PARDOE G.I. (1973) Agglutinins from fish ova defining blood groups B and P. *Vox Sang.*, **25**, 347–360.

636 CANN GILLIAN B. (1971) The study of a haemagglutinating substance extracted from the albumin gland of the snail *Helix aspersa*. M.Sc. thesis, Bristol University.

637 BIZOT M. (1971) Hémagglutination des Globules Rouges par les Extraits de Gastéropodes Terrestres. Thesis, Faculty of Pharmacy, University of Montpellier.

638 WATKINS WINIFRED M. (1972) The biochemical basis of human blood group ABO and Lewis polymorphism. Review article in Annual Report, The Lister Institute of Preventive Medicine, 12–29.

639 WIENER A.S., SOCHA W.W. and GORDON E.B. (1972) The relationship of the *H* specificity to the ABO blood groups. II. Observations on Whites, Negroes and Chinese. *Vox Sang.*, **22**, 97–106.

640 VOAK D. and LODGE T.W. (1968) The role of H in the development of A. *Vox Sang.*, **15**, 345–352.

641 YAMAKAWA T. and SUZUKI S. (1952) The chemistry of the lipids of post-hemolytic residue or stroma of erythrocytes. III. Globoside, the sugar containing lipid of human blood stroma. *J. Biochem., Tokyo*, **39**, 393.

642 KOSCIELAK J. (1963) Blood group A specific glycolipids from human erythrocytes. *Biochim. biophys. Acta*, **78**, 313–328.

643 HAKOMORI S. and STRYCHARZ G.D. (1968) Investigations on cellular blood-group substances. I. Isolation and chemical composition of blood-group ABH and Le^b isoantigens of sphingoglycolipid nature. *Biochemistry*, **7**, 1279.

644 WATKINS W.M., KOSCIELAK J. and MORGAN W.T.J. (1964) The relationship between the specificity of the blood-group A and B substances isolated from erythrocytes and from secretions. *Proc. Ninth Congr. Int. Soc. Blood Transfusion* (Mexico, 1962), p. 213.

645 HEARN V.M., SMITH Z.G. and WATKINS W.M. (1968) An α-N-acetylgalactosaminyltransferase associated with the human blood-group A character. *Biochem. J.*, **109**, 315.

646 TUPPY H. and SCHENKEL-BRUNNER H. (1969) Occurrence and assay of alpha-N-acetyl-galactosaminyltransferase in the gastric mucosa of humans belonging to blood-group A. *Vox Sang.*, **17**, 139–142.

647 KOBATA A., GROLLMAN E.F. and GINSBURG V. (1968) An enzymatic basis for blood type A in humans. *Arch. Biochem. Biophys.*, **124**, 609.

[648] SAWICKA T. (1971) Glycosyltransferases in human plasma. *FEBS Letters*, **16**, 346.

[649] HEARN V.M., RACE CAROLINE and WATKINS WINIFRED M. (1972) α-N-acetylgalactos-aminyl- and α-galactosyltransferases in human ovarian cyst epithelial linings and fluids. *Biochem. biophys. Res. Commun.*, **46**, 948.

[650] RACE CAROLINE, ZIDERMAN DIANE and WATKINS WINIFRED M. (1968) An α-D-galactosyl-transferase associated with the blood group B character. *Biochem. J.*, **107**, 733–735.

[651] KOBATA A., GROLLMAN E.F. and GINSBURG V. (1968) An enzymatic basis for blood type B in humans. *Biochem. biophys. Res. Commun.*, **32**, 272.

[652] PORETZ R.D. and WATKINS WINIFRED M. (1972) Galactosyltransferases in human sub-maxillary glands and stomach mucosa associated with the biosynthesis of blood group B specific glycoproteins. *Eur. J. Biochem.*, **25**, 455.

[653] SHEN LAURA, GROLLMAN EVELYN F. and GINSBURG V. (1968) An enzymatic basis for secretor status and blood group substance specificity in humans. *Proc. Nat. Acad. Sci.*, **59**, 224–230.

[654] SCHACHTER H., MICHAELS M.A., TILLEY CHRISTINE A., CROOKSTON MARIE C. and CROOK-STON J.H. (1973) Qualitative differences in the N-acetyl-D-galactosaminyltransferases produced by human A^1 and A^2 genes. *Proc. nat. Acad. Sci., USA*, **70**, 220–224.

[655] BOETTCHER B. (1967) ABO blood group agglutinins in saliva. *Acta haemat.*, **38**, 351–360.

[656] JAKOBOWICZ RACHEL and GRAYDON J.J. (1968) Association of hererospecific pregnancies and the presence of saliva antibodies. *Vox Sang.*, **14**, 357–362.

[657] BELL C.E. and FORTWENGLER H.P. (1971) Salivary anti-A and anti-B activity of group O males. *Vox Sang.*, **21**, 493–508.

[658] FELLOUS M., BILLARDON C., DAUSSET J. and FRÉZAL J. (1971) Linkage probable entre les locus 'HLA' et 'P'. *C. r. hebd. Séanc. Acad. Sci., Paris*, **272**, 3356–3359.

[659] FELLOUS M., TESSIER C., GERBAL A., SALMON C., FRÉZAL J. and DAUSSET J. (1972) Genetic dissection of P biosynthesis pathway. *Bull. Eur. Soc. Hum. Genet.*, 31.

[660] DZIERZKOWA-BORODEJ WANDA, CHUDZIK JADWIGA and LESKIEWICZ ALDONA (1972) Six-month serological observation in a case of A_1B-like phenomenon. *Arch. Immunol. Ther. Exp.*, **20**, 861–868.

[661] BUSH MIRIAM and SABO BERNICE (1973) Three generations of AB antigens in cis position. *Transfusion, Philad.*, **13**, 362.

[662] WITEBSKY E. and KLENDSHOJ N.C. (1941) The isolation of an O specific substance from gastric juice of secretors and carbohydrate-like substances from gastric juice of non-secretors. *J. Exp. Med.*, **73**, 655–667.

[663] POSKITT T.R. and FORTWENGLER P. (1973) A study of weak subgroups of blood group A with an antiglobulin-latex test. *Transfusion, Philad.*, **13**, 347.

[664] MARSH W.L., FERRARI MARY, NICHOLS MARGARET E., FERNANDEZ GLORIA and COOPER K. (1973) B_m^H: a weak B antigen variant. *Vox Sang.*, **25**, 341–346.

[665] MOHN J.F., CUNNINGHAM R.K., PIRKOLA ANNA, FURUHJELM U. and NEVANLINNA H.R. (1973) An inherited blood group A variant in the Finnish population. I. Basic characteristics. *Vox Sang.*, **25**, 193–211.

[666] SALMON C., LOPEZ M., GERBAL A., BOUGUERRA A. and CARTRON J.P. (1973) Current genetic problems in the ABO blood group system. *Biomedicine*, **18**, 375–386.

[667] DUCOS J., MARTY Y. and RUFFIÉ J. (1974) A new case of A_x phenotype transmitted by A_2B subjects. *Vox Sang.*, in the press.

[668] WIENER A.S. and CIOFFI A.F. (1972) A group B analogue of subgroup A_3. *Amer. J. clin. Path.*, **58**, 693–697.

[669] DUCOS J. (1958) Technique de groupage du foetus 'in utero'. *Revue fr. Etud. clin. biol.*, **3**, 1109–1110.

[670] TIPPETT PATRICIA and TEESDALE PHYLLIS (1973) Limited blood group tests on samples from two coelacanths (*Latimeria chalumnae*). *Vox Sang.*, **24**, 175–178.

[671] NEVANLINNA H.R. and PIRKOLA ANNA (1973) An inherited blood group A variant in the Finnish population. II. Population studies. *Vox Sang.*, **24**, 404–416.

[672] RUBINSTEIN P., ALLEN F.H. and ROSENFIELD R.E. (1973) A dominant suppressor of A and B. *Vox Sang.*, **25**, 377–381.

[673] SSEBAI E.C.T. (1973) Fluctuation of natural anti-A and anti-B in high-titre Ugandans. *Vox Sang.*, **24**, 472–476.

[674] SPRINGER G.F. and TEGTMEYER HERTA (1974) Absence of B antibody in a blood group A_1 person. *Vox Sang.*, **26**, 247–258.

[675] HOLBURN A.M. and MASTERS CAROLE A. (1974) The radioimmunoassay of serum and salivary blood group A and Le^a glycoproteins. *Brit. J. Haemat.*, **28**, 157–167.

Chapter 3
The MNSs Blood Groups

At a time when only the ABO groups were known Landsteiner and Levine, seeking other antigenic differences, injected rabbits with different samples of human red cells and absorbed the resulting rabbit immune serum with other red cell samples until they found what they were looking for—antibodies which would distinguish between blood in a way that was cutting across the known ABO distinctions.

In the first brief announcement in 1927, Landsteiner and Levine[1] describe M, and in a second short[2] note we are introduced to N and P and the inheritance of M is established. Frequencies were reported in two more papers[3,4]. The latter paper[4] is instructive as a pattern of the type of reasoning by which advances in blood group knowledge are made; in it Landsteiner and Levine give the detailed results of testing 64 families with 286 children, and discuss the possible manner of inheritance of the MN groups. The two-allele theory was put forward as the most likely solution. According to the theory there are two alleles M and N, either of which determines the presence of the corresponding antigen on the red cells. Thus there are three genotypes MM, MN and NN and three corresponding phenotypes M, MN and N.

The theory was soon confirmed by Schiff[5], who tested 42 families and by Wiener and Vaisberg[6] who tested 131 families, and by thousands of families tested since. (The present tendency to think of N as a basic substance acted on by two alleles M and m makes no practical difference to the description of the system: if the tendency should prove to be correct the time may come when N will be changed to m. See page 121.)

During the following third of a century several rare antigens were identified: some could be attributed to alleles of M and N and some could not—though they obviously belonged to the MN system. The most important step was made when, in 1947, Walsh and Montgomery[24] found a 'new' antibody at first thought to bear no relation to any of the known systems of blood groups. The serum was kindly sent to the authors and it soon became apparent[25,29] that, although the antibody was not anti-M or anti-N, it was recognizing an antigen associated with M and N and it was called S. When the serum had been tested against 190 English blood samples the following 2 × 2 table made the association clear:

92

		M+MN	N	
Anti-S	+	93	15	108
	−	52	30	82
		145	45	190

$$\text{for } \chi^2 = \frac{[(93 \times 30) - (52 \times 15)]^2 \times 190}{145 \times 45 \times 108 \times 82} = 13, \text{ for 1 d.f.}$$

which corresponds to a probability of less than 0·001.

The recognition of the association of the 'new' antibody with the MN system was entirely due to the habit of resolving blood group problems into 2×2 tables[26,27]. On the other hand, no association between the reactions of anti-S and the antigens of the A_1A_2BO, P, Rh, Lutheran, Kell, Lewis, Duffy or Kidd systems emerged.

S could be shown not to be an allele of *M* and *N*—it was evidently related to M and N as C, D and E are related in the Rh system. It was calculated that anti-s, when it was found, would react with 88% of English bloods. When, in 1951, Levine, Kuhmichel, Wigod and Koch[28] found the first example of anti-s it reacted with 89% of English bloods.

Table 7 shows the genetical interpretation of the reactions which was, at an early stage, supported by phenotype frequencies and family evidence[25,29-31]. It has been confirmed by all subsequent work on white people.

Table 7. Genetical interpretation of the reactions of anti-M, anti-N, anti-S and anti-s sera

Anti- M N S s	All 4 sera: genotype	First 3 sera: genotype or phenotype
+ − + −	*MS/MS*	*MM.S*
+ − + +	*MS/Ms*	
+ − − +	*Ms/Ms*	*Ms/Ms*
+ + + −	*MS/NS*	
+ + + +	*MS/Ns*	*MN.S*
	Ms/NS	
+ + − +	*Ms/Ns*	*Ms/Ns*
− + + −	*NS/NS*	*NN.S*
− + + +	*NS/Ns*	
− + − +	*Ns/Ns*	*Ns/Ns*

The next advance was the recognition[50] that rather less than 1% of negro blood samples lack both S and s.

MNSs FREQUENCIES IN WHITE PEOPLE

Innumerable series of tests have been reported from many parts of the world. The earlier work was, of necessity, confined to tests with anti-M and anti-N but in recent series anti-S, with or without anti-s, has been included. In case they might be useful some references to earlier work not mentioned in this chapter but noted in the 5th edition have been left amongst the references (7 to 11).

In white people the complication of U and S^u can for most purposes be ignored. The gene frequencies can be calculated from the results of tests with the three antisera, anti-M, -N, -S, with or without those given by the fourth antiserum, anti-s. J.H. Edwards (cited by Cleghorn[75]) estimates that 1,000 samples tested with the three antisera give as much information as 800 tested with the four antisera.

Table 8 shows the gene frequencies calculated from four series of tests on people of Northern European extraction: the agreement between the four estimates is so close that any of them may, according to taste, be taken as the standard frequencies at this level of discrimination.

Table 8. Frequencies of the *MNSs* gene complexes in some people of Northern European extraction

Gene complex	a 1,419 British	b 1,000 British	c 1,400 Canadian	d 3,895 Swiss
MS	0·2472	0·2371	0·2546	0·2447
Ms	0·2831	0·3054	0·3043	0·2915
NS	0·0802	0·0709	0·0607	0·0790
Ns	0·3895	0·3866	0·3804	0·3829
				0·0019*

a. Tested with anti-M, -N, -S. Pooled data of Walsh and Montgomery[24], Sanger and Race[25], Pickles[32], Race *et al.*[33], Bertinshaw *et al.*[34]. Calculations by R.A. Fisher.
b. Tested with anti-M, -N, -S, -s. Cleghorn[75]. Calculations, slightly modified since the first publication, by J.H. Bennett[12] and by J.H. Edwards[45].
c. Tested with anti-M, -N, -S, -s. Chown, Lewis and Kaita[46].
d. Tested with anti-M, -N, -S, all s+ samples tested with anti-s, Metaxas *et al.*[199].
* Includes rarer gene complexes, see pages 104–106.

The calculation of the frequencies of the *MNSs* gene complexes usually requires specialist help. Fisher used his maximum likelihood method originally designed for Rh[37,38]. Edwards designed a computer programme for the purpose. Chown and his colleagues[46] were able, very ingeniously, to circumvent the higher mathematics because their 1,400 people were parents, all but 50 of whose genotypes were made clear by their offspring: the 50 *MNSs* were distributed in proportion to the known *MS/Ns* and *Ms/NS* and the gene complexes could then simply be counted.

Other methods of calculating the *MNSs* gene frequencies are described by Boyd[39–41], by Mourant[42], by Wiener[43], by de Groot and Li[76] and by Morton and Miki[200].

The gene frequencies once calculated can be recombined to give the expected incidence in the genotype classes. Cleghorn's series is used for this purpose in Table 9 where the fit between calculated and observed incidence is very close, as it was when the other three series of Table 8 were similarly treated.

Table 9. One thousand random English bloods tested with anti-M, anti-N, anti-S and anti-s. (After Cleghorn[75], 1960)

	Expected proportion	Expected absolute	Observed absolute	χ^2
MS/MS	0·0562	56·2	57	0·01
MS/Ms	0·1448	144·8	140	0·16
Ms/Ms	0·0933	93·3	101	0·64
MS/NS	0·0336	33·6	39	0·87
MS/Ns *Ms/NS*	0·2266	226·6	224	0·03
Ms/Ns	0·2362	236·2	226	0·44
NS/NS	0·0050	5·0	3	0·80
NS/Ns	0·0548	54·8	54	0·01
Ns/Ns	0·1495	149·5	156	0·28
Total	1·0000	1,000·0	1,000	3·24 for 5 d.f. P = about 0·7

Table 9 may also help in the often troublesome question—how many degrees of freedom? To lighten our darkness Fisher took Table 9 as an example and, in a letter from Adelaide, wrote:

DEGREES OF FREEDOM

Nine counts constitute the data   9

To compare with the data we use expectations, but the expectations in this case, as also usually, are constructed from the data to which they are to be compared. In this reconstruction we use

(i) Total size of sample
(ii) Proportion M
(iii) Proportion S
(iv) Proportion MS

However listed, there are only 4 constraints linking the reconstruction to the data with which it is to be compared

D.F. = 9 − 4 = 5

So the degrees of freedom in Table 9 are 5. When only anti-M, -N, -S are used the degrees of freedom are 6 − 4 = 2.

Hints we have picked up about the number of degrees of freedom in other blood group situations are to be found on page 482 (and p. 118 of our 5th ed.)

The approximate frequencies in Table 10 may help in practical problems of identifying antibodies by the use of cells from people of Northern European extraction.

Table 10. Some approximate phenotype frequencies in the MNSs
system for people of Northern European extraction

| | | Positive reactions with | |
		anti-S	anti-s
All samples		55%	89%
M samples	28%	72%	78%
MN samples	50%	56%	92%
N samples	22%	31%	97%

INHERITANCE OF MNSs IN WHITE PEOPLE

The recognition of the antigens S and s greatly increased the genetical interest of
the MN groups; and here is one way of illustrating the advance in discrimination:

Antisera	Phenotypes	Genotypes	Phenotypically distinct matings	Genotypically different matings
anti-M, -N	3	3	6	6
anti-M, -N, -S	6	10	21	55
anti-M, -N, -S, -s	9	10	45	55

The antigens M, N, S and s are inherited as dominant characters. As we have
already said, the *MNSs* gene complex is like that of *Rh*. The antigens M and N
behave as if controlled by allelic genes and so do the antigens S and s. Whether
the mutational site or sites for *M* and *N* are in the same cistron as those for *S* and *s*
or whether they are thought of as being in closely adjacent cistrons really makes no
difference. One thing is certain, their sites are very close together: were recombination between them other than a very rare event the ratio *MS*: *Ms* would be the
same as *NS*: *Ns*, which it is not.

Previous editions of this book had tables showing the calculated frequency of
the mating types and the children expected therefrom; but, not having found these
tables useful ourselves, we left them out this time.

Vast numbers of families must have been tested with anti-M, -N and anti-S.
Anti-s is still rather precious and tends to be used on families presenting some
problem connected with the MNSs system. The use of anti-s, in white families
at any rate, is often withheld if the reactions of anti-S are negative.

The following are the only substantial *series* of unselected white families
tested with anti-M, -N, -S, -s that we know of: Blood Group Unit[30,44], English,
101 families with 203 children. Chown, Lewis and Kaita[46], Canadian, 700 families
with 1977 children. Heiken[66], Swedish, 81 families with 174 children. These
families have been analysed for MNSs as a whole and also for MN and Ss separately: the agreement between the observed and expected distribution of matings
and children therefrom was very close.

Amongst many hundreds tested in our Unit we can remember only two unselected white families in which S^u (see below), or a gene indistinguishable in

effect, has to be invoked to explain the Ss reactions: we know of several other such white families (Dr T.E. Cleghorn, personal communication, Giblett et al.[86], Chown et al.[46], Heiken[66], Krauland and Smerling[201,266], Polesky et al.[202]). S^u has been proved to be the cause of a false appearance of exclusion of paternity in white families (Hrubiško, two 3 generation families, personal communication; Metaxas and Metaxas-Bühler[268]).

The sometime disarray of the S, s and U reactions in the Rh_{null} condition is referred to on page 225.

Pedigrees illustrating the inheritance of the *MNSs* gene complexes will be found on pages 98, 110 and 512.

Anti-S makes the MNS system only slightly less efficient than the Rh system in distinguishing between two samples of blood; if anti-s is used as well, MNSs becomes the most discriminating of all systems. Fisher[47] has used the MNSs groups as a model for his 'Standard calculations for evaluating a blood group system', which will be referred to on page 507.

Evidence for recombination within the complex locus

The evidence that recombination between the sites for MN and for Ss can occur, as a great rarity, is substantial. Before a case can be made for recombination, illegitimacy, or accidental interchange of babies, has to be ruled out. This can be done with a high degree of probability by the application of the whole range of blood groups, serum groups and biochemical genetical markers. On occasion rare inherited abnormalities can provide overwhelming evidence against illegitimacy or interchange and this is illustrated in the very important family reported by Gedde-Dahl, Grimstad, Gundersen and Vogt[94]. Mutation can always be invoked as an alternative to recombination, but if mutation be the explanation of Gedde-Dahl's family it would show that *S* or *s* can mutate independently of *M* or *N* and this would give evidence, from a different direction, of the separateness of the mutational sites.

Figure 6 shows the pedigree of the family investigated by Gedde-Dahl and his colleagues[94]. II-1 is undoubtedly of the genotype *MS/NS*: this is shown by the reactions of his cells and is confirmed by the groups of his wife and children and re-affirmed by the groups of his grandchildren. The parents of II-1 are, however both *MS/Ns*: this is established by the informative sibs of II-1. The possibility that II-1 is extra-marital has been eliminated: all his other red cell and serum groups fit and, even more significant, he has a variant form of epidermolysis bullosa just like his father. Realizing the importance of excluding affected relatives of I-1 as possible fathers of II-1, Gedde-Dahl and his colleagues exonerated the only two candidates, both now dead, by the MNSs groups of their many children. Furthermore, Parish Registers allowed the calculation that II-1 was probably conceived during the 3rd week after the wedding of I-1 and I-2.

So the choice lay between recombination and mutation, and Gedde-Dahl and

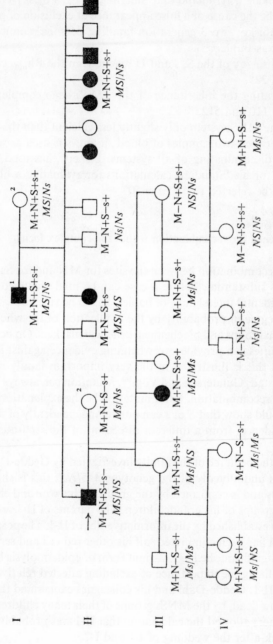

Fig. 6. The most likely explanation of the genotype of II-1 is that there has been crossing-over between *MN* and *Ss* at the first meiotic division of spermatogenesis in his father or oogenesis in his mother. Black = epidermolysis bullosa. The birth order is not that of the original pedigree—it has been re-arranged for convenience. (From Gedde-Dahl *et al.*[94], 1966)

his colleagues decided in favour of recombination after considering frequency estimates of mutation and recombination. In an Appendix they analyse MNSs families taken from the literature or gathered by enquiry from certain laboratories: these families gave information about 1,538 meiotic divisions with respect to crossing-over and six other possible recombinations were present. Three of these had not been re-tested and will not be considered here. Some notes about the three remaining cases follow.

Chown, Lewis and Kaita[112] were the first to report a family giving evidence of recombination between *MN* and *Ss*. The phenotypes of this Dutch Canadian family were: father Ns, mother MNSs, three children Ns, three MNSs (all of which fix the genotype of the parents as *Ns/Ns* and *MS/Ns*) while one child, the fifth, is MNs. The legitimacy of this fifth child was virtually proved by other red cell groups, by serum groups and by biochemical genetical markers. Recombination at oogenesis was considered the most likely explanation.

Another white family investigated by Chown, Lewis and Kaita (personal communication, and cited by Gedde-Dahl *et al.*[94]) was of the same mating type as their previous family: father Ns and mother MNSs; one daughter was Ns (with MNs and Ns children) and the other was MNs (with Ns, Ms and MNs children).

Another good example is pointed out by Gedde-Dahl *et al.*[94] in a series of families tested by Scholz and Murken[113]. The results were confirmed on repeat samples using several examples of anti-M, -N, -S, -s (Scholz, and Murken[197]). The phenotype of the father is MNSs and his genotype, proved by his mother and sibs, is *MS/Ns*; the mother is MNSs, the son is Ns (*Ns/Ns*) and the daughter MNS (*MS/NS*). Father and daughter both have a rare dominant condition causing cartilaginous exostoses. Red cell and serum groups and other tests strongly favoured the legitimacy of the son.

Thus there are three well established cases that can best be explained by recombination between *MN* and *Ss* sites. If mutation were the cause we should surely by now have examples of children having M or N or S or s which both their parents lack. Incidentally, if mutation does occur it must be an extremely rare event in the ABO system for in spite of the vast number of families tested there is no record that we know of where a case is made for mutation.

The only apparent example of mutation happening at a blood group locus was in a family extensively studied by Henningsen and Jacobsen[23] in 1954: an N child was born, at home, to an M mother. The mother and child were retested in 1963 by Dr Henningsen and by Dr and Mrs Metaxas: M^g was not the explanation, and M^k was ruled out because both mother and child have S and s. The mother's cells gave a clear double dose of M but the child's cells only a single dose of N, confirmed by their not reacting with a special anti-N serum[134] which reacts only with homozygotes. Whether the explanation is, as Dr Metaxas suggests, some sort of mutational loss to an *M* allele, or whether some as yet unknown recessive inhibitor of M is at work remains a puzzle. (An account of rare alleles that may give the appearance of exceptions to the orderly inheritance of the MNSs groups will be found on page 104 *et seq.*)

MNSs IN NEGROES: THE PROBLEM OF U

In 1953 Wiener, Unger, Gordon and Cohen[48,49] described an antibody, anti-U, which agglutinated the red cells of all of 1,100 white people tested, but which failed to agglutinate the red cells of 12 out of 989 New York Negroes. These investigators were able to test the blood of relatives of four of the twelve negative persons and concluded: 'Presumably, the factor is inherited by a pair of allelic genes U and u, where gene U determines the presence of the factor and gene u its absence.'

A second example of anti-U was found a year later by Greenwalt, Sasaki, Sanger, Sneath and Race[50]. During the investigation it was observed that the two available examples of blood not agglutinated by anti-U were not agglutinated by anti-S or by anti-s. All samples of blood previously tested with anti-S and anti-s had been agglutinated by one or the other, or by both of these two antisera. (All subsequent U negative samples tested have been S–s–.) Anti-U could most easily be thought of as anti-S+anti-s, or, rather, anti-Ss since attempts to split the antibody into two components by absorption or elution were unsuccessful. (This was confirmed by Hackel[95].) However, the reactions of anti-U no longer exactly fit those expected of a hypothetical anti-Ss, as will be seen from what now follows.

The next step was the recognition that not all S–s– samples are U–. This complication was first recorded in our 4th edition in which we wrote:

> though all the 20 or more U– samples from unrelated people that we have tested have been S–s– not all the S–s– have been U–. Through the kindness of Miss Betty Francis, Mr D. Hatcher, Dr Cahan, Dr Greenwalt and Dr Cleghorn we have had the opportunity to test six samples of negro blood which, though clearly S–s–, do react, relatively weakly, with anti-U: the six samples vary in the strength of their reaction and in the number of anti-U sera with which they react. Absorption and elution tests show that the reaction is truly due to anti-U. None of these aberrant types of S–s– has made anti-U; all MN groups are represented amongst them.
>
> The families of two of these less common S–s– people were studied in collaboration with Miss Francis and Mr Hatcher. In one family a sib of the propositus is S–s– and gives exactly the pattern of reactions with different anti-U sera given by the propositus. In another family a sib of the propositus gives a pattern identical with that of the propositus; but, more illuminating, a grand-daughter of this sib is S–s– and again gives the family pattern with anti-U sera and so demonstrates that the idiosyncrasy of behaviour is a heterozygous effect (though, of course, the S–s– reaction is a homozygous effect).

Since then the relative frequencies of the two types of S–s– in random Negroes have been recorded by Allen, Madden and King[114] and by Francis and Hatcher[115]: about 84% are U– and 16% U+.

A further step was the observation by Allen and his collaborators[110,114] that cells of the phenotype M S–s–U– or M S–s–U+ do not contain the small amount of N which is to be found in, as far as is known, all other M cells.

Possible backgrounds for the S–s–U– phenotype were discussed by Greenwalt and his colleagues[50,35,96]; they were:

1   An allele of Ss,S^u.
2   A 'built-in' inhibitor gene suppressing the action of S or s in *cis*. (At the time we thought this 'far fetched' but later Morton, Mi and Yasuda[116] pointed out that this was no longer so in the light of the work of Jacob and Monod.)
3   An unlinked suppressor locus. This was ruled out by family tests quoted in our fourth edition; other families confirming this are to be found in the data of Goldstein[129] and of Morton *et al.*[116]
4   Absence of genetic material. This is difficult to rule out but was probably made unlikely by the observation that some S–s– people are U+.

So we are left with a choice between 1 and 2, but from the point of view of analysis they come to the same thing. We will continue to use the symbol S^u to represent the allele or alleles responsible for the S–s– phenotype, at any rate in the following calculations, for it makes no difference for this purpose whether or not the S–s– phenotype be heterogeneous.

It is satisfying to be able to make preliminary analysis of data in the laboratory without the help of mathematician or computer, and we have taken pleasure in the following homespun way of dealing with anti-S and anti-s results in Negroes. An example is given in Table 11.

The frequency of the allele S^u was taken as the square root of the proportion of S–s– in the sample (0·0151) which is 0·1229. Using this figure and the proportion of S–s+, which is 0·6817, an estimate of the frequency of the allele s may be had from the quadratic equation

$$s = \frac{-(2 \times 0\cdot1229) + \sqrt{\{(2 \times 0\cdot1229)^2 + 4(0\cdot6817)\}}}{2} = 0\cdot7118$$

and the frequency of $S = 1 - S^u - s = 0\cdot1653$.

These three gene frequencies are recombined to give the expected distribution in the four phenotype classes in Table 11. The agreement between observed and expected is close enough and the theory that the gene or genes responsible for the

Table 11. Tests with anti-S and anti-s on samples from 1322 American Negroes: expectations based on a three-allele interpretation. (Taken from the data of Francis and Hatcher[115], Crawford[198] and Issitt, Haber and Allen[147])

Anti-S s	Observed	Interpretation	Expected proportion	Expected absolute	χ^2
– –	20	$S^u S^u$	0·0151	20·0	0·00
+ –	78	$\begin{cases} SS^u \\ SS \end{cases}$	$\begin{matrix} 0\cdot0406 \\ 0\cdot0273 \end{matrix}$	89·8	1·55
+ +	323	Ss	0·2353	311·1	0·46
– +	901	$\begin{cases} sS^u \\ ss \end{cases}$	$\begin{matrix} 0\cdot1750 \\ 0\cdot5067 \end{matrix}$	901·2	0·00
	1,322		1·0000	1322·1	2·01

for 1 d.f.
P = 0·18

S—s— phenotype are allelic to *S* and *s* is supported by the data. Some earlier tests were analysed in this way in our 4th edition.

At this stage some MNSs phenotype frequencies for American Negroes may be helpful; those in Table 12 are taken from the same three series used in Table 11.

Table 12. The MNSs phenotype frequencies observed in samples from 1322 American Negroes. (Figures from the data of Francis and Hatcher[115], Crawford[198] and Issitt, Haber and Allen[147])

	S—s—	S+s—	S+s+	S—s+	Total
M	0·4%	2·1%	7·0%	15·5%	25·0%
MN	0·4%	2·2%	13·0%	33·4%	49·0%
N	0·7%	1·6%	4·5%	19·2%	26·0%
Total	1·5%	5·9%	24·5%	68·1%	

Different examples of anti-S and anti-s sera agree in giving a clear picture of reactions, −−, +−, ++ and −+, and the results can be analysed as above, and, no doubt, in other more complicated ways too. The reactions of anti-U sera, on the other hand, are difficult to analyse: all examples of the antiserum agree that S+s−, S+s+ and S—s+ samples are positive, but when it comes to the one new and useful distinction they can make, that between S—s—U— and S—s—U+, their performance is disappointingly varied. Using strong anti-U sera 16% or more of S—s— samples give positive reactions[114,115,198]. Attempts to distinguish qualitatively between these reactions[130,129] do not seem to us too hopeful: they recall attempts to distinguish qualitatively between the reactions of various anti-D sera with the spectrum of D^u antigens. The postulation of two kinds of anti-U, anti-U^a and anti-U^b (Brice and Hoxworth[130], Goldstein[129], Goldstein and Hoxworth[203]), does not to us seem to explain adequately the grades of reactions: Issitt, Haber and Allen[147], on the other hand, think it could cope with discrepant frequencies of reaction of different anti-U sera[204] and their thoughtful paper should be read.

Though *S*, *s* and S^u can be distinguished and dealt with separately from *M* and *N* they can, even allowing for the evidence that recombination may on very rare occasions occur between the loci for their two series of alleles, be considered as part of the same gene complex. Table 13 shows the frequencies of these complexes calculated from two series of extensive tests. In both series the M_1 distinction was made (see page 107). The asterisk denotes an allele which produces no S or s antigen but may or may not produce U. We do not like the asterisk for the S—s— alleles: it is untypeable on our machines and starts a fruitless search for a footnote. Since the S—s— condition can be thought of as being due to an allele of *S* and *s* we prefer the old fashioned symbol S^u, but with the clear understanding that it is heterogeneous.

Many S—s— families must now have been tested with anti-M, -N, -S, -s, -U but only a few are reported[35,114,116,129]. Those that are, however, agree in showing

Table 13. The *MNSs* gene frequencies of two series of American Negroes: a. 322 from Houston (Francis and Hatcher[115], 1966; calculations by Yasuda[115]). b. 500, mostly from New Jersey (Issitt, Haber and Allen[147], 1968; calculations by Morton and Miki[200], 1968)

	Houston	New Jersey
M_1S	0·03188	0·02672
M_1s	0·07612	0·09776
MS	0·06631	0·07060
Ms	0·25951	0·25143
NS	0·07285	0·06752
Ns	0·38006	0·38072
$M_1{}^*$	0·01803	0·00681
M^*	0·04320	0·03368
N^*	0·05204	0·06476

that S−s− people do not have S+s+ parents or children, that is to say, as we have already said, S−s− is not caused by an unlinked suppressor gene. Goldstein[129] in her thesis described dosage tests on appropriate members of 15 negro families with S−s− propositi, but no clear effect could be shown in any of the members though the anti-s serum in use was making a clear distinction between *S*s and *ss* samples from white people.

We still have not heard of an S−s− white person. Neither Greenwalt nor his colleagues[96] found an example of U− in testing nearly 10,000 Milwaukee Whites. However, as mentioned on page 96, the allele S^u, or something like it, has had to come to the rescue to reconcile the MNSs reactions in several European families.

But the phenotype S−s−U− has been found outside people of African extraction: Moores[205] describes four such sibs in an Indian family living in Natal. There was no known consanguinity between the parents. There was no sign in the family, serological or physical, of African admixture. No further example of the phenotype was found in testing a further 1,000 Natal Indian blood donors.

As would be expected, the phenotype U− is more frequent in Africans than in American Negroes. The record is still held by the Congo Pygmies: Fraser, Giblett and Motulsky[193] found 35% of 126 samples to be U−. At the other extreme, Lowe and Moores[280] found no example in 1,000 Bantu.

The antigen U is present in neutrophil leucocytes but M, N, S and s are not (Marsh *et al.*[276] 1974).

FURTHER VERSATILITY OF THE SYSTEM

The main skeleton of the MNSs system, the antigens M, N, S, s and the phenotype S^u, having been outlined there remains a rather bewildering crop of exostoses to be dealt with. A collection of jig-saw pieces of serological knowledge is piling up and we guess that chemical knowledge of the system will have to be very far advanced before most of the pieces are seen to fall into any grand pattern. But the pieces taken by themselves are interesting serologically and genetically and are sometimes of practical use.

The antigen M^g

This antigen, representing an allele of M and N, which was discovered in Boston by Allen, Corcoran, Kenton and Breare[87] (1958), is of interest out of all proportion to its frequency which seems to be one of the lowest (outside Switzerland and Sicily) of all the known blood group antigens. The M^g propositus was a patient and by chance the serum of his proposed donor contained anti-M^g. Part of the family of the patient is given in Figure 7. The antigen M^g does not react with anti-M or anti-N.

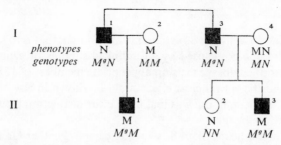

Fig. 7. The discovery of M^g, a rare allele of M and N: the antigen M^g does not react with anti-M or with anti-N but it does react with anti-M^g. Black = antigen M^g present, white = M^g absent. (Part of the pedigree from Allen, Corcoran, Kenton and Breare[87] 1958.)

Blood representing the genotype $M^g M$ if tested with only anti-M and anti-N gives the reaction of M, but it gives only the single dose reaction when tested against titrations of anti-M sera. Similarly, blood representing $M^g N$ tested only with anti-M and anti-N appears to be N, but gives only a single dose reaction against anti-N.

In Figure 7 it is of interest to note that the use alone of anti-M and anti-N would have appeared to exclude I-1 from being the father of II-1, and to exclude I-3 from being the father of II-3. Anti-M^g, on the other hand, proves that the fathers of these two children are indeed the fathers—for they all have an extremely rare antigen.

The antigen M^g is certainly rare in the United States and in England. Up to 1965 the Blood Grouping Laboratory in Boston had tested approximately 44,000 random people and Cleghorn, up to 1964, had tested 61,128 English donors (personal communications cited by Metaxas et al.[140]) without finding a single example of the antigen.

But in 1961 Metaxas and his colleagues[132] struck gold in Switzerland and have since opened up a mine of M^g there. This made possible very thorough studies[132,140,141,199] of the frequency and inheritance of M^g and of certain serological aspects. The frequency of the antigen M^g in Switzerland[132, 140] was found to be 10 in 6,530 tests or 0·153%. Twenty-one families of the mating type $M^g+ \times M^g-$, with 51 children, confirmed the original view that M^g is an allele of M and N. In all these families, as in the original Boston family, the gene complex was $M^g s$, and the s antigen appeared normal. A second Boston family[142], again not random but selected by cross-matching difficulty, also showed the alignment $M^g s$.

Metaxas and his colleagues[140] even found a family in which both parents had M^g: husband $M^g s/Ns$, wife $M^g s/MS$. The only child was MS/Ns, and, on arrival[141], the eagerly awaited second child fulfilled all hopes by being homozygous for M^g, $M^g s/M^g s$: the first person, out of hundreds of thousands tested, to be M–N–; or very nearly M–N–, for Metaxas-Bühler and her colleagues[141] found that $M^g M^g$, like MM, does result in a little detectable N antigen. In fact M^g results in a little more N than does M.

The first family in which M^g was shown to be aligned with S was found by Brocteur[206] in Belgium; the family was Sicilian. Brocteur then began a systematic search and by 1972 had tested close to 43,000 samples including approximately 6,300 from Italian immigrants, of whom 1,889 were estimated to be of Sicilian origin[207]: four more examples of M^g were found, all from immigrants, one from the mainland of Italy, with the alignment $M^g s$ and three, not known to be related to each other, from Sicily—all three with the alignment $M^g S$. It looks as if the antigen M^g is as frequent in Sicily as in Switzerland and, within the narrow limit of present knowledge, that the alignment $M^g S$ is diagnostic of Sicilian extraction.

No example of M^g was found in 320 Copper Eskimos[13] nor in 1,350 citizens of Prague[143], nor in 433 Thais[144]. Two examples of M^g were found in Bombay[208] in a total of just over 9,000 samples: the alignment was $M^g s$ in one family but undisclosed in the other.

Further interest in the M^g condition was stimulated in 1969 when Nordling et al.[209] found it to be associated with certain physicochemical changes to the red cell surface. This aspect will be dealt with in the chapter on En (page 470).

M^k, an allele producing no M,N,S or s antigen

Metaxas and Metaxas-Bühler[149] in 1964 made an observation of considerable interest. They described a Swiss family in which three members had an allele which produced no M or N antigen nor M^g antigen. The family did not show whether the new allele, M^k, produced any S or s antigen. The propositus was recognized when her cells though apparently N gave a single dose with anti-N: later one of her three children was found to be M.

Henningsen[150] then found a Danish family in which the same allele was segregating: it produced the same effect, no M or N: but the family groups fortunately gave more information and made clear that the new allele produced no S or s either. The family illustrates remarkably well the effect the allele can have on a pedigree: in no less than three successive generations the established MNSs groups appear to exclude the maternity of children, five in all. (An M S−s+ grand-mother has an N S−s+ daughter married to an M S+s+ man and they have an M S+s− and two M S−s+ daughters, one of whom has an N S−s+ child.)

Seven more M^k families have since been reported: two of them, one Swedish[151] and one Chinese[210], found by apparent discrepancies in family MNSs groups, and five of them, all Swiss-Germans, found by dosage mesaurements[199,211]. Analysis of these hard-won families, by Metaxas and his colleagues[211], established the dominance of the M^k character.

The only estimate of the frequency of the gene M^k is to be found in the admir-able paper by Metaxas, Metaxas-Bühler and Edwards[199]: it is 0·00064, based on tests of 3,895 Swiss blood donors. The importance of the condition is out of all proportion to its frequency.

The M^k allele results in no M, N, S or s antigens. At first it was thought to pro-duce an M^k antigen (page 125) but more recent work by Nordling et al.[209], dis-cussed in the En chapter (page 463), has shown that what appeared to be an antigen is much more likely a reflection of the marked shortage of sialic acid on the surface of the cells of M^k heterozygotes.

As one of us wrote[212] 'Incidentally M^k may not exactly be a true allele of MNSs: its relationship might be that of an operator gene at the complex locus which has switched off all activity at the adjacent MN and Ss structural sites.' And, along the same lines, Metaxas, Metaxas-Bühler and Romanski[211] suggest that M^k may be 'an amorph whose presence at the MNSs locus leaves unconverted a basic substance from which the MNSs antigens normally arise' and liken it to the amorphic type of Rh_{null} (page 220) and the K_0 condition (page 292).

Weak M and N antigens associated with direct positive antiglobulin reaction

The surprising observation that the direct positive antiglobulin reaction could be an inherited character was made first by Jakobowicz, Bryce and Simmons[19,20]. The reaction was inherited in a family together with a variant of M antigen. (A second child with the two conditions was born after the publications cited[21].) Two further families with an inherited direct antiglobulin reaction, this time travelling with a weak N variant, were reported by Jensen and Freiesleben[136] and by Jeannet, Metaxas-Bühler and Tobler[137,138]. A fourth family was found by Funfhausen and Velhagen (personal communication, 1970): the cells of a mother and son gave a direct positive antiglobulin reaction but gave normal M reactions. This subject will be returned to in the chapter on En (page 472) where blood group antigens having special effects on the red cell membrane are collected.

A qualitative variant of M had been described as early as 1938 by Friedenreich and Lauridsen[18]. In 1935 a weak N antigen had been found by Crome[14], and another by Friedenreich[15] who named it N_2 having shown that it was inherited as an allele of M and N. (Other references to N_2: 16, 8, 17.) It is not easy to place these earlier M and N variants in the present range defined by a greater choice of group-ing reagents.

The antigen M_1, a subdivision of M

There is a component of some human anti-M sera called anti-M_1 (see page 123) which divides the M antigen into two groups in a qualitative way, not merely into stronger M or weaker M (Jack, Tippett, Noades, Sanger and Race[98]). The antigen which reacts is called M_1 and is a somewhat graded character; it is commoner in Negroes than in Whites.

The original estimate of M_1 frequencies in Whites and American Negroes was confirmed by tests on much larger series (Francis and Hatcher[115], Issitt, Haber and Allen[147], Le Roux and Shapiro[213]) and the frequency in Bantu[213] was found to be twice as high as that in American Negroes. Phenotype frequencies are given in Table 14 and gene frequencies for American Negroes in Table 13 (page 103). The proportion of M genes that are M_1 is, in Whites 3%, in American Negroes 26% and in Bantu 50%.

Table 14. Summary of potentially useful polymorphisms within the main MNSsS^u system: those known to distinguish 2% or more of a population

Phenotype	Whites	American Negroes	Certain Africans	Certain Asiatics
M_1+	4%	24%	47%	
Tm+ Sj+	2%	4%		
Tm+ Sj−	24%	28%		
Hu+	<1%	7%	22%	
He+	<1%	3%	3 to 14%	
Mi.III (Mur+)	<1%	<1%		5 to 10%
St(a+)	<1%			6%

The alignment of M_1 with S, s or S^u does not differ from that of the rest of M genes[145,115,147]. We found the N antigen to be, on the average, weaker in M_1N than in other negro MN: this was shown by human, rabbit and plant anti-N alike. Le Roux and Shapiro[213] found the average strength of M_1 higher in Bantu than in Whites.

From the time of its recognition in 1965 all the work on M_1 was done with anti-sera from N people and they contained anti-M+anti-M_1. It was hoped[204] that if an anti-M_1 made by an MN person, and presumably therefore free from anti-M, were to be found it would give a clearer definition of M_1. Such an antiserum has recently been detected by Giles and Howell[275] in a white British patient. From tests on 280 negro people it was calculated that 16·7% of their M genes were M_1, considerably lower than the earlier estimate, and very likely nearer the truth. As the authors wrote, 'it is possible that the difference may be reflecting the unknown quantitative effect of the anti-M component in anti-M+M_1 sera'.

It is a great pity that this apparently very hopeful polymorphism has not to our knowledge been consolidated by family tests. Not until this has been done can the implications of the exceptional inheritance in the family reported by Richmond and Innella[214] be properly appreciated.

The antigens Tm and Sj

In 1965, Issitt, Haber and Allen[146] reported an antibody, anti-Tm, which reacted with the cells of about 20 % of white people and about 30 % of New York Negroes: most positive reactors possessed N. The Tm antigen was found to be very variable in strength. Another antibody, called anti-Sj was later separated[147] from the same serum: all Sj+ people, about 2 % of Whites and 4 % of Negroes, have so far been Tm+.

In an important survey Issitt and his collaborators[147] tested the blood of 500 Whites and 500 American Negroes with a wide range of antisera belonging to the MNSs system, anti-Tm and anti-Sj included (for some approximate phenotype frequencies see Table 14). The results were put to the computer by Morton and Miki[200] and frequencies for 28 gene complexes emerged, from which may be extracted the following:

	Whites	Negroes
genes producing Tm and Sj	0·0111	0·0192
genes producing Tm but not Sj	0·1229	0·1525
genes producing neither Tm nor Sj	0·8660	0·8283

Tm and Sj, therefore, promised really useful genetical applications; but, as far as we know, only two informative families have been tested[147], in one *Tm* was travelling with *NS* and in the other with *Ns*. The reasons for this shortage of genetic information are the same as those noted for M_1. Issitt *et al.*[147] report that the antigens Tm and Sj tend to be labile on storage and that this applies also to anti-Tm.

The antigens Hu and He

Hu was the first antigen to be found related to M and N, the first of a very long procession. In 1934 Landsteiner, Strutton and Chase[57] injected several rabbits with the blood of a Negro, Mr Hunter. One of the rabbits responded by making an antibody to an antigen, Hu, present in about 7 % of American Negroes[8] and about 22 % of West Africans[59]. It occurs, but is rare, in Europeans. The association of the antigen with the MN system was disclosed by the early finding that all the blood samples giving 'distinct, positive reactions' belonged to group N or MN.

Issitt *et al.*[147] noticed that Hu+ people were too often Tm+. In their American Negro series of 500 they found 36 Hu+, a frequency of 7·2 % which agrees very well with the 7 % of the earlier work. Though the anti-Hu sera we have worked with never gave reliable results it is obvious that given the right conditions a series of random samples can be properly grouped. Hu seems to be like M_1 and Tm in that the antigen has never proved to be a useful genetic marker.

Another negro antigen, He, identified by Ikin and Mourant[58] has proved to be a useful genetic marker as well as giving much anthropological information. The antibody, anti-He, was present in a rabbit anti-M serum. It was later made intentionally by injecting rabbits with the blood of a positive Nigerian, Mr Henshaw (Chalmers, Ikin and Mourant[59]). The antigen He was found in 38 (2·7%) of 1,428 West Africans: it was not found in 1,500 Whites. The antigen was shown to belong to the MNSs system when most of the positives were found to have the antigens N and S as well, the coincidence of the three antigens being highly significant.

Subsequent work has shown the antigen He to be associated in New York Negroes[99] (1,000 tested, 3·2% positive) predominantly with *NS*, in Papua[60] with *Ns*, in Congo Negroes[60] with *MS*, in the Hottentots[61] with *MS*, and in 'Cape Coloureds'[62] with *Ms*. Shapiro[62] tested 4,000 South African Bantu and found that the distribution of He was random in respect of MNSs as did Issitt *et al.*[147] in testing 500 American Negroes (2·0% positive). In testing 4,510 Milwaukee Negroes, Greenwalt[97] found 139 (3·08%) He positive.

Chalmers, Ikin and Mourant[59] tested some Nigerian families possessing the antigens Hu or He and the results suggested that both antigens were Mendelian characters, but did not show whether the antigens were allelic to each other or not.

A fine study of the inheritance of He was made by Shapiro[62] who gives details of seven very large families. In different families the antigen is seen segregating with *Ms*, with *Ns* and with *MS*. No doubt is left that the gene *He* is closely, if not absolutely, linked to the *MNSs* genes.

Rosenfield, Haber, Schroeder and Ballard[100] report a negro family in which one gene complex is apparently transmitting the antigens N, S, Hu *and* He: it all depends on the legitimacy of one child in a sibship which contains one child known to be illegitimate. If this finding be confirmed it means that Hu and He are not 'allelic' antigens. The anti-Hu was made by injecting rabbits with the blood of Mr Hunter some 25 years after he had given blood to Landsteiner, Strutton and Chase.

Wiener and Rosenfield[133] describe a rabbit anti-M which also reacts with N, He+ cells: from the results of absorption and elution tests they postulate the existence of M^e, a 'factor' common to M and He.

The Miltenberger series of antigens

The beginning of this complicated story was the recognition in 1954 by van der Hart, Bosman and van Loghem[56] that Vw, an antigen of low incidence which was being investigated, was closely or absolutely linked to the *MNSs* locus (Figure 8). Subsequently Vw was realized to be related to two low incidence antigens previously reported but not seen to belong to the MNSs system—Gr (Graydon[102]) and Mi[a] (Levine, Stock, Kuhmichel and Bronikovsky[55]). Related but not identical antisera and antigens were found and the subject was in confusion

5

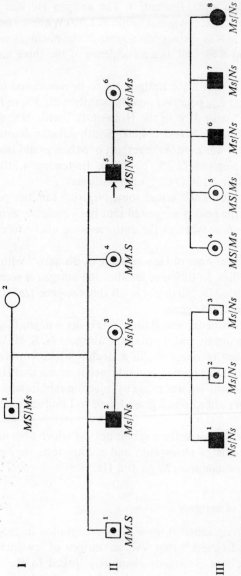

Fig. 8. A Dutch family showing that the gene for the antigen Vw is linked to the *MNSs* genes. (After van der Hart, Bosman and van Loghem[56].) Black = presence of the antigen Vw; dot = its absence; arrow = propositus. I-2 is dead, but her children show that she must have had *Ns*; this gene complex has been inherited by II-2, II-5, III-1, III-6, III-7 and III-8 and these are the only members of the family who have received the gene *Vw*, which must also have come from I-2 since the antigen Vw is a dominant character and I-1 lacks it. Antisera used: anti-Vw, anti-M, anti-N, anti-S and (on most of the samples) anti-s.

for some years until, in 1966, Cleghorn[154] decided that something should be done to bring it to order.

Cleghorn's approach was to collect samples of blood from the original cases and to test the serum and cells against a range of cells and sera known to be involved in what he called the sub-system. The results were described in terms of the donors' names rather than in names given to the antibodies thought to be present.

Cleghorn called the sub-system 'Miltenberger' because the serum of Mrs Miltenberger contained the first example of the antibody now known to be the most comprehensive in its reactions. He began his demolition and reconstruction work thus: 'I. Four different distinctive type-sera have been identified in women immunized by Miltenberger-positive pregnancy: (i) Verweyst[56] (ii) Miltenberger[55] (iii) Murrell[103] (iv) Hill[155]'; he went on to list the four types of cell samples then recognized, using the earliest propositi as examples. This is illustrated in Table 15 together with the addition of a fifth class of cells. Class V cells were first found in an English family described by Crossland et al.[215] in 1970.

In Table 15 it can be seen that the antigens of Classes I–IV are rare in Whites, though Metaxas (personal communication, 1973) found Class I to be more frequent in the Grisons, S.E. Switzerland (22, or 1·43%, of 1,541 donors) than in Zürich (4, or 0·09%, of 4,418 donors). Class V must be rare in England for Cleghorn had found none in his tests on over 50,000 donors. However, Metaxas and Metaxas-Bühler[216] found 3 in only 6,202 Swiss donors and Metaxas et al.[217] found 2 more in Swedish affiliation cases.

Class III has a remarkably high frequency in Asiatics. Amongst 2,500 Thai blood donors Chandanayingyong and Bejchandre[218] found 241 to be Class III (9·6%); of 268 American Chinese on the eastern coast[195] and 211 of the Los Angeles area[274] 5% were Mur+. Thus the antigen is potentially a good genetic tool in parts of Asia. Earlier anthropological work on the Miltenberger system disclosed no positive amongst Papuans[102], Australian aborigines[102], Japanese[106,219], Copper Eskimos[13], Alaskan Eskimos and Indians[107]. Two positives were found in 609 American Negroes[104] and, subsequently, twenty in one large Japanese family[158] ascertained through the sole positive found in testing 3,350 unrelated Japanese people with the type (ii) serum. One positive was found in 324 Seneca Indians[220] and one in many thousand Indians in Middle and South America[221].

The inheritance of the cell classes and the alignment of the corresponding genes with MS, Ms, NS or Ns has been well worked out. References to these family investigations are given in the last column of Table 15.

The MNSs genes when aligned with one of the Miltenberger series may express themselves normally or they may not; when there is some abnormal reaction it involves only the cis alignment. Here we meet the need for gene symbols for the series: Metaxas et al.[217] suggest that when the alignment is known the gene complexes may be written, for example, $Ms^{Mi.III}$, $Ns^{Mi.V}$ etc., which seems a good idea. (For phenotype symbols they suggest Mi.I, Mi.II etc.)

Table 15. The Miltenberger complex of antigens. (Following Cleghorn[154], 1966)

Class	Early propositi	Ver-weyst (i)	Milten-berger (ii)	Murrell (iii)	Hill (iv)	Hut (v)	Approximate frequency in random Whites	Alignment, in decreasing order of frequency (in Whites)	References to family studies (all races)
I	Dr Graydon[102] Mr Miltenberger[55] Mr Verweyst[56]	+	+	−	−	−	1 in 1,755 (52,635 tested)	*Ns, NS, Ms, MS*	56, 108, 65, 101 103, 156, 154
II	Mr Hutchinson[64,65]	−	+	−	−	+	1 in 1,552 (32,591 tested)	*MS, Ns, Ms*	65, 103, 157, 158
III	Mr Murrell[103]	−	+	+	+	+	1 in 10,020 (50,101 tested)	*Ns, Ms*	103, 154, 191, 210
IV	Mr Hopper[154]	−	+	+	−	+	1 in 50,101 (50,101 tested)	*NS*	154
V	Mrs R.[215]	−	−	−	+	−	see text	*Ns, Ms*	215, 217

Notes about the four types of antisera:

(i) Verweyst, usually called anti-Vw, has caused haemoylytic disease of the newborn stimulated by the cells of class I[56]; it is common in the serum of patients with acquired haemolytic anaemia and is found in the serum of approximately 1% of random healthy white people (see page 126). Cleghorn[154] suggests the notation anti-Gr.

(ii) Miltenberger, usually called anti-Mi^a, has caused haemolytic disease stimulated by cells of class I or class II[154]; it is common in the serum of patients with acquired haemolytic anaemia but has not yet been found in the serum of random healthy people. These antisera are of variable complexity, see Cleghorn[154] and Mohn and Macvie[194].

(iii) Murrell, once called anti-Mu, now called anti-Mur (because Mu was later used for another purpose). Several examples have now been found, the first caused haemolytic disease of the newborn.

(iv) Hill, called anti-Hil, the only known example[154,155] caused haemolytic disease of the newborn.

(v) Anti-Hut, originally separated from a class ii serum, Hutchinson, by absorption with class I cells[154,65,194], but straight examples exist which have caused haemolytic disease of the newborn[263,264]. (Often mistaken for anti-Mur when class II cells are not available for testing.)

The frequencies in classes I and II are those given in our last edition, the majority from Cleghorn[103], but some from other sources[55,56,65,101,102,104,105]; those for classes III and IV are Cleghorn's for South London.

Classes I and II (Mi.I and Mi.II). No defective M, N, S or s reactions have been reported.

Class III (Mi.III). In a Chinese family with the alignment $Ms^{Mi.III}$ Cleghorn[154] observed that the resulting s antigen did not react with all anti-s sera and that there was more N antigen than a normal M gene usually lets through. $Ms^{Mi.III}$ had exactly the same effect in a large Canadian family of Portugese-Indian descent[191] and in a large Chinese family in America[210].

In a Philippino family, where $Ms^{Mi.III}$ stimulated anti-Mur, which caused haemolytic disease of the newborn, the groups of the father's family showed that he and one of his sisters were homozygous $Ms^{Mi.III}/Ms^{Mi.III}$: both their parents were $Ms^{Mi.III}/Ns$ and some sibs were $Ms^{Mi.III}/Ns$ and others Ns/Ns. The anti-Mur did not show a convincing dosage effect[267].

Mi.III antigen has caused haemolytic disease due to anti-Mur (immunizing antigen $Ns^{Mi.III}$, mother Ms/Ns in one family[103], immunizing antigen $Ms^{Mi.III}$, mother MS/Ms in another[267]) and to anti-Hut (immunizing antigen $Ms^{Mi.III}$, mother Ms/Ms in one family[263]).

Class IV (Mi.IV). In the only family tested[154] the alignment was $Ns^{Mi.IV}$ and the S antigen was peculiar in reacting with some but not all anti-S sera.

Class V (Mi.V). Crossland et al.[215] noted in their original family, in which the alignment was $Ns^{Mi.V}$, that the N antigen was weakly expressed. This was confirmed when Metaxas et al.[217] found three families with the same alignment, and they further observed that the s reactions were exaggerated. The same workers found one family with the alignment $Ms^{Mi.V}$ and here the M antigen was depressed and, again, the s antigen exalted. It was further recorded[216] that Mi.V cells showed some of the signs of a surface change (page 471) like En and M^k and M^g.

As a further contribution to this very involved subject Cleghorn[103] recorded a family (later retested and confirmed) in which a daughter (MS/Ns) and her child (MS/Ms) have Mi.I, the alignment being $MS^{Mi.I}$, but neither the daughter's father (MS/MS) nor her mother (Ns/Ns) have any Miltenberger antigen. Very extensive tests (red cell groups, serum groups and biochemical markers) failed to give any evidence of illegitimacy. Cleghorn was left wondering whether Mi.I in this family cannot be expressed in the genotype MS/MS; however, it was pointed out that no example of the antigen was found in testing many relatives of the father, so his possible carrier state could not be demonstrated.

The antigen M^v

In 1966 Gershowitz and Fried[152] told a fascinating story of five years' work with a serum, 'anti-M^v', which behaved like anti-N but declared its special quality by reacting with 1 in about 400 M samples from white people. The antibody was evidently the result of immunization of an MM woman by an MM^v foetus. The anti-N and anti-M^v components in the serum could not be separated, but the admirable analysis achieved in spite of this difficulty was shown to have been perfectly correct when, in 1970, anti-M^v without the anti-N component was

Table 16. 'Satellite' antigens attendant on the MNSs system

Antigen	Reference	Incidence in unrelated people	Alignment clearly with
Vr (Verdegaal)	v.d. Hart et al.[109], 1958	3 in 1,200 Dutch	Ms in 3 families
Ri^a (Ridley)	Cleghorn[159], 1962	3 in 17,013 English	MS in 1 family
St^a (Stones)	Cleghorn[159], 1962	20 in 17,013 English (2 related)	Ns in 9 families NS in 2 families Ms in 1 family Ms or MS in 1 family
St^a (Stones)	Madden et al.[160], 1964	14 in 220 Japanese 6 in 420 Chinese 0 in 386 Mexicans	
St^a (Stones)	Metaxas, pers. comm., 1973	5 in 1,435 Swiss (Zürich)	
Mt^a (Martin)	Swanson and Matson[161], 1962	28 in 11,907 Whites	Ns in 1 family
Mt^a (Martin)	Konugres et al.[162], 1965		Ns in 2 families
Mt^a (Martin)	Chandanayingyong et al.[144], 1967	3 in 318 Thais	
Mt^a (Martin)	Metaxas, pers. comm., 1973	6 in 1,435 Swiss (Zürich)	
Cl^a (Caldwell)	Wallace and Izatt[163], 1963	0 in 11,000 Scottish	Ms in 2 families
Cl^a (Caldwell)	Metaxas, pers. comm., 1973	0 in 1,541 Swiss (Grisons)	
Ny^a (Nyberg)	Ørjasaeter et al.[164,165], 1964	10 in 5,931 Norwegians	Ns in 12 families
Ny^a (Nyberg)	Cleghorn, 1964, pers. comm. to Nakajima et al.[223]	0 in 800 British 0 in 300 'coloured'	
Ny^a (Nyberg)	Matson, 1964, pers. comm. to Nakajima et al.[223]	0 in 210 American Indians	
Ny^a (Nyberg)	Ørjasaeter, 1966, pers. comm. to Nakajima et al.[223]	0 in >1,000 Boston Whites 0 in 350 Boston Negroes	
Ny^a (Nyberg)	Nakajima et al.[223], 1967	0 in 3,281 Japanese 0 in 1,032 Chinese 0 in 1,041 Ryukyuans 0 in 1,236 Taiwan aborigines	
Ny^a (Nyberg)	Pineda and Taswell[224], 1969	0 in 7,400 S.E. Minnesotans	

Table 16—continued

Ny^a (Nyberg)	Metaxas, pers. comm., 1973	1 in 1,541 Swiss (Grisons) 0 in 7,994 Swiss (Zürich)	Ns in 1 family
Ny^a (Nyberg)	Schimmack et al.[225], 1971	0 in 20,000 Germans	
Ny^a (Nyberg)	Kornstad et al.[226], 1971	8 in 3,746 Norwegians 0 in 305 Lapps	Ns in 7 families
M^v	Gershowitz and Fried[152], 1966	See page 113	Ms in 10 kindred MS in 2 kindred
M^v	Crossland et al.[215], 1970	14 in 2,371 English	Ms in 4 families
Sul	Konugres and Winter[166], 1967	0 in 4,935 many races	Ns in 1 family
Sul	Metaxas, pers. comm., 1973	0 in 6,456 Swiss (Zürich)	
Far	Cregut et al.[227,228], 1968, 1974	0 in 14,273 French	Ns in 1 family

found by Crossland, Pepper, Giles and Ikin[215] in, of all places, a supposedly inert control AB serum. The original serum can now be thought of as anti-M^{v}N.

Crossland *et al.*[215] found that 14 (0·6%) of 2,371 English donors in Leeds were M^v positive: the identity of the M^v in all 14 donors was confirmed by absorption tests using American M^v control cells. An estimate of the M^v gene frequency in English people is therefore 0·0030, very close to the original estimate of 0·0025 for American Whites[152].

In a genetic investigation on a magnificent scale Gershowitz and Fried[152] showed that M^v was, as expected, a dominant character and they found the gene M^v in alignment with S and with s. When aligned with s the resulting s antigen was weaker than normal; and this was confirmed in the four English families tested[215] in all of which the alignment was $M^v s$.

The particular interest of M^v is that in some respects it is like M, in others like N. M^v produces an antigen which behaves like M in being agglutinated by anti-M but not by anti-N sera: however, an $M^v M$ foetus stimulated an antibody in a MM mother which behaved like anti-N except that it also reacted with the rare $M^v M$ cells (anti-M^{v}N). M^v is more like N in the frequency of its alignment with s and S (Table 16).

The antigens Vr, Ri^a, St^a, Mt^a, Cl^a, Ny^a, Sul and Far

All these antigens are recognized by specific antibodies and are not yet known to be perplexingly interrelated like those of the Miltenberger series. We found it convenient to refer to them as satellite antigens, though doubt whether a special name is justified. They are all dominant characters. With one exception nothing peculiar has so far been suspected of the M, N, S or s antigens with which they segregate. The exception is St^a: it may have an effect on an M antigen with which it travels, because 2 odd M types, called M^z and M^r, were both found to be St(a+)[222]. This can hardly be a coincidence because of the rarity of St^a, especially in the company of M.

St^a is further set apart[216] from this group of antigens because its presence is accompanied by detectable changes to the cell surface, like M^k, M^g and Mi.V (see page 471).

The main facts about this group of antigens, together with those for M^v, are collected in Table 16. It can be seen that St^a is potentially a useful genetic tool in Japan.

M^c, M^r, M^z, N$_2$, M^a, N^a

None of these phenotypes has a specific antibody: they were distinguished by their unusual reactions with anti-M or anti-N or both.

M^c

In 1953, Dunsford, Ikin and Mourant[22] described an antigen which reacted with the majority of anti-M and the minority of anti-N rabbit sera: it was called M^c and considered to be intermediate between M and N; it was found in three members of an English family. By distributing samples of M^c red cells the Sheffield Blood Transfusion Service has with the help of this family made possible, for over 20 years, the classification of anti-M and anti-N reagents into reactors or non-reactors with M^c, and also the distinction from M^c of later variants.

Metaxas and his colleagues[222] found two more M^c propositi, one of French Basque and one of German origin and, later but unpublished, a further two, one French and one Italian: in three of these propositi the alignment is, as in the original family, $M^c s$, but in the German it is $M^c S$.

It can hardly be a coincidence, considering the relative infrequency of M_1 in Whites, that the original[204] and the four subsequent $M^c N$ propositi tested by Dr Metaxas are all M_1 positive. However, M^c is not the same as M_1, for $M_1 N$ cells can react well with anti-M sera which fail to react with M^c cells.

Metaxas and his colleagues[222] point out that M^c, unlike other M alleles, though producing some N antigen when measured by rabbit and human reagents, produces none when measured by *Vicia graminae* extract: this is true of all $M^c M$ samples they have since tested and should be remembered when considering 'N_{VG}' as a precursor of N (page 121).

M^r and M^z

Both these variants are very rare; they were found by Metaxas, Metaxas-Bühler and Ikin[222] (1968) amongst donors giving unexpected M or N dosage reactions.

M^z results in an antigen which, like M^c, reacts with a majority of anti-M and a minority of anti-N sera, but the reactions do not coincide. M^z further distinguishes itself from M^c by not reacting with anti-M_1 and by reacting with anti-M'. In the only known family the alignment is $M^z s$.

M^r also results in an antigen which reacts with most anti-M and some anti-N sera, but it reacts with neither anti-M_1 nor anti-M'. M^r has been found in the alignment $M^r s$ and $M^r S$.

Both M^z and M^r cells are St(a+) and both, like M^g etc., have some alteration of the cell surface (page 471). Given the special antisera the three similar conditions may be distinguished thus:

$$M^c \text{ cells are } M_1+, M'-, St(a-)$$
$$M^z \text{ cells are } M_1-, M'+, St(a+)$$
$$M^r \text{ cells are } M_1-, M'-, St(a+)$$

Dr and Mrs Metaxas tell us that all further samples they have tested since 1968 involving the $M.St^a$ complex are M^r and the original M^z family remains the only exception. They emphasize a striking feature common to M^r and M^z is that they both, especially M^r, 'let through' a lot more N antigen than does normal M; the M produced by M^r is almost normal while that produced by M^z is somewhat depressed.

5*

N_2

Metaxas and his colleagues in their great series[222] came across two propositi and their families with simple uncomplicated weak N antigens. The gene symbol N_2 was justifiably used, though it should be distinguished from the weak N associated with a direct positive antiglobulin reaction (page 472) which is sometimes called N_2.

M^a

Konugres, Brown and Corcoran[148] found anti-M in the serum of a child of group MN, whose paternity was in dispute; this anti-M did not react with the child's own cells which evidently lacked some facet of the normal M antigen. A parallel was drawn with the anti-D present in the serum of some people who have the antigen D. The child's antigen was denoted M^a and her antibody anti-M^A.

A similar case was reported by Schmidt and Taswell[229], again an MN person with anti-M in his serum: the anti-M did not react with his own cells, nor with the cells of those of his children who had inherited his M (his wife was N). Samples were no longer available from the child described by Konugres *et al.* so it could not be said whether the same piece of M was missing in the two cases. Howard and Picoff[230] found another example of non-auto anti-M in a MN patient.

N^a

In two healthy Melanesian blood donors Booth[231] found an anti-N, as proved by the cells of white people, which failed to agglutinate between 10% and 30% of *NN* Melanesians of different ethnic groups. The antiserum was called anti-N^A, and N cells which reacted positively, N^A, and negatively, N^a. The testing of Melanesian families[232] showed N^A to be dominant over N^a. The proportion of N genes which were N^A varied in different New Guinea populations from more than half to less than half.

Ss variants

S^u, the allele that produces neither S nor s antigen, has been described above; and so has M^k, perhaps an operator gene, which prevents the expression of the M, N, S and s antigens. We have also recorded how several of the genes responsible for the Miltenberger series of antigens can affect the expression of the S or s antigens.

S_2, on the other hand, so far appears to be a straightforward allele of S and s: it produces a weak S antigen and there was no evidence that the difference was qualitative. The antigen was found in 12 members of a white family (Hurd, Jacox, Swisher, Cleghorn, Carlin and Allen[153]). The alignment in this family was MS_2 and the resulting M antigen appeared normal.

Booth[233] in a most pregnant paper describes an antigen Z associated with S and s. Only one example of anti-Z has been found, 'naturally occurring' in the serum of a Papuan male blood donor. Z was found to be less common in Melanesians (36%) than in Europeans (61%). Among 263 Europeans Booth found S+Z+ 135, S+Z− 1, S−Z+ 25, S−Z− 102. The phenotype S+Z− is more common in Melanesians, 26 in 890. Tests on 42 Melanesian families confirmed the association with S, for Z was travelling with S in all the informative families. No doubt by the time this edition is printed more will be known about this potentially very useful antibody. At present, it seems to us that there is nothing to prove that anti-Z is not an anti-S which is recognizing a variant of S in Melanesians together with unseparable[233] anti-Tm or some other antibody which reacts with about 20% of European samples.

OTHER NOTES ABOUT THE MNSs SYSTEM

Dosage effects

The dosage effect of the *MN* genes was observed soon after their discovery. In 1927 Landsteiner and Levine[2] wrote that 'the reactions for N seem to be strong in most cases where M is absent'. This was a happy choice of words: it means that two *N* genes in the classical sense make more detectable N antigen than does one; but it is also a true statement if we think of N, as many now do, as a background substance, made by unknown genes, which *M* converts into M antigen and which *m* (our *N*) lets through unconverted.

The dosage effect can be dramatic: it was particularly well demonstrated by a horse anti-M serum sent to us by Dr Levine: in titrations against 18 M samples and 32 MN samples (all taken on the same day) we found that 17 of the M scored between 30 and 32, one M scored 23 and all MN scored between 13 and 21. This serum contained no anti-M_1 component. Some sera which are very sensitive to the M_1 distinction have failed to detect M dosage. A strong reaction does not always indicate a quantitative effect: during this quantitative work we found one out of 7 N samples from Whites to give outstandingly strong reactions with all anti-N sera, even with one that showed no dosage effect.

The average dosage effect of the *S* gene is definite[30, 51] but has not yet proved of great diagnostic use in individual cases.

The dosage effect of the *s* gene was observed by Levine and his collaborators[28]. In our experience the effect is so marked with some sera that it is usually possible from an anti-s result to forecast correctly the reaction of the sample with anti-S.

Dosage measurements with anti-M, -N, -S, -s have been very useful in the unravelling of most of the newer alleles of the system, particularly M^g and M^k. With the finding of the, so far, unique $M^g M^g$ homozygote, Metaxas-Bühler and her colleagues[141] were able to show that three out of six anti-M^g sera gave a striking dosage effect.

Dosing anti-M and anti-N sera were used to great effect in detecting possible variants of MNSs, candidates for further investigation (Metaxas et al.[222], 1968).

Lawler and her colleagues[167] point out some of the difficulties facing attempts to use MNSs dosage measurements in various trisomies in the hope of assigning the locus to a particular autosome.

Development of the antigens

The antigens M and N are well developed in the newborn and are constant throughout life (Schiff and Boyd[52]). Moureau[53] grouped, without difficulty, 17 foetuses of various ages, the youngest being nine weeks.

The antigen S is well developed at birth, and we found it in three foetuses (two '17 weeks' and one '12 weeks'). Indeed, Lawler, Marshall and Shatwell[167] found MN cord cells to be somewhat stronger in M than adult cells, and Ss cord cells to be definitely stronger in S than adult Ss cells.

We find s well developed in cord samples and Speiser[111] found it in a 27 mm. foetus.

The antigen U is certainly developed at birth for it has caused haemolytic disease of the newborn[168]. We do not know about the development of the weaker U reaction of the rare S−s−U+ Negroes.

The rare antigen M^g is now known to be well developed at birth[141] and so are Mt^a, Cl^a, Ny^a, Far and the antigens of the Miltenberger series. The antigen Tm, on the contrary, is not well developed at birth[147].

Offspring from the mating MN × MN

During thirty years much has been written about an excess of MN children from the mating MN×MN to be found in many reports. In the 5th edition of this book we gave powerful reasons for agreeing with the opinion of Wiener[8] that the apparent excess is due to grouping errors. We think the subject is better forgotten: however, papers in which it is at least mentioned are to be found under the following reference numbers: 7, 8, 10, 11, 36, 54, 169 and 234.

Reaction of anti-N with M cells

In 1928 Landsteiner and Levine described how rabbit anti-N sera can be deprived of almost all antibody by absorption with M cells though antibody is not removed from anti-M sera by absorption with N cells. The anti-N of *Vicia graminea* behaves like the rabbit anti-N (Levine, Ottensooser, Celano and Pollitzer[78], 1955). Human anti-N also behave like rabbit anti-N (Hirsch, Moores, Sanger and Race[77], 1957). The latter authors found that the 'cross-reaction' between M and anti-N was increased by lowering the temperature or by treatment of the cells with trypsin (on the other hand, the reaction was much weakened by papain). Allen, Corcoran and Ellis[110] (1960) attribute all these findings not to cross-reaction but to the production of some N antigen by the *M* gene. They made the very interesting observation that M S−s−U− cells do not react with anti-N. We confirmed this, and during quantitative tests on cells all taken on the same day found that the ability of M to react with anti-N is affected by the SsS^u genes in such a way that the strength of the reaction falls off in this order: MS, Ms, MS^u; the M_1 status does not seem to influence the reaction. Figur and Rosenfield[174] also confirmed the work of Allen et al.[110]. Allen, Madden and King[114] later reported that M S–s–U+ cells behave like M S–s–U– cells in not reacting with anti-N.

Metaxas-Bühler, Cleghorn, Romanski and Metaxas[141] show that M^g produces more N than does ordinary M: this was fairly apparent from the behaviour of M^g heterozygotes and confirmed by the reactions of the single known M^gM^g homozygote.

This production of N by M^g cannot be put down to the surface changes in M^g cells for these changes are less marked than are those resulting from M^k and $Ms^{Mi.V}$ neither of which produces any N antigen[149, 217].

A further complication was mentioned in previous editions: we found a MS^u/NS^u sample which gave outstandingly low scores with two human anti-N but normal scores with rabbit and Vicia graminea anti-N.

If we prefer to think of N as a precursor substance this section can be adjusted by changing the occasional 'produces N' to 'lets through N'.

Chemistry of MN and theoretical pathways

In 1954, Hohorst[175] had separated an MN active preparation from human red cells but work on the chemistry of MN seems really to date from 1958 when Springer and Ansell[235] in Philadelphia and Mäkelä and Cantell[236] in Helsinki independently reported that neuraminidases from influenza viruses and from Vibrio cholerae inactivated the MN activity of human cells with the release of sialic acid (N-acetylneuraminic acid, NANA). It was concluded[236] 'that sialic acid is an essential part of the M and N receptors'.

Subsequent work in the schools of Springer, Uhlenbruck, Baranowski and Romanowska on separated substances and tests on intact cell with enzymes has resulted in a vast literature which we are incompetent to write about. However, the following references may be some help to introduce a new student to the subject: 176 to 182, 117, 118, 196, and, more recently, 237 to 242.

The M and N antigens are glycoproteins and are dependent on the presence of sialic acid in appropriate linkages: we think it is safe for us to go this far. According to Springer and Huprikar[242] there is 'no information on the structures differentiating M and N specificity', but there is more β-D-galactopyranosyl in N than in M.

Uhlenbruck, cited by Prokop and Uhlenbruck[176, 182], first applied the scheme of genetical pathways leading toward the ABO, secretor, Lewis characters to thought about MN. Over the years the pathway has become increasingly elaborate but Uhlenbruck[238] and Springer and his colleagues[241, 242] appear to be in agreement that the antigen which reacts with Vicia graminea, 'N_{VG}', is a precursor of N and that N, in its turn, is acted on by the M gene to make M antigen; the allele of

M is seen as an amorph. The observation[222] that the product of the rare allele M^c does not react with *Vicia graminea* (page 117) is difficult to fit into this pathway scheme. Wiener *et al.*[281] extended the scheme to take in apes as well as man.

Two steps towards the pathway were the old recognition that the M antigen has some N activity, and the newer observation that the anti-N activity of *Vicia* is not destroyed by neuraminidase and therefore the antigen it recognizes is, unlike M and N (as measured by human antisera), not dependent on sialic acid.

There are observations which do not yet seem to fit easily into the scheme. Allen *et al.*[110] found that M cells lacking S, s and U do not contain some N antigen as do ordinary M cells, and this was confirmed when substances prepared from such MS^u/MS^u cells failed to show N activity[181,180], unlike preparations from ordinary M cells. The *Ss* alleles would, of course, be expected to play some part in the scheme. A further observation that needs to be fitted into any pattern is that the antigen M^g, produced by a reputable allele of MN, is not inactivated by neuraminidase[237].

The basis of such schemes for MNSs would gain strong support if a family turned up showing that the locus producing N is not genetically linked to M, as certain 'Bombay' families showed that H was not linked to ABO.

The red cell membrane upset associated with the En(a−) state and its relation to the MN antigens is referred to in Chapter 22.

ANTIBODIES OF THE MNSs SYSTEM

About 30 different antibodies have so far been recognized. It still seems possible to make some division into those found in man and those made in rabbits though the distinction is becoming blurred by successful efforts to make anti-M^g, anti-Mt^a and anti-Ny^a in rabbits. Assuming that all the antigens of the system are controlled by the many mutational sites of one or more cistrons (if more than one cistron is involved it must be closely linked to its fellow, or fellows) it is curious that a classification into man-made and rabbit-made still seems to have something in it. No doubt this will eventually find an explanation in chemical terms.

Anti-M

Anti-M (and anti-N) sera are usually made by injecting rabbits with appropriate human red cells. Though theoretically simple, the preparation of reliable antisera (particularly anti-N) has proved to be a difficult task. In the first two editions of this book we gave in detail the method used by Dr Elizabeth Ikin, of the Medical Research Council Blood Group Reference Laboratory. Dr Ikin has kindly provided us with all our rabbit anti-M and anti-N sera. Davidsohn and his co-workers[67,68] gave a detailed account of their method.

Both the horse[119] and the cow[131] have proved useful sources of anti-M.

Anti-M in human serum was first identified by Wolff and Jonsson[69], in 1933. Since the dawn of the Rh era and the investigation of human sera on a large scale many hundred examples must have been found. (Dunsford[183], for example, referred to 90 in the Sheffield collection alone.) The antibody can be 'naturally occurring' or frankly immune[70,89,120], or even passive[71]; it has caused haemolytic disease of the newborn[121-124,243], and has been found as an auto-antibody[244,245, and 270,272,273].

Anti-M^A, found in MN people, is referred to on page 118.

Lectins

Hyland Laboratories of Los Angeles discovered[271] a surprising source of anti-M in the seeds of *Iberis amara* (candy tuft species). No less surprisingly Nakajima and his colleagues[246,247] found anti-M in extracts of the seeds of four varieties of the Japanese radish and one variety of turnip.

Anti-M$_1$ and anti-M'

Anti-M$_1$ was found to be a component of six out of 20 human anti-M sera[98]: it was not found in the anti-M serum from eight rabbits or from one horse; it was not found in an extract of *Iberis amara*. We did not find anti-M$_1$ in testing 41 rabbit and four human anti-N sera or in a wide range of other antisera. So far, all examples of anti-M$_1$ have been found in the sera of N people, in which anti-M is detectable at lower temperatures: absorption of these sera by M cells which are negative with anti-M$_1$ results in a gradual removal of anti-M$_1$.

Anti-M$_1$ detects a qualitative difference in the M antigen, it is not merely detecting strong M, for our two best anti-M$_1$ sera were insensitive to the greater amount of M known to be present in cells representing the genotype *MM* than in those representing *MN*; and, conversely, because two anti-M sera in our collection which were particularly sensitive to this dosage difference made no distinction between M$_1$ and ordinary M.

Beattie and Zuelzer[184] found the optimum pH for the detection of naturally occurring anti-M to be 6·5. When working on the M$_1$ antigen we found that a powerful human anti-M serum reacted at pH 6·2 very much more strongly than at pH 8·2; however, the anti-M$_1$ component withstood the higher pH better than the rest of the anti-M complex and the serum became an almost diagnostic reagent, making distinctions nearly as clear as those of more specific anti-M$_1$ sera.

Another qualitative difference between anti-M$_1$ and anti-M was found by Le Roux and Shapiro[213]: a splendid anti-M$_1$ from a Bantu woman was not denatured by treatment with 2-mercaptoethanol as was a control human anti-M.

The making of the M:M$_1$ distinction should become easier with the finding, by Giles and Howell[275], of an anti-M$_1$ without an anti-M component.

Anti-M' was found by Metaxas and his colleagues[222] in the serum of a healthy male donor of group N. Anti-M' is like anti-M$_1$ in its lack of clear cut reactions with some samples, and the only difference between the two antisera is that anti-M' fails to react with M^c cells and does react with M^z cells, the reverse of the reactions of anti-M_1.

Anti-N

Anti-N is usually made in rabbits, as stated above. The first report of its presence in human serum is that of Iseki, Fukao and Suzuki[72], written in Japanese. Many examples have now been found though it is much rarer than anti-M. Anti-N may be 'naturally occurring'[77,125] or frankly immune[73,74] or auto[248,249,270].

Anti-N was found in the serum of three healthy MN donors[134,185,250]. The antisera gave a clear dosage effect; the first [134] was helpful in the Zürich M^g work and was instrumental in the elucidation there of the rare allele M^k; two of them[134,250] reacted more strongly with O than with A_1 cells.

Anti-N^A, found in two healthy MN Melanesians[231], which differs from the anti-N of the previous paragraph[269], is referred to on page 118.

It has been shown[77,125] that human anti-N, though specific for N at certain temperatures, will react with M cells when the temperature is reduced or when the cells are treated with enzymes. Human anti-M, on the other hand, is faithful to M cells. Rabbit[3,110] anti-N and seed[78] anti-N behave like human anti-N in giving some reaction with M cells; this is discussed on page 120.

Lectins

The observation, made by Ottensooser and Silberschmidt[251] in 1953, that extracts of the seeds of the South American plant *Vicia graminea* agglutinate cells containing N much more strongly than those lacking it, was a major contribution to the subject: at once there was provided a splendid research tool and routine reagent.

Seven other, less satisfactory, sources of anti-N were found by the Mäkeläs[252-254]; three of them also belonged to the tribe *Viciae* and four to the genus *Bauhinea*. However, very useful extracts were prepared from *Bauhinea purpurea*[255] and *Bauhinia variegata*[256]; we found the latter extract particularly useful in work on the En system.

A surprising extract of the seeds of *Moluccella laevis* behaved as anti-N, but only with O and B cells[257]: all A cells having N were agglutinated and the agglutinin, which was unsplittable, evidently had the specificity anti-(A+N).

Anti-M^g

This is possibly the commonest antibody belonging to the MNSs system: in the original paper Allen *et al.*[87] report that four examples were found in testing the sera of 500 normal people in Boston. Dr Allen kindly sent us samples of M^g cells and with the help of Dr R.A. Zeitlin we found 23 examples of the antibody in testing the serum of 703 normal people. Incidentally, ABO grouping discrepancies led to the recognition of anti-M[g] in three routine anti-A sera[140,206,208]. The antibody has been made in rabbits[186].

Anti-S

Many examples of human anti-S have now been found: the first[24,25] is described on page 92. The antibody may be 'naturally occurring'[79-82] or frankly immune[32,51,83,258]. It has not yet been made by a rabbit.

Anti-s

This expected antibody was found[28] four years after anti-S. Many examples have been found since and some of them have been published[84,85,88,126,127,187,279]. Anti-s has been the cause of haemolytic disease of the newborn[88,187,278]. All examples so far found were considered to be immune in origin. Anti-s was successfully induced in 2 out of 22 injected rabbits[259].

Anti-U

The first person known to make the antibody[48] died of it after a transfusion. The second example[50] of anti-U was caused by pregnancy, and all since have been considered immune: one was the cause of stillbirth due to haemolytic disease[168]. Acquired haemolytic anaemia has several times been attributed to auto-anti-U[260-262], with [262] or without Rh overtones. Auto-anti-U was found in the serum of a patient with myasthenia gravis[277].

Apart from the auto examples anti-U has been made only by immunized S–s– people, all, as far as we know, Negroes except for one Indian[205]. Anti-U sera vary in their ability to react with cells of the rare phenotype S–s–U+ (see page 102), just as anti-D sera vary in their ability to react with D[u] cells.

'Anti-M[k]'

Weak specific anti-M[k] was thought to exist[63], but this is now realized to reflect the interaction of immune antisera in general with the changed surface properties of M[k] cells (page 470).

Anti-Tm and anti-Sj

The original anti-Tm and anti-Sj were found in the same serum[146,147]. Anti-Tm is not uncommon but is difficult to work with and tends to 'go off' both *in vivo* and *in vitro*[147,204]: its specificity, however, makes it potentially a very useful antibody. No frankly immune example has been reported. Of the examples we have had the chance to test three were from *MS/Ms* people and two from MNSs so the antibody has yet to be found in an N person.

Anti-Sj seems to be more stable[147] than anti-Tm.

Anti-Hu and anti-He

These antibodies are made by rabbits in response to injections of red cells of Negroes; anti-He does not seem difficult to make[59]. Only one example of anti-He in human serum has been reported, in a girl who was pregnant but who had not been transfused; Macdonald and his colleagues[189] thought that the antibody was probably 'naturally occurring'. We have had the opportunity of checking two further examples of human anti-He.

Anti-Mi[a], -Vw (or -Gr), -Mur, -Hil, -Hut

These antibodies to the Miltenberger series of antigens have been found only in human sera. Examples of all types have caused haemolytic disease of the newborn (see legend to Table 15), but anti-Vw, at any rate, is more often 'naturally occurring': this was first realized by Darnborough[108], and when 7,248 samples of normal serum had been tested[108,128,103,101,156] no less than 73, or 1 %, contained anti-Vw. Cleghorn[103] found six anti-Mi[a] and three anti-Vw in testing the serum of only 16 patients suffering from acquired haemolytic anaemia. In testing 101 other 'pathological' sera he found no anti-Mi[a] but 13 anti-Vw. Several examples of anti-Mur have been found[154,190,191,266], some in normal sera, but still only one example of anti-Hil is known[154].

Anti-Hut was first isolated by absorbing anti-Mi[a] with Vw+ Mi(a−) cells[65,154,194] but several straight examples have been found since[263,264], all of which had been the cause of haemolytic disease of the newborn.

Anti-M[V]

The antibody which recognizes the M[V] antigen was first reported[188] as 'an unusual anti-N', which indeed it appeared to be, for its anti-N and anti-M[V] aspects could not be separated. Its positive reactions descended in order of strength from M[V]N, N, M[V]M, MN to negative with ordinary M cells. The antibody was almost certainly immune[152]. Testing for M[V] was made easier when a 'pure' anti-M[V] without the anti-N component was found[215], presumably 'naturally occurring', in a control AB serum.

Anti-Vr, -Ri[a], -St[a], -Mt[a], -Cl[a], -Ny[a], -Sul, -Far

The original example[109] of anti-Vr was almost certainly immune; two further examples were found in anti-S sera (one of them had anti-Vw and anti-M[g] as well); no example was found in 202 normal sera.

Anti-Ri[a] and anti-St[a] were found together[159] in one serum, which also contained anti-Wr[a] and anti-Sw[a]: all four antibodies were separable by appropriate absorption. Further examples of anti-St[a] were found[160], but not of anti-Ri[a] in testing about 1,000 normal sera[190] with Ri(a+) cells.

The first example of anti-Mt^a was thought to be 'naturally occurring'. No further example was found in 3,500 normal sera[161]; however, it has caused haemolytic disease of the newborn and was successfully produced in rabbits[192].

Anti-Cl^a turned up in an anti-B serum and was then found to be present in the serum of 24, or 0·45%, of 5,326 random Glasgow and London donors[163].

Anti-Ny^a was found in the serum of a normal donor; subsequently four examples were found in testing 3,693 random Norwegian donors[164,165], and tens of thousands of normal sera have been tested since[225]. The antibody was made in rabbits[165].

Anti-Sul was found in the sera of two normal donors; the antibody is relatively common, for four further examples were found in testing 119 normal Bostonian sera[166].

Anti-Far resulted from foeto-maternal immunization[227].

The MNSs system distinguishes more efficiently between random people of most races than does any other blood group system: it is therefore outstanding in its usefulness when applied to human genetics.

REFERENCES

[1] LANDSTEINER K. and LEVINE P. (1927) A new agglutinable factor differentiating individual human bloods. *Proc. Soc. exp. Biol. N.Y.*, **24**, 600–602.

[2] LANDSTEINER K. and LEVINE P. (1927) Further observations on individual differences of human blood. *Proc. Soc. exp. Biol. N.Y.*, **24**, 941–942.

[3] LANDSTEINER K. and LEVINE P. (1928) On individual differences in human blood. *J. exp. Med.*, **47**, 757–775.

[4] LANDSTEINER K. and LEVINE P. (1928) On the inheritance of agglutinogens of human blood demonstrable by immune agglutinins. *J. exp. Med.*, **48**, 731–749.

[5] SCHIFF F. (1930) Die Vererbungsweise der Faktoren M und N von Landsteiner und Levine. *Klin. Wchnschr.*, **2**, 1956–1959.

[6] WIENER A.S. and VAISBERG M. (1931) Heredity of the agglutinogens M and N of Landsteiner and Levine. *J. Immunol.*, **20**, 371–388.

[7] TAYLOR G.L. and PRIOR AILEEN M. (1939) Blood Groups in England. III. Discussion of the family material. *Ann. Eugen., Lond.*, **9**, 18–44.

[8] WIENER A.S. (1943) *Blood Groups and Transfusion*, 3rd edition, Thomas, Springfield.

[9] HALDANE J.B.S. (1948) The formal genetics of man. *Proc. Roy. Soc. B.*, **135**, 147–170.

[10] WIENER A.S. (1951) Heredity of the M-N types; analysis of twenty years' work. *Amer. J. hum. Genet.*, **3**, 179–183.

[11] WIENER A.S., DI DIEGO N. and SOKOL S. (1953) Studies on the heredity of the human blood groups. I. The M-N types. *Acta Genet. Med. Gemell.*, **2**, 391–398.

[12] BENNETT J.H. (1965) Estimation of the frequencies of linked gene pairs in random mating populations. *Amer. J. hum. Genet.*, **17**, 51–53.

[13] CHOWN B. and LEWIS MARION (1959) The blood group genes of the Copper Eskimo. *Amer. J. phys. Anthrop.*, **17**, 13–18.

[14] CROME W. (1935) Uber Blutgruppenfragen: Mutter M, Kind N. *Dtsch. Ztschr. gerichtl. Med.*, **24**, 167–175.

[15] FRIEDENREICH V. (1939) Ein erblicher defekter N-Receptor, der wahrscheinlich eine bisher unbekannte Blutgruppeneigenschaft innerhalb des MN-Systems darstellt. *Dtsch. Ztschr. gerichtl. Med.*, **25**, 358–368.

[16] ANDRESEN P.H. (1947) Reliability of the exclusion of paternity after the MN and ABO systems as elucidated by 20,000 mother-child examinations and its significance to the medico-legal conclusion. *Acta. path. microbiol. scand.*, **24**, 545–552.

[17] ANDRESEN P.H. (1948) *Menneskets Blodtyper Anvendelsen i Retsmedicinen*, Munksgaard, Copenhagen.

[18] FRIEDENREICH V. and LAURIDSEN A. (1938) On a variety of human type-antigen M and its relation to other M antigens. *Acta. path. microbiol. scand.*, supp. **38**, 155–157.

[19] JAKOBOWICZ RACHEL, BRYCE LUCY M. and SIMMONS R.T. (1949) The occurrence of unusual positive Coombs reactions and M variants in the blood of a mother and her first child. *Med. J. Austral.*, **2**, 945–948.

[20] JAKOBOWICZ RACHEL, BRYCE LUCY M. and SIMMONS R.T. (1950) The occurrence of unusual positive Coombs reactions and M factors in the blood of a mother and her first baby. *Nature, Lond.*, **165**, 158.

[21] BRYCE LUCY M. (1952) Personal communication.

[22] DUNSFORD I., IKIN ELIZABETH W. and MOURANT A.E. (1953) A human blood group gene intermediate between M and N. *Nature, Lond.*, **172**, 688–689.

[23] HENNINGSEN K. and JACOBSEN T. (1954) A probable mutation within the MN blood group system. *Acta. path. microbiol. scand.*, **35**, 240–248.

[24] WALSH R.J. and MONTGOMERY CARMEL (1947) A new human isoagglutinin subdividing the MN blood groups. *Nature, Lond.*, **160**, 504.

[25] SANGER RUTH and RACE R.R. (1947) Subdivisions of the MN blood groups in man. *Nature, Lond.*, **160**, 505.

[26] FISHER R.A. (1946) *Statistical Methods for Research Workers*, 10th edition, Oliver and Boyd, Edinburgh, p. 96.

[27] MATHER K. (1943) *Statistical Analysis in Biology*, Methuen, London, p. 193.

[28] LEVINE P., KUHMICHEL A.B., WIGOD M. and KOCH ELIZABETH (1951) A new blood factor, s, allelic to S. *Proc. Soc. exp. Biol. N.Y.*, **78**, 218–220.

[29] SANGER RUTH, RACE R.R., WALSH R.J. and MONTGOMERY CARMEL (1948) An antibody which subdivides the human MN blood groups. *Heredity*, **2**, 131–139.

[30] SANGER RUTH and RACE R.R. (1951) The MNSs blood group system. *Amer. J. hum. Genet.*, **3**, 332–343.

[31] RACE R.R. and SANGER RUTH (1954) *Blood Groups in Man*, 2nd edition, Blackwell Scientific Publications, Oxford, p. 71.

[32] PICKLES MARGARET M. (1948) A further example of the anti-S agglutinin. *Nature, Lond.*, **162**, 66.

[33] RACE R.R., SANGER RUTH, LAWLER SYLVIA D. and BERTINSHAW DOREEN (1949) The inheritance of the MNS blood groups: a second series of families. *Heredity*, **3**, 205–213.

[34] BERTINSHAW DOREEN, LAWLER SYLVIA D., HOLT HELENE A., KIRMAN B.H. and RACE R.R. (1950) The combination of blood groups in a sample of 475 people in a London hospital. *Ann. Eugen., Lond.*, **15**, 234–242.

[35] SANGER RUTH, RACE R.R., GREENWALT T.J. and SASAKI T. (1955) The S, s and S^u blood group genes in American Negroes. *Vox Sang.*, **5**, 73–81.

[36] MORTON N.E. and CHUNG C.S. (1959) Are the MN blood groups maintained by selection? *Amer. J. hum. Genet.*, **11**, 237–251.

[37] FISHER R.A. (1946) The fitting of gene frequencies to data on *rhesus* reactions. *Ann. Eugen., Lond.*, **13**, 150–155.

[38] FISHER R.A. (1947) Note on the calculation of the frequencies of *rhesus* allelomorphs. *Ann. Eugen., Lond.*, **13**, 223–224.

[39] BOYD W.C. (1953) Estimation of gene frequencies from MNS data. *Science*, **118**, 756.

[40] BOYD W.C. (1954) Maximum likelihood method for estimation of gene frequencies from MNS data. *Amer. J. hum. Genet.*, **6**, 1–10.

[41] BOYD W.C. (1956) The 'accuracy' of estimates of MNS gene frequencies. *Acta Genet. Med. Gemell.*, **5**, 234–237.

[42] MOURANT A.E. (1954) *The Distribution of the Human Blood Groups*, Blackwell Scientific Publications, Oxford, p. 358.

[43] WIENER A.S. (1954) Serology genetics and nomenclature of the M-N-S types. *Acta Genet. Med. Gemell.*, **3**, 314–321.

[44] RACE R.R., SANGER RUTH and THOMPSON JOAN S. (1953) Quoted in 2nd edition of this book but not elsewhere published.

[45] EDWARDS J.H. (1966) Personal communication.

[46] CHOWN BRUCE, LEWIS MARION and KAITA HIROKO (1967) The inheritance of the MNSs blood groups in a Caucasian population sample. *Amer. J. hum. Genet.*, **19**, 86–93.

[47] FISHER R.A. (1951) Standard calculations for evaluating a blood-group system. *Heredity*, **5**, 95–102.

[48] WIENER A.S., UNGER, L.J. and GORDON EVE B. (1953) Fatal hemolytic transfusion reaction caused by sensitization to a new blood factor U. *J. Amer. med. Ass.*, **153**, 1444–1446.

[49] WIENER A.S., UNGER L.J. and COHEN LAURA (1954) Distribution and heredity of blood factor U. *Science*, **119**, 734–735.

[50] GREENWALT T.J., SASAKI T., SANGER RUTH, SNEATH JOAN and RACE R.R. (1954) An allele of the S(s) blood group genes. *Proc. nat. Acad. Sci. Wash.*, **40**, 1126–1129.

[51] LEVINE P., FERRARO L.R. and KOCH ELIZABETH (1952) Hemolytic disease of the newborn due to anti-S. *Blood*, **7**, 1030–1037.

[52] SCHIFF F. and BOYD W.C. (1942) *Blood Grouping Technic*, Interscience Publishers, New York.

[53] MOUREAU P. (1935) Contribution a l'étude des facteurs d'individualisation du sang humain et leur applications en médecine légale. 2e memoire. Les groupes M et N d'hémo-agglutination de Landsteiner et Levine. *Rev. belge. Sci. méd.*, **7**, 540–588.

[54] MATSUNAGA E. (1962) Some evidence of heterozygote advantage in the polymorphism of MN blood groups. *Proc. 8th Congr. int. Blood Transf.*, Tokyo 1960, 126–130.

[55] LEVINE P., STOCK A.H., KUHMICHEL A.B. and BRONIKOVSKY N. (1951) A new human blood factor of rare incidence in the general population. *Proc. Soc. exp. Bio. N.Y.*, **77**, 402–403.

[56] HART MIA V. D., BOSMAN HÉLÈNE and LOGHEM J.J. VAN (1954) Two rare human blood group antigens. *Vox Sang.*, **4**, 108–116.

[57] LANDSTEINER K., STRUTTON W.R. and CHASE M.W. (1934) An agglutination reaction observed with some human bloods, chiefly among Negroes. *J. Immunol.*, **27**, 469–472.

[58] IKIN ELIZABETH W. and MOURANT A.E. (1951) A rare blood group antigen occurring in Negroes. *Brit. Med. J.*, **i**, 456–457.

[59] CHALMERS J.N.M., IKIN ELIZABETH W. and MOURANT A.E. (1953) A study of two unusual blood-group antigens in West Africans. *Brit. med. J.*, **ii**, 175–177.

[60] NIJENHUIS L.E. (1953) The Henshaw bloodgroup (He) in Papuans and Congo Negroes. *Vox Sang.*, **3**, 112–114.

[61] ZOUTENDYK A. (1955) The blood groups of South African natives with particular reference to a recent investigation of the Hottentots. *Proc. 5th Congr. int. Blood Transf.*, 247–249.

[62] SHAPIRO M. (1956) Inheritance of the Henshaw (He) blood factor. *J. forensic Med.*, **3**, 152–160.

[63] METAXAS M. N., METAXAS-BÜHLER M., ROMANSKI J. and BÜTLER R. (1967) The frequency of M^k in Swiss blood donors and its inheritance in five independent families. *Proc. 11th Congr. int. Soc. Blood Transf.*, Sydney 1966. 399–404.

[64] WALLACE J., MILNE G.R., MOHN J., LAMBERT R.M., ROSAMILIA H.G., MOORES PHYLLIS, SANGER RUTH and RACE R.R. (1957) Blood group antigens Miᵃ and Vw and their relation to the MNSs system. *Nature, Lond.*, **179**, 478.

[65] MOHN J.F., LAMBERT R.M., ROSAMILIA H.G., WALLACE J., MILNE G.R., MOORES PHYLLIS, SANGER RUTH and RACE R.R. (1958) On the relationship of the blood group antigens Mi^a and Vw to the MNSs system. *Amer. J. hum. Genet.*, **10**, 276–286.

[66] HEIKEN A. (1965) A genetic study of the MNSs blood group system. *Hereditas, Lund.*, **53**, 187–211.

[67] DAVIDSOHN I. and ROSENFELD I. (1939) The preparation of anti-M and anti-N testing fluids. *Am. J. clin. Path.*, **9**, 397–413.

[68] MENOLASINO N.J., DAVIDSOHN I. and LYNCH DOROTHY E. (1954) A simplified method for the preparation of anti-M and anti-N typing sera. *J. Lab. clin. Med.*, **44**, 495–498.

[69] WOLFF E. and JONSSON B. (1933) Studien uber die Untergruppen A$_1$ und A$_2$ mit besonderer Berucksichtigung der Paternitätsuntersuchungen. *Dtsch. Ztschr. gerichtl. Med.*, **22**, 65–85.

[70] BROMAN B. (1944) The blood factor Rh in man. *Acta paediatrica*, supplementum **2**, 1–178 (page 128).

[71] JAKOBOWICZ RACHEL and BRYCE LUCY M. (1951) A note on a placenta-permeating anti-M agglutinin. *Med. J. Aust.*, **i**, 365–367.

[72] ISEKI S., FUKAO T. and SUZUKI J. (1937) On the Anti-N agglutinin found in normal human serum. *Hanzaigaku-Zasshi*, **11**, 245–242 (Japanese).

[73] SINGER E. (1943) Isoimmunization against blood factor N. *Med. J. Austral.*, **ii**, 29.

[74] CALLENDER SHEILA T. and RACE R.R. (1946) A serological and genetical study of multiple antibodies formed in response to blood transfusion by a patient with lupus erythematosus diffusus. *Ann. Eugen., Lond.*, **13**, 102–117.

[75] CLEGHORN T.E. (1960) MNSs gene frequencies in English blood donors. *Nature, Lond.*, **187**, 701.

[76] DE GROOT M.H. and LI C.C. (1960) Simplified method of estimating MNS gene frequencies. *Ann. hum. Genet.*, **24**, 109–115.

[77] HIRSCH W., MOORES PHYLLIS, SANGER RUTH and RACE R.R. (1957) Notes on some reactions of human anti-M and anti-N sera. *Brit. J. Haemat.*, **3**, 134–142.

[78] LEVINE P., OTTENSOOSER F., CELANO M.J. and POLLITZER W. (1955) On reactions of plant anti-N with red cells of chimpanzees and other animals. *Amer. J. phys. Anthrop.*, **13**, 29–36.

[79] COOMBS H.I., IKIN ELIZABETH W., MOURANT A.E. and PLAUT GERTRUDE (1951) Agglutinin anti-S in human serum. *Brit. med. J.*, **i**, 109–111.

[80] RACE R.R., HOLT HELENE A., GORIUS L. and BESSIS M. (1949) Une agglutinine anti-S à la suite de transfusions répétées. *C. r. Soc. Biol.*, **143**, 980.

[81] VOGEL P. and ROSENFIELD R.E. (1950) Personal communication.

[82] CONSTANTOULIS N.C., PAIDOUSSIS M. and DUNSFORD I. (1955) A naturally occurring anti-s agglutinin. *Vox Sang.* (o.s.) **5**, 143–144.

[83] CUTBUSH MARIE and MOLLISON P.L. (1949) Haemolytic transfusion reaction due to anti-S. *Lancet*, **ii**, 102–103.

[84] SANGER RUTH, RACE R.R., ROSENFIELD R.E. and VOGEL P. (1953) A serum containing anti-s and anti-Jk^b. *Vox Sang.* (o.s.), **3**, 71.

[85] FUDENBERG H. and ALLEN F.H. (1957) The blood group antibody anti-s: a third example. *Vox Sang.*, **2**, 133–137.

[86] GIBLETT ELOISE R., GARTLER S.M. and WAXMAN S.H. (1963) Blood group studies on the family of an XX/XY hermaphrodite with generalized tissue mosaicism. *Amer. J. hum. Genet.*, **15**, 62–68.

[87] ALLEN F.H., CORCORAN PATRICIA A., KENTON H.B. and BREARE NANCY (1958) M^g, a new blood group antigen in the MNS system. *Vox Sang.*, **3**, 81–91.

[88] GIBLETT ELOISE, CHASE JEANNE and CREALOCK F.W. (1958) Hemolytic disease of the newborn resulting from anti-s antibody. *Amer. J. clin. Path.*, **29**, 254–256.

[89] FREIESLEBEN E. and KNUDSEN ELSE E. (1957) A human incomplete immune anti-M. P.H. Andresen Festskrift, Munksgaard, Copenhagen, 26–31.

90 LINNET-JEPSEN P., GALATIUS-JENSEN F. and HAUGE M. (1958) On the inheritance of the Gm serum group. *Acta. genet.*, **8**, 164–196.

91 GALATIUS-JENSEN F. (1958) On the genetics of the haptoglobins. *Acta genet.*, **8**, 232–247.

92 GALATIUS-JENSEN F. (1960) *The Haptoglobins. A Genetical Study.* Dansk Videnskabs Forlag, København, pp. 117.

93 LEWIS MARION, KAITA HIROKO and CHOWN B. (1957) The blood groups of a Japanese population. *Amer. J. hum. Genet.*, **9**, 274–283.

94 GEDDE-DAHL T., GRIMSTAD A.L., GUNDERSEN S. and VOGT E. (1967) A probable crossing over or mutation in the MNSs blood group system. *Acta genet.*, **17**, 193–210.

95 HACKEL E. (1958) Elution of anti-U from SS and ss cells. *Vox Sang.*, **3**, 92–93.

96 GREENWALT T.J., SASAKI T., SANGER RUTH and RACE R.R. (1958) S^u, an allele of S and s. *Proc. 6th Congr. int. Soc. Blood Transf.*, 104–106.

97 GREENWALT T.J. (1961) Conspectus of the red cell blood groups in *Progress in Hematology*, 3rd edition, edited by L.M. Tocantins.

98 JACK J.A., TIPPETT PATRICIA, NOADES JEAN, SANGER RUTH and RACE R.R. (1960) M$_1$ a subdivision of the human blood-group antigen M. *Nature, Lond.*, **186**, 642.

99 POLLITZER W.S. (1956) The Henshaw blood factor in New York city Negroes. *Amer. J. phys. Anthrop.*, **14**, 445–447.

100 ROSENFIELD R.E., HABER GLADYS V., SCHROEDER RUTH and BALLARD RACHEL (1960) A Negro family revealing Hunter-Henshaw information, and independence of the genes for Js and Lewis. *Amer. J. hum. Genet.*, **12**, 143–146.

101 SIMMONS R.T., ALBREY J.A. and McCULLOCH W.J. (1959) The duplication of the Gr (Graydon) blood group by Vw (Verweyst). *Vox Sang.*, **4**, 132–137.

102 GRAYDON J.J. (1946) A rare iso-haemagglutinogen. *Med. J. Aust.*, **ii**, 9–10.

103 CLEGHORN T.E. (1961) *The Occurrence of Certain Rare Blood Group Factors in Britain.* M.D. Thesis, University of Sheffield.

104 MOHN J.F., LAMBERT R.M. and ROSAMILIA H.G. (1961) Incidence of the blood group antigen Mi^a in the Caucasian and Negro populations of Western New York. *Transfusion, Philad.*, **1**, 392–393.

105 WALKER MARY E., TIPPETT PATRICIA A., ROPER JUDITH M., OSTHOLD MARGARETHE D., MUNN MARILYN J., MATHESON ANNE, LEWIS SHEILA J., KRABBE SISSEL M.R., GILLIS MARY, FARRENKOPF CLARE F., DOWNS JUNE M., CRAWCOUR PAMELA, CORCORAN PATRICIA A., CASPERSEN KARI, VON BERCKEN TRAUTE, BALL RITA and ALLEN F.H. (1961) Tests with some rare blood-group antibodies. *Vox Sang.*, **6**, 357.

106 ISEKI S., MASAKI S., FURUKAWA K., MOHN J., LAMBERT R.M. and ROSAMILIA H.G. (1958) Diego and Miltenberger blood factor in Japanese. *Gunma J. med. Sci.*, **7**, 120–126.

107 CORCORAN PATRICIA, ALLEN F.H., ALLISON A.C. and BLUMBERG B.S. (1959) Blood groups of Alaskan Eskimos and Indians. *Amer. J. phys. Anthrop.*, **17**, 187–193.

108 DARNBOROUGH J. (1957) Further observations on the Verweyst blood group antigen and antibodies. *Vox Sang.*, **2**, 362–367.

109 HART MIA V.D., VEER MARGA V.D., LOGHEM J.J. VAN, SANGER RUTH and RACE R.R. (1958) Vr, an antigen belonging to the MNSs blood group system. *Vox Sang.*, **3**, 261–265.

110 ALLEN F.H., CORCORAN PATRICIA A. and ELLIS F.R. (1960) Some new observations on the MN system. *Vox Sang.*, **5**, 224–231.

111 SPEISER P. (1959) Ueber die bisher jüngste menschliche Frucht (27 mm/2.2 g), an der bereits die Erbmerkmale A₁, M, N, s, Fy(a+), C, c, D, E, e, Jk(a+?) im Blut festgestellt werden Konnten. *Wien. klin. Wschr.*, **71**, 549–551.

112 CHOWN B., LEWIS MARION and KAITA HIROKO (1965) An anomaly of inheritance in the MNSs blood groups. *Amer. J. hum. Genet.*, **17**, 9–13.

113 SCHOLZ W. and MURKEN J-D. (1963) Koppelungsuntersuchungen bei Familien mit multi plen cartilaginären Exostosen. *Z. menschl. Vererb. -u. Konstit. -Lehre*, **37**, 178–192.

114 ALLEN F.H. JR., MADDEN HELEN J. and KING R.W. (1963) The MN gene *MU*, which produces M and U but no N, S or s. *Vox Sang.*, **8**, 549–556.

[115] FRANCIS BETTY J. and HATCHER D.E. (1966) MN blood types. The S–s–U+ and the M_1 phenotypes. *Vox Sang.*, **11**, 213–216.

[116] MORTON N.E., MI M.P. and YASUDA N. (1966) A study of the S^u alleles in northeastern Brazil. *Vox Sang.*, **11**, 194–208.

[117] UHLENBRUCK G. (1960) Neuraminsäurehaltige Mucoide aus menschlichen Erythozyten und ihr Verhalten gegenüber verschiedenen Enzymen. *Zbl. Bakt.*, **177**, 559–581 or 197–219.

[118] KLENK E. and UHLENBRUCK G. (1960) Über neuraminsuärehaltige Mucoide aus Menschenerythrocytenstroma, ein Beitrag zur Chemie der Agglutinogene. *Hoppe-Seyl. Z.*, **319**, 151–160.

[119] LEVINE P., CELANO M.J., LANGE S. and BERLINER V. (1957) On anti-M in horse sera, *Vox Sang.*, **2**, 433–439.

[120] SPEISER P. (1956) Serologische Studien an fünf menschlichen Anti-M-Körpern. *Z. Immun-Forsch.*, **113**, 165–170.

[121] BOMCHIL G. (1951) Isoinmunizacion por el antigeno M. Nuevo causa de enfermedad hemolitica neonatal. *Hematologia y Hemoterapia*, **3**, 104–109.

[122] STONE B. and MARSH W.L. (1959) Haemolytic disease of the newborn caused by anti-M. *Brit. J. Haemat.*, **5**, 344–347.

[123] SIMMONS R.T., KRIEGER VERA I and JAKOBOWICZ RACHEL (1960) Anti-M antibody as a rare cause of haemolytic disease of the new-born. *Med. J. Aust.*, **ii**, 337–338.

[124] FREIESLEBEN E. and JENSEN K.G. (1961) Haemolytic disease of the newborn caused by anti-M. The value of the direct conglutination test. *Vox Sang.*, **6**, 328–335.

[125] STERN K., ELLIS F.R. and MASAITIS LILLIAN (1957) Report on an anti-N agglutinin having characteristics of a natural anitbody. *Amer. J. clin. Path.*, **27**, 635–638.

[126] ALBREY J.A. and SIMMONS, R.T. (1958) Anti-s of the MNSs blood group system. *Med. J. Aust.*, **i**, 630–633.

[127] O'RIORDAN J. and CANN J. (1959) Potent anti-s in pregnancy. *Vox Sang.*, **4**, 242–246.

[128] ZEITLIN R.A., SANGER RUTH and RACE R.R. (1958) Unpublished observations.

[129] GOLDSTEIN ELEANOR I. (1966) *Investigation of the inheritance of the U factors: emphasis on dosage studies of S and s and studies with anti* $-U^A$ *and* U^B. Master of Science Thesis, University of Cincinnati.

[130] BRICE CHARMAINE L. and HOXWORTH P.I. (1965) *Some unusual observations in the search for rare donors*. Paper read at American Association of Blood Banks, Miami.

[131] STONE W.H. and ANDERSON C.W. (1963) The preparation of human blood typing fluids from cattle normal and immune sera. *Proc. 2nd int. Congr. hum. Genet.*, Rome 1961, **2**, 889–893.

[132] METAXAS M.N., MATTER M., METAXAS-BÜHLER M., ROMANSKI Y. and HÄSSIG A. (1964) Frequency of the M^g blood group antigen in Swiss blood donors and its inheritance in several independent families. *Proc. 9th Congr. int. Soc. Blood Transf.*, Mexico 1962, 206–209.

[133] WIENER A.S. and ROSENFIELD R.E. (1961) M^e, a blood factor common to the antigenic properties of M and He. *J. Immunol.*, **87**, 376–378.

[134] METAXAS-BÜHLER MARGRIT, IKIN ELIZABETH W. and ROMANSKI J. (1961) Anti-N in the serum of a healthy blood donor of group MN. *Vox Sang.*, **6**, 574–582.

[135] RACE R.R. and SANGER RUTH (1962) *Blood Groups in Man*, 4th edition, Blackwell Scientific Publications, Oxford, p. 91.

[136] JENSEN K.G. and FREIESLEBEN E. (1962) Inherited positive Coombs' reaction connected with a weak N-receptor (N_2). *Vox Sang.*, **7**, 696–703.

[137] JEANNET M., METAXAS-BÜHLER M. and TOBLER R. (1963) Anomalie héréditaire de la membrane érythrocytaire avec tests de Coombs positif et modification de l'antigène de groupe N. *Schweiz. med.Wschr.*, **93**, 1508–1509.

[138] JEANNET M., METAXAS-BÜHLER M. and TOBLER R. (1964) Anomalie héréditaire de la membrane érythocytaire avec test de Coombs direct positif et modification de l'antigène de groupe N. *Vox Sang.*, **9**, 52–55.

139 HEIKEN A. and IKIN ELIZABETH W. (1964) An inherited N_2 antigen of different strengths in mother and child. *Acta genet.*, **14**, 57–62.

140 METAXAS M.N., METAXAS-BÜHLER M. and ROMANSKI J. (1966) Studies on the blood group antigen M^g. I. Frequency of M^g in Switzerland and family studies. *Vox Sang.*, **11**, 157–169.

141 METAXAS-BÜHLER M., CLEGHORN T.E., ROMANSKI J. and METAXAS M.N. (1966) Studies on the blood group antigen M^g. II. Serology of M^g. *Vox Sang.*, **11**, 170–183.

142 WINTER NANCY M., ANTONELLI GLORIA, WALSH ELIZABETH A. and KONUGRES ANGELYN A. (1966) A second example of blood group antigen M^g in the American population. *Vox Sang.*, **11**, 209–212.

143 KOUT M. (1962) The incidence of the C^w, M^g and Wr^a agglutinogens in the population of Prague. *Vox Sang.*, **7**, 242–244.

144 CHANDANAYINGYONG D., SASAKI T.S. and GREENWALT T.J. (1967) Blood groups of the Thais. *Transfusion, Philad.*, **7**, 269–276.

145 RACE R.R. and SANGER RUTH (1962) *Blood Groups in Man*, 4th edition, Blackwell Scientific Publications, Oxford, p. 93.

146 ISSITT P.D., HABER JANE M. and ALLEN F.H. JR. (1965) Anti-Tm, an antibody defining a new antigenic determinant within the MN blood-group system. *Vox Sang.*, **10**, 742–743.

147 ISSITT P.D., HABER JANE M. and ALLEN F.H. JR. (1968) Sj, a new antigen in the MN system, and further studies on Tm. *Vox Sang.*, **15**, 1–14.

148 KONUGRES ANGELYN A., BROWN LINDA S. and CORCORAN PATRICIA A. (1966) Anti-M^A, and the phenotype M^aN, of the MN blood-group system (A new finding). *Vox Sang.*, **11**, 189–193.

149 METAXAS M.N. and METAXAS-BÜEHLER M. (1964) M^k: an apparently silent allele at the MN locus. *Nature, Lond.*, **202**, 1123.

150 HENNINGSEN K. (1966) Exceptional MNSs- and Gm-types within a Danish family. Causal relationship or coincidence? *Acta genet.*, **16**, 239–241.

151 HEIKEN A., IKIN ELIZABETH W. and MÅRTENSSON L. (1967) On the M^k allele of the MNSs system. *Acta Genet.*, **17**, 328–337.

152 GERSHOWITZ H. and FRIED K. (1966) Anti-M^v, a new antibody of the MNS blood group system. I. M^v, a new inherited variant of the M gene. *Amer. J. hum. Genet.*, **18**, 264–281.

153 HURD J.K., JACOX R.F., SWISHER S.N., CLEGHORN T.E., CARLIN SANDRA and ALLEN F.H. JR. (1964) S_2, a new phenotype in the MN blood group system. *Vox. Sang.*, **9**, 487–491.

154 CLEGHORN T.E. (1966) A memorandum on the Miltenberger blood groups. *Vox Sang.*, **11**, 219–222.

155 WORLLEDGE SHEILA, GILES CAROLYN M. and CLEGHORN T.E. (1963) Unpublished finding.

156 KORNSTAD L., ØRJASAETER H. and LARSEN A.M. (1966) The blood group antigen Vw and anti-Vw antibodies: some observations in the Norwegian population. *Acta genet.*, **16**, 355–361.

157 LEWIS MARION, KAITA HIROKO and UCHIDA IRENE (1963) Segregation of Mi^a with Ms. *Vox Sang.*, **8**, 245.

158 MOHN J.F., LAMBERT R.M., ISEKI S., MASAKI S. and FURUKAWA K. (1963) The blood group antigen Mi^a in Japanese. *Vox Sang.*, **8**, 430–437.

159 CLEGHORN T.E. (1962) Two human blood group antigens, St^a (Stones) and Ri^a (Ridley), closely related to the MNSs system. *Nature, Lond.*, **195**, 297–298.

160 MADDEN HELEN J., CLEGHORN T.E., ALLEN F.H. JR., ROSENFIELD R.E. and MACKEPRANG MURIEL (1964) A note on the relatively high frequency of St^a on the red blood cells of orientals, and report of a third example of anti-St^a, *Vox Sang.*, **9**, 502–504.

161 SWANSON JANE and MATSON G.A. (1962) Mt^a, a 'new' antigen in the MNSs system. *Vox Sang.*, **7**, 585–590.

162 KONUGRES ANGELYN A., FITZGERALD HELEN and DRESSER ROBERTA (1965) Distribution and development of the blood factor Mt^a. *Vox Sang.*, **10**, 206–207.

163 WALLACE J. and IZATT MARIAN M. (1963) The Cl^a (Caldwell) antigen: a new and rare human blood group antigen related to the MNSs system. *Nature, Lond.*, **200**, 689–690.

164 ØRJASAETER H., KORNSTAD, L., HEIER A.M., VOGT E., HAGEN P. and HARTMANN O. (1964) A human blood group antigen, Ny^a (Nyberg), segregating with the *Ns* gene complex of the MNSs system. *Nature, Lond.*, **201**, 832.

165 ØRJASAETER H., KORNSTAD L. and HEIER ANNA-MARGRETHE (1964) Studies on the Ny^a blood group antigen and antibodies. *Vox Sang.*, **9**, 673–683.

166 KONUGRES ANGELYN A. and WINTER NANCY M. (1967) Sul, a new blood group antigen in the MN system. *Vox Sang.*, **12**, 221–224.

167 LAWLER SYLVIA D., MARSHALL RUTH and SHATWELL HELEN S. (1964) Trisomy and titrations with particular references to the MN system. *Vox Sang.*, **9**, 455–462.

168 BURKI U., DEGNAN TH. J. and ROSENFIELD R.E. (1964) Stillbirth due to anti-U. *Vox Sang.*, **9**, 209–211.

169 CHUNG C.S., MATSUNAGA E. and MORTON N.E. (1961) The MN polymorphism in Japan. *Jap. J. Genet.*, **6**, 1–11.

170 LEWIS MARION, CHOWN B. and KAITA HIROKO (1963) Inheritance of blood group antigens in a largely Eskimo population sample. *Amer. J. hum. Genet.*, **15**, 203–208.

171 GREUTER W., HESS M., RENAUD N., SCHMITTER M. and BÜTLER R. (1963) Beitrag zur genetik des Gm- und Gc-serumgruppensystems anhand von untersuchungen an schweizerfamilien. *Arch. Klaus-Stift. VerebrForsch.*, **38**, 77–92.

172 MOHR J. (1966) Genetics of fourteen marker systems: association and linkage relations. *Acta genet.*, **16**, 1–58.

173 STEINBERG A.G., SHWACHMAN H., ALLEN F.H., JR and DOOLEY R.R. (1956) Linkage studies with cystic fibrosis of the pancreas. *Amer. J. hum. Genet.*, **8**, 162–176.

174 FIGUR A.M. and ROSENFIELD R.E. (1965) The crossreaction of anti-N with type M erythrocytes. *Vox Sang.*, **10**, 169–176.

175 HOHORST H.J. (1954) Zur Kenntnis der Natur der M- und N-Substanz menslicher Erythrocyten. *Z. Hygiene*, **139**, 561–564. (Not seen, cited by HOTTA K., and SPRINGER G.F. (1965) *Proc. 10th Congr. int. Soc. Blood Transf.*, Stockholm 1964, 505–509.)

176 PROKOP O. and UHLENBRUCK G. (1966) *Lehrbuch der menslichen Blut- und Serumgruppen*, 2nd edition, Thieme, Leipzig, pp. 924. English translation: Prokop O. and Uhlenbruck G. (1969) *Human Blood and Serum Groups*, pp. 891, Maclaren, London.

177 ROMANOWSKA ELZBIETA (1964) Reactions of M and N blood group substances natural and degraded with specific reagents of human and plant origin. *Vox Sang.*, **9**, 578–588.

178 UHLENBRUCK G. (1965) Immunochemical studies on erythrocyte mucoids: the nature of the M and N specific substances. *Proc. 10th Congr. int. Soc. Blood Transf.*, Stockholm 1964, 476–482.

179 HOTTA K. and SPRINGER G.F. (1965) Isolation and partial characterization of blood group N. Specific haptens from human blood group M and N substances. *Proc. 10th Congr. int. Soc. Blood Transf.*, Stockholm 1964, 505–509.

180 UHLENBRUCK G. and KRÜPE M. (1965) Cryptantigenic Nv$_g$ receptor in mucoids from Mu/Mu cells. *Vox Sang.*, **10**, 326–332.

181 STALDER K. and SPRINGER G.F. (1962) Serological characterization of isolated receptors of the MN erythrocyte system. *Proc. 8th Congr. europ. Soc. Haemat.*, Vienna 1961, paper no. 489.

182 PROKOP O. and UHLENBRUCK G. (1963) *Lehrbuch der menslichen Blut- und Serumgruppen*. Thieme, Leipzig, p. 349.

183 DUNSFORD I. (1964) Anti-M in neoplastic disease. *Vox Sang.*, **9**, 212–213.

184 BEATTIE KATHRYN M. and ZUELZER W.W. (1965) The frequency and properties of pH, dependent anti-M. *Transfusion, Philad.*, **5**, 322–326.

185 GREENWALT T.J., SASAKI T. and STEANE E.A. (1966) Second example of anti-N in a blood donor of group MN. *Vox Sang.*, **11**, 184–188.

186 IKIN ELIZABETH W. (1966) The production of anti-M^g in rabbits. *Vox Sang.*, **11**, 217–218.

[187] LUSHER J.M., ZUELZER W.W. and PARSONS P.J. (1966) Anti-s hemolytic disease: a case report. *Transfusion, Philad.*, **6**, 590–591.

[188] GERSHOWITZ H. (1964) An unusual human anti-N serum. *Proc. 2nd int. Congr. hum. Genet.*, Rome 1962, 833–835.

[189] MACDONALD K.A., NICHOLS MARGARET E., MARSH W.L. and JENKINS W.J. (1967) The first example of anti-Henshaw in human serum. *Vox Sang.*, **13**, 346–348.

[190] CLEGHORN T.E. (1966) Personal communication.

[191] CORNWALL SHEILA, WRIGHT J. and MOORE B.P.L. (1968) Further examples of the antigen Mur (Murrell), a rare blood group associated with the MNSs system. *Vox Sang.*, **14**, 295–298.

[192] KONUGRES ANGELYN A., HUBERLIE MARY M., SWANSON JANE and MATSON G.A. (1963) The production of anti-Mt^a in rabbits. *Vox Sang.*, **8**, 632–633.

[193] FRASER G.R., GIBLETT E.R. and MOTULSKY A.G. (1966) Population genetic studies in the Congo. III. Blood groups (ABO, MNSs, Rh, Js^a). *Amer. J. hum. Genet.*, **18**, 546–552.

[194] MOHN J.F. and MACVIE SHEILA (1967) Serologic studies on the relationship of the Mi^a and Vw blood group antigens. Unpublished observations.

[195] MADDEN HELEN J., CLEGHORN T.E. and ALLEN F.H. (1964) Unpublished observations.

[196] SPRINGER G.F., NAGAI Y. and TETGMEYER HERTA (1966) Isolation and properties of human blood-group NN and meconium-Vg antigens. *Biochemistry*, **5**, 3254–3272.

[197] SCHOLZ W. and MURKEN J.-D. (1967) Beobachtung eines Faktorenaustausches zwischen des Blutgruppen-Genorten MN und Ss. *Hum. Genet.*, **4**, 268–273.

[198] CRAWFORD MARY, N. (1967) 500 Philadelphia Negroes tested with anti-M, -N, -S, -s, -U. Personal communication, quoted in *Blood Groups in Man*, 5th edition.

[199] METAXAS M.N., METAXAS-BÜHLER M. and EDWARDS J.H. (1970) MNSs frequencies in 3,895 Swiss blood donors. *Vox Sang.*, **18**, 385–394.

[200] MORTON N.E. and MIKI CAROLINE (1968) Estimation of gene frequencies in the MN system. *Vox Sang.*, **15**, 15–24.

[201] KRAULAND W. and SMERLING M. (1970) Reinerbigkeitsausschlüsse SS/ss. *Ärztl. Lab.*, **16**, 98–99.

[202] POLESKY H.F., MOULDS J. and SMITH R. (1972) Anomalous inheritance of Ss in a Caucasian family. Abstracts AABB and ISH Meeting, Washington, p. 12.

[203] GOLDSTEIN E.I. and HOXWORTH P.I. (1969) Investigation of the inheritance of the U^A and U^B specificities of the U blood-group factor. *Transfusion, Philad.*, **9**, 280–281. (Abstract.)

[204] RACE R.R. and SANGER RUTH (1962) *Blood Groups in Man*, 4th edition, Blackwell Scientific Publications, Oxford.

[205] MOORES PHYLLIS (1972) Four examples of the S–s–U-phenotype in an Indian family. *Vox Sang.*, **23**, 452–454.

[206] BROCTEUR J. (1969) The M^gS gene complex of the MNSs blood group system, evidenced in a Sicilian family. *Human Hered.*, **19**, 77–85.

[207] BROCTEUR J. (1972) Confirmation of the M^gS gene complex found in 3 new Sicilian families. Abstracts AABB and ISH Meeting, Washington, p. 12.

[208] JOSHI S.R., BHARUCHA Z.S., SHARMA R.S. and BHATIA H.M. (1972) The M^g blood group antigen in two Indian families. *Vox Sang.*, **22**, 478–480.

[209] NORDLING S., SANGER RUTH, GAVIN JUNE, FURUHJELM U., MYLLYLÄ G. and METAXAS M.N. (1969) M^k and M^g: some serological and physicochemical observations. *Vox Sang.*, **17**, 300–302.

[210] STURGEON P., METAXAS-BÜHLER M., METAXAS M.N., TIPPETT PATRICIA and IKIN E.W. (1970) An erroneous exclusion of paternity in a Chinese family exhibiting the rare MNSs gene complexes M^k and Ms^{III}. *Vox Sang.*, **18**, 395–406.

[211] METAXAS M.N., METAXAS-BÜHLER M. and ROMANSKI Y. (1971) The inheritance of the blood group gene M^k and some considerations on its possible nature. *Vox Sang.*, **20**, 509–518.

[212] SANGER RUTH (1970) Genetics of blood groups. In: *Blood and Tissue Antigens*, ed. D. Aminoff, New York, Academic Press Inc., pp. 17–31.

[213] ROUX MARJORIE E. le and SHAPIRO M. (1969) The antigen M_1. *J. Foren. Med.*, **16**, 135–138.

[214] RICHMOND R.S. and INNELLA FILOMENA (1968) Anomalous expression of the M_1 antigen of the MN system in an American Negro family. *Vox Sang.*, **15**, 463–466.

[215] CROSSLAND J.D., PEPPER M.D., GILES C.M. and IKIN E.W. (1970) A British family possessing two variants of the MNSs blood group system, M^v and a new class within the Miltenberger complex. *Vox Sang.*, **18**, 407–413.

[216] METAXAS M.N. and METAXAS-BÜHLER M. (1972) The detection of MNSs 'variants' in serial tests with incomplete Rh antisera in saline. *Vox Sang.*, **22**, 474–477.

[217] METAXAS M.N., METAXAS-BÜHLER M., HEIKEN A., VAMOSI M., IKIN E.W. and BULL W. (1972) Further examples of Miltenberger cell class V, one of them inherited with a depressed M antigen. *Vox Sang.*, **23**, 420–428.

[218] CHANDANAYINGYONG D. and BEJCHANDRE S. (1972) The incidence of blood group antigen 'Mi^a' in the Thai people. Abstracts AABB and ISH Meeting, Washington, p. 10.

[219] MURAKAMI S. (1967) The rare blood types and variants in Japanese. *Act. Crim. Japon.*, **33**, 138–145.

[220] DOEBLIN T.D. and MOHN J.F. (1967) The blood groups of the Seneca Indians. *Amer. J. Hum. Genet.*, **19**, 700–712.

[221] MATSON G.A. and SWANSON J. (1965) Distribution of hereditary blood antigens among Indians in middle America. *Am. J. Phys. Anthrop.*, **23**, 413–426.

[222] METAXAS M.N. METAXAS-BÜHLER M. and IKIN E.W. (1968) Complexities of the *MN* locus. *Vox Sang.*, **15**, 102–117.

[223] NAKAJIMA H., OHKURA K., ØRJASAETER H. and KORNSTAD L. (1967) The Ny^a blood group antigen among Japanese, Ryukyuan and Chinese and the mountainous Aborigines in Taiwan. *Jap. J. Hum. Genet.*, **11**, 263–265.

[224] PINEDA A.A. and TASWELL H.F. (1969) First example of Ny^a blood group antigen in American population. *Vox Sang.*, **17**, 459–461.

[225] SCHIMMACK L., MÜLLER I. and KORNSTAD L. (1971) A contribution to the Ny^a problem. *Human Hered.*, **21**, 346–350.

[226] KORNSTAD L., LARSEN A.M. HEIER and WEISTER O. (1971) Further observations on the frequency of the Ny^a blood-group antigen and its genetics. *Am. J. Hum. Genet.*, **23**, 612–613.

[227] CREGUT R., LEWIN D., LACOMME M. and MICHOT O. (1968) Un cas d'anasarque foeto-placentaire par iso-immunisation contre un antigène 'privé'. *Rev. franc. Transf.*, **11** 139–143.

[228] CREGUT R., LIBERGE G., YVART J., BROCTEUR J. and SALMON C. (1974) A new rare blood group antigen, 'FAR', probably linked to the MNSs system. *Vox Sang.*, **26**, 194–198.

[229] SCHMIDT A.P. and TASWELL H.F. (1969) Coexistence of MN erythrocytes and apparent anti-M antibody. *Transfusion, Philad.*, **9**, 203–204.

[230] HOWARD P.L. and PICKOFF R.C. (1972) Another example of anti-M in an M-positive patient. *Transfusion, Philad.*, **12**, 59–61.

[231] BOOTH P.B. (1971) Anti-N^A. An antibody sub-dividing Melanesian N. *Vox Sang.*, **21**, 522–530.

[232] BOOTH P.B., HORNABROOK R.W. and MALCOLM L.A. (1972) The red cell antigen N^A in Melanesians: family and population studies. *Hum. Biol. Oceania*, **I**, 223–228.

[233] BOOTH P.B. (1972) A 'new' blood group antigen associated with S and s. *Vox Sang.*, **22**, 524–528.

[234] MORTON N.E., KRIEGER H. and MI M.P. (1966) Natural selection on polymorphisms in Northeastern Brazil. *Am. J. Hum. Genet.*, **18**, 153–171.

[235] SPRINGER G.F. and ANSELL NORMA J. (1958) Inactivation of human erythrocyte agglutinogens M and N by influenza viruses and receptor-destroying enzyme. *Proc. nat. Acad. Sci., Wash.*, **44**, 182–189.

236   MÄKELÄ O. and CANTELL KARI (1958) Destruction of M and N blood group receptors of human red cells by some influenza viruses. *Ann. Med. exp. Fenn.*, **36**, 366–374.

237   SPRINGER G.F. and STALDER K. (1961) Action of influenza viruses, receptor-destroying enzyme and proteases on blood group agglutinogen M^g. *Nature, Lond.*, **191**, 187–188.

238   UHLENBRUCK G. (1969) Possible genetical pathways in the MNSsUu system. *Vox Sang.*, **16**, 200–210.

239   SPRINGER G.F. (1970) Role of human cell surface structures in interactions between man and microbes. *Naturwissenschaften*, **57**, 162–171.

240   COHEN E., ROBERTS S.C., NORDLING S. and UHLENBRUCK G. (1972) Specificity of *Limulus polyphemus* agglutinins for erythrocyte receptor sites common to M and N antigenic determinants. *Vox Sang.*, **23**, 300–307.

241   SPRINGER G.F., TEGTMEYER HERTA and HUPRIKAR S.V. (1972) Anti-N reagents in elucidation of the genetical basis of human blood-group MN specificities. *Vox Sang.*, **22**, 325–343.

242   SPRINGER G.F. and HUPRIKAR S.V. (1972) On the biochemical and genetic basis of the human blood-group MN specificities. *Haematologia*, **6**, 81–92.

243   MACPHERSON C.R. and ZARTMAN E.R. (1965) Anti-M antibody as a cause of intrauterine death. A follow-up. *Am. J. clin. Path.*, **43**, 544–547.

244   FLETCHER J.L. and ZMIJEWSKI C.M. (1970) The first example of auto-anti-M and its consequences in pregnancy. *Transfusion, Philad.*, **10**, 282. (Abstract of *Int. Arch. Allerg.* 37, 586.)

245   HYSELL J.K., BECK M.L., GRAY J.M. and OBERMAN H.A. (1972) Auto anti-M. Abstracts AABB and ISH Meeting, Washington, p. 63.

246   NAKAJIMA H. and NAKAYAMA T. (1968) Anti-M lectin of *Iberis amara L.* Reports of the Japanese National Research Institute of Police Science, **21**, 111–115.

247   OKADA T. and NAKAJIMA H. (1970) Anti-M lectin of Japanese radish. *Reports of the Japanese National Research Institute of Police Science*, **23**, 207–209.

248   HOWELL ELEANOR D. and PERKINS H.A. (1972) Anti-N-like antibodies in the sera of patients undergoing chronic hemodialysis. *Vox Sang.*, **23**, 291–299.

249   BOWMAN H., MARSH W., SCHUMACHER H., OYEN, R. and REIHART, J. (1972) Auto anti-N immunohemolytic anemia in infectious mononucleosis (IM). Abstracts AABB and ISH Meeting, Washington, p. 63.

250   MOORES P., BOTHA M.C. and BRINK S. (1970) Anti-N in the serum of a healthy type MN person—a further example. *Am. J. Clin. Path.*, **54**, 90–93.

251   OTTENSOOSER F. and SILBERSCHMIDT K. (1953) Haemagglutinin anti-N in plant seeds. *Nature, Lond.*, **172**, 914.

252   MÄKELÄ O. and MÄKELÄ PIRJO (1956) Some new blood group specific phytagglutinins. *Ann. Med. exp. Fenn.*, **34**, 402–404.

253   MÄKELÄ O. (1957) Studies in hemagglutinins of Leguminosae seeds. Thesis, supplement No. 11, *Ann. Med. exp. Fenn.*, **35**, 1–133.

254   MÄKELÄ O. and HAUTALA TUULA (1958) Reactions of plant anti-N agglutinins with red cells treated with proteolytic enzymes. *Ann. Med. exp. Fenn.*, **36**, 323–327.

255   BOYD W.C., EVERHART D.L. and MCMASTER MARJORIE H. (1958) The anti-N lectin of *Bauhinia purpurea. J. Immunol.*, **81**, 414–418.

256   FLETCHER GAY (1959) The anti-N phytagglutinin of *Bauhinia variegata. Aust. J. Sci.*, **22**, 167.

257   BIRD G.W.G. and WINGHAM JUNE (1970) Agglutinins for antigens of two different human blood group systems in the seeds of *Moluccella laevis. Vox Sang.*, **18**, 235–239.

258   BRIZARD C.P., SELVE A. la and PETIT J.C. le (1969) Isoimmunisation foeto-maternelle anti-S: maladie hémolytique du nouveau-né chez les deux descendants. *Rev. franc. Transf.* **12**, 249–257.

259   PUNO C.S. and ALLEN F.H. JR. (1969) Anti-s produced in rabbits. *Vox Sang.*, **16**, 155–156.

260   BLAJCHMAN M.A., HUI Y.T., JONES T.E. and LUKE K.H. (1971) Familial autoimmune

hemolytic anemia with autoantibody demonstrating U specificity. Program, AABB
Meeting, p. 82.

[261] NUGENT MARY E., COLLEDGE KATHERINE I. and MARSH W.L. (1971) Auto-immune hemolytic anemia caused by anti-U. *Vox Sang.*, **20**, 519–525.

[262] MARSH W.L., REID MARION E. and SCOTT E. PATRICIA (1972) Autoantibodies of U blood
group specificitiy in autoimmune haemilytic anaemia. *Brit. J. Haemat.*, **22**, 625–629.

[263] HART MIA v.d. (1971) Unpublished observations.

[264] SAUSAIS LAIMA and MANN JULIA (1971) Unpublished observations.

[265] FIELD T.E., WILSON T.E., DAWES B.J. and GILES C.M. (1972) Haemolytic disease of the
newborn due to anti-Mt^a. *Vox Sang.*, **22**, 432–437.

[266] SMERLING M. (1971) S^u in der weissen Bevölkerung (Bericht über Familienuntersuchungen).
Beitr. gericht. Med., **28**, 237–239.

[267] BERGREN MILDRED (1972) Unpublished observations.

[268] METAXAS M.N. and METAXAS-BÜHLER M. (1971) Die Bedeutung von MNSs-Varianten in
Fällen von Umstrittener Vaterschaft. 3. Tagung der Gesellschaft für forensische Blut-
gruppenkunde e.V., Mainz.

[269] BOOTH P.B. and MOORES PHYLLIS (1973) The non-identity of anti-N^A and anti-N in the serum
of an MN person. *Vox Sang.*, **25**, 374–376.

[270] PERRAULT R. (1973) Naturally-occurring anti-M and anti-N with special case: IgG anti-N
in a NN donor. *Vox Sang.*, **24**, 134–149.

[271] ALLEN NANCY K. and BRILLIANTINE LAURA (1969) A survey of hemagglutinins in various
seeds. *J. Immunol.*, **102**, 1295–1299.

[272] TEGOLI J., HARRIS J.P., NICHOLS M.E., MARSH W.L. and REID M.E. (1970) Autologous
anti-I and anti-M following liver transplant. *Transfusion, Philad.*, **10**, 133–136.

[273] HYSELL J.K., BECK M.L. and GRAY J.M. (1973) Additional examples of cold autoagglutinins with M specificity. *Transfusion, Philad.*, **13**, 146–149.

[274] STURGEON P. (1973) Personal communication.

[275] GILES C.M. and HOWELL P. (1974) An antibody in the serum of an MN patient which reacts
with M$_1$ antigen. *Vox Sang.*, **27**, 43–51.

[276] MARSH W.L., ØYEN R., NICHOLS M.E. and CHARLES H. (1974) Studies of MNSsU antigen
activity of leukocytes and platelets. *Transfusion, Philad.*, **14**, 462–466.

[277] BECK M.L., BUTCH S.H., ARMSTRONG W.D. and OBERMAN H.A. (1972) An autoantibody
with U-specificity in a patient with myasthenia gravis. *Transfusion, Philad.*, **12**, 280–283.

[278] DRACHMANN O. and BROGAARD HANSEN K. (1969) Haemolytic disease of the newborn due
to anti-s. *Scand. J. Haemat.*, **6**, 93–98.

[279] LALEZARI P., MALAMUT DOROTHY C., DREISIGER MARTHA E. and SANDERS C. (1973) Anti-s
and anti-U cold-reacting antibodies. *Vox Sang.*, **25**, 390–397.

[280] LOWE R.F. and MOORES PHYLLIS P. (1972) S–s–U– red cell factor in Africans of Rhodesia,
Malawi, Mozambique and Natal. *Hum. Hered.*, **22**, 344–350.

[281] WIENER A.S., GORDON EVE B., MOOR-JANKOWSKI J. and SOCHA W.W. (1972) Homologues
of the human M-N blood types in gorillas and other non-human primates. *Haematologia*,
6, 419–432.

Chapter 4
The P Blood Groups

The discovery of the P groups in 1927 by Landsteiner and Levine[1] resulted from the same brilliant immunization experiments which also unveiled the existence of the MN groups. The sera of certain rabbits which had been immunized with human red cells were found, after absorption of the species agglutinins, to agglutinate some samples of blood, but not others. The distinction could not be explained on the basis of the ABO or MN systems. The two types of blood were called P+ and P−.

The same antibody, anti-P, was found soon after in the serum of a human being[2], and in normal, non-immune, sera from horses, rabbits, pigs and cattle[3].

Owing to the existence of blood samples which reacted weakly to the early anti-P sera the frequency of the two groups could not at first be established with certainty[4], but that there were racial differences was recognized[1,5], and the P antigen was shown to be inherited in all probability as a Mendelian dominant character[2,3].

The most important subsequent addition to knowledge was the discovery of the antigen Tj[a] by Levine, Bobbitt, Waller and Kuhmichel[6] coupled with the recognition by Sanger[7] that this antigen is, in fact, part of the P system: suddenly it became clear that P− people, far from lacking an antigen of the system, share a powerful one with P+ people: a third, and extremely rare, group is defined in which this antigen is lacking. The discovery entirely altered our way of thinking of the P system and required a modification of the original notation:

the phenotype P+ became P_1
the phenotype P− became P_2
anti-P became anti-P_1

A further important step was the recognition of the antigen P^k (Matson, Swanson, Noades, Sanger and Race[59], 1959). This rare red cell antigen, almost unique amongst blood groups in the manner of its inheritance, gives a glimpse of the complexity of the genetic background of the P system.

FREQUENCIES

In our second edition we gave a long list of results of tests with anti-P_1 on the blood of 'Caucasians'. The frequency of negatives varied from 18% to 30%. Such differences reflect serological difficulties and not anthropological differences. The lower frequencies of P_2 are often due to the presence of anti-A_1 in the anti-P_1 sera and the higher frequencies are due to the anti-P_1 sera being weak ones.

From the literature it still seems that the best work in distinguishing P_1 and P_2 was done in Scandinavia, notably by Henningsen[8-10] using the technique of Jonsson. Henningsen's figures are:

Total tested	P_1	P_2
2,345	1,849	496
	78·85%	21·15%

The frequencies of the genes responsible for the P groups are obtained thus: the frequency of the gene P_2 in any population is the square root of the proportion of people who are P_2. The frequency of the gene P_1 is $1 -$ frequency of P_2. These calculations depend on the antigen P_1 being inherited as a Mendelian dominant character, which, as will be seen later, is the case.

The frequencies of the genotypes in a population are obtained from the gene frequencies thus:

Phenotypes	Genotypes	Frequency
P_1	P_1P_1	$(P_1)^2$
	P_1P_2	$2(P_1P_2)$
P_2	P_2P_2	$(P_2)^2$

Applying these formulae to Henningsen's results we have:

gene $P_2 = 0\cdot4599$
gene $P_1 = 0\cdot5401$
genotype $P_1P_1 = 0\cdot2917$ or $0\cdot3699$⎫ of all
genotype $P_1P_2 = 0\cdot4968$ or $0\cdot6301$⎭ P_1
genotype $P_2P_2 = 0\cdot2115$

INHERITANCE

Landsteiner and Levine[2,3] showed that the P_1 antigen was inherited and that the manner of inheritance was probably that of a dominant Mendelian character. This has been supported by all subsequent work.

From the genotype frequencies given above the expected frequency of the six genotypically and three phenotypically different matings can be calculated, together with the children expected therefrom (Table 17).

In Table 18 the calculated phenotype frequencies are applied to a series of families tested by Henningsen. The agreement between observed and expected children is remarkably close and leaves no doubt of the correctness of Landsteiner and Levine's views on the inheritance of the P groups. However, such agreement

Table 17. The expected distribution of the P groups in European parents and offspring

Genotypes				
Matings		**Children**		
Type	Frequency	P_1P_1	P_1P_2	P_2P_2
$P_1P_1 \times P_1P_1$	0·0851	0·0851	—	—
$P_1P_1 \times P_1P_2$	0·2898	0·1449	0·1449	—
$P_1P_2 \times P_1P_2$	0·2468	0·0617	0·1234	0·0617
$P_1P_1 \times P_2P_2$	0·1234	—	0·1234	—
$P_1P_2 \times P_2P_2$	0·2102	—	0·1051	0·1051
$P_2P_2 \times P_2P_2$	0·0447	—	—	0·0447
	1·0000			

Phenotypes			
Matings		**Proportion of children from each mating**	
Type	Frequency	P_1	P_2
$P_1 \times P_1$	0·6217	0·9008	0·0992
$P_1 \times P_2$	0·3336	0·6850	0·3150
$P_2 \times P_2$	0·0447	—	1·0000
	1·0000		

has not been achieved by other workers, all using less rigorous tests than did Henningsen. With only a few exceptions other family series[12-19,43,44,50,68,69,71,76,77] contain too many P_2 children from the matings $P_1 \times P_1$ and $P_1 \times P_2$.

Hoping to forestall the building of formidable theories we hasten to give our explanation: families often include young children with a somewhat weak P_1 antigen, and anti-P_1 sera are often not very strong, so, as a result, a proportion of P_1 children are scored as P_2.

Table 18. The P groups of 304 Danish families with their 803 children (After Henningsen[11], 1950)

Matings			Children				
	Number			P_1		P_2	
Type	obs.	exp.	Total	obs.	exp.	obs.	exp.
$P_1 \times P_1$	194	189·0	524	471	472·0	53	52·0
$P_1 \times P_2$	93	101·4	240	169	164·4	71	75·6
$P_2 \times P_2$	17	13·6	39	1*	0·0	38	39·0

* Extra-marital also according to the Rh groups.

6

One of the series from our Unit[20] may be pilloried as an example, a series of 306 English families with 700 children (Table 19). The expectations are based on gene frequencies calculated from the 612 parents: $P_1 = 0.5841$ and $P_2 = 0.4519$.

Table 19. The P groups of 306 English families and their 700 children
(Race, Sanger and Thompson[20], 1953)

	Matings			Children					
	Number					P_1		P_2	
Type	obs.	exp.	χ^2	Total	obs.	exp.	obs.	exp.	χ^2
$P_1 \times P_1$	190	193.8	0.07	440	384	397.4	56	42.6	4.67
$P_1 \times P_2$	107	99.5	0.57	243	163	167.4	80	75.6	0.37
$P_2 \times P_2$	9	12.8	1.13	17	0	0.0	17	17.0	
			1.77						5.04
			for 2 d.f.						for 2 d.f.
			P = 0.4						P = 0.08

Although in the children's compartment of Table 19 the total χ^2 is not too bad, the 4.67 (for 1 d.f.) of the first row is. So these families call for further analysis; and since another method is available, which has to be described somewhere, here it is.*

Fisher's method for analysing the blood groups of families

Professor Sir Ronald Fisher pointed out certain objections to the method used in Table 19, which had almost become the standard way of verifying unifactorial inheritance. The mating $P_1 \times P_1$ is genotypically of three kinds, and the mating $P_1 \times P_2$ of two kinds. Children from, say, the phenotype mating $P_1 \times P_2$ are not independent samples from a homogeneous population, with an expectation of 0.6888 P_1 to 0.3112 P_2, and should not be treated as independent in calculating goodness of fit. That the method does in fact usually give a very good fit is probably due to the shortage of large families in the data.

In 1939 Fisher suggested that account should be taken separately of the totals yielded by the group of families containing recessive children, and of the individual sizes of families containing none. This method was applied to the A_1A_2BO groups by Taylor and Prior[21] (1939) and by Race, Ikin, Taylor and Prior[22] (1942), and to he Duffy groups by Race and Sanger[23] (1952).

The number of families observed to contain no recessive children, irrespective of size, is compared with the number expected, taking account of the estimated gene frequency and of the sizes of all families observed.

* Those about to skip this section should remember that a method exists, and one which they will be able to apply with an effort very trifling compared with that of collecting the data they wish to analyse. Smith[78] (1956) has also devised a method for analysing the observed segregation of a character in family data.

Details of the 306 families to be analysed are given in Table 20: this compact way of giving a lot of information was suggested to us by Professor C.D. Darlington. The gene frequencies to be used in the analysis are once again those derived from the 612 parents.

Table 20. Details of the 306 families and 700 children of Table 19

Mating			Children		Mating			Children	
Father	Mother	No.	P_1	P_2	Father	Mother	No.	P_1	P_2
P_1 × P_1		52	1	–	P_1 × P_2		4	–	1
		49	2	–			5	1	1
		29	3	–			7	–	2
		7	4	–			3	1	2
		7	5	–			2	2	1
		3	6	–			1	2	2
		1	8	–			1	3	1
P_1 × P_1		6	–	1			1	3	3
		14	1	1			1	6	3
		5	–	2	P_2 × P_1		4	–	1
		9	2	1			16	1	1
		1	1	3			2	–	2
		3	3	1			3	1	2
		1	2	3			2	2	1
		1	3	2			1	1	3
		1	6	2			1	3	1
		1	5	4			1	4	1
P_1 × P_2		10	1	–			1	3	3
		10	2	–	P_2 × P_2		3	–	1
		3	3	–			4	–	2
		2	4	–			2	–	3
		1	5	–					
P_2 × P_1		8	1	–					
		9	2	–					
		7	3	–					
		1	4	–					

The formulae given by Taylor and Prior[21] for the matings B × O and B × B can be directly applied to matings P_1 × P_2 and P_1 × P_1. These formulae are also applicable to family studies of the Lutheran, Kell, Duffy and Kidd groups where:

    a represents the gene frequency of P_1 (or Lu^a, K, Fy^a or Jk^a)
  and *b* represents the gene frequency of P_2 (or Lu^b, k, Fy^b or Jk^b)

Of course, if the antithetical antibody (anti-Lu^b, anti-k, anti-Fy^b or anti-Jk^b) has been used as well in the tests then no such elaborate analysis as that to follow is needed.

The explanation given below is almost a direct transcription from Taylor and Prior's lucid account of the method, with the necessary change of symbols.

Mating $P_1 \times P_2$

The P_1 parent can be one of two genotypes, P_1P_1, the frequency of which is a^2, or P_1P_2 with the frequency of $2ab$. The frequency of the phenotype P_1 in the population is therefore $a^2 + 2ab$; hence the probability of a P_1 person being P_1P_1 is

$$\frac{a^2}{a^2 + 2ab} \quad \text{or} \quad \frac{a}{a + 2b}, \quad \text{and of being } P_1P_2 \text{ is } 1 - \frac{a}{a + 2b}$$

From the mating $P_1P_1 \times P_2P_2$ all children will be P_1, from the mating $P_1P_2 \times P_2P_2$ some children may be P_2. The probability of a child of the mating $P_1P_2 \times P_2P_2$ being of the phenotype P_1 is $\frac{1}{2}$, of two children being both P_1 is $(\frac{1}{2})^2$ and of n children all P_1 is $(\frac{1}{2})^n$. The occurrence of a P_2 child is at present the only means of knowing that the P_1 parent is heterozygous, hence in the mating $P_1 \times P_2$ the families are divided into two groups, those with all children P_1, and those with some children P_2.

All children P_1

Families of 1 child. Probability of this child being P_1 = probability of the P_1 parent being $P_1P_1 + \frac{1}{2} \times$ (probability of the P_1 parent being P_1P_2) =

$$\frac{a}{a + 2b} + \tfrac{1}{2}\left(1 - \frac{a}{a + 2b}\right).$$

Therefore the expected number of families with one child, this child being P_1

$$= \begin{bmatrix} \text{observed number of } P_1 \times \\ P_2 \text{ families with one child} \end{bmatrix} \times \left[\frac{a}{a + 2b} + \tfrac{1}{2}\left(1 - \frac{a}{a + 2b}\right)\right].$$

Since a = the frequency of the gene P_1 = 0·5481, and b = the frequency of the gene P_2 = 0·4519 and the total number of 1 child families of the mating type $P_1 \times P_2$ is 26, then the expected number of such families with 1 child, this child being P_1, is 26 × 0·68875 or 17·91; 18 were observed.

Families of n children. Probability of all n children being

$$P_1 = \frac{a}{a + 2b} + (\tfrac{1}{2})^n\left(1 - \frac{a}{a + 2b}\right).$$

As above, to get the expected number of such families this figure must be multiplied by the observed number of families of n children with parents $P_1 \times P_2$.

Applying these formulae to the matings $P_1 \times P_2$, shown in Table 20, the expectations for the number of families in which all children are P_1 are as shown in Table 21.

Table 21. Analysis of families of the mating type $P_1 \times P_2$

Family size	Total families	Number of families with only P_1 children	
		exp.	obs.
1	26	17·91	18
2	49	26·12	19
3	20	9·11	10
4	7	2·91	3
5	2	0·79	1
6	2	0·77	0
9	1	0.38	0
Total	107	57·99	51

Some children P_2

The expected number of families with P_2 children is obtained by subtracting the expected number of families whose children are all P_1 from the total number of observed families of the type $P_1 \times P_2$. Applying this to the present investigation we find that the expected number of such families is $107 - 57·99$ or $49·01$, while 56 were observed.

Mating $P_1 \times P_1$

In this mating also the parents can be of two genotypes P_1P_1 or P_1P_2 and the families are again divided into two groups, those with all children P_1, and those with some children P_2.

Probability of one parent being $P_1P_2 = \dfrac{2b}{a+2b}$.

Probability of both parents being $P_1P_2 = \left(\dfrac{2b}{a+2b}\right)^2$.

Thus the probability of at least one parent being $P_1P_1 = 1 - \left(\dfrac{2b}{a+2b}\right)^2$.

All children P_1

Families of 1 child. Probability of this child being P_1 = the probability of at least one parent being $P_1P_1 + \frac{3}{4} \times$ (the probability of both parents being

$$P_1P_2) = 1 - \left(\frac{2b}{a+2b}\right)^2 + \tfrac{3}{4}\left(\frac{2b}{a+2b}\right)^2.$$

Therefore the expected number of families with 1 child, this child being P_1

$$= \begin{bmatrix} \text{observed number of } P_1 \times P_1 \\ \text{families with 1 child} \end{bmatrix} \times \left[1 - \left(\frac{2b}{a+2b}\right)^2 + \tfrac{3}{4}\left(\frac{2b}{a+2b}\right)^2\right].$$

Families of n children. Probability of all children being

$$P_1 = 1 - \left(\frac{2b}{a+2b}\right)^2 + (\tfrac{3}{4})^n \left(\frac{2b}{a+2b}\right)^2.$$

Applying these formulae to the matings $P_1 \times P_1$ shown in Table 20, the expectations for the number of families in which all children are P_1 are as given in Table 22.

Table 22. Analysis of families of the mating type $P_1 \times P_1$

Family size	Total families	Number of families with only P_1 children	
		exp.	obs.
1	58	52·38	52
2	68	56·47	49
3	38	29·49	29
4	11	8·09	7
5	9	6·34	7
6	3	2·04	3
8	2	1·30	1
9	1	0·64	0
Total	190	156·75	148

Some children P_2

The expected number of families with P_2 children will be the difference between the total number of observed families of the type $P_1 \times P_1$ and the expected number of such families whose children are all P_1. In the present example the expected number of such families is $190 - 156·75$ or $33·25$, while 42 were observed.

A summary of the results of analysing the 306 families by Fisher's method is given in Table 23. The families come reasonably up to expectation: $P = 0·1$; which means that such a divergence from the ideal, or a greater one, would be

Table 23. Summary of the analysis by Fisher's method of the 306 families

Class of mating	Class of family	Number of families		χ^2	d.f.
		exp.	obs.		
$P_1 \times P_1$	all children $\quad$ P_1	156·75	148	2·79	1
	some children P_2	33·25	42		
$P_1 \times P_2$	all children $\quad$ P_1	57·99	51	1·84	1
	some children P_2	49·01	56		
				4·63	2
				$P = 0·1$	

found once in very ten such investigations. But, knowing that nearly all other workers find too many P_2 children, when we observe a deviation in the same direction we can be confident that our results appear not to be significantly upset only because there are too few of them.

This misclassification of a relatively small proportion of children does not call in question the practical use of anti-P_1 in linkage work or in affiliation tests. In affiliation tests a child can be excluded only if it is P_1 and both supposed parents are P_2. In the various series of families referred to above we counted 133 matings $P_2 \times P_2$ with 380 children: all but six were P_2 and four of these were stated to be extra-marital, from information beyond the P groups.

A rare inhibitor of P_1 and other antigens

In 1974, Crawford, Tippett and Sanger[148] found that the rare dominant inhibitor of the antigens Lu^a, Lu^b and Au^a inhibits also, almost out of recognition, the antigen P_1. The inhibitor locus called *In(Lu)* is not linked to the *Lutheran* or *P* loci. Unlike P_1, the antigen P is not involved in the inhibition. It was anticipated that in Lu(a–b–) families a mating of the phenotype $P_2 \times P_2$ might be found with a P_1 offspring, and an example soon presented itself in a Sardinian family (Contreras and Tippett[149], 1974).

The subject of In(Lu) is discussed in the chapters on Lutheran and on Auberger.

Linkage and syntenic relations of the *P* locus

They are dealt with in the chapter on autosomal mapping. There is some evidence[142] that *P* is linked to *ADA* (adenosine deaminase).

Fellous and his colleagues[126–128] found that the antigens P and P_1 are detectable on fibroblasts, and furthermore their mouse-man hybrid cell cultures suggested that *P* and *HL-A* were syntenic. There is only slight evidence that *P* and *HL-A* may be linked (Edwards *et al.*[142]). However, since *HL-A* is generally believed to be on chromosome No. 6 and *ADA* on No. 20, the relation of *P* to these two loci is rather at hazard.

VARIATIONS IN STRENGTH OF THE P_1 ANTIGEN

Landsteiner and Levine, in their first communication[1] on the P groups, spoke of two grades of P_1 blood samples; one reacting strongly, and the other weakly, with anti-P_1 sera. In a later paper[5] they recorded their results in four categories which they properly called an 'arbitrary arrangement'. Several workers since have tackled the P_1 antigen quantitatively[8,17,24,25]. From the varying frequencies they report it is clear that the divisions of strength are indeed arbitrary.

Using a modification of Jonsson's titration method, Henningsen[8] found that it was not possible to subdivide P_1 blood samples into distinct categories: the results showed a normal curve of distribution. Similar results were obtained when the antigen strength was measured by the absorption method. Henningsen was not able to detect any suggestion of qualitative antigenic differences. The weakest antigen would remove all the agglutinin from an anti-P_1 serum.

The antigen strength was found to be considerably weaker in children, which agreed with the results of most previous workers.

The inheritance of the grades of strength of the P_1 antigen

Moharram[14] classified the P_1 members of his 12 families with 42 children into two grades and the results suggested that the strength was inherited.

Henningsen[9, 10] made a fine quantitative study of 221 families with 616 children (all included in Table 18). The P_1 members were divided arbitrarily into three classes, P_1 strong, P_1 medium and P_1 weak. When not masked by homozygosity each P_1 class was found to be inherited without significant variation. Henningsen concludes that 'offspring from a $P_1 \times P_2$ mating cannot have a receptor strength of greater potency than that of the positive parent, provided that a difference of at least two titration steps between the receptor strength of parent and offspring is claimed for the difference to be significant.'

Professor Sir Ronald Fisher after studying Henningsen's paper considered that this fine body of material deserved further analysis; Dr Henningsen therefore sent him the complete details of the 221 families.

Fisher's very subtle analysis must be consulted in the original[26]. From the nine mating classes involving a P_1 parent Fisher used the presence of P_2 children and the size of families without them to estimate the proportions of heterozygotes (P_1P_2) and homozygotes (P_1P_1) in P_1 strong, P_1 medium and P_1 weak parents. These estimates agreed closely with those calculated simply from the proportion of P_2 amongst the parents. As it seems that almost the last word on the subject is given in Fisher's summary we quote it in full.

An analysis of Henningsen's family data, in which parents are classified as Strong, Medium and Weak reactors to anti-P [anti-P_1] serum shows that these three phenotypic classes contain very unequal proportions of heterozygotes.

Subject to errors of random sampling, the proportions are estimated to be

Strong	..	33·597 per cent heterozygous
Medium	..	70·162 per cent heterozygous
Weak	..	100·000 per cent heterozygous

The total number of homozygotes estimated in this way, 123·9, agrees closely with the number 122·6, estimated from the proportion of Negative parents.

Of the total number enumerated it appears that the homozygotes are about equally divided between the Strong and Medium phenotypes; while of the heterozygotes about 14 per cent are Strong, 67 per cent Medium and 19 per cent Weak.

Homozygosity is therefore a well-established cause of the variation of reactive strength. As to the residual causes, it would appear premature yet to infer even that these are of genetic origin, still less that they can be ascribed to a series of recognizable alleles at the P locus.

THE ENLARGEMENT OF THE P SYSTEM

Though its birth had been so illustrious the P system for 28 years seemed rather puny because we knew only of the weaker of its antibodies. But, when the antigen Tj^a, present in the vast majority of people[6], and the corresponding antibody anti-Tj^a were seen[7] to be part of P the system emerged as a strong system with regularly occurring antibody, like anti-A and anti-B in the ABO system, but more violent than anti-A or anti-B in haemolytic power.

The recognition[59,60], in 1959, of the antigen P^k showed the P groups to be at least as complicated as ABO: but when the Luke serum was found[79], the reactions of which were influenced by the P *and* the ABO groups, we began to feel lost in amazement at the complexity of the P system.

The phenotype p

This rare phenotype, originally called Tj(a−), was described by Levine, Bobbitt, Waller and Kuhmichel[6] in 1951. In the next four years four more examples were found[34−37]: all the propositi and all of their compatible sibs had anti-Tj^a in their serum.

Samples of blood from three unrelated Tj(a−) persons were tested by one of us[7] and all three were negative with anti-P$_1$. This was startling, for only one white person in five is negative. Excited scrutiny of published work then showed that the P groups of three other unrelated Tj(a−) persons and of one sib had been recorded and all four were negative with anti-P$_1$. The probability that six consecutive unrelated Tj(a−) persons should be negative with anti-P$_1$ merely by chance was too remote to be entertained.

It was then found that if anti-Tj^a sera were absorbed by P$_2$ cells anti-P$_1$ was left behind. Thus both the antigen Tj^a and the antibody anti-Tj^a behaved as if they

Table 24. The expanded P system. (After Sanger[7], 1955)

Phenotypes					Approximate European frequencies
Anti-PP$_1$	Anti-P$_1$	Symbol	Antigens	Genotypes	
+	+	P$_1$	P P$_1$	P_1P_1	29%
				P_1P_2	50%
				P_1p	0%
+	−	P$_2$	P	P_2P_2	21%
				P_2p	0%
−	−	p	none detected	pp	0%

Anti-PP$_1$ is the antibody once called anti-Tj^a, Anti-P$_1$ is the antibody once called anti-P. P$_1$ is the phenotype once called P+. P$_2$ is the phenotype once called P−. p is the phenotype once called Tj(a−).

6*

belonged to the P system. All subsequent examples of Tj(a−) have, when tested, been found to be negative with anti-P_1.

The P system as it appeared in 1955 is summarized in Table 24. We thought of p as a recessive character controlled by a third allele, p, at the P_1P_2 locus.

The P system shows remarkable parallels to the A_1A_2O system (Table 25) which are useful at least as an aid to remembering the details of P. The usefulness of the analogy is limited by uncertainty about the serological relationship of A_1 to A_2.

Table 25. The P system and the A_1A_2O model. (After Sanger[7], 1955)

Presence of antigens and antibodies			
Red cell phenotype	Antibodies in serum	Red cell phenotype	Antibodies in serum
O	always anti-A+A_1	p	always anti-P+P_1
A_2	sometimes anti-A_1	P_2	sometimes anti-P_1
A_1	none	P_1	none

Behaviour of antigens and antibodies	
Anti-A+A_1	Anti-P+P_1
Absorption by A_2 cells leaves anti-A_1. Eluate from absorbing cells reacts more strongly with A_1 than with A_2 cells. Absorption by A_1 cells removes all antibody. Anti-A_1 is the last component to be removed.	Absorption by P_2 cells leaves anti-P_1. Eluate from absorbing cells reacts more strongly with P_1 than with P_2 cells. Absorption by P_1 cells removes all antibody. Anti-P_1 is the last component to be removed.

Frequency of p

In Table 26 are listed all the p propositi we know of: they come from many parts of the world. All the earlier examples had selected themselves out of unknown millions because of trouble caused by the antibody in their serum: no random p person had been found when more than 36,000 white people had been tested[6,34−36,40,80,81]. Vastly greater numbers of people had, in fact, been screened for p during the serum checks of routine ABO grouping or in cross-matching tests, in which the presence of anti-PP_1 would have led to further investigation.

However, in 1966 Dr Bertil Cedergren, working at the University Hospital, Umeå, began to find that p people were less rare in the county of Västerbotten in North Sweden. Because of this, the figures for North Sweden and for the rest of the world will be considered separately.

Outside North Sweden

No random p person having been found, we attempted to get some idea of the frequency of the phenotype using the Lenz-Dahlberg formula given on page 483.

Table 26. A summary of p people and their relatives

Reference	Propositus and country	Sibs p	Sibs P₁	Sibs P₂	Spouse	Children P₁	Children P₂	Parents Father	Parents Mother	Parents Consanguinity
Levine et al.[6]	Mrs Jay. (U.S.A.)	1		2		0	4			1st cousins
	her p sib		not p							
Zoutendyk et al.[34]	Mrs Mc. (S. Africa)					7	0			no information
Hirszfeld et al.[35]	Frau Z. (Poland)							P₂	P₁	no information
Walsh et al.[36]	Mrs Y. (Australia)	1	4 not p			0	2			not related
Levine et al.[37]	Mrs E.E. (U.S.A.)	1	0	1				P₂	P₂	1st cousins
Davidsohn et al.[38] Blood Group Res. Unit[89]	Mrs El. (Canada, now England)	0	1	0	P₂		2		P₁	not related
Iseki et al.[41,39]	Mrs Rit. Ho. (Japan)	3	0	1		1	0	P₂		not related
Sanger et al.[40]	Herr K. (Germany)									not related
McNeil et al.[42]	Mr T.C. (U.S.A.)	1	0	0					P₁	1st cousins
Broman[51]; Cedergren[80]	Fru X. (or G.W.) (N. Sweden)	0	0	1	P₂			P₂	P₂	not related
Yasuda et al.[52,53]	Mrs A.K. (Japan)	0	0	1		0		P₂	P₂	not related
Friedlander et al.[54]	Mr Or. (U.S.A.)	1	0	3			2		P₂	not related
Stern and Busch[55]	Mrs L.L. (U.S.A.)	5	1	3				P₁	P₂	1st cousins†
Catino et al.[82]	her p cousin, A*	0	0	5						1st cousins
	her p cousin, D*	0	0	5						1st cousins
	her p cousin, E*	0	4	1				P₂	P₁	1st cousins once removed
Woods et al.[56]	Mr F.H. (U.S.A.)	0	2 not p							not related
Ryttinger[57]	Fru E.K. (Sweden)	0	1	0						not related
Waller[72]	Mr M.H. (U.S.A.)	0				0	3		P₁	1st cousins†

Table 26—continued

Reference	Propositus and country	Sibs p	Sibs P_1	Sibs P_2	Spouse	Children P_1	Children P_2	Parents Father	Parents Mother	Consanguinity
Salmon et al.[73]	Mme Mag. (France) her p sib	1	0	1	P_1	1	0	P_2	P_2	not related
Fisher and Cahan[83]	Mr M.K. (U.S.A.)									no information
Rosenfield et al.[84]	Snra Cav. (Italy)	0	3	0	P_1	3	1	P_1	P_1	no information
Cedergren[80]	Fröken S.L. (N. Sweden)	1	2	1				P_2	P_2	2nd cousins
	her p cousin, Fru T.A.									1st cousins
Cedergren[80]	Fru G.N. (N. Sweden)	2	0	4	P_2	0	3	P_2	P_1	2nd cousins
Cedergren[80]	Fru A.J. (N. Sweden)	0	3	0	P_1	0	2			not related
Cedergren[80]	Herr A.K. (N. Sweden)	0	1	0	P_1	0	1		P_1	not related
Cedergren[80]	Fru U.W. (N. Sweden)	0	1	0	P_1	1	1		P_1	not related
Cedergren[80]	Herr D.N. (N. Sweden)	0	1	0				P_1	P_1	3rd cousins
Broman[85], Cedergren[80]	Fru V.I.S. (N. Sweden)				P_1			P_2	P_1	not related
Hornstein and Pinkas-Schweitzer[86]	Mrs N.P. (Israel, Moroccan)	1	1 not p	0						not related
dos Santos et al.[87]	Mr N.Y. (Barbados)	0	1	0		3	0		P_1	no information
Tovey and Crossland[88]	Mrs P.W. (England)	0	0	3				P_2	P_2	not related
Molthan and M. Levine[114]	Mr R.S. (Philadelphia, Negro)									no information
Hayashida et al.[115]	Mrs S.S. (Taiwan)	0	0	1	P_1	0	1			not related
Cedergren[80]	Herr M.M. (N. Sweden)	0	0	3	P_1	1	0	P_2	P_1	not related
Cedergren[80]	Fru S.La (N. Sweden)	2	1	3	P_1	0	1	P_1	P_2	not related
Cedergren[80]	Herr H.J. (N. Sweden)	2	4	0						1st cousins
Cedergren[80]	Herr E.G. (N. Sweden)	1	0	1				P_2	P_2	2nd cousins
Cedergren[80]	Herr P.F. (N. Sweden)	0	5	0						not related
Cedergren[80]	Fru B.A. (N. Sweden)				P_1	1	0	P_1	P_1	not related
Cedergren[80]	Fröken D.E. (N. Sweden)	0	0	2				P_2	P_2	not related

Table 26—*continued*

| Reference | Propositus and country | Sibs | | | Spouse | Children | | Parents | | |
		p	P₁	P₂		P₁	P₂	Father	Mother	Consanguinity
Cedergren[80]	Fru M.L. (N. Sweden)	1	0	0		0	2	P₁		not related
Cedergren[80]	Fru C.O. (N. Sweden)				P₂				P₂	not related
Guévin et al.[116]	Mlle G.H. (Canada)	2	2	3				P₂	P₁	1st cousins
Bidet et al.[117]	Mons E.H. (France)				P₂	0	3			not related
Metaxas[118]	Snra A.P. (Italy)	1	0	0	P₁					not related
Levene and Izakson[119]	Mrs A.T. (Israel, Moroccan, 1st cousin of N.P. above)*	0	1	1	P₂	0	1			not related
Bitz and Ehrke[138]	Mrs D.K. (Turkey)									no information
Speiser[143]	Frau E.J. (Austria)	1	1	0	P₁	1	0		P₂	2nd cousins
Tomita and Nakajima[144]	Mr N.F. (Japan)	0	3	1				P₂		not related
Yokota and Nakajima[147]	Miss T.N. (Japan)									not related
Yamaguchi et al.[145]	Mr Miy. (Japan)*	2	0	1				p**	P₂	not related
Miwa et al.[146]	Mr H.S. (Japan)*	0	0	1					p	2nd cousins
	his p mother*	1	0	0						not related
Salmon and Gerbal[121]	Mons J.M. (France)	1	2	1						no information
Salmon and Gerbal[121]	Mme S.B. (Tunisia)	1	0	0						no information
Salmon and Gerbal[121]	Mons C.T. (Armenia)	0	2	0					P₁	no information
Battaglini and Melis[150]	Mme H.J. (Tunisia)	1	4	3	P₂ 2nd cous.	3p	5	P₂	P₁	6th cousins
Cleghorn[151]	Mr A.L. (England)	1	1	2				P₁	P₂	not related

* Not included in the sib count in the text.
** Parents probably related, they came from the same island in the Inland Sea.
† Originally thought to be unrelated.
Some more recent p propositi (3 from U.S.A. and 5 from Tunisia or Algeria) for whom there is no family information are not included in this table.

We guessed the first cousin marriage rate in the countries involved to be 0·01: the first cousin marriage rate of the parents of the non-Northern Swedish propositi of Table 26 is 0·21. From this the formula gives the frequency of the gene p as 0·0024 and of the phenotype as 5·8 in a million.

In Northern Sweden

Cedergren[139] describes the systematic screening of 40,149 blood donors, pregnant women and patients with a variety of diseases living in the Västerbotten county: 8 p people were found. After some allowance had been made for coefficients of inbreeding, a p gene frequency of 0·0119 was arrived at, and a phenotype frequency of 141 in a million. This observed incidence of p people in Västerbotten is about 24 times that roughly estimated for people elsewhere.

Inheritance of the phenotype p

Table 26 contains all the useful information we can extract from the literature or from correspondence about p people and their relatives.

We assume that the phenotype p reflects a homozygous genetic background for two main reasons. First, of the sibs of the propositi in Table 26 about a quarter are p: of the 119 sibs 32 are p and 87 not p, very close to the incidence expected if p were a recessive character. Second, the high consanguinity rate of the parents of these propositi again directly points to a recessive homozygous background.

But for what is the p phenotype homozygous? There are two obvious possibilities: p people may be homozygous for (i) a third allele at the P_1P_2 locus, p; or, for what is practically the same thing, a suppressor gene built into the P_1 or P_2 gene complex: (ii) an allele at some other, not attached, locus—a 'regulator' allele with the faculty to prevent the P_1 and P_2 genes expressing themselves as antigens.

If (i) were correct, the parents of p people would have to be heterozygous P_1p or P_2p and we would expect the phenotype distribution of these parents to match the P_1P_2 gene frequencies appropriate to their racial groups. A count of parents from Table 26 (leaving out the Japanese, who have a very high incidence of the phenotype P_2, and the Barbadian family, and counting only the first two parents in the curiously inbred family reported by Stern and Busch) comes to 20 P_1 and 25 P_2. This is close to the approximate 50:50 gene frequency expected of Europeans in general and closer still to the somewhat higher rate of the gene P_2 in parts of Sweden[140] and the distinctly higher rate in Finland[67].

If (ii) were correct, the parents would be heterozygous at the unlinked 'regulator' locus and should have the normal P phenotype distribution appropriate to their racial groups: the observed 20 P_1 and 25 P_2 represent a significant excess of P_2 parents, far removed from the normal P phenotypes, even of Scandinavians[67].

The P groups of the children of p people also favour p being due to homozygosity for an allele p rather than for an unlinked suppressor or 'regulator' gene:

of all 17 children of 5 P_2 × p matings none is P_1; of 15 children of 10 P_1 × p matings 8 are P_1 and 7 P_2.

We realize that these calculations concerning the precise genetical background of the recessive character p are somewhat unsatisfactory: the propositi come from different countries and even within a country there may be isolates with different frequencies of P_1 and P_2. In addition, the high abortion rate in p mothers (see Table 29, page 170) may introduce another complication. However, excepting Africans and Japanese as we have done, we think the P frequencies in the parts of the world from which the propositi came are near enough alike to give a lot of weight to our argument that p is an allele of P_1 and P_2.

We are greatly indebted to Dr Cedergren for generously contributing so many hard won and so far unpublished facts to Table 26.

Possible existence of an antigen p

In 1971 Engelfriet and his colleagues in Amsterdam[129] investigated the blood of a 72-year-old woman, suffering from pulmonary fibrosis, who had had a bout of jaundice. Her red cells were P_1. Her serum contained an antibody which was probably anti-p though the authors were not dogmatic about this.

Three samples of her serum were tested and the following antibodies reported in the first sample '(1) agglutinins, the reaction of which was best at lower temperatures and much stronger with pp than with P_1 or P_2 cells; (2) warm haemolysins, only reactive with enzyme treated pp cells; (3) biphasic haemolysins, reacting well with non-enzyme treated cells and much stronger with pp than with P_1 or P_2 cells'. In the second sample there were: '(1) cold agglutinins, only reactive with pp and not with P_1, P_2 or P_1^k cells; (2) warm haemolysins, also only reacting with pp cells; (3) biphasic haemolysins, the titre of which with pp cells had remained unchanged, but now no reaction was obtained with P_1, P_2 or P_1^k cells.' The activity of this second sample was removed by absorption with p but not with P_1 or the patient's own cells. In the third sample no antibody apart from her anti-B was found. In the investigation 5 different examples of p cells and 2 of P_1^k were used.

If anti-p exists, as it probably does, then the schemes for the P system as a whole (pages 161–163) will need extension, and p could no longer be thought of as an amorph.

Another phenotype

A 'new' phenotype belonging to the P system was found by Mrs M.L. Darrah of Ravenna, Ohio and Mr A.G. Gelb of East Brunswick, New Jersey, who kindly let us join in the investigation. Anti-PP_1P^k was found in the serum of a white woman, Mrs O.H., aged 79, whose cells, unexpectedly, were not p: she had never been transfused. Mrs O.H.'s cells, which are P_2 (and negative with anti-P^k) reacted with 8 out of 12 anti-PP_1P^k sera from p people and with all of 9 anti-P sera from P^k people: the reactions were much weaker than those given by control P_2 cells and the four sera which failed to react were the weakest in our collection. The cells of

Mrs O.H. did not react with the anti-Luke serum (page 163) nor with an anti-P from a case of paroxysmal cold haemoglobinuria (page 171).

The anti-PP$_1$P^k in Mrs O.H.'s serum reacted strongly with all P$_1$, P$_2$ and P^k cells tested but did not react with any of 16 p samples or with her own cells: hydatid cyst fluid inhibited the antibody reaction for P^k but not for P$_1$ or P$_2$ cells.

The P groups of Mrs O.H.'s relatives are normal: both of her surviving sibs are P$_1$: her two daughters are P$_2$, and all four are Luke (+). Her parents were said not to be consanguineous.

This interesting family has not been included in Table 26 since Mrs O.H. is not p. There is nothing in her history to suggest an environmental cause and her cells and serum did not change in their behaviour in several samples taken over a period of ten months; the antibody had evidently been present five years previously when cross-matching difficulty prevented her having a transfusion. If, as seems likely, her phenotype is reflecting her true genotype then a gene allelic to P$_1$, P$_2$ and p is perhaps the best guess.

A perhaps similar phenotype in a Puerto Rican woman was recently described by Allen et al.[134]: her antibody (page 168) however differed in that it reacted only weakly with i cells and it had no anti-P^k component.

The red cell phenotype P^k

Though extremely rare, even in Finland, the red cell antigen P^k is of extraordinary interest because, unlike practically all other blood group antigens, it is not inherited as a straightforward dominant character, and because of the light it should be able to throw on the P system as a whole and because of the startling detection of the antigen in cultured fibroblasts (page 161).

The phenotype P^k was realized to be associated with the P system when a sample of blood was found to contain an anti-Tj^a-like antibody though the cells did not give the expected negative reaction with antibodies from p people (Matson, Swanson, Noades, Sanger and Race[59], 1959).

Reactions of P^k

The positive reaction of P^k cells with the serum of p people (previously thought to contain only two antibodies, anti-P$_1$ and anti-P) showed that a third antibody component was present, anti-P^k. Isolated anti-P^k can be left in the serum of some p people by absorption with P$_1$ cells.

The antibody which occurs regularly in the serum of P^k people is anti-P, one of the antibodies in the serum of p people.

All P^k people have the antigen P^k and lack the antigen P: the majority have the antigen P$_1$ (phenotype P$_1^k$) but some lack P$_1$ (phenotype P$_2^k$). Different examples of P$_1^k$ cells vary in the strength of their reaction with anti-P$_1$, just as P$_1$ cells do. On the other hand all examples of P$_1^k$ or P$_2^k$ cells we have tested reacted equally strongly with anti-P^k.

The interactions of the system are summarized in Table 27. Serological intricacies are dealt with by Kortekangas, Kaarsalo, Melartin, Tippett, Gavin, Noades, Sanger and Race[90].

Table 27. The P groups defined by the three antibodies anti-P_1, anti-P and anti-P^k

Approximate frequency	Phenotype	Anti-P_1 P_2 people or animals	Anti-PP_1P^k (anti-Tj^a) p people	Anti-P P^k people	Anti-P^k Anti-PP_1P^k absorbed by P_1 cells
75%	P_1	+	+	+	−
25%	P_2	−	+	+	−
v. rare	p	−	−	−*	−
v. rare	P_1^k	+	+	−	+
v. rare	P_2^k	−	+	−	+

* Some examples of anti-P do react weakly.

Frequency of the antigen P^k

Even in Finland the antigen P^k must be very rare: Kaarsalo, Kortekangas, Tippett and Hamper[67] found no sample negative with anti-P in testing 571 unrelated people, nor did Nevanlinna and Furuhjelm[91] in testing 28,677 more. That the antigen is very rare is certain, for the accompanying anti-P would disclose itself in cross-matching tests and serum checks in the routine ABO grouping of donors. Dr Darnborough tells us that in Cambridge they have tested 39,939 donors with anti-P from two P^k sisters without finding a single negative.

Over 20 P^k propositi have so far been found (Table 28) and no relationship has been traced between them; their relatives provide further examples. Eleven of the families are Finnish. The original descriptions will be found in Matson et al.[59] and Kortekangas et al.[60,61,90]. These papers deal with the families of the first five propositi. The cases following Rouva Usk in Table 28 are mostly unpublished and we are grateful to the investigators for the details given in that table.

Inheritance of the red cell antigen P^k

The P^k families of Table 28 were investigated more energetically than were the p families of Table 26. Of the first eight propositi found in Finland no fewer than 366 relatives were tested.

P^k is highly unusual amongst blood group antigens in not being inherited as a straightforward dominant character. The antigen must reflect a recessive, homozygous, background for the following reasons. (i) All the parents so far tested of P^k people have lacked the antigen (Figure 9 and Table 28). (ii) A count of the sibs of the P^k propositi in Table 28 is 15 P^k and 35 not P^k, which is close to the $1:3$ ratio expected of a recessive character. (iii) Five of 23 P^k propositi have definitely consanguineous parents and others may have.

The gene responsible for P^k is not an allele, recessive in effect, at the P_1P_2 locus. This is shown by the following observations. (i) The children of P^k people have the normal Finnish distribution of P_1 or P_2 phenotypes (there are 25 P_1 and 11 P_2 Finnish children in Table 28): were P^k an allele the phenotypes of these children should be distributed in proportion to the gene frequencies of P_1 and P_2 in Finland,

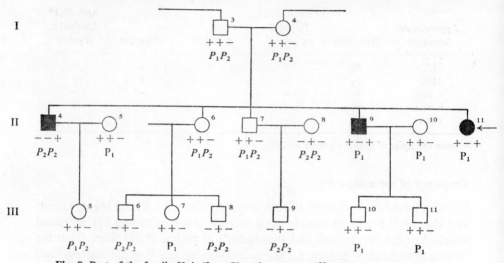

Fig. 9. Part of the family Koi. (from Kortekangas *et al.*[90], 1965) illustrating the inheritance of the red cell antigen P^k, and its genetical independence of the P_1P_2 locus.

Black $= P^k$, hollow $=$ absence of P^k. The $+$ and $-$ signs represent the agglutination reactions of the red cells with anti-P_1, anti-P and anti-P^k, in that order. The P groups are given as phenotypes or, when disclosed by parents or offspring, as genotypes.

which is near to $50:50$ P_1 and P_2. (ii) A family was found in which a P^k mother and a P_2 father had one P_1 and three P_2 children (Kortekangas *et al.*[90]).

From the realization[89,90] that P^k people had ordinary P_1 or P_2 genes it followed that the phenotype P_2^k should exist, and, after several years wait, the first example was found (II-4 in Figure 9: more have since disclosed themselves[93,94,122]).

If it be allowed that P^k is a homozygous condition, the family in Figure 9 confirms that the locus responsible for P^k is not part of the P locus and further it shows that the P^k locus is not closely linked to the P locus: if P^k were due to an allele at the P locus, or to genes at an adjacent locus, then all the P^k children of I-3 and I-4 should have the same P phenotype but this is not so: the cells of II-4 do not react with anti-P_1 while those of II-9 and II-11 do. (Another family showing the genetical independence of the two loci was later to be found by Yokota and Nakajima[147].)

Table 28. A summary of P^k people and their relatives

| | | Relatives of propositi | | | | | | | | | |
| | | Sibs | | | | | Children | | Parents | | |
Reference	Propositus and country	P_1^k	P_2^k	P_1	P_2	Spouse	P_1	P_2	Father	Mother	Consanguinity
Matson et al.[59]	Mrs Mys. (U.S.A., Finnish)	1	0	3	0	P_2	3	2		P_1	not related
	her P_1^k sib						0	3			
Kortekangas et al.[60]	Rouva Pel. (Finnish)	1	0	6	0	P_2	0	1	P_1	P_1	not related
	her P_1^k sib					P_1	2	0			
Kortekangas et al.[90]	Rouva Rain. (Finnish)	0	0	2	0	P_1	3	0			not related
	her mother's sibs	3	0	0	0						not related
	her mat. uncle					P_1	2	1			
	her mat. uncle						1	1			
	her mat. aunt					P_2	1	3			
Kortekangas et al.[90]	Rouva Koi. (Finnish)	1	1	2	0	P_1	1	0	P_1	P_1	not related
	her P_2^k sib					P_1	2	0			
	her P_1^k sib					P_1					
Kortekangas et al.[90]	Rouva Usk. (Finnish)	0	0	2	0	P_1	2	0		P_1	not related
Nevanlinna and Furuhjelm[91]	Herra Vaa. (Finnish)	0	0	2	0				P_2	P_1	not related*
Kaarsalo et al.[92]	Herra Tam. (Finnish)	0	0	1	0	P_1	4	0	P_1	P_2	not related
Nevanlinna and Furuhjelm[91]	Rouva Vei. (Finnish)	1	0	2	0	P_1	4	0	P_1	P_1	not related*
Stroup et al.[93]	Mrs Hea. (U.S.A., Scottish-Irish)	0	0	1	1	P_1	1	0		P_1	1st cousins

Table **28**—*continued*

		Relatives of propositi									
		Sibs				Spouse	Children		Parents		
Reference	Propositus and country	P_1^k	P_2^k	P_1	P_2		P_1	P_2	Father	Mother	Consanguinity
Stroup et al.[93]	Miss Hoc. (U.S.A., white, not Finnish)										not related
Kaarsalo[92]	Rouva Ahl. (Finnish)										not related
Miki and Hayashida[94]	Mrs Sug. (Japanese)	0	1	0	3	P_2					1st cousins
Schneider et al.[120]	Herr G.R. (German)	1	0	1	0				P_1		not related
Salmon and Gerbal[121]	Mons Sto. (French)									P_1	not related
Salmon and Gerbal[121]	Mme Dab. (French) her P_1^k sib	1	0	0	1		2 / 1	1 / 1		P_1	2nd cousins
Stevenson[123]	Mrs M.S. (U.S.A., white)	1	0	1	0					P_1	uncle:niece
Klossner[122]	Herra A.L. (Finnish)										not related*
Brueton and Giles[136]	Mr H.P. (English) his P_1^k sib	3	0	1	1		3	0		P_1	not related
van der Hart[137]	Mrs W.B-K. (Dutch)	0	0	1	0						no information
van der Hart[137]	Mrs L.K.-L. (Dutch)	0	0	2	1						no information
Yokota and Nakajima[147]	Mr H.K. (Japanese)	0	0	0	1	P_1	2	0			not related
Yamaguchi et al.[145]	Mr Mae. (Japanese)	0	0	0	1				P_1	P_2	1st cousins

All propositi are P_1^k except Miss Hoc., Mrs Sug., Herra A.L. and Mr Mae. who are P_2^k.
* But their paternal and maternal ancestors lived in the same area.

We therefore thought of the antigen P^k as due not to an allele at the P locus but to genes somewhere in the dark background of the P system which will now be discussed.

Attempts to relate the inheritance of the phenotypes P_1, P_2, p and P^k

We do not believe that a blood group antigen can be a recessive character in the simple sense that a double dose of an allele is needed before the antigen can appear. We prefer to think along the lines of the Morgan-Watkins-Ceppellini approach to the interactions of the ABO, H, secretor and Lewis genes (Figure 22, page 342). According to this scheme an antigen that may appear to be recessive is seen as an earlier substance along an assembly line, a substance which would, in the presence of a gene dominant in effect, be converted into something else: two genes recessive in effect do not mould the substance but let it through unchanged—give it a bye into the next round.

We have attempted two such schemes[95, 90] both of which foundered on then uncharted facts, but, undaunted, we tried a third (Figure 10) which, as will be seen in the next paragraph, has probably met the same fate. The scheme, however, does illustrate the general course on which we expected the solution to be found and it may help to remember the facts, which lie to the east in the figure.

P^k on fibroblasts of all but p people

At a meeting of the European Society of Human Genetics in Amsterdam in 1972 Fellous, Tessier, Gerbal, Salmon, Frézal and Dausset[130] in a notable paper gave the astonishing news that the antigen P^k, so extremely rare on red cells, could be demonstrated on the cultured fibroblasts of all of 9 P_1 and 10 P_2 people tested but not on the fibroblasts of 7 p people.

As a possible explanation of absence of P^k from the red cells of ordinary people yet presence in their fibroblasts Fellous and his colleagues proposed that P^k is an almost universal 'public' gene which is prevented from expressing itself on red cells by the genotypes Ff or FF: the Ff locus, unlinked to P^k, having the same sort of control over the red cells as the $Sese$ locus over the secretion of ABH in the saliva. The genotype ff, which allows P^k to be expressed on the red cells, would have to be very rare indeed.

Fellous and his colleagues[152] then turned attention to the results of their mouse-man hybrid cultures involving samples from P_1 or P_2 people. Fifty clones were examined for the PP_1 and P^k antigens with the following results:

		PP_1	
		+	−
P^k	+	16	0
	−	15	19

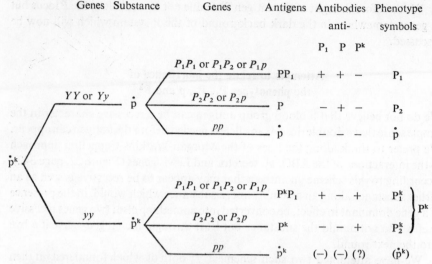

Fig. 10. A very tentative interpretation of the genetic background of the P system. p^k represents a hypothetical precursor substance which is acted on successively by a gene Y, converting p^k to p, and by P_1 and P_2, converting p to PP_1 and P respectively. p is considered an amorph which makes no conversion of p substance. The gene y is also considered an amorph, making no conversion of p^k substance which then becomes exposed to the action of P_1 and P_2, and these genes convert p^k into P^kP_1 and P^k respectively. The facts would not allow the P_1P_2p locus to be closely linked to the hypothetical Yy locus.

The reactions in the columns headed antibodies are those of the three clearly defined antibodies with cells of the phenotypes of the last column. The existence of a phenotype p^k is theoretical only, and this is indicated by brackets: even if it can exist its rarity should be such that it might never be encountered.

Note: In this figure p̊ is used in place of the roman p in order to distinguish it more clearly from P, a helpful suggestion of our printers for the purpose of this figure only. In this fount roman p can be distinguished from P if lined up as in the text, but in the wide separation of such a diagram it scarcely can: the italic p and P do not present such a difficulty. We had no intention that p̊ should be used as symbol for p as it has once or twice been taken to be.

P^k could depart from a clone whether PP_1 remained or not; and this was taken to confirm that P^k is genetically independent of the P locus. On the other hand P^k did not remain when PP_1 had departed; and this suggested that in the biosynthetic pathway the PP_1 genes act earlier than the P^k genes. They pointed out that if the pathway of Figure 10 were correct, had p^k substance preceded the action of the P genes, the hybrid clones should have fallen out thus:

		PP_1	
		+	−
P^k	+	n.1	n.2
	−	0	n.3

As a result of their work on fibroblasts in simple and in hybrid culture Fellous and his colleagues proposed the scheme shown in Figure 11, which is, no doubt nearer the truth than ours in Figure 10. (If, however, an antigen p does exist, page 155, it will call for some modification of either scheme, because the gene *p* could no longer be thought of as an amorph.)

Looking at the scheme in Figure 11, *F* may be considered a dominant inhibitor of P^k on the red cells, just as *In(Lu)* is a dominant inhibitor of Lu^a and Lu^b (page 267). It is perhaps surprising that *F* does not also inhibit P$_1$ in the red cells, since

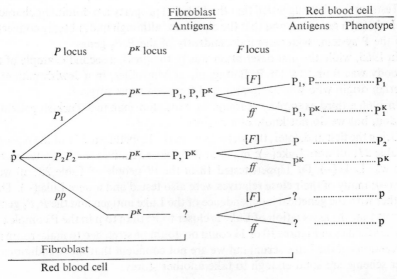

Fig. 11. A model for the biosynthesis of the P system antigens (from Fellous *et al.*[152], 1974). 'ṗ represents an hypothetical precursor which is acted upon, first by the *P*, and second by the *P^k* locus; the genes *P$_1$* or *P$_2$* transform this ṗ substrate into the PP$_1$ and P specificity, respectively, the *p* allele which is considered an amorph at the locus, does not cause any conversion of the substrate. *P^k* is a very frequent public gene which transforms the P antigen to the P^k specificity. Moreover the *Ff* system acts on the biosynthesis pathway only in the red cell and mature lymphocyte. The *f* allele is considered an amorph.'

P^k and P$_1$ are so alike in their inhibition reactions. It is to be hoped that this fascinating work will continue: it would be interesting to know, for example, whether P is to be found on the fibroblasts of people with P^k on their red cells, as the scheme appears to require.

The Luke phenotypes

A further complication of the P system was introduced in 1965 when Tippett, Sanger, Race, Swanson and Busch[79] reported an agglutinating system which they called Luke. The agglutinin was found in the serum of a Negro, Mr Luke P. who had never been transfused and was suffering from Hodgkin's disease. The problem was kindly referred by Dr W.T. Snoddy of Oklahoma City.

The Luke antibody is like anti-P in that it fails to react with the cells of p and P^k people but unlike anti-P in that it further fails to react with the cells of about 2% of P_1 and P_2 people.

The antibody gave three grades of reaction (+), (w) and (−). A further complication was that the (w) and (−) reactions were very significantly more common with P_2 than with P_1 cells, and with A_1 and A_1B cells than with O, A_2, A_2B and B cells.

Tests on families suggested that the Luke(+) property is a dominant character and Luke(−) a recessive, and that the character, although undoubtedly connected with the P system, segregates independently of the P_1P_2 genes.

In 1965, while the first description was in the press, a second example of the antibody was found by Dr P. Battaglini, of Marseilles, in a Jewish patient of Algerian origin who was being prepared for open heart surgery.

In 1966 a third example was found by Miss Boorman in a Turkish patient in London, but we do not know of any since.

Using the first and, later, the second serum Dr Tippett tested 18 of the p people of Table 27: all were Luke(−); many of their close relatives were also tested but none was Luke(−). Dr Tippett tested 18 of the P^k people of Table 28: all were Luke(−); many of their close relatives were also tested and 6 were Luke(−). This, together with the genetical independence of the Luke antigen and the P_1P_2 genes, suggests that the association of Luke is closer to P^k than to p in the P complex.

The schemes in Figures 10 or 11 could no doubt be stretched to make room for the reactions of the Luke serum but we are not confident that the foundations of either scheme are solid enough to take another storey.

OTHER NOTES ABOUT THE P SYSTEM

Development of the P antigens

In its development the P_1 antigen again reflects the behaviour of the A_1 antigen. Henningsen[8] studied this problem and his results showed quite clearly that P_1 (like A_1) is usually not fully developed at birth. We[74] tested the blood of two '17 weeks' and one '12 weeks' foetus and were somewhat surprised to see that the cells of all three were agglutinated by anti-P_1 (human). This was later realized to be a rather general phenomenon: Ikin, Kay, Playfair and Mourant[75] found that younger foetuses were more frequently and more strongly P_1 than were older foetuses.

We tested the cord blood of a child who is of the genotype P_2p: the antigen P was well developed. No P^k person has yet been tested at birth. The Luke antigen is well developed in cord blood[79].

The development of the antigen P_1 in infancy was particularly studied by Heiken[77] who concluded: 'The results of the family investigations indicate that the age for the complete development of the P_1 receptor might be as high as seven years or higher.'

Racial differences in distribution of P_1

There are marked differences which may possibly be useful in checking hypotheses about the P system: West Africans are over 95% P_1; Japanese[58] are only about 41% P_1. Most Europeans are about 78% P_1 but the frequency is somewhat lower in Finland[66,67], about 70% P_1. The Finnish gene frequencies[67] may be useful in thinking about P^k: $P_1 = 0.456$, $P_2 = 0.544$.

The identity of P_1 and Q

Henningsen established[27,28] that the blood group antigen reported from Japan and called Q is indeed the antigen P_1 of Landsteiner and Levine. The Q groups have been investigated by Furuhata and others since 1935, or earlier[24,29-33].

P_1- and P^k-like substances

Hydatid cyst fluid

The finding of a strong anti-P_1 in two patients suffering from hydatid disease led Cameron and Staveley[45] (1957) to the extraordinary discovery that the fluid from hydatid cysts of sheep's livers (provided they contain scolices) will inhibit anti-P_1 sera. The fluid also inhibits in part anti-P+P_1 sera (Staveley and Cameron[46]). Anti-P^k, like anti-P_1, is strongly inhibited, but anti-P is inhibited only weakly or not at all[59,60].

The P_1-like antigen in hydatid cyst fluid was used by Levine, Celano and Staveley[62,63] with some success to produce anti-P_1 in rabbits by injection of tanned human P_2 cells, or rabbit cells, which had been exposed to cyst fluid of sheep and human origin. Prokop and Oesterle[64] and Kerde, Fünfhausen, Brunk and Brunk[65], report the very successful immunization of goats with hydatid cyst fluid from pigs. In correspondence, Professor Prokop told us that they later thought that the response should have been attributed mainly to traces of pig substance in the cyst fluid. We have found the resulting anti-P_1 very useful indeed, especially in detecting weak P_1. Watkins and Morgan[96] were successful in producing powerful anti-P_1 in rabbits by injecting a phenol insoluble, water soluble preparation of P_1 substance made from sheep hydatid cyst fluid; the substance was coupled with the conjugated protein of the O somatic antigen of *Shigella shigae*.

The question whether P_2 people are more likely to get hydatid disease was studied by Gonano[97], in Sardinia, who found that the $P_1:P_2$ distribution in 86 cases did not differ significantly from the distribution in the normal population. On the other hand de Tapia[98] reports the finding of anti-P_1 in the serum of 8 out of

20 hydatid patients in Buenos Aires, which suggests a high frequency of P_2 (the P groups of the eight are not given).

Worms

Prokop and Schlesinger[99,100] provided the next surprise: *Lumbricus terrestris* caught freshly, gaily or briskly (according to our German–English dictionary) then cut up, dried, pulverized and extracted with saline, will inhibit anti-P_1 and also anti-B and anti-H. Extracts of other worms, including *Ascaris suum*, inhibit these antibodies too[100,101].

Prokop and Schlesinger[100] discuss the possibility that the anti-P_1 in P_2 people and the anti-PP_1P^k in p people may be the result of past immunization by ascaris or other parasites.

During an outbreak of liver fluke disease, Bevan *et al.*[124] reported that of 19 patients 5 were P_2 and had powerful anti-P_1 in their serum.

Chemistry of the P_1 substance

The discovery of P_1 substance in hydatid cyst fluid enabled Morgan and Watkins[96,102] to begin work on its chemistry. Having partially purified the P_1 component they showed it to be a glycoprotein, chemically similar to the ABH and Lewis substances, and that α-D-galactosyl units evidently played an important part in P_1 specificity. (And see Addenda.)

Marcus[135] isolated a substance with P_1 activity from red cell stroma and found it to be a galactose-containing glycosphingolipid which was, in view of the red cell ABH antigens, not surprising. (And see Addenda.)

Judging by straightforward inhibition of the anti-P^k:P^k red cell reaction Voak *et al.*[125] concluded that P^k is also α-galactose specific.

Antibodies of the P system

The interactions of the various antibodies and antigens of the system (excepting Luke) are shown in Table 27, page 157. In general the P antibodies are saline agglutinins and react more strongly at temperatures lower than 37°C.: some, especially anti-PP_1P^k, tend to announce themselves as haemolysins.

Anti-P_1

The first anti-P_1 sera were produced by rabbits stimulated by human red cells. Then it was recognized that anti-P_1 could occur naturally in human serum and did occur frequently in non-immune sera of animals of several different species. Excellent anti-P_1 sera have been made in goats and rabbits (see section above on hydatid cyst fluid).

A very surprising source of anti-P_1 was found by Schnitzler *et al.*[141] in extracts of the roe of *Rutilis rutilis* (Roach). The extract also had anti-B specificity which could not be separated from the anti-P_1.

Henningsen[8] observed that if anti-P_1 is sought for with a suitably sensitive technique it is found in the serum of P_2 persons with a regularity approaching that of the agglutinins of the ABO system: nevertheless, examples of the human antibody sufficiently powerful to be useful as reagents are rare.

As already mentioned, the antibody recognizes a wide range of strength of the P_1 antigen in P_1 and P_1^k cells.

The reaction of anti-P_1 with P_1 and with P_1^k cells is inhibited by hydatid cyst fluid and this can be a useful diagnostic tool.

Evidence that on rare occasions anti-P_1 can be stimulated by transfusion was given by Wiener and Peters[47] and by Wiener[48]. Moureau[49] reported a case in which a fatal haemolytic transfusion reaction was attributed to anti-P_1.

Mollison and Cutbush[70] described how about 50% of P_1 cells labelled with ^{51}Cr were rapidly eliminated from the circulation of a patient whose serum contained anti-P_1: the rest of the cells were eliminated very slowly.

Anti-PP_1P^k (anti-Tj^a)

The rare p people regularly have this antibody, or rather, these antibodies, in their serum. Absorption of anti-PP_1P^k sera by P_2 cells usually leaves anti-P_1 and anti-P^k. Absorption by P_1 cells sometimes leaves anti-P^k and sometimes does not: absorption of the serum of Mrs El. and of Mme Mag. (Table 26) by P_1 cells does leave avid specific anti-P^k. Absorption of the latter two sera by P_1^k cells leaves the expected pure anti-P; absorption by P_2^k cells, also as expected, leaves anti-P, but, unexpectedly, no anti-P_1 (as judged by subsequent negative reactions with P_1^k cells). This paradoxical ability of P_2^k cells to remove anti-P_1 from anti-PP_1P^k but not from ordinary anti-P_1 was a little further investigated by Kortekangas et al.[90], but no comforting explanation emerged. Voak et al.[125] suggest, as a possible explanation of this paradoxical observation, that certain anti-PP_1P^k sera may contain anti-P and anti-P_1^k, the hypothetical anti-P_1^k component being a cross-reacting antibody which reacts with P_1 cells and with P_1^k or P_2^k cells.

Mixed with hydatid cyst fluid the antibody behaves in the way expected of its supposed component parts: that is to say the anti-P_1 and anti-P^k are inhibited while the anti-P is not.

According to Wurzel et al.[131] 'It has previously been reported that anti-Tj^a antibodies are primarily IgM antibodies', but they had found two examples primarily IgG in nature.

Anti-P

This is present, apparently pure, in the serum of all known P^k people. (As mentioned above it can be isolated from some anti-PP_1P^k sera by absorption with P^k cells.) Anti-P reacts equally strongly with P_1 as with P_2 cells, and the reaction is not inhibited by hydatid cyst fluid. Most anti-P do not react with p cells though a minority do give a weak reaction[90].

Anti-P^k

Anti-P^k has not been found unaccompanied by other P antibodies. As noted above, avid and specific anti-P^k can be isolated from some, but not all, anti-PP_1P^k sera by absorption with P_1 cells.

Anti-P^k has given equally strong reactions with all P^k cells, whether P_1^k or P_2^k, so far tested. The reaction is completely inhibited by hydatid cyst fluid.

Miss Stroup and Mrs Gellerman, of Ortho, told us of their finding anti-P^k in the serum of a P_1 woman with autoimmune haemolytic anaemia. Dr Salmon (personal communication) found anti-P^k in the serum of one of 55 sufferers from autoimmune haemolytic anaemia and in 2 of 60 sufferers from biliary cirrhosis.

Luke antibody

Three examples of this antibody have been found (see page 155). In failing to react with p or P^k cells the Luke antibody declares its allegiance to the P system, but the nature of its loyalty is not clear. The original example gave (+), (w) and (−) reactions and the (w) reactions were sufficiently frequent for 2×2 tables to demonstrate that the antibody was sensitive to the A_1A_2BO groups as well as to the P_1 or P_2 groups of the cells. This sensitivity to the P and ABO groups was probably demonstrable because the antibody was a saline agglutinin (its reactions with (+) and (w) cells were stepped up proportionally if enzymes were used). Dr Tippett has not been able to show such sensitivity in the reactions of the second serum, perhaps because it is not a characteristic of all Luke sera or perhaps because the second antibody is not a straightforward agglutinin: it reacts best, after the addition of complement, by the antiglobulin test using trypinized cells, and the distinction between Luke (+) and Luke (w) is not easily made.

Anti-p

A serum probably containing this antibody[129] is described on page 155.

Anti-IP_1, anti-I^TP_1 and anti-IP

Just as I is related in some way not yet understood to the ABH antigens so it is to P_1. Issitt et al.[132] reported four antibodies apparently anti-P_1 but which did not react with P_1 i cells: and recently Miss Mia van der Hart told us this is a not uncommon finding. Booth[133] described an antibody in a Melanesian which at first appeared to be anti-P_1 but the strength of its reaction with P_1 cells was related to the I^T strength of the cells (see page 454). Allen et al.[134] reported an antibody of the specificity anti-IP: it was a reminder of the curious case of Mrs O.H. (page 155).

P antibodies and disease

Anti-P_1 seldom causes any trouble in transfusion. It is fortunate that anti-PP_1P^k and anti-P are very rare for, being powerful antibodies, they cause trouble in cross-matching and in ante-natal blood grouping.

Anti-PP_1P^k and early abortions

Anti-Tj^a, as it used to be called, was thought to be a cause of abortion early in pregnancy (Iseki, Masaki and Levine[39]; Levine and Koch[103]). However, the association was questioned[104]: it could be held that the relationship between antibody and abortion was apparent only, and simply due to the fact that people who have abortions are more likely than normal people to have their serum examined and so become candidates for recognition as owners of the antibody.

In several earlier editions of this book we were quite confident in our opinion that the apparent association could be attributed to ascertainment and that removal of propositi tested because they had had abortions left the rest with a more or less normal abortion rate. But now that the list of 'the rest' is longer, mainly due to the researches of Dr Cedergren, there is little doubt that Dr Iseki, Dr Levine and their colleagues were right all the time. In Table 29 there are now 31 p mothers who were recognized for reasons other than having had abortions: they have had 57 live children and 49 abortions, an abortion rate of 46%, much higher than that usually estimated for European people. It should be mentioned that 10 of the 49 abortions were provided by one N. Swedish kindred, possibly a warning that we may be running into some effect of stratification rather than association. Nevertheless, it does seem that the regular presence of anti-PP_1P^k in p females is a potent cause of abortion, and we would guess that it is the anti-P component which is responsible. The groups of the mothers and live children in this upper list of Table 29 do not suggest that ABO incompatibility is additionally involved.

Auto-anti-Tj^a and threatened abortion

A transient anti-Tj^a-like antibody was found in the serum of about one-third of Western Australian women in the Perth area who threatened to abort for the second time (Vos et al.[105], 1964; Vos[106–108]). The patients are of ordinary P groups, P_1 or P_2. (The antibody was not found in similar patients in Canada[105], the United States[105] or Hungary[109].)

The antibody reacted with all cells tested save p (we can find no reference to the testing of P^k cells). Though of the same, or similar, specificity, the antibody does not behave quite like the anti-PP_1P^k of p people: it haemolyses but does not agglutinate nor does it give an antiglobulin reaction. The antibody is heat labile: it is inactivated by heating at 56°C. for 30 minutes. Activity is not restored by adding complement. In fact, the antibody does not require complement[107].

As for the cause of the antibody, Vos et al.[105] wondered whether it might lie in environmental factors, such as 'viruses, diet, immunization, etc.'. Prokop and

Table 29. Ascertainment of p mothers with anti-PP_1P^k (anti-Tj^a) in their serum

	Live children	Abortions	Reason for serum examination
Mrs Jay.	4	0	pre-op. cross match
Her sister	7	0	sib of a propositus
Mrs Y.	2	1	a blood donor
Mrs El.	2	0	pre-op. cross match
Mrs R.	1	2	sib of a propositus (Mr T.C.)
Mrs Con.	0	4	sib of a propositus (Mr Or.)
Mrs L.L.	2	3	pre-op. cross match
Fru E.K.	0	1	pre-op. cross match
Mme Val.	1	0	sib of a propositus (Mme Mag.)
Snra Cav.	4	0	Ante-natal test
Fru A-M.B.	0	3	sib of a propositus (S.L.)
Fru G.N.	4	2	ante-natal test
Fru A.J.	2	0	transfusion complication
Fru U.W.	2	0	transfusion complication
Mme Mag.	1	0	cross-match, ectopic gestation
Mrs P.W.	0	1	ante-natal test
Mrs S.S.	1	0	child had h.d.n.
Fru T.A.	0	7	1st cousin of a propositus (S.L.)
Fru K.W.	0	1	sib of a propositus (G.N.)
Fru S.La.	1	1	cross-match, hypertonia
Fru G.L.	0	1	sib of a propositus (S.La.)
Fru B.A.	2	0	ante-natal test
Snra A.P.	3	0	post-partum cross-match
Fru M.L.	2	2	ante-natal test
Frau E.J.	1	3	ante-natal test
Frau H.F.	1	1	sib of a propositus (E.J.)
Mrs ?	1	0	sib of a propositus (Mr Miy.)
Mrs S.S.	2	1	mother of a propositus (Mr H.S.)
Mrs S.H.	1	7	sib of a propositus (Mrs S.S.)
Mme H.J.	9	3	ante-natal test
Mrs A.T.	1	5	pre-op. cross-match
	57	49	
Mrs Mc.	0	4	abortions
Frau Z.	0	4	abortions
Mrs E.E.	0	3	abortions
Mrs Rit.Ho.	0	6	abortions
Fru X. (or G.W.)	1	3	abortions
Mrs A.K.	0	9	abortions
Mrs N.P.	1	7	abortions
Fru V.I.S.	0	4	abortions
Fru C.O.	0	3	abortions
Mrs D.K.	0	10	abortions
	2	53	

The references to the papers describing these cases are to be found in Table 26 (page 151).

Schlesinger[100] suggest that infestation by nemathelminthes might possibly be the stimulus. But they remain a puzzle, do those eclectic aborters of Perth.

Auto-anti-P in paroxysmal cold haemoglobinuria

In 1963, Levine, Celano and Falkowski[110] found that the serum of six PCH patients would haemolyse P_1 and P_2 cells but not p or P^k cells, and this was confirmed by van der Hart and her colleagues[111] on a further two cases and by Worledge and Rousso[112] on eleven more. All patients so far tested are of the phenotype P_1 or P_2.

Unlike the antibody in the serum of the threatened aborters of Perth the PCH antibody gives a strong antiglobulin reaction with cells that have survived haemolysis. Again unlike the Perth antibody, sensitization at low temperature is a necessary preliminary to haemolysis.

Weiner, Gordon and Rowe[113] point out that the PCH antibody is not always anti-P.

Though p and P^k are extremely rare red cell phenotypes, the recognition of their existence brought about a revolution in the P groups which, from being the least, emerged as one of the most interesting of the systems.

REFERENCES

1   LANDSTEINER K. and LEVINE P. (1927) Further observations on individual differences of human blood. *Proc. Soc. exp. Biol. N.Y.*, **24**, 941–942.
2   LANDSTEINER K. and LEVINE P. (1930) On the inheritance and racial distribution of agglutinable properties of human blood. *J. Immunol.*, **18**, 87–94.
3   LANDSTEINER K. and LEVINE P. (1931) The differentiation of a type of human blood by means of normal animal serum. *J. Immunol.*, **20**, 179–185.
4   LANDSTEINER K. and LEVINE P. (1928) On individual differences in human blood. *J. exp. Med.*, **47**, 757–775.
5   LANDSTEINER K. and LEVINE P. (1929) On the racial distribution of some agglutinable structures of human blood. *J. Immunol.*, **16**, 123–131.
6   LEVINE P., BOBBITT O.B., WALLER R.K. and KUHMICHEL A. (1951) Iosimmunization by a new blood factor in tumor cells. *Proc. Soc. exp. Biol. N.Y.*, **77**, 403–405.
7   SANGER RUTH (1955) An association between the P and Jay systems of blood groups. *Nature, Lond.*, **176**, 1163–1164.
8   HENNINGSEN K. (1949) Investigations on the blood factor P. *Acta path. microbiol. scand.*, **26**, 639–654.
9   HENNINGSEN K. (1949) On the heredity of blood factor P. *Acta path. microbiol. scand.*, **26**, 769–785.
10   HENNINGSEN K. (1952) *Om Blodtypesystemet P.* M.D. Thesis. Dansk Videnskabs Forlag A/S, Copenhagen, 95 pp.
11   HENNINGSEN K. (1950) Etude d'ensemble du facteur sanguin P. *Rev. Hémat.*, **5**, 276–284.
12   DAHR P. (1942) Ueber die bisher im Kölner Hygienischen Institut gewonnen Untersuchungsergebnissen über das Blutmerkmal P. *Z. ImmunForsch.*, **101**, 346–355.
13   JUNGMICHEL G. (1942) *Ztschr. gerect. Med.*, **36**, 259. Not consulted in the original, but quoted from Henningsen.[8]

[14] MOHARRAM I. (1942) The blood group factor P in Egypt. *Laboratory and Medical Progress*, **3**, 1–8.

[15] SANGER RUTH, LAWLER SYLVIA D. and RACE R.R. (1949) L'hérédité des groupes sanguins P chez 85 familles angalises. *Rev. Hémat.*, **4**, 28–31.

[16] GROSJEAN R. (1950) Sur l'hérédité de l'agglutinogène P. *C. r. Soc. Biol., Paris*, **144**, 1011.

[17] GROSJEAN R. (1952) Nouvelles recherches sur l'agglutinogène P (2ᵉ Memoire). *Sang.*, **23**, 490–507.

[18] BRENDEMOEN O.J. (1952) P blood group in 89 families. *Acta path. microbiol. scand.*, **31**, 71–72.

[19] WIENER A.S. (1953) Personal communication.

[20] RACE R.R., SANGER RUTH and THOMPSON JOAN S. (1953) Quoted in the 2nd, 3rd and 4th editions of this book but not elsewhere published.

[21] TAYLOR G.L. and PRIOR AILEEN M. (1939) Blood groups in England. III. Discussion of the family material. *Ann. Eugen., Lond.*, **9**, 18–44.

[22] RACE R.R., IKIN ELIZABETH W., TAYLOR G.L. and PRIOR AILEEN M. (1942) A second series of families examined in England for the A_1A_2BO and MN blood group factors. *Ann. Eugen., Lond.*, **11**, 385–394.

[23] RACE R.R. and SANGER RUTH (1952) The inheritance of the Duffy blood groups: an analysis of 110 English families. *Heredity*, **6**, 111–119.

[24] CAZAL P. and MATHIEU M. (1950) Recherches sur les groupes sanguins du système PQ. *Sang.*, **21**, 717–727.

[25] SPEISER P. and WEIGL BERTA (1952) Das Blutfaktorensystem P in der Wiener Bevolkerung (1951), ausgewertet mit einem menschlichen, natürlichen anti-P-serum. *Z. klin. Med.*, **7**, 54–61.

[26] FISHER SIR RONALD (1953) The variation in strength of the human blood group P. *Heredity*, **7**, 81–89.

[27] HENNINGSEN K. (1954) The relationship between blood factors P and Q. *Proc. 5th Congr. int. Soc. Blood Transf., Paris*, 215–218.

[28] HENNINGSEN K. and JACOBSEN T. (1955) Relationship between blood factors P and Q. *Nature, Lond.*, **176**, 1179.

[29] FURUHATA T. and IMAMURA S. (1935) The heredity of the new factor Q in human bloods. *Jap. J. Gen.*, **11**, 91–98. (In Japanese.)

[30] FURUHATA T. and MURAKAMI T. (1948) On the blood types (ABO, MN, Qq) of a quadruplet. *Proc. imp. Acad. Japan*, **24**, 1–2.

[31] FURUHATA T. and IMAMURA S. (1949) On the heredity of anti-Q agglutinin. *Proc. imp. Acad. Japan*, **25**, 71–75.

[32] TANAKA K. (1951) Linkage relation between Q agglutinogen and anti-Q agglutinin. *Kyushu Memoirs of Medical Sciences*, **2**, 103–112.

[33] TANAKA K. (1951) An apparent linkage of the ABO blood groups with the Q agglutinogen. *Kyushu Memoirs of Medical Sciences*, **2**, 95–102.

[34] ZOUTENDYK A. and LEVINE P. (1952) A second example of the rare serum anti-Jay (Tjᵃ). *Amer. J. clin. Path.*, **22**, 630–633.

[35] HIRSZFELD L. and GRABOWSKA MARIA (1952) Über individuelle Bluteigenschaften. *Experientia*, **8**, 355–357.

[36] WALSH R.J. and KOOPTZOFF OLGA (1954) The human blood group Tjᵃ. *Aust. J. exp. Biol. med. Sci.*, **32**, 387–392; and personal communication.

[37] LEVINE P., ROBINSON ELIZABETH A., PRYER BETTY and MICHEL O. (1954) Anti-Tjᵃ in second pair of U.S. sibs with observations on the original sibs. *Vox. Sang.* (O.S.), **4**, 143–148.

[38] DAVIDSOHN I. and KING A. Personal communication to Levine P., and Koch Elizabeth (1954) *Science*, **122**, 239.

[39] ISEKI S., MASAKI S. and LEVINE P. (1954) A remarkable family with the rare human isoantibody anti-Tjᵃ in four siblings; anti-Tjᵃ and habitual abortion. *Nature, Lond.*, **173**, 1193–1194.

40 SANGER RUTH, RACE R.R. and VOIGT G. (1955) Über ein anti-Tjᵃ im Serum eines Blut-
    spenders. *Blut*, 1, 292–295.
41 ISEKI S. and MASAKI S. (1953) A new human blood group antibody. *Gunma J. Med. Sci.*, 2,
    293–294.
42 McNEIL C., TRENTELMAN E.F. and THOMAS M. (1957) Anti-Tjᵃ—another family example.
    Vox Sang., 2, 114–116.
43 MOHR J. (1966) Genetics of fourteen marker systems: associations and linkage relations.
    Acta genet., 16, 1–58.
44 V.D. WEERDT CHRISTINA M. (1965) *Platelet Antigens and Isoimmunization.* Doctoral Thesis,
    'Aemstelstad', Amsterdam, pp. 108.
45 CAMERON G.L. and STAVELEY J.M. (1957) Blood Group P substance in hydatid cyst fluids.
    Nature, Lond., 179, 147–148.
46 STAVELEY J.M. and CAMERON G.L. (1958) The inhibiting action of hydatid cyst fluid on
    anti-Tjᵃ sera. *Vox Sang.*, 3, 114–118.
47 WIENER A.S. and PETERS H.R. (1940) Hemolytic reaction following transfusions of blood of
    the homologous group, with three cases in which the same agglutinogen was responsible.
    Ann. Int. Med., 13, 2306–2322.
48 WIENER A.S. (1942) Hemolytic transfusion reactions. iii. Prevention, with special reference
    to the Rh and cross-match tests. *Am. J. clin. Path.*, 12, 302–311.
49 MOUREAU P. (1945) Les réactions post-transfusionnelles. *Rev. belge, Sci. med.*, 16, 258–300.
50 GALATIUS-JENSEN F. (1960) *The Haptoglobins. A Genetical Study*, pp. 117, Dansk. Viden-
    skabs Forlag, Copenhagen.
51 BROMAN B. (1955) Personal communication.
52 YASUDA J. and YOKOYAMA M. (1960) A case of anti-Tjᵃ in Japan. *Proc. 8th Congr. int. Soc.
    Blood Transf.*, II-a-20.
53 YOKOYAMA M., YASUDA J. and AKAGI M. (1960) A further Japanese example of anti-P+P₁
    (Tjᵃ). *Amer. Ass. Blood Banks Bull.*, October, pages 1–3 in offprint.
54 FRIEDLANDER S., JACK J.A. and CAHAN A. (1960) Personal communication.
55 STERN K. and BUSCH SHIRLEY (1963) Report on a family with six Tjᵃ-negative siblings.
    Transfusion, Philad., 3, 105–113.
56 WOODS A.H. and BOTTOMLEY SYLVIA S. (1960) Characterization of the rare isohemagglu-
    tinin anti-Tjᵃ (anti-P+P₁). *Clin. Res.*, 8, 55 (Abstract).
57 RYTTINGER L. (1960) Personal communication.
58 LEWIS MARION, KAITA HIROKO and CHOWN B. (1957) The blood groups of a Japanese
    population. *Amer. J. hum. Genet.*, 9, 274–283.
59 MATSON G.A., SWANSON JANE, NOADES JEAN, SANGER RUTH and RACE R.R. (1959) A 'new'
    antigen and antibody belonging to the P blood group system. *Amer. J. hum. Genet.*, 11,
    26–34.
60 KORTEKANGAS A.E., NOADES JEAN, TIPPETT PATRICIA, SANGER RUTH and RACE R.R.
    (1959) A second family with the red cell antigen Pᵏ. *Vox Sang.*, 4, 337–349.
61 KORTEKANGAS A.E., KAARSALO E., TIPPETT PATRICIA, HAMPER JEAN, SANGER RUTH and
    RACE R.R. (1962) Blood group antigen Pᵏ. *Acta path. microbiol. scand.*, suppl. 154, 359–
    360.
62 LEVINE P., CELANO M. and STAVELEY J.M. (1958) The antigenicity of P substance in
    Echinococcus cyst fluid coated on to tanned red cells (1958). *Vox Sang.*, 3, 434–
    438.
63 LEVINE P. and CELANO M.J. (1959) Antigenicity of P substance in Echinococcus cyst fluid
    coated on to tanned rabbit cells. *Fed. Proc.*, 18.
64 PROKOP O. and OESTERLE P. (1958) Zur Frage der P-Antigenität von Echinokokkenflüssig-
    keit aus Schweinelebern. *Blut*, 4, 157–158.
65 KERDE C., FÜNFHAUSEN G., BRUNK RE, and BRUNK RU. (1960) Über die Gewinnung von
    hochwertigen Anti-P-Immunseren durch Immunisierung mit Echinokokkenzystenflüssig-
    keit. *Z. ImmunForsch.*, 119, 216–224.

7

66 ANTTINEN E.E. (1953) Occurrence of blood group P in Finland. *Ann. Med. exp. Fenn.*, **31**, 285–290.

67 KAARSALO E., KORTEKANGAS A.E., TIPPETT PATRICIA A. and HAMPER JEAN (1962) A contribution to the blood group frequencies in Finns. *Acta path. microbiol. scand.*, **54**, 287–290.

68 LEWIS MARION, KAITA HIROKO and CHOWN B. (1957) The blood groups of a Japanese population. *Amer. J. hum. Genet.*, **9**, 274–283.

69 STEINBERG A.G., SHWACHMAN H., ALLEN F.H. and DOOLEY R.R. (1956) Linkage studies with cystic fibrosis of the pancreas. *Amer. J. hum. Genet.*, **8**, 162–176.

70 MOLLISON P.L. and CUTBUSH MARIE (1955) The use of isotope-labelled red cells to demonstrate incompatibility *in vivo*. *Lancet*, **i**, 1290–1295.

71 GREUTER W., HESS M., RENAUD N., SCHMITTER M. and BÜTLER R. (1963) Beitrag zur Genetik des Gm- und Gc-Serumgruppensystems anhand von Untersuchungen an Schweizerfamilien. *Arch. Klaus-Stift. VererbForsch.*, **38**, 77–92.

72 WALLER MARION (1961). Unpublished observations.

73 SALMON C., REVIRON J., CREGUT R. and LIBERGE G. (1962) Deux soeurs de phébotype Tj(a–). *Transfusion, Paris*, **5**, 267–271.

74 RACE R.R. and SANGER RUTH (1954 and 1958) Second and third editions of this book.

75 IKIN ELIZABETH W., KAY H.E.M., PLAYFAIR J.H.L. and MOURANT A.E. (1961) P_1 antigen in the human foetus. *Nature, Lond.*, **192**, 883.

76 PRICE EVANS D.A., DONOHOE W.T.A., BANNERMAN R.M., MOHN J.F. and LAMBERT R.M. (1966) Blood group gene localization through a study of mongolism. *Ann. hum. Genet.*, **30**, 49–67.

77 HEIKEN A. (1966) Observations on the blood group receptor P_1 and its development in children. *Hereditas, Lund.*, **56**, 83–98.

78 SMITH C.A.B. (1956) A test for segregation ratios in family data. *Ann. hum. Genet.*, **20**, 257–265.

79 TIPPETT PATRICIA, SANGER RUTH, RACE R.R., SWANSON JANE and BUSCH SHIRLEY (1965) An agglutinin associated with the P and the ABO blood group system. *Vox Sang.*, **10**, 269–280.

80 CEDERGREN B. (1968 et seq.) Unpublished observations.

81 CLEGHORN T.E. (1965) Unpublished observations.

82 CATINO MARY LU, BUSCH SHIRLEY, HUESTIS D.W. and STERN K. (1965) Transmission of the blood group genotype *pp* (Tj^a-negative) in a kinship with multiple consanguineous marriages. *Amer. J. hum. Genet.*, **17**, 36–41.

83 FISHER NATHALIE and CAHAN A. (1963) Personal communication.

84 ROSENFIELD R.E. and PIOMELLI S. (1964) Unpublished observations.

85 BROMAN B. (1963) Unpublished observations.

86 HORNSTEIN LEA and PINKAS-SCHWIETZER RACHEL (1969) Anti-Tj^a, a rare human isoantibody. First finding in Israel. *Israel J. Med. Sci.*, **5**, 114–116.

87 DOS SANTOS W.A. and GILES CAROLYN (1967) Personal communication.

88 TOVEY L.A.D. and CROSSLAND J.D. (1967) Personal communication.

89 RACE R.R. and SANGER RUTH (1962) *Blood Groups in Man*, 4th edition, Blackwell Scientific Publications, Oxford.

90 KORTEKANGAS A.E., KAARSALO E., MELARTIN LIISA, TIPPETT PATRICIA, GAVIN JUNE, NOADES JEAN, SANGER RUTH and RACE R.R. (1965) The red cell antigen P^k and its relationship to the P system: the evidence of three more P^k families. *Fox Sang.*, **10**, 385–404.

91 NEVANLINNA H. and FURUHJELM U. (1966) Unpublished observations.

92 KAARSALO E. (1965–1967) Unpublished observations.

93 STROUP MARJORY, MACILROY MIJA, SUGGS GOLDYE and MORGAN P. (1964) Two additional examples of rare pp (Tj^a–) individuals who are Pk+. Paper to Amer. Ass. Blood Banks.

94 MIKI T. and HAYASHIDA YOSHIKO (1967) In preparation.

95 RACE R.R. and SANGER RUTH (1964) Some complications in the dominant inheritance of blood group antigens. *Proc. 2nd int. Congr. hum. Genet.*, Rome 1961, 812–817.

96 WATKINS W.M. and MORGAN W.T.J. (1964) Blood-group P_1 substance: (II) Immunological properties. *Proc. 9th Congr. int. Soc. Blood Transf.*, Mexico 1962, 230–234.

97 GONANO F. (1962) Studio su eventuali correlazioni tra gruppo 'P' ed echinococcosi in sardegna. *Atti Ass. genet. ital.*, 7, 90–93.

98 DE TAPIA G.M. (1964) Aglutinas anti-P en enfermos portadores de quiste hidático. *Proc. 9th Congr. int. Soc. Blood Transf.*, Mexico 1962, 731–734.

99 PROKOP O. and SCHLESINGER D. (1965) Über das Vorkommen von P_1-Blutgruppensubstanz oder einer 'P_1-like-substance' bei Lumbricus terrestris. *Acta biol. med. germ.*, 15, 180–181.

100 PROKOP O. and SCHLESINGER D. (1965) Über das Vorkommen von P_1-Blutgruppensubstanz bei einigen Metazoen, insbesondere Ascaris suum und Lumbricus terrestris. *Z. ImmunForsch.*, 129, 344–353.

101 PROKOP O. and SCHLESINGER D. (1965) Über das Vorkommen von P_1-Blutgruppensubstanz in Ascaris suum. *Dte. GesundhWes.*, 1584.

102 MORGAN W.T.J. and WATKINS W.M. (1964) Blood group P_1 substance: (I) Chemical properties. *Proc. 9th Congr. int. Soc. Blood Transf.*, Mexico 1962, 225–229.

103 LEVINE P. and KOCH ELIZABETH A. (1954) The rare human isoagglutinin anti-Tj^a and habitual abortion. *Science*, 120, 239–241.

104 SANGER RUTH (1958) The P and Jay systems of blood groups. *Proc. 6th Congr. int. Soc. Blood Transf.*, Boston 1956, 110–113.

105 VOS G.H., CELANO M.J., FALKOWSKI F. and LEVINE P. (1964) Relationship of a hemolysin resembling anti-Tj^a to threatened abortion in Western Australia. *Transfusion, Philad.*, 4, 87–91.

106 VOS G.H. (1965) A comparative observation of the presence of anti-Tj^a-like hemolysins in relation to obstetric history, distribution of the various blood groups and the occurrence of immune anti-A or anti-B hemolysins among aborters and nonaborters. *Transfusion, Philad.*, 5, 327–335.

107 VOS G.H. (1966) The serology of anti-Tj^a-like hemolysins observed in the serum of threatened aborters in Western Australia. *Acta haemat.*, 35, 272–283.

108 VOS G.H. (1967) A study related to the significance of hemolysins observed among aborters, nonaborters and infertility patients. *Transfusion, Philad.*, 7, 40–47.

109 HORVÁTH E. and PAISZ IDA (1966) Absence of anti-Tj^a-like hemolysin in pregnant aborters in Budapest. *Transfusion, Philad.*, 6, 499–500.

110 LEVINE P., CELANO M.J. and FALKOWSKI F. (1963) The specificity of the antibody in paroxysmal cold hemoglobinuria (P.C.H.). *Transfusion, Philad.*, 3, 278–280.

111 V.D. HART MIA, V.D. GIESSEN M., V.D. VEER MARGA, PEETOOM F. and V. LOGHEM J.J. (1964) Immunochemical and serological properties of biphasic haemolysins. *Vox Sang.*, 9, 36–39.

112 WORLLEDGE SHEILA M. and ROUSSO C. (1965) Studies on the serology of paroxysmal cold haemoglobinuria (P.C.H.), with special reference to its relationship with the P blood group system. *Vox Sang.*, 10, 293–298.

113 WEINER W., GORDON E.G. and ROWE D. (1964) A Donath-Landsteiner antibody (nonsyphilitic type). *Vox Sang.*, 9, 684–697.

114 MOLTHAN LYNDALL and LEVINE M. (1968) Letter to the Editor. *Transfusion, Philad.*, 8, 196.

115 HAYASHIDA YOSHIKO and WATANABE A. (1968) A case of p Taiwanese woman delivered of an infant with hemolytic disease of the newborn. *Jap. J. legal Med.* 22, 10–15.

116 GUÉVIN R.M., TALIANO V., HAREL P. and GAUTHIER J. (1970) Trois nouveaux exemples d'anti-Tj^a dans une famille Canadienne. *Un. méd. Can.*, 99, 1255–1259.

117 BIDET J.M., LAGET R. and SALMON C. (1968) Personal communication.

118 METAXAS M. (1970) Personal communication.

119 LEVINE C. and IZAKSON M. (1973) Personal communication.

120 SCHNEIDER W., TIPPETT PATRICIA and GOOCH ANN (1969) The antigen P^k in a German family. *Vox Sang.*, **16**, 67–68.

121 SALMON C. and GERBAL A. (1973) Personal communication.

122 KLOSSNER MARJA-LIISA (1971) Unpublished observations

123 STEVENSON MABEL M. (1973) Unpublished observations

124 BEVAN B., HAMMOND W. and CLARKE R.L. (1970) Anti-P_1 associated with liver-fluke infection. *Vox Sang.*, **18**, 188–189.

125 VOAK D., ANSTEE D. and PARDOE GRACE (1973) The α-galactose specificity of anti-P^k. *Vox Sang.*, **25**, 263–270.

126 FELLOUS M., BILLARDON C., DAUSSET J. and FRÉZAL J. (1971) Étude de linkage en culture de cellules. II. Marqueurs antigéniques. Abstracts *4th Int. Congr. Hum. Genet., Paris.* Excerpta Medica No. 233, pp. 66–67.

127 FELLOUS M., BILLARDON C., DAUSSET J. and FRÉZAL J. (1971) Linkage probable entre les locus 'HLA' et 'P'. *C. R. Acad. Sci., Paris*, **272**, 3356–3359.

128 FELLOUS M., COUILLIN P., NEAUPORT-SAUTES C., FRÉZAL J., BILLARDON C. and DAUSSET J. (1973) Studies of human alloantigens on man-mouse hybrids: possible synteny between HL-A and P systems. *Eur. J. Immunol.*, **3**, 543–548.

129 ENGELFRIET C.P., BECKERS DO, VON DEM BORNE, A.E.G.KR., REYNIERSE, E. and VAN LOGHEM J.J. (1971) Haemolysins probably recognizing the antigen p. *Vox Sang.*, **23**, 176–181.

130 FELLOUS M., TESSIER C., GERBAL A., SALMON C., FRÉZAL J. and DAUSSET J. (1972) Genetic dissection of P biosynthesis pathway. *Bull. Europ. Soc. Hum. Genet.*, Nov., p. 31. And Fellous M. personal communication.

131 WURZEL H.A., GOTTLIEB A.J. and ABELSON NEVA M. (1971) Immunoglobulin characterization of anti-Tj^a antibodies. AABB program, Chicago, 103–104.

132 ISSITT P.D., TEGOLI J., JACKSON VALERIE, SANDERS C.W. and ALLEN F.H. (1968) Anti-IP_1: antibodies that show an association between the I and P blood group systems. *Vox Sang.*, **14**, 1–8.

133 BOOTH P.B. (1970) Anti-I^TP_1: an antibody showing a further association between the I and P blood group systems. *Vox Sang.*, **19**, 85–90.

134 ALLEN F.H., MARSH W.L., JENSEN LEILA and FINK J. (1974) Anti-IP: another antibody defining a product of interaction between the genes of the I and P blood group systems. *Vox Sang.*, **27**, 442–446.

135 MARCUS D.M. (1971) Isolation of a substance with blood-group P_1 activity from human erythrocyte stroma. *Transfusion, Philad.*, **11**, 16–18.

136 BRUETON N. and GILES CAROLYN M. (1970) Unpublished observations.

137 VAN DER HART MIA (1973) Unpublished observations.

138 BITZ H. and EHRKE K. (1973) Unpublished observations.

139 CEDERGREN B. (1973) Population studies in northern Sweden. IV. Frequency of the blood type p. *Hereditas*, **73**, 27–30.

140 BECKMAN L. (1959) A contribution to the physical anthropology and population genetics of Sweden. *Hereditas*, **45**, 1–189.

141 SCHNITZLER S., MÜLLER G. and PROKOP O. (1967) Ein 'neuer' Antikörper: Anti-P_{rut}, aufgefunden im Rogen von Rutilus rutilus. *Z. Immun. Allerg.-Forsch.*, **134**, 45–53.

142 EDWARDS J.H., ALLEN F.H., GLENN K.P., LAMM L.U. and ROBSON E.B. (1973) The linkage relationships of HL-A.

143 SPEISER P. (1973) Unpublished observations.

144 TOMITA K. and NAKAJIMA H. (1972) An example of the antibodies of P-Tj^a found after incompatible blood transfusions. *J. Jap. Soc. Bld. Transf.*, **19**, 33–40. (In Japanese with English summary.)

145 YAMAGUCHI H., OKUBO Y., TANAKA M., MURAKAMI W. and HONKAWA T. (1973) In preparation.

[146] MIWA S., MATUHASI T. and YASUDA J. (1974) The p phenotype in two successive generations of a Japanese family. *Vox Sang.*, **26**, 565–567.

[147] YOKOTA T. and NAKAJIMA H. (1972 and 1973) Unpublished observations.

[148] CRAWFORD M.N., TIPPETT P. and SANGER R. (1974) Antigens Au^a, i and P_1 of cells of the dominant type of Lu(a−b−). *Vox Sang.*, **26**, 283–287.

[149] CONTRERAS MARCELA and TIPPETT PATRICIA (1974) The Lu(a−b−) syndrome and an apparent upset of P_1 inheritance. *Vox Sang.*, **27**, 369–371.

[150] BATTAGLINI P. and MELIS CHRISTINA (1973) Unpublished observations.

[151] CLEGHORN T.E. and JOHNSON PAULINE (1974) Personal communication.

[152] FELLOUS M., GERBAL A., TESSIER C., FRÉZAL J., DAUSSET J. and SALMON C. (1974) Studies on the biosynthetic pathway of human P erythrocyte antigens using somatic cells in culture. *Vox Sang.*, **26**, 518–536.

Chapter 5
The Rh Blood Groups

The discovery of the Rh groups by Landsteiner and Wiener[1] in 1940, with which must be associated the work of Levine and Stetson[2] in 1939, was undoubtedly the most important event in the blood group field since the discovery of the ABO system forty years before.

When Wiener and Peters[3] recognized that anti-Rh could be a cause of haemolytic reaction to transfusion it showed that the new groups were of some clinical importance; but when Levine, Katzin, Vogel and Burnham[4-6] demonstrated that incompatibility of these groups between mother and child was the cause of erythroblastosis foetalis, or haemolytic disease of the newborn, it became clear that a great contribution had been made to the science of medicine.

HISTORY

In 1939 Levine and Stetson[2] published their historic paper describing how the mother of a stillborn foetus suffered a severe haemolytic reaction to the transfusion of her husband's blood. Then it was found that the mother's serum agglutinated the cells of her husband and those of 80 out of 104 ABO compatible donors. The antigen responsible was shown to be independent of the ABO, MN and P groups and an unsuccessful attempt was made to immunize rabbits against it.

Levine and Stetson's interpretation of the case is now known to have been entirely correct. They said that the mother who lacked the 'new' antigen had become immunized by her foetus which possessed this antigen, having inherited it from the father. When the husband's blood was transfused the maternal antibody reacted with this same antigen on the red cells of the father.

Had Levine and Stetson given a name to the blood group system which they had discovered, it, and not Rh, would have been found in the title of this chapter and of a thousand other publications.

In 1940 Landsteiner and Wiener[1], having immunized rabbits and guinea-pigs with the blood of the monkey *Macacus rhesus*, made the very surprising discovery that the resulting antibodies agglutinated not only the monkey red cells but also the red cells of about 85 per cent of white people in New York. The 85% whose red cells were agglutinated by the rabbit anti-rhesus serum the authors called Rh positive, the remaining 15% Rh negative.

The next step was the demonstration by Wiener and Peters[3] that the antibody anti-Rh, apparently the same as that made by the rabbit against monkey cells, could be found in the serum of certain people who had incompatible transfusion reactions following transfusion of blood of the correct ABO group.

The antibody discovered in Levine and Stetson's case of 1939 was then found also to be indistinguishable from the rabbit anti-rhesus antibody. So the idea of 1939 that this antibody had been stimulated by foetal immunization could be translated into terms of Rh, and in 1941 Levine and his associates Burnham, Katzin and Vogel[4-6] showed that erythroblastosis foetalis was the result of Rh blood group incompatibility between mother and child.

In 1941 Landsteiner and Wiener[10] published a full account of their work: the Rh antigen was found to be present in about 85 % of white people and tests on 60 families showed it to be a dominant character.

Many years later it came to be realized that the rabbit anti-rhesus and the human anti-Rh antibodies are not the same. The vast literature which had accumulated made it impossible to change the name of the human antibody from anti-Rh, and the suggestion of Levine that the rabbit anti-rhesus antibody should be called anti-LW, in honour of Landsteiner and Wiener, has been widely adopted.

Almost all subsequent work on Rh has been done with human antisera which are immune in origin. ('Naturally occurring' examples are relatively rare and references may be found in Harrison[434] and Mollison[435].)

The recognition of complexity

As early as 1941 it was realized that the Rh groups were not as simple as they seemed at first[10-19]. By 1943 the Americans[18] had three antisera and had defined six alleles, while the British[17] had four antisera and had defined seven alleles.

Fisher's synthesis

At the end of 1943 Fisher[20], studying the results of the British work with four antisera, noticed that the reactions of two of them were antithetical and he supposed that the antigens, and the genes, recognized by these two antibodies, were 'allelic' and called them C and c. The reactions of the remaining two sera were not antithetical; the antigens which they were recognizing Fisher called D and E and supposed that they also had 'allelic' forms, d and e, which would be capable in favourable circumstances of stimulating their own antibodies, anti-d and anti-e.

Fisher assumed that the three genes, if separable, must be very closely linked, for no crossing-over had been observed[21]. Furthermore, if crossing-over could occur at all freely the frequencies would differ very greatly from those observed.

An Rh gene complex could therefore be assembled in eight different ways: *CDe, cDE, cde, cDe, cdE, Cde, CDE* and *CdE*. Seven of these assemblages could be identified in the alleles already known, the eighth, *CdE*, remained to be found.

Confirmation

The first step in the confirmation of the theory was taken when two unknown re-actions of *CDE* were shown to be as predicted[22]. Then in 1945 anti-e was found by Mourant[23] and all the anticipated interactions were confirmed at the time, or, in the case of *CdE*, later.

It is now almost certain that the postulated anti-d does not exist: three early reports[24-26] have not stood up to the criticism of the years.

The first conclusive example of *CdE* was demonstrated by van den Bosch[27] and many examples have since been found[89-94], even homozygotes in two families[260, 316].

Now that the groups seem so clear (at any rate as defined by anti-D, -C, -c, -E and -e), it must be difficult to realize how obscure they appeared before Fisher illuminated them. Such successful prediction must be rare in biology.

We still think of C, D and E as representing certain lengths of genetic material but, since the work of the bacterial geneticists on the fine structure of genes, we have pictured not three but perhaps many mutational sites involved in Rh. This will be returned to on page 240.

The crossing-over idea

Noticing that in the English population there were three orders of frequency of the gene complexes, *CDe*, *cde* and *cDE* 12% or over, then *cDe*, *cdE*, *Cde* and *CDE* less than 3% and finally *CdE* with a frequency so low that it had not at that time been found, Fisher[130-132] suggested that the rarer combinations might be main-tained by occasional crossing-over from the common heterozygotes. For example, a cross-over happening between C and D in *CDe/cde* would produce *cDe* and *Cde*. All four second order combinations could be produced in this way, but not the third order *CdE*. The production of *CdE* would require a cross-over from a heterozygote, e.g. *cDE/Cde*, involving a second order complex *Cde*, itself accord-ing to the theory, a cross-over. This would doubtless be a very rare event. The theory thus offered a very satisfactory explanation of the then puzzling absence of *CdE*.

Fisher[130, 131] carried this brilliant idea a step further in suggesting that the order of sites is such that *C* lies between *D* and *E*. The reason is that the frequency ratio of *cdE* to the heterozygote *cDE/cde*, which represents a cross-over between *D* and *E*, is considerably larger than the ratios of *Cde* to *CDe/cde* (cross-over between *C* and *D*) and of *CDE* to *CDe/cDE* (cross-over between *C* and *E*).

It should be made clear that the crossing-over hypothesis did not pretend to offer an explanation of the frequent alignments in any population, but, given the frequent combinations, it might explain the less frequent.

It was hoped that the testing of populations which differ sharply from the English might, by the infrequent gene complexes revealed, provide a clear con-firmation or refutation of the crossing-over idea, but this has not happened: some series have been strikingly for and some against.

Subsequent work, such as that on the gene complex $-D-$, on the combined antigens ce, Ce, etc., and on G, persists in associating C with E and D with C, but nothing, with one possible exception (page 203), has turned up so far to connect D with E: that is the order DCE still seems to hold.

Phylogeny

Other blood group systems were gradually recognized to be constructed on the same complex pattern as Rh; MNSs next, then Kell, then Lutheran. The usual explanation for such piling together of loci involved in the same sort of activity is that in the development of the species a locus has duplicated itself along the line of its chromosome as the result of a rare accident of unequal crossing-over at meiosis. (Unequal crossing-over was discovered in 1925 by Sturtevant[484] when working on the eye condition in Drosophila called double-Bar.) The idea is that later in the history of the species a mutation happens at the duplicated locus and the mutant produces something along the general lines of, but different from, the products of the ancestral locus. In 1935 Bridges commented[485] that the main interest in duplications 'lay in their offering a method of evolutionary increase in lengths of chromosomes with identical genes which could subsequently mutate separately and diversify their effects'.

The incomplete antibody

During the first four years of Rh many workers were puzzled by the fact that mothers of children with haemolytic disease, but in whose serum no anti-Rh could be found, were Rh negative to significant excess. Anti-Rh should have been present in their serum, yet it could not be found.

Early in 1944 Diamond[205] reported that a preparation of concentrated globulin from an Rh antiserum showed a prozone effect, and moreover was capable of inactivating serum containing an anti-Rh agglutinin of high titre. Later in 1944 Race[184] and Wiener[206] independently observed the phenomenon and elucidated its nature. Hidden anti-D was present which Race called incomplete antibody, and Wiener blocking antibody.

Race[184] showed that the presence of the incomplete anti-D could be detected by its inhibitory effect on an agglutinating anti-D, and also by its direct effect on Rh positive cells. If Rh positive cells were suspended in a serum containing incomplete anti-D, the mixture centrifuged and the cells washed and resuspended in saline, then these treated cells were no longer agglutinable by agglutinating anti-D though they were as agglutinable as before by anti-c, anti-C and anti-E. Thus the blocking was specific. The incomplete antibody was looked upon as being defective in that it was not a suitable partner for the second stage of the antigen-antibody reaction. It was noted that if Rh positive cells were exposed to a mixture of agglutinating and incomplete anti-D the incomplete antibody 'seemed to win the race for antigen'. An example was given of D cells absorbing preferentially incomplete anti-D from a mixture of incomplete and agglutinating anti-D.

7*

Wiener's[206] findings were identical. He considered that the blocking antibody was monovalent, and that it was probably of greater clinical significance in the causation of erythroblastosis than the agglutinating antibody.

The interest taken in these observations soon brought to light examples of earlier work showing the same phenomenon[207-211]. Various serological aspects of incomplete anti-D were thereupon studied[212-216].

The observation of Baar[217], that incomplete anti-Rh could be found in cord blood of infants suffering from haemolytic disease much more frequently than agglutinating anti-Rh, suggested that the former antibody had greater powers of permeating the placenta.

Tests for the detection of the incomplete antibody more efficient than the original method were soon developed. Diamond and his colleagues, Abelson[218,219], Denton[220] and Cameron[221] introduced protein solutions as suspending fluids for the red cells: the fluid of choice was 20 per cent bovine albumin.

A different approach to the investigation of the nature and the detection of the presence of the incomplete antibody was opened by the antiglobulin test of Coombs, Mourant and Race[228-230] (1945). Red cells sensitized by incomplete anti-Rh antibodies and then washed free from serum were agglutinated on exposure to the serum of a rabbit previously immunized against human globulin or against human serum.

This test has proved of great clinical importance particularly in its 'direct' form in which it demonstrates that cord blood has been sensitized *in utero*. The test made an early contribution to knowledge when it demonstrated the existence of the Kell system[230] of blood groups, and it has revealed practically all the subsequent systems.

Soon after the test had been developed Coombs made the much more difficult discovery that Moreschi[231] had, in 1908, used the same method in a goat anti-rabbit-red cell system.

The next important step was the discovery by Pickles[232] that enzyme treatment of D cells made them agglutinable by incomplete anti-D. The first activating fluid was a filtrate of a culture of cholera vibrio; then Morton and Pickles[233] found that treatment with trypsin had the same result.

During the last 30 years the literature devoted to the antiglobulin reaction and to the effect of various enzymes on red cells has become so immense that we have had no difficulty in persuading ourselves that these subjects lie outside the scope of this book.

More recent history

The spade work on Rh had been completed in the forties. It was followed by a fairly luxurious flowering of variant phenotypes and new antibodies. To our minds, by far the most important recent advance was the distinguishing between anti-D and the rabbit anti-rhesus antibody now called anti-LW, a distinction which has altered our way of thinking of the genetical background of Rh.

Notation

Neither the CDE nor Dr Wiener's Rh-Hr notations found it easy to digest the surfeit of more recent complex antibodies and antigens.

In 1962, Rosenfield, Allen, Swisher and Kochwa[322] developed a numerical notation originally proposed by Murray[81,82] in 1944 (in a simple form appropriate to the time). The notation is based on observed reactions and is free from any genetical implications (e.g. that E is allelic to e, or C to c). This is surely the way to store information for the future and probably better for computers too; but, just for the present generation, the notation does make it impossible to read a paper which has not one of the other notations in brackets (which most of them fortunately have).

Rosenfield, Allen and Rubinstein[438], in their herculean 1973 paper on a genetic model for the Rh groups, give the most recent glossary of numbers for Rh antigens that we know of, and these are shown in Table 30. Many of the antibodies to the antigens of Table 30 must be heterogeneous, notably in our experience anti-D, -C, -e, -V and -VS, though the red cell samples needed to show the heterogeneity are rare.

Though in favour of the numerical notation for recording Rh reactions, we are not using it in this chapter because we feel that we should try to communicate something intelligible to people who, like ourselves, are ill at numbers and who find most of the pleasure of blood groups to lie in their genetics.

Table 30. Numerical Rh notation: the CDE and Rh-Hr synonyms

	CDE	Rh-Hr		CDE	Rh-Hr	CDE	Neutral	Rh-Hr
Rh1	D	Rh_0	Rh13	*	Rh^A	Rh25	LW	
Rh2	C	rh'	Rh14	*	Rh^B	Rh26	'Deal'	
Rh3	E	rh"	Rh15	*	Rh^C	Rh27	cE	
Rh4	c	hr'	Rh16	*	Rh^D	Rh28		hr^H
Rh5	e	hr"	Rh17	†	Hr_0	Rh29	'Total Rh'	
Rh6	f, ce	hr	Rh18		Hr	Rh30	Go^a	
Rh7	Ce	rh_i	Rh19	‡	hr^s	Rh31	‡	hr^B
Rh8	C^w	rh^{w1}	Rh20	VS, e^s		Rh32	$\overline{R}^N$	
Rh9	C^x	rh^x	Rh21	C^G		Rh33	$R^{0\ Har}$	
Rh10	V, ce^s	hr^v	Rh22	CE		Rh34	Bas	
Rh11	E^w	rh^{w2}	Rh23	Wiel, D^w		Rh35	1114	
Rh12	G	rh^G	Rh24	E^T				

* Corresponding to some of the apparent anti-D made in D people (page 190).
† Corresponding to an antibody made by $-D-/-D-$, etc. people (page 215).
‡ See apparent anti-e made in e people (page 209).

THE Rh GROUPS AT THE LEVEL OF GENERAL USE

In this section we attempt to give an account of the groups at the level at which they are commonly used—at the level of the antisera anti-D, -C, -c, -E, -e and anti-C^w. The antigen C^w, 'allelic' to C and c, will be described more fully in a later section (page 195) and so will D^u, the name given to a series of antigens which give some but not all the reactions of D (page 189).

Frequencies

There are wide racial differences in the frequencies of the Rh gene complexes: a large collection will be found in Dr Mourant's books[77,461].

Estimates of the frequencies of the gene complexes in Whites are given in Table 31. Those for England were based on a series of 2,000 samples tested 27 years ago (Race, Mourant, Lawler and Sanger[80], 1948): the calculations were done by Sir Ronald Fisher who devised a maximum likelihood method for the purpose[78,79]. The Swedish estimates (Heiken and Rasmuson[88], 1966) were based on a series of 8,297 children to which Fisher's method was applied. (Other ways of calculating the Rh gene frequencies are available[84,77,85-87].) In the English tests 'high grade' D^u were classified as D. Since 'low grade' D^u were not at that time recognized they will mostly be hidden amongst Cde/cde and cdE/cde. In the Swedish tests both high and low grade D^u were classified as D. The gene frequencies for Canada were based on tests of 2,000 parents: they were arrived at by an ingenious method of simple counting (Lewis, Kaita and Chown[460], 1971). D^u was counted as D.

Hässig, Rosin and Rothlin[94] estimated the frequency of CdE in Switzerland to be 0·00014: there are no English, Swedish or Canadian estimates.

The 12 gene complexes of Table 31 can be paired in (12/2) (12 + 1) or 78 different ways. We can therefore say that 78 different genotypes exist even ignoring D^u and the very many variant alleles to be described later in this chapter.

Table 31. Frequencies of the *Rh* gene complexes in England, Sweden and Manitoba (After Race, Mourant, Lawler and Sanger[80], 1948, Heiken and Rasmuson[88], 1966 and Lewis, Kaita and Chown[460], 1971)

Gene complex		England	Sweden	Manitoba
Fisher	Wiener			
CDe	R^1	0·4076	0·40356	0·3946
cde	r	0·3886	0·38205	0·3912
cDE	R^2	0·1411	0·16701	0·1602
cDe	R^0	0·0257	0·01855	0·0218
C^wDe	R^{1w}	0·0129	0·01983	0·0144
cdE	r″	0·0119	0·00295	0·0060
Cde	r′	0·0098	0·00489	0·0108
CDE	R^z	0·0024	0·00082	0·0008
C^wde	r'^w	—	0·00034	—
CdE	r^y	—	—	—
C^wDE	R^{zw}	—	—	—
C^wdE	r^{yw}	—	— —D—	0·0002
		1·0000	1·00000	1·0000

Table 32 shows the phenotypes observed by Heiken and Rasmuson[88] in their tests on the 8,297 unrelated Swedish children. From these were calculated the gene frequencies of Table 31 which were recombined to give the expected incidence of genotypes and phenotypes (there are 45 genotypes because the data disclosed only 9 gene complexes). The 33 further genotypes involving the very infrequent complexes CdE, C^wDE and C^wdE are left out because their inclusion in the table would complicate it unnecessarily.

In Table 32 ordinary anti-C is called anti-CC^w. As will be explained later most anti-C sera have some anti-C^w specificity. A few of them are pure anti-C. The use of pure anti-C serum splits off only two rare groups, C^wDe/C^wDe and C^wde/C^wde, beyond those already distinguished by the use of the other antisera. When anti-C is mentioned in the literature it can generally be understood to be anti-CC^w. The point is not of great practical importance.

We use the CDE notation in problems concerning Rh: when the Rh groups have been done, along with other groups, in investigations not specifically concerning Rh we use a short notation. Until recently our short notation differed slightly from that given in the phenotype column of Table 32: we used R′ for r′, R″ for r″, and R′^{w} for r′^{w}: but we have now, in common with most workers, changed to the lower case r when D is absent—a practice long advocated by Dr Wiener.

When the problem specifically concerns Rh it is our custom to give the results as 'most probable genotype' and this usually involves the use of judgment. For example blood reacting with anti-D and anti-c but not with anti-C or anti-E (row 2 of Table 32) might represent the genotype cDe/cde or cDe/cDe. If the donor be Swedish we say his probable genotype is cDe/cde, because the chances are 142 to 3 (about 50 to 1) that this is his genotype: if, on the other hand, the donor be an American Negro then no useful guess can be made because the two genotypes have more or less the same frequency.

The errors involved in making the various guesses can be judged from Table 32. These apply only to random people and not to fathers of children with haemolytic disease in whom the known preponderance of DD homozygotes affects the calculation[83]. The genotype can, of course, often be established beyond any doubt by tests on relatives.

It must be emphasized that the use of the phrase 'probable genotype' does not mean hopeless uncertainty but that the blood belongs to one of two, or three or four, perfectly clearly defined genotypes. These alternatives are, of course, allowed for in assessing, for example, the children possible from the various matings; they do not in any way invalidate the use of the Rh groups in, for example, cases of disputed paternity.

Inheritance

The theme of inheritance runs through the rest of this chapter but, at the level so far described, the genetics of Rh may be said to be simple. The gene complexes are

Table 32. Rh frequencies in Sweden: tests on 8,297 children (Heiken and Rasmuson[88], 1966)

Reactions with anti-						Phenotypes	Observed Number	Observed %	Expected %	Genotypes		Expected %
CC^w	C^w	c	D	E	e							
−	−	+	−	−	+	rr	1,236	14·897	14·596	*cde/cde*	rr	14·5962
−	−	+	+	−	+	R_0r	123	1·482	1·452	*cDe/cde*	R^0r	1·4174
										cDe/cDe	R^0R^0	0·0344
−	−	+	−	+	+	$r''r$	18	0·217	0·225	*cdE/cde*	$r''r$	0·2254
−	−	+	−	+	−	$r''r''$	0	0	0·001	*cdE/cdE*	$r''r''$	0·0009
−	−	+	+	+	−	R_2R_2	256	3·085	2·888	*cDE/cDE*	R^2R^2	2·7892
										cDE/cdE	R^2r''	0·0985
−	−	+	+	+	+	R_2r	1,037	12·499	13·392	*cDE/cde*	R^2r	12·7612
										cDE/cDe	R^2R^0	0·6196
										cDe/cdE	R^0r''	0·0110
+	−	+	−	−	+	$r'r$	32	0·386	0·374	*Cde/cde*	$r'r$	0·3736
+	−	+	+	−	+	R_1r	2,715	32·723	32·351	*CDe/cde*	R^1r	30·8360
										CDe/cDe	R^1R^0	1·4972
										cDe/Cde	R^0r'	0·0181
+	+	+	+	−	+	R_1^wr	120	1·446	1·590	*C^wDe/cde*	$R^{1w}r$	1·5152
										C^wDe/cDe	$R^{1w}R^0$	0·0735
										C^wde/cDe	r^wR^0	0·0013
+	−	+	−	+	+	$r'r''$	0	0	0·003	*Cde/cdE*	$r'r''$	0·0029
+	−	+	+	+	+	R_1R_2	1,200	14·463	13·947	*CDe/cDE*	R^1R^2	13·4797
										CDe/cdE	R^1r''	0·2381
										Cde/cDE	$r'R^2$	0·1633
										CDE/cde	R^zr	0·0627
+	−	+	+	+	−	R_zR_2	4	0·048	0·028	*CDE/cDe*	R^zR^0	0·0030
										CDE/cDE	R^zR^2	0·0274
										CDE/cdE	R^zr''	0·0005

Table 32—continued

CCw	Cw	c	D	E	e	Phenotype	Obs. Number	Obs. %	Exp. %	Genotype	Symbol	Exp. %
+	+	+	+	+	+	$R^{1w}R_2$	55	0·663	0·685	C^wDe/cDE	$R^{1w}R^2$	0·6624
										C^wDe/cdE	$R^{1w}r''$	0·0117
										C^wde/cDE	r'^wR^2	0·0113
+	+	+	−	+	+	r'^wr''	0	0	0·000	C^wde/cdE	r'^wr''	0·0002
+	+	+	−	−	+	r'^wr	2	0·024	0·026	C^wde/cde	r'^wr	0·0260
+	−	−	−	−	+	$r'r'$	0	0	0·002	Cde/Cde	$r'r'$	0·0024
+	−	−	+	−	+	R_1R_1	1,341	16·163	16·681	CDe/CDe	R^1R^1	16·2861
										CDe/Cde	R^1r'	0·3947
+	+	−	−	−	+	r'^wr'	0	0	0·000	C^wde/Cde	r'^wr'	0·0003
										C^wde/C^wde	$r'^wr'^w$	0·0000
+	+	−	+	−	+	$R_1^wR_1$	154	1·856	1·688	C^wDe/CDe	$R^{1w}R^1$	1·6005
										C^wDe/Cde	$R^{1w}r'$	0·0194
										C^wDe/C^wDe	$R^{1w}R^{1w}$	0·0393
										C^wde/CDe	r'^wR^1	0·0274
										C^wde/C^wDe	r'^wR^{1w}	0·0014
+	−	−	+	+	+	R_zR_1	4	0·048	0·067	CDE/CDe	R^zR^1	0·0662
										CDE/Cde	R^zr'	0·0008
+	+	−	+	+	−	R_zR_z	0	0	0·000	CDE/CDE	R^zR^z	0·0001
+	+	−	+	+	+	$R_1^wR_z$	0	0	0·003	C^wDe/CDE	$R^{1w}R^z$	0·0033
										C^wde/CDE	r'^wR^z	0·0001
						Total	8,297	100·000	99·999			99·9999

inherited in a straightforward way and families may be analysed in terms of the separate antigens D, D^u or their absence (d), in terms of C, C^w and c and in terms of E and e. This is manageable and in our previous editions we analysed an increasingly large number of families in this way. Alternatively, families may be analysed in terms of the whole gene complex, but this presents formidable printing difficulties. (For example, the observed phenotypes in Table 32 alone represent 120 possible phenotype matings and, of course, very many more genotypically different matings: the phenotypic mating $R_1r \times R_1r$ includes six genotypically different matings with the combined possibility of ten genotypically different children.)

A strong element of selection comes into most of the earlier series of families since so many of them were tested for special reasons, notably haemolytic disease of the newborn. References are: 10, 13, 8, 21, 28, 108–123, 126.

Unselected series are fewer; they mostly appear in accounts of searches for linkage between blood groups and rare autosomal characters. Some references are: 7, 9, 124–125, 323–329, but a splendid collection of families *per se* is published by the Winnipeg group[460,462].

Claims for recombination or fresh mutation

Evidence is mounting that either crossing-over or even mutation has, on very rare occasions, been caught happening at the *MNSs* complex locus. Whether crossing-over or mutation be the answer it would seem that the separateness of mutational sites controlling MN and Ss has been demonstrated. No doubt many sites are involved. The problem, which applies to Rh also, is discussed on pages 97 to 99.

In Rh two examples have been claimed. In 1965 Steinberg[107] described a family: father *CDe/cde*, mother *cde/cde*, four exemplary children *cde/cde* and three more *CDe/cde* but one child, the sixth born, is *Cde/cde*. Though the exception is against the father, illegitimacy was ruled out by the peculiar customs of the sect involved (and, incidentally, made unlikely by blood and serum groups). Steinberg considered a recessive suppressor of D to be an improbable explanation and thought that the choice lay between recombination and mutation. However, several recessive suppressors of Rh are now known which to our minds provide the more likely explanation.

In 1971, Chown, Lewis and Kaita[463] attributed a very unusual Rh complex (page 205), in the eldest of seven children, to mutation: recombination could be excluded. The children were products of a cousin mating.

A well investigated blood group system, very like Rh, is known in pigs. Following gonadal X-irradiation of the sire, a mating produced a litter of which twelve were of the two expected genotypes and one was not. From the same mating type all of 1,357 offspring fell into one or the other expected genotype. Andresen[136] (1967) considers the exception to represent either a recombinant or a mutation or the effect of a modifying gene.

Linkage relations of Rh and assignment to autosome No. 1

The second autosomal linkage to be established in man was between Rh and elliptocytosis: this and later linkages involving Rh, and the story of the triumphant assigning of the *Rh* locus to autosome No. 1, are described in Chapter 27, particularly on pages 561, 562 and 568.

SOME 'ALLELIC' ANTIGENS

Six antibodies in rather general use have already been mentioned but there are about 30 more and, to make further complication, not all the antibodies in a class are of identical specificity. The possible variations of the Rh antigens sometimes appear to be almost unlimited, though, fortunately from the clinical point of view, most of the variants are rare.

These antigens have to be classified somehow and we shall continue to collect them under 'allelic antigens' and 'compound antigens' though such packaging may be thought to be no longer justified. An alternative possibility would have been to divide them into antigens found in Whites and antigens found in Negroes, but here also there would be overlapping.

Two of the further complications, C^w and D^u, have already been briefly mentioned; more details will be given below.

Antigens attributed to alleles of *D*

The antigens D^u

In 1946 Stratton[35] described a new Rh antigen, called D^u, which was agglutinated by some anti-D sera and not by others. The antigen was shown to be inherited[35-37].

The D^u antigen was then studied intensively and independently by Stratton and Renton[38], and by Race, Sanger and Lawler[39,36], with almost completely concordant results.

Both groups of workers found different grades of the D^u antigen; cells of the 'higher' grade being agglutinated by certain anti-D sera while cells of the lowest grade were only distinguishable from *Cde/cde* or *cdE/cde* by a positive indirect antiglobulin test with incomplete anti-D sera. Tests against a battery of anti-D sera[39,36] showed that many varieties of D^u exist—hardly any two being quite alike, unless they were from related people. It is now known that some of the 'high grade' D^u are not due to an allele D^u but to a position effect exerted by *Cde* on an ordinary *D* in the opposite gene complex (Ceppellini[40]; Ceppellini, Dunn and Turri[41]; see Figure 17, page 234).

Estimates in Europeans of the proportion of apparent *Cde/cde* that are really CD^ue/cde vary from 31 to 44% and of the *cdE/cde* that are really cD^uE/cde from

7 to 34% [42,37,43-45,393], and of the apparent cde/cde that are really cD^ue/cde from 0.07 to 0.5% [43-45].

Other papers on the subject of D^u are listed in the references [46-50,76,100] and [262,178-181,171,172,234,394].

The subject is of practical importance because D^u is common in Negroes, because D^u can stimulate anti-D in a dd person [164,173,174] and because some D^u variant people have made anti-D.

Strong D

At the other end of the scale, strong D antigens were reported 20 years ago [53,54]: it seems reasonable to expect the strength of the antigen to vary for reasons unknown, but of certain strong Ds something of the background is known, as will be mentioned later in the chapter: the D of $-D-$ is one example and the D of En(a−) cells another.

Subdivisions of the D antigen

It has been known since the paper by Argall, Ball and Trentelman [175] appeared in 1953 that exceptional people with some kind of D could make anti-D. As they were not suffering from acquired haemolytic anaemia it had to be supposed that they lacked some part of the normal D and that they had made antibody to the missing part.

More examples were reported [176,51,52,182,183,185,194-196,198,222,235] and there was enough cross-testing between cells and sera of the various propositi to show that the situation though complex did not appear to be beyond all unravelling.

The subject has been studied and reviewed by Unger and Wiener [223-227,236] who name component parts of what we call the D antigen, A, B, C and D, and indicate missing components by a small letter, for example Rh_1^c, Rh_1^{cd}, Rh_2^b etc. Unger, Wiener and Katz [227], found that D samples in Negroes and in Whites very seldom lacked A, B or C components but that about half D^u samples lacked one or more components.

In 1962 Tippett and Sanger [266] summarized their findings on D people who had anti-D in their serum: a table giving the interactions between cells and serum of 18 such people showed that there were six separate categories of D antigen.

In 1963 Tippett [169] added a further 11 propositi without having to increase the number of categories. A fairly detailed summary of her findings was given in our last edition, together with notes on how the categories fitted with other published examples.

Since 1963 Dr Tippett has tested many more examples and they continue to be accommodated within the six broad categories of Table 33 though there is heterogeneity within some of them, as will be noted below. It should be said that these D variants are not D^u, not merely a weak kind of D: this is excluded before classification, by tests against ordinary anti-D sera from *dd* people. (D^u variants belonging to these categories no doubt exist but need not confuse the picture.) The same five antisera of Table 33 have been used since 1960, some by Löw's papain method, others by ficin tests.

Table 33. Interaction between cells and serum of people with D on their cells and anti-D in their serum: primary classification (after Tippett[169], 1963)

Cells	Sera					Approximate percentage of 'normal' anti-D positive
Categories	II McI.	III D.S.	IV Rog.	V J.N.	VI Sor. Kem.	
I	+	+	+	+	+	100%
II	−	+	+	+	+	100%
III	+	−	+	+	+	100%
IV	+	w	−	+	+	96%
V	+	−	+	−	±	74%
VI	−	−	+	−	−	35%

For notes on the various categories and their subdivisions see text.
Cells of Negroes from Category IV are Go(a+).
Cells of members of Category V are D^w (Wiel+).

The following notes on the various categories are taken from Dr Tippett's published[266,169] and unpublished work.

Category I

A heterogeneous class, so far all Whites. Red cells react with all anti-D sera, whether from D+ or D− people, except their own. The anti-D in all so far tested is too weak to give reliable results. The *D* responsible for this variety was seen to be travelling with *Ce* in the one informative family[198] tested.

Category II

So far a homogeneous class, but it still contains only three unrelated (two white, one unspecified) propositi. Serum of founder member, McI., used in primary classification. The *D* variant is travelling with *Ce* in the two families tested.

Category III

The serum, D.S., used in primary classification is the original anti-Rh^D of Sacks et al.[195] and people in this category have been classified[195,236] as Rh$_0^d$. Most, but not all, members of this class are Negroes and, so far, three subdivisions can be made:

a)   Like the founder member, D.S., all are Negroes: many have *cDe* the product of which reacts with anti-VS sera but not with one of two anti-V sera. The *D* variant is travelling with this peculiar *ce* in the several families tested.

b)   Again all are Negroes, those tested in our Unit being from South Africa; they differ from subgroup a) in that their cells lack G. Their serum reacts with the cells of subgroups a) and c) of Category III, presumably due to the presence of anti-G.

c)   Two white propositi (V-J. and Zol.), differ from the above two subgroups in that they are C+, G+, V−, VS−.

Cape Coloured and Bantu kindreds with Category III type of D (Rh$_0^d$) and with various e variants (hr^H, hr^B) are recorded by Shapiro and his colleagues[245,437].

Category IV

The serum used in primary classification, Rog., is one of four founder members and more avid than that of Cor., the first one reported[51]. Another founder member was classified[236] as Rh$_1^a$rh. The *D* variant is travelling with *ce* in all families tested. Most members are Negroes, a few are Whites. The category was thought to be homogeneous till the finding that negro Category IV people are Go(a+) and that Go^a segregated with Category IV D (see page 194). So far it seems:

negro Category IV members are Go(a+);
white Category IV members are Go(a−).

Selected anti-D sera show Go(a+) Category IV members to have elevated D.

Category V

The founder member, J.N., was classified[222] as Rh$_1^{cd}$: her serum, shown in Table 33, was called anti-Rh^C. The category contains both negro and white members. The *D* variant is travelling with *ce* in some families and with *Ce* in others. The cells of all members of the category react with anti-D^w, and *D^w* segregates with the unusual *D* (see page 193).

Category VI

The cells of one member of this category were classified as $\mathfrak{Rh}_1^{ac}$, two as $\mathfrak{Rh}_1^{aBcd}$, two as $\mathfrak{Rh}_1^{abcd}$ but Tippett was unable to distinguish these five people by any reactions: however, she agrees the class is somewhat heterogeneous as judged by reactions with anti-D sera. All of many members are white. Usually the *D* variant travels with *Ce*, but it has been found with *cE*, and with *ce*.

Category VI people without anti-D in their serum are sometimes recognized when having been classed as *Cde/cde* donors they are later found to be apparently normal *CDe/cde*. This is because the majority of anti-D sera do not react with Category VI D. We once wondered whether Category VI cells were indeed *Cde/cde* with an unusual form of the G antigen; but in our last edition we gave

Tippett's[169] reasons for concluding that the antibody for Category VI cells and anti-G are certainly not the same antibody but are likely to occur in the same 'hyperimmune' sera.

Category VI cells are often called Rh^B (or D^B). We find this misleading since Wiener et al.[227] showed Rh^B to be a normal component of what we call the D antigen, and about two thirds of our 'routine' anti-D sera (and a greater proportion of unselected anti-D sera[237]) failed to react with D^{VI}. cells.

Chown et al.[238] and Macpherson et al.[239] reported two puzzling cases of D positive men (one probably Category VI and the other Category V) who, at a time when they were making anti-D in response to transfusion, developed direct positive antiglobulin reactions. Interesting also is the case of an apparent D with anti-D, the D positiveness of whose cells was an artefact eventually explained by the Matuhasi-Ogata phenomenon: the anti-D sera used to group them also contained Bg antibodies (Wilkinson et al.[453]).

The patterns of reactions of people who lack part of the D antigen do seem to have some limit; the crispness of the reactions is in pleasant contrast to the gradation of D antigen strength shown by D^u people.

The antigen D^w

In 1962, Chown, Lewis and Kaita[319] reported a 'new' Rh antigen, at first called Wiel and later D^w. The antibody defining the antigen was found in a serum, Bill., which contained also separable anti-C and anti-C^w: the antigen travelled with what appeared to be cD^ue, in two families.

Cells of the propositus Wiel. were found in London[169,319] to give the reactions of Category V (Table 33). Tippett[169] tested four more members of Category V and all were, like Mrs Wiel., positive with the anti-D^w serum (Bill.).

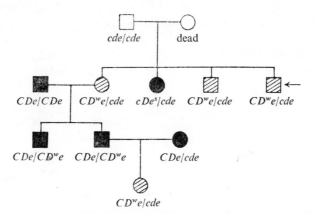

Fig. 12. Showing D^w inherited with an unusual D antigen. (From Tippett[169] and Cleghorn.) Black = normal D antigen; hatched = unusual D antigen, peculiar to Category V of Table 33. Two members of the third generation give normal reactions because of D in *trans*.

Chown and his colleagues[319, 240, 241] found D^w in the alignment cD^we in three families (two negro, one white) and in CD^we in one (white). Tests with anti-D^w showed[240] the antigen to be more frequent in Negroes than in Whites: no random D^w person was found in testing 13,000 Whites while nine were found among 235 Negroes.

Cleghorn, using the Canadian serum, found three more examples of D^w: two of them could be shown to belong to Category V, but the third could not be so classified because of a normal D in *trans*. The pedigree of one of these donors is shown in Figure 12.

As far as we know no other example of anti-D^w has been found.

The antigen Goᵃ, D^{Cor}, or Rh30

Anti-Goᵃ, the cause of mild haemolytic disease of the newborn in a Puerto Rican family, was briefly reported in 1962 (Alter, Gelb and Lee[454]) but a comprehensive account of a lot of work on this antigen, a negro character, appeared five years later (Alter, Gelb, Chown, Rosenfield and Cleghorn[455], 1967, in which paper there is a misleading mistake in the reported Rh group of III-3, family Go.). Soon afterwards Lewis, Chown, Kaita, Hahn, Kangelos, Shepeard and Shackelton[456] showed Goᵃ to be part of the Rh system.

Alter *et al.*[455] found the antigen in 1·86% of 1,560 Negroes, mostly American, but in none of more than 3,000 British and Canadian people. Lovett and Crawford[457] found 2·8% of American Negroes to be Go(a+) and noticed the distribution of Go(a+) supported an association with Rh.

Chown *et al.*[458] by testing two large negro families presented overwhelming evidence that Goᵃ was segregating with Rh and, further, that it is a definitive antigen of Category IV. A family with seven children, tested by Dr Tippett, which added to the proof is shown in Figure 13. All subsequent tests in our and other laboratories[459] have confirmed that anti-Goᵃ is reacting with the facet of D missing from D^{IV}.

Other examples of anti-Goᵃ, sometimes the cause of severe haemolytic disease, have been found though not, as far as we know, published.

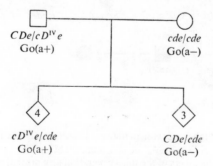

Fig. 13. A negro family showing Goᵃ segregating with Category IV D.

Antigens attributed to alleles of C and c

The antigen C^w

The existence of an antigen 'allelic' to C and c was described in 1946, by Callender and Race[28]. The specific antibody was found in the serum of a CDe/CDe patient who had been transfused with blood of a genotype which came to be called C^wDe/CDe. The antibody has since been found on many occasions, and some examples have been published[186-191,168]; for some there was no known stimulus[190,192,129]. Tests for the antigen C^w are included in routine Rh investigations in some laboratories: the frequencies are given in Tables 31 and 32. The allele responsible has been found in the following alignments besides the common one, C^wDe: C^wde[28,96,97]; C^wdE[95,432]; C^wDE[144-146]; C^wD^ue[98]; and C^wD-[102,261] which will be discussed on page 215.

The original anti-C^w was found to give a marked dosage effect when titrated againt C^wDe/CDe and C^wDe/C^wDe cells[28]: the homozygous cells reacted much more strongly than the heterozygous. More modern examples of anti-C^w have behaved in the same way.

The highest incidence of the antigen C^w (7 to 9 %) so far found is in Latvians[147], in Lapps[148-150] and in Finns[151]. Rare depressions of C^w will be noted later.

The antigen C^x

Stratton and Renton[29] (1954) reported an antibody for a rare antigen called C^x. C^xc blood when tested with a battery of anti-C sera gives some, but not all, the reactions expected of Cc blood. The antigen C^x was found in 4 out of 3,931 unrelated people. The alignment was always C^xDe until, after 20 years, the anticipated C^xde disclosed itself[490].

Further examples were soon found[193,153]. Anti-C^x has caused haemolytic disease of the newborn, in the first example[29] the mother was CDe/cDE and in a later case[433] the mother was CDe/CDe. Cleghorn[154] found that the antibody is quite common, together with such antibodies as anti-Wr^a, anti-Sw^a and anti-Mi^a, in the serum of people suffering from acquired haemolytic anaemia.

Other variants of C and c

In 1948 Race, Sanger and Lawler[30-32] described what appeared to be two more alleles of C. One of them, c^v, was later found[152] not to be an allele of C but the expression of C in the alignment CDE (see page 200). The antigen C^u was present in the genetic alignment C^uDe and distinguished itself by giving some but not all the reactions of C. C^u may, in view of recent advances, be an example of a depressed Rh antigen (see pages 217-219).

A sample of blood was found by Huestis, Catino and Busch[160] to be original in that it reacted with all available anti-c sera save one (and that a good one). Two further propositi were found in testing 1,900 random C positive people. Two of the propositi proved to be related and all three to be of Italian descent. Tests on the three families showed the peculiar c antigen to be regularly inherited; the genetic alignment was with d and e in each family. But for the one eclectic anti-c serum the cells of all three propositi would have been called CDe/cde. However, their reaction with ordinary anti-c (and with anti-ce) was somewhat weaker than that expected of CDe/cde cells. The odd anti-c was given the number anti-Rh26 (Table 30): a second example of the antibody has yet to be found.

The antigen C^G

This is the name given by Levine, Rosenfield and White[299] to that antigenic component of $r^G r^G$ or $r^G r$ cells by virtue of which they react with some anti-C sera (see Table 34, page 201). There is no specific anti-C^G serum, only anti-CC^G. In their synoptic scheme for Rh (page 241) Rosenfield, Allen and Rubinstein[438] attach great importance to C^G (Rh21) and make it, rather than C, the keystone for their model. However, C^G is difficult to define and anti-C^G may perhaps be likened to anti-D sera which are capable of reacting with the weakest of D^u cells.

Antigens attributed to alleles of E and e

The antigen E^w

In 1955 Greenwalt and Sanger[55] described the antigen E^w. The antibody defining the antigen and gene had been the cause of haemolytic disease in a family in which the mother was CDe/cde and the father $C^w De/cDE^w$; the affected child was CDe/cDE^w. Cells containing E^w react with anti-E^w; they are agglutinated by some but not by all anti-E sera. No further example of the antigen was found in testing the blood of 721 unselected white Americans, of 578 English persons and of 69 unselected American Negroes.

Three other families in which cDE^w is segregating were subsequently reported, one nine, one eleven and one sixteen years after the first. Two propositi[161,162] drew attention to themselves in the first place when their cells reacted only with some anti-E sera, the third[436] suffered from haemolytic disease of the newborn due to anti-E^w. All were confirmed using the original anti-E^w.

E^u, a variant of E

This antigen was found in the complex cDE^u (Ceppellini, Ikin and Mourant[56], 1950): it distinguished itself by giving some but not all the reactions expected of E. A very fine family study (Ceppellini[57]) showed the antigen to be inherited in a straightforward way. Examples from Switzerland[58] and from Wales gave the same pattern of reactions with the antisera used on the Italian family. From just three examples it may be rash to suggest that perhaps E^u is a more uniform difference than is D^u or C^u. A further example of E^u, not tested with the European antisera, has been described in an American Negro[59]. Two Irish families are reported (O'Riordan et al.[163]) in which cdE^u is segregating.

E^u may, like C^u, be an example of a depressed Rh antigen (see page 217).

We found variants of E to be not uncommon in non-Ashkenazi communities in Israel.

The antigen E^T

Anti-E^T, apparently a 'naturally occurring' antibody, was found in the serum of an Australian aboriginal of the genotype CDe/cDE (Vos and Kirk[165]). So far, all white people tested who have E have the antigenic component E^T, but not so the Australian aborigines: in the Western Desert about one-third of those with E lack the E^T component. The variant was shown to be inherited straightforwardly.

Examples of weak E antigens, perhaps related to E^T, had been reported by Sanger et al.[166] in Australian aborigines and by Nijenhuis[167] in Papuans, Javanese, Ambonese and Surinam Indians.

The antigens e^s and hr^H

In 1960, we and our colleagues Noades, Tippett, Jack and Cunningham[156] gave the name e^s or VS to an antigen present more frequently in samples from Negroes than from Whites. The antibody defining the antigen was found in the serum of Mrs V.S.: it sensitized the cells of people with the predominantly negro phenotypes V and r's. Absorption and elution tests strongly suggested that only one antibody was present in the serum. Other examples of anti-VS were soon found, usually in the company of other antibodies. As noted in Table 48 in our third edition, and as shown by Tippett[169] in her thesis, not all anti-VS sera proved to have identical specificity. Shapiro[245] working with three examples showed the heterogeneity very clearly in Bantu people: he suggests that the original anti-VS serum was of double specificity, anti-hr^v (anti-V) plus anti-hr^H. Certainly the alleles of C and E appear to be even more bewildering in Negroes than in Whites: the subject is returned to on page 209.

The factor hr^s

In the important paper describing the recognition and analysis of anti-hr^s Shapiro[158] uses the notation of Dr Wiener and, in order to attempt a summary without making implications which Dr Shapiro would probably not wish to be made, we must use the same notation. We look on hr^s as a variant of e (see page 209). That the superscript s was used for both e^s and hr^s in papers that came out almost simultaneously was an unlucky accident, for e^s and hr^s are not the same thing.

The serum of a Bantu woman, Mrs Shabalala, of the Rh phenotype $\mathfrak{Rh}_0^v$ (the germanic letter denotes D^u) who had been immunized by pregnancy, was found to react with all of 1,858 samples from Whites and 1,749 samples from Bantus. Two antibodies were distinguished, one, called anti-Hr, could be removed by absorption with Rh_2Rh_2 cells leaving the other, anti-hr^s.

The anti-hr^s serum, free of anti-Hr, reacted with all but 21 out of 1,390 Bantu samples. The samples lacking hr^s were of the following phenotypes: $\hat{R}h_0$ 1, $\mathfrak{Rh}_0$ 1, $Rh_2\hat{r}h$ 11 and Rh_2Rh_2 8. Of 1,779 white samples 39 lacked hr^s; 3 were of the phenotypes Rh_2rh and 36 Rh_2Rh_2. The caret was used to indicate the absence of the hr^s factor in gene complexes that have e.

Shapiro estimates that about 6% of the Bantu gene complexes are of the hr^s deficient kind. All three white Rh_2rh samples were found to be of the genotype $R^2\hat{R}_0$ and this suggested that the hr^s deficiency 'is not shared proportionately by all agglutinogens containing hr″, as might be expected if hr^s was a subsidiary blood factor "associated" with hr″.'

Extensive family groupings showed the inheritance of the hr^s deficiency to be straightforward, that is to say it was detectable in the homozygous state and when its fellow gene complex was R^2 (no example coupled with $r″$ has yet been found).

Anti-hr^s appears to be a component of the great majority of anti-hr″ sera.

Shapiro considers that the agglutinogen Rh_0^u of Wiener, Gordon and Cohen[101], outstanding by being negative with anti-rh″ and anti-hr″ was negative with the latter serum because the example in use happened to contain anti-hr^s and no anti-hr″. The gene complex R^{0u} Shapiro would denote $\hat{R}_0$.

Shapiro stresses the considerable importance of restraint in interpreting the anti-hr″ results in paternity tests involving Negroes.

Another example of anti-hr^s was reported by Grobbelaar and Moores[170].

We have found a number of variants of e in Negroes (see page 209): there is a general feeling, in which Shapiro shares, that they are analogous to the various kinds of D possessed by the rare Rh+ people who make anti-D.

The factor hr^B

Shapiro, le Roux and Brink[437] (1972) described anti-hr^B which, like anti-hr^s, defines another 'blood factor' associated with hr″. It was found in the serum of a South African negro woman (Mrs Bas.) who is $\hat{R}h_1^{ndH}$ and shown by a beautiful family study to be one of the genotype $\hat{r}'^{nH}\hat{R}^{odH}$ (no doubt oversimplifying, we would call her $Cde^s/cD^{III}e$). After absorption of Mrs Bas.' serum with R^2R^2 (cDE/cDE) cells anti-hr^B remains and this is directed at what we would call a negro e variant. Shapiro et al.[437] designate the gene complexes lacking hr^B as R^2, $\hat{r}'^{nH}$, $\hat{R}^{odH}$, $\hat{R}^0$ and $\hat{r}$.

As will be pointed out later there seems to be an almost infinite variety of e variants in Negroes.

Rosenfield, Allen and Rubinstein[438] give hr^B the number Rh31: they have also named the antibody present in Mrs Bas.' serum before absorption with R^2R^2 cells anti-Rh34, Rh34 being the 'total immune response of Mrs Bas.': no doubt there is a good reason for this, but here we are out of our depth.

The antigen e^i

In a small group of Columbian Indians called Ica, Layrisse and his colleagues[159,177] found that about 20 per cent of the gene complexes were of a 'new'

THE Rh BLOOD GROUPS

kind to which the label cDe^i is given. The homozygotes are very like $cD-/cD-$ from which they are distinguished by giving weak reactions with some anti-e sera and, more decisively, by giving positive reactions with sera from immunized $-D-/-D-$ people (which do not react with $cD-/cD-$ cells). Further, the D in cDe^i, though weaker than that corresponding to $cD-$, is stronger than the D which results from negro cDe.

COMPOUND AND OTHER COMPLEX ANTIGENS

The idea of a combined antigen produced only when c and e are in *cis* but not in *trans* was considered, though not favoured by the authors, in the original paper on f, in 1953. Since that time the interpretation of f as ce and the idea that certain other antigens are the combined effect of C and E alleles (in *cis*) has gained support from several investigations.

The antigens described here may not stay neatly tucked into their allotted sections; however, even if the interpretation as compound is not the final answer, it is at present the best way of communicating something about them.

The antigen f, or ce

The antibody defining this antigen was found in the serum of a much transfused white man of the genotype CDe/cDE (Rosenfield, Vogel, Gibbel, Sanger and Race[68, 69], 1953). Anti-f reacted with a product of the gene complexes cde, cDe and cD^ue. All the other gene complexes known at the time were investigated and were found to lack f.

Trying to fit in f, we at first favoured the possibility that it represented a fourth series of allelic genes but we also considered the possibility that it was a 'blended' antigen produced by c and e in *cis*. This latter idea was championed by other workers[70], but it was the interpretation, by Rosenfield and Haber[269], of the reactions of certain anti-C sera, described below, which converted us to thinking of anti-f as anti-ce.

The inheritance of f is that expected of an Rh antigen: 47 families were reported in the first publication[69], two soon after[70] and very many more families have now been tested.

Anti-f is seldom used outside special Rh problems, for it makes few useful distinctions beyond those made by the more readily available Rh antisera—the most useful distinction is between CDe/cDE (f negative) and CDE/cde (f positive).

Other examples of anti-f

In the original paper it was stated that anti-f was present in most anti-c and anti-e sera[69, 70]. The presence of anti-f in these sera could obviously confuse any dosage effect they might give. An example is recorded[267] of a weak anti-c with a strong anti-f (to the anti-f was attributed the haemolytic disease of a newborn in this family). It was eight years before another example[268] of anti-f was found in a *CDe/cDE* person—a much transfused Negress.

Difficulties

There are several difficulties about anti-f being simply anti-ce:

1   The gene complex *cD–* produces about half a dose of the antigen f when we would expect it to produce none[290].

2   The gene complex r^L, to be described below, is represented by very weak c and e antigens but by a full-blooded f antigen. Also a gene complex '*cde*', investigated by the late Dr Dunsford and ourselves, which resulted in an abnormal c antigen, reacting only with about half anti-c sera, nevertheless had a normal f antigen.

3   The fact that cells of the genotype *cDE/Cde^s* react with anti-f is not so surprising now that it has been proved that *Cde^s*, or *r'^s*, produces c as well as C antigen (see below).

The antigens Ce or rh₁, and CE and cE

By using certain chosen anti-C and anti-E sera a difference was demonstrated in the C and E reactions of the red cells of donors whose genotypes contain the same Rh genes, *C, D, E*, etc., but in different alignments (Race, Sanger, Levine, McGee van Loghem, van der Hart and Cameron[76], 1954). The effect may be summarized thus:

	C antigen	E antigen
genotype *CdE/cde*	a little	a lot
genotype *Cde/cdE*	a lot	a little
genotype *CDE/cDe*	a little	a lot
genotype *CDe/cDE*	a lot	a little

In our third edition we wrote: 'The rule seems to be that when *C* and *E* are in the *cis* position the antigen C is inhibited, and when *C* and *E* are in the *trans* position E is inhibited. The word "inhibited" is used in terms of eclectic antisera: with certain other antisera the antigens C and E appear to be present in much the same strength in all the samples.'

The interpretation which we now prefer is that put forward in 1958 by Rosenfield and Haber[269] who proposed that when *C* and *e* are in *cis* they produce a compound antigen which they called rh₁ (Ce): when *C* and *e* are in *trans* they do not produce this antigen. One must suppose that different anti-C sera have different proportions of anti-C and anti-Ce. The eclectic anti-C sera cited above would be mainly anti-Ce in constitution and have but little anti-C.

The anti-E reactions can be interpreted in the same way by postulating a compound antigen CE and supposing that anti-E sera have variable amounts of anti-CE. The eclectic sera mentioned above would have more anti-CE than anti-E in their constitution.

A good example of the antibody anti-CE was found by Dunsford[242] in a serum which also contains some anti-Ce. (Some of the reactions of this serum are given by Tippett, Sanger, Dunsford and Barber[270].) Another anti-CE serum was found by Dr P. B. Booth (personal communication).

Keith, Corcoran, Caspersen and Allen[243] (1965) consolidated the existence of the antibody anti-cE, the loom of which had already been logged by Gold, Gillespie and Tovey[244] (1961) and a third example is on record[397]. Keith *et al.*[243] prefer to think of the antibody as anti-'$R^{-2,3}$' (which, could be translated as anti-E without C) rather than anti-cE. (We do not know whether it could equally well be called anti-'$R^{4,-5}$' or anti-c without e.)

It must be said that the reactions of anti-C sera (containing no anti-D or anti-G) cannot completely be interpreted in terms of anti-C, anti-Ce and anti-CE components. The heterogeneity of these sera is illustrated in Table 34: six patterns of reaction were distinguished when our battery of antisera was tested against the exotic cells of the table. However, anti-Ce and anti-CE, like anti-ce, are useful in distinguishing certain genotypes: *CDE/cde* or *CDE/cDe* from *CDe/cDE* and *CdE/cde* from *Cde/cdE*.

Table 34. The heterogeneity of anti-C sera (without anti-D or anti-G) illustrated by the reactions with a remarkable collection of cell samples

Cells	Patterns of reaction of anti-C sera					
	1	2	3	4	5	6
Cde/cde, CDe/cDE, CDe/cde	+	+	+	+	+	−
C^wDe/cDE	+	+	+	+	−	−
C^wDe/C^wDE	+	+	+	+	−	+
CDE/cde, CDE/CDE	+	+	+	−	−	+
C^wdE/cde	+	+	−	−	−	+
Cde^s/cde	+	+	−	−	−	−
r^Gr^G	+	−	−	−	−	+
cde/cde, cDe/cde, cDE/cDE, C^wD−/C^wD−	−	−	−	−	−	−

The 6th category was represented by only one serum (Jarvis anti-CE from which a weak anti-Ce had been removed). Each of the other categories was represented by several sera. The two positive reactions of *r^Gr^G* cells would be attributed by Levine *et al.*[299] to an anti-C^G component in sera of type 1 and type 6.

The antigen G

The antigen G may not be a compound antigen but its description here is convenient. In a very important paper Allen and Tippett[279] (1958) described the reactions of the red cells of Mrs Crosby, a white Boston blood donor: though apparently Rh negative, her cells reacted with most 'anti-CD' sera. This was explained by postulating an antigen G present in Mrs Crosby's cells but normally present only in cells possessing the antigens D or C; Mrs Crosby's genotype was written $r^G r$, and 'anti-CD' sera were assumed to have an anti-G component and probably to be heterogeneous—anti-D+G, anti-C+G, anti-D+C+G.

Allen and Tippett isolated anti-G by sensitizing the $r^G r$ cells of Mrs Crosby with various 'anti-CD' sera and making eluates. Using a successful eluate they were able to show that all the common gene complexes except cde and cdE give rise to the antigen G.

The recognition of the existence of G explained several puzzles of the past. It explained how cde/cde women, immunized by pregnancy but never transfused, could make apparent anti-CD although their husbands lacked C: they were in fact making anti-D+G. It also illuminated the comparable finding, by Jacobowicz and her colleagues[280,247], of apparent anti-CD in the serum of two cde/cde mothers made in response to their Cde/cde foetuses: the antibody is, in fact, anti-C+G.

G also explained curious absorption results of 'anti-CD' sera which had puzzled many workers. For example, in our second edition (1954, page 189), from one 'anti-CD' serum absorption by cDe/cde was even more effective at removing the 'anti-C' component than the anti-D, while absorption by Cde/cde removed the 'anti-C' but not the anti-D: in the light of Allen and Tippett's observations we would now call such an antiserum anti-D+G.

G also could explain why 'C' appeared to be so ineffective an antigen to cDE/cde recipients, yet so effective to cde/cde recipients: cDE/cde recipients, having G, cannot make anti-G and the apparent anti-C component of 'anti-CD' sera is often anti-G.

Vos[281] using anti-G eluates ('anti-CD' eluted from Cde/cde and re-eluted from cDe/cde) showed that D^u(with or without C) reacted relatively weakly with anti-G. We confirmed this by testing comparable $cD^u e/cde$ and cDe/cde samples from white people against titrations of two anti-C+G sera: the pooled score for the former was 35 and for the latter 67.

Allen and Tippett[279,282] in elaborate blocking tests found that their anti-G eluate blocked, to a varying degree depending on the indicator system, the antigen e as well as C and D: these results were confirmed by Nijenhuis[248] in blocking tests with an incomplete 'anti-CD', which presumably contained anti-G. This is a puzzle.

Stern and Berger[317] achieved a useful anti-G containing no anti-D and very little anti-C, by injecting $r^G r$ cells into a rr man.

That anti-G was recognizing a distinct Rh antigen and was not anti-'C or D' was clear from the start, but it was five years before any sample having D or C but lacking G was reported. Then, in 1963, Stout, Moore, Allen and Corcoran[249] found in three generations of a white Canadian family a complex cDE which did not produce G: the propositus, cDE/cde, was brought to notice because her serum contained what turned out to be anti-C and anti-G; her D antigen was thoroughly explored with exotic anti-D sera and appeared normal. Then Shapiro[245] found five out of seven Rh_0^d propositi (either Bantu or Cape Coloured) to lack G, and Zaino[250] reported a *cDe/cde* negro woman who lacked G and had made anti-G during pregnancy.

The converse situation, in which people who lack C and D have G, was encountered in three unrelated *cdE/cde* people, who were otherwise normal in their reactions (Tippett[169]; two of the samples were recognized by Dr Rosenfield). Dr Giles and Dr Tippett have been sent other examples over the years: in some the G antigen is weaker than in others. Case[448] showed this rare *cdE* which does produce G is inherited, as expected, straightforwardly and, when partnered with *CDe* it was seen to make normal c antigen.

The antigens corresponding to the gene complex r^G are discussed on page 217 in the section on depressed antigenic complexes, where is mentioned also the weaker G (sometimes called G^u) of negro r^G.

The antigen Rh33 or R_0^{Har}

In 1971 Giles, Crossland, Haggas and Longster[466] described an interesting Rh antigen which unlike any previously found appears to be associated with a variant of D and depression of e, and which is defined by a specific antibody, anti-Rh33. (This is, incidentally, the only Rh number we can remember without referring to a key such as Table 30.)

The antigen was first found in a German donor, who was apparently homozygous for the corresponding gene complex, but no family was available. The same antigen was recognized in an English blood donor (Har. H.) at first thought to be Rh negative, but his cells reacted with a minority of anti-D and anti-CD sera: anti-D could be eluted from Har. H.'s cells when sensitized with reacting anti-D sera, but not when 'sensitized' with non-reacting anti-D. An antibody specific for Har. H. and the German's cells, anti-Rh33, was separable from one reactive anti-D serum but not from others; no further Rh:33 person was found among 1,060 donors in Leeds.

The family of Har. H. was informative: the *cDe* complex producing the Rh33 antigen produced apparently normal c, unusual D, very weak e, weak ce, no G, and, as judged by the presumed homozygous German cells, no Hr or hr^s.

As far as we know only the one example of anti-Rh33 *separable* from anti-D has been found: the owner of the antibody is *Cde/cde*, has never been transfused and, although she has made incomplete anti-D in response to five pregnancies, her saline reacting anti-Rh33 is negative with her husband's *CDe/cDE* cells.

Since 1971 Dr W. Schneider of Hagen has sent us seven samples, from apparently unrelated donors, which reacted with anti-Rh33: all were brought to notice by giving discrepant reactions with anti-D sera and they represent the testing of approximately 14,000 Rh negative donors. Dr W. Orth of Giessen likewise sent us two examples: the family of one of them again showed Rh33 to be inherited straightforwardly, through three generations, the gene complex producing the antigen again being *cDe*.

Whether Rh33 is commoner in Germany than elsewhere is debatable, for it seems possible that the anti-D sera used there are more eclectic. Whether the rare Rh33 will always be associated with the complex cDe cannot be certain; for their ascertainment has so far depended upon the rigorous testing afforded to Rh negative blood donors.

Rh33 does not, so far, comfortably couch itself in the CDE pattern for it seems that the products of the D and E loci are unusual while leaving those of C unscathed. Rosenfield, Allen and Rubinstein[438], less worried by this, place R^{33} at the 'main regulatory locus' of Rh where it 'can be used for an abnormal expression of all structurally specified antigens with coincidental emergence of a rare and otherwise unobserved antigen, Rh33'—which cannot lightly be gainsaid.

The antigen Be^a (Berrens)

The powerful antibody anti-Be^a was described by Davidsohn, Stern, Strauser and Spurrier[478] in 1953; it had been the cause of haemolytic disease of the newborn and, in a later pregnancy, of stillbirth (Stern et al.[479]). The cells of the father, Mr Berrens, were used successfully to stimulate anti-Be^a in two volunteers[479]: Be^a was evidently a strong antigen. The antiserum was widely distributed to many workers but no random Be(a+) person was found in testing more than 25,000 donors of various races. However, after 20 years, haemolytic disease in two more families led to the recognition of other Be(a+) people. The Berrens are of East German extraction and the recent families both have Polish names: the Klep. family was described by McCreary et al.[480] (1973) and the Koz. family by Ducos et al.[481] (1974).

It is the Koz. family who demonstrate that Be^a belongs to the Rh system, and they do it by serological reactions rather than by the evidence of genetical linkage, which is the usual way of demonstrating such assignments. In three generations of the family there are five Be(a+) members and all four who were appropriately tested have an unusual cde complex producing weak e, c and ce antigens, whereas in two Be(a−) members and controls no such abnormality was detected. This association of Be^a with a cde-like allele is not contradicted by the two previous families, and, indeed, as long ago as 1957 we found the ce (f) antigen of Mr Berrens to be unusually weak, but did not report it for the observation was not confirmed elsewhere.

Anti-Be^a has been made by CDe/CDe, cDe/cde and cDE/cde mothers whose husbands appeared to be cde/cde, and by CDe/CDe and cde/cde volunteers.

The phenotypes $\bar{\bar{R}}^N$ and (C)D(e)

Gene complexes were long known which distinguished themselves only by the weak C and e antigens they produced, but some of them have now further distinguished themselves by producing an antigen for which specific antibody exists. There are two main classes, the negro $\bar{\bar{R}}^N$ and the white (C)D(e), the brackets denoting weakness.

$\bar{\bar{R}}^N$

In 1960 Rosenfield *et al.*[273] described a negro family in which a gene complex causing weak C and e antigens was segregating. The complex was named $\bar{\bar{R}}^N$: the D antigen was not exalted, as it is in $-D-$.

It was soon realized that the negro $\bar{\bar{R}}^N$ and the white $(C)D(e)$, though producing phenotypically similar antigens, could not be identical, for Dr Tippett found they showed a different pattern of reactions with her battery of anti-C and anti-e sera.

In our last edition (page 209) we mentioned that antibodies specific for antigens produced by $\bar{\bar{R}}^N$ but not by the white $(C)D(e)$ were being investigated in several laboratories (Chown, Allen, Cleghorn, Giles and Tippett, personal communications). The antibody came to be called anti-$\bar{\bar{R}}^N$, though nothing was published for more than three years, probably because of lack of, or occasionally discrepancy in, family studies: eventually Chown, Lewis and Kaita[463] summarized some findings of several laboratories and $\bar{\bar{R}}^N$ was allotted[464] a number, Rh32.

$\bar{\bar{R}}^N$ is thought of as a negro gene complex (perhaps about 1% of American Negroes possesses it[463]) but it does occur as a rarity in Whites. Though none was found in testing 906 random Whites, $\bar{\bar{R}}^N$ was found by Dr Allen and Miss Corcoran in a Spanish American family[463] and another as 'an anomaly of inheritance, probably due to mutation' in a Canadian Mennonite family. (That we would not like to blame mutation, especially when so few families with $\bar{\bar{R}}^N$ have been tested, takes nothing away from the fascinating account given by Chown, Lewis and Kaita[463].)

That $\bar{\bar{R}}^N$ can be inherited straightforwardly was beautifully demonstrated in a white Swiss family investigated by Dr Drescher, Dr Müller and Miss Kaczmarski, who kindly shared the samples with Dr Tippett: 4 of 8 sibs had the $\bar{\bar{R}}^N$ gene complex and these 4 sibs had 5 children with, and 7 without, $\bar{\bar{R}}^N$. In some family members $\bar{\bar{R}}^N$ was partnered by CDe and this gave Dr Tippett the opportunity to show that $\bar{\bar{R}}^N$, unlike r'^s, does not produce any c antigen.

> Although all seven anti-$\bar{\bar{R}}^N$ sera in our collection behave alike with negro and white samples they appear to differ in immunological background: some are frankly immune and some cannot have been stimulated by $\bar{\bar{R}}^N$ cells. Anti-$\bar{\bar{R}}^N$ has been made by Negroes and Whites of various Rh groups, CDe/cDE, CDe/cde, cDE/cde and cDe/cDe (or cDe/cde).

In 1968 Dr Salmon and his colleagues sent us a sample from a Senegalese man, at first thought to be $(C)D-/(C)D-$, which Dr Tippett found to react with some anti-e sera, with anti-$\bar{\bar{R}}^N$ sera, and to give all the reactions expected of $\bar{\bar{R}}^N\bar{\bar{R}}^N$.

Dr Holman, Dr Ata and Mr Dobson were faced with the problem of a negro mother, from the Gambia, with antibody incompatible with all cells tested except $-D-/-D-$, and, subsequently, Rh_{null}. Dr Tippett found the mother's cells to give the reactions expected of $\bar{\bar{R}}^N\bar{\bar{R}}^N$: both children's cells reacted with anti-$\bar{\bar{R}}^N$.

Rosenfield, Allen and Rubinstein[438] think of $\bar{\bar{R}}^N$ as an 'operator or promoter' depressing C and e products which 'leads to the expression, perhaps as a direct

8

consequence, of the rare antigen Rh32', but it is easier, and lazier, to think of it as a compound antigen produced by some unusual *Ce* complex.

(C)D(e)

In 1963, Broman, Heiken, Tippett and Giles[265] found six examples of the complex (*C*)*D*(*e*) in unrelated Swedish people. Relatives of all six propositi were tested and the gene complex shown to be inherited in the normal way. Further examples were reported by Heiken and Giles[264], who showed the Swedish (*C*)*D*(*e*) to be heterogeneous, one producing normal and the other elevated D antigen. Then, in 1971, Giles and Skov[465] found an antibody specific for the product of (*C*)*D*(*e*) without enhanced D: it was present in a routine anti-C^w+Wr^a serum, and was later, we believe, given the number anti-Rh35.

The antigen V, or ce^s

Anti-V was reported in 1955 (DeNatale, Cahan, Jack, Race and Sanger[71]): it was found in the serum of a *cde*/*cde* recipient of many transfusions. The predominantly negro antigen V was found only in people possessing the gene complexes *cDe* or *cde*. V was later found[271], as expected, also in the complex *cD^{u}e*.

Table 35 shows the frequency of the antigen V in various peoples: in Africa the *ce* gene complexes carrying V are, as expected, more frequent than in American Negroes. From the Rh groups of the New York, West African and Seattle Negroes it was clear that V accompanies *cDe* at least twice as often as it does *cde* in these people.

It is rather interesting, and illustrative of the diagnostic power of anti-V, that the two people with V among the 444 New York Whites were found, on inquiry, to be Puerto Ricans: there were only five Puerto Ricans amongst the 444. In the families of the two English donors with V there was no sign or history of African ancestry.

Table 35. The antigen V: frequency in Negroes and other peoples

		Number tested	V+ obs.	%
DeNatale *et al.*[71]	Whites in London	407	2*	0·49
DeNatale *et al.*[71]	Whites in New York	444	2*	0·45
Giblett *et al.*[72]	Whites in Seattle	514	1	0·19
DeNatale *et al.*[71]	Negroes in New York	168	45	26·79
Giblett *et al.*[72]	Negroes in Seattle	327	94	28·75
DeNatale *et al.*[71]	W. Africans in Lagos and Accra	150	60	40·00
Shapiro[245]	Bantu in S. Africa	511	170	33·27
Giblett *et al.*[72]	Orientals	272	1	0·37
Giblett *et al.*[72]	American Indians	174	2	1·15

* See text.

In the original paper[71], tests on 15 negro families and one large white family showed V to be a dominant character, always travelling with *ce* (*cDe* or *cde*): many other families have now been tested, some of them published[271–273,245].

Two more examples of anti-V were soon found[72]. As far as we know, all examples so far are from transfused people and none has been blamed for haemolytic disease of the newborn.

In our hands anti-V sera are not all precisely alike, but so far have only disclosed their heterogeneity when tested with the cells of some of the rare e people with anti-e-like antibodies in their serum: amongst these are the famous Shabalala[158] and Santi[303] often mentioned in the literature.

In the original paper we said that we could not exclude the possibility that *V* was an allele of *f*, and when the anti-VS serum (anti-e^s) was found to react with all V+ samples and with 'negro r''' samples, this seemed to be supported, for V could be interpreted most easily as a combined antigen, ce^s, which could be considered 'allelic' to f(ce).

This interpretation was, however, severely criticized by Shapiro[245]. Furthermore, Rosenfield, Allen and Rubinstein[438] consider V to be a product of the *Ee* structural locus rather than a *cis* product involving also *c*; in their glossary they, rather unfortunately we think, use e^s as a synonym for V though we had used e^s for VS, as will be seen below, if the reader gets so far.

If V were a product of the *Ee* structural locus rather than a *cis* product involving also *c*, then a gene complex producing C and V might be expected to exist. And perhaps this has been found by Miss Charmaine Brice, of Knoxville, in a sample from Mr Ink., a white man, whose blood has been tested in many laboratories, but never reported.

Mr Ink. is *C^{w}De/CDe* and his cells react with most, but not all, anti-V and anti-VS sera: the cells of his sister, *CDe/cde*, give similar unusual V and VS reactions which are presumably the product of her *CDe* gene complex since her son is *cDE/cde* and V–VS–.

So we are probably wrong in thinking of V as ce^s; though this is how V manifests itself in all but the exceptional sample.

The antigen VS and the gene complex *r'^{n}*, *r'^{s}* or *Cde^s*

We do not, at present, look on this antigen as a member of the compound series but its close relationship to V makes its description convenient here.

That the reactions of most apparent *Cde/cde* samples from Negroes are variable with anti-C sera had been common experience for some time. Sturgeon, Fisk, Wintler and Chertock[274,275] cleared the air by showing that the majority of *Cde/cde* negro samples reacted with anti-C but not with anti-Ce sera. This was attributed to a difference in Ce which was represented by the symbol C^n. At about the same time, Zoutendyk and Teodorsuk[276,277] observed, from tests with anti-C and anti-Ce sera, that the Bantu were relatively rich in this unusual *Cde*.

The finding of the antibody anti-VS (anti-e^s) mentioned on page 197, led Sanger and her colleagues[156] to prefer to think of the predominantly negro type of r' as due to a difference in e rather than in C. The symbol e^s rather than e^n was chosen, with apologies to Dr Sturgeon and his collaborators, because considerable objection had arisen to the use of the n which was considered to be a racial label.

The reactions of anti-VS are shown in Table 36: it sensitizes all normal V+ samples and most negro r' samples. Our interpretation is given in Table 37. The hypothesis would adumbrate the existence of an antibody anti-Ce^s: it certainly explains neatly the negative or weak reactions of r'^{s}r (Cde^s/cde) cells with anti-Ce sera. Family tests would be needed to demonstrate CDe^s—if its exists.

Table 36. Results of testing the red cells of 262 unrelated but often selected people with the serum of Mrs V.S. (From Sanger, Noades, Tippett, Race, Jack and Cunningham[156], 1960)

	Negroes				Whites			
	V	r'^{s}	r'	Others	V	r'^{s}	r'	Others
VS+	28	13	0	0	3	2	0	0
VS−	0	0	1	50	0	0	80	85*

* Includes one example of $r^G r$ and representatives of almost all the the known Rh genotypes.

Table 37. One interpretation of the haploid reactions given by V and r'^{s}

		Antibodies			
		anti-V	anti-VS	anti-C	
				some	others
dCe^s	r'^{s}	−	+	+	−
					or w
dce^s	r^v	+	+	−	−
dCe	r'	−	−	+	+
dce	r	−	−	−	−
		anti-ce^s	anti-e^s	anti-C	anti-Ce

Inside the border are the known reactions: outside is the interpretation. (After Sanger, Noades, Tippett, Race, Jack and Cunningham[156], 1960.)

One difficulty about r'^{s} is that it should not be written as Cde^s but as $Ccde^s$. Rosenfield et al.[273] noticed, and we did too[278], that Cde^s/cde (r'^{s}r) cells react more strongly with anti-f (anti-ce) than do cells representing a single dose of ce in cis and, demonstrating the point more clearly, that cells of the genotype Cde^s/cDE (r'^{s}R$_2$) do react with anti-f. Furthermore, these cells, Cde^s/cDE, do react, sometimes rather weakly, with most anti-e sera. This, at any rate, could be comfortably understood if the antigen e^s cross-reacts with anti-e in the way we have had to suppose that anti-C cross-reacts, relatively weakly, with the antigen C^w.

Sturgeon *et al.*[274] from the results of absorption and titration of an anti-c serum concluded that Cde^s/cde ($r'^s r$) cells have slightly less than double but more than a single dose of c antigen. Rosenfield *et al.*[273] found such cells to give a double dose and we find that they give a double, a single or one and a half doses, depending on the anti-c used.

Rosenfield, Haber and Degnan[246] showed conclusively that Cde^s or r'^s does indeed produce some c antigen as well as some C antigen: they found that the cells of the CDe/Cde^s father of two Cde^s/cde children reacted with anti-c.

We have noticed that the r'^s gene complex has a depressing effect on a *trans* D analogous to that produced by r' (page 233): it was observed in the genotype Cde^s/cDE.

Another allele which produces both C and a weak c and which also produces weak E, was detected in a Brazilian family by Morton and Rosenfield[391]. The allele was called r^{yn} because it echoes r'^n (or r'^s) in its production of C and c: it does not produce VS(e^s) or f (ce) or Ce.

Other examples of anti-VS(-e^s) soon turned up, very often accompanied by other Rh antibodies. Although these examples gave uniform reactions with the ordinary run of negro red cell samples, it soon became clear (Table 48 of our third edition, and Tippett[169]) that not all examples of anti-VS were of identical specificity.

Shapiro[245] in reporting a fine study of Bantu bloods asserts that some anti-VS are anti-hr^H and others, like the original, are anti-hr^v (anti-V) plus anti-hr^H. For many years we have been using the same anti-VS as Dr Shapiro (provided by Miss Jean P. Harris of New York) and we agree that rare negro people exist whose cells are V+VS− and others whose cells are C−V−VS+. Those interested in negro Rh must read Shapiro's paper[245]: in it our interpretation is roundly criticized, so Table 37 should not be taken as gospel. However, V and VS, though their interpretation is so difficult, are very useful and straightforward genetic markers.

Other e variants in Negroes

Many of the Rh problems peculiar to Negroes seem to hinge on variants of e. Through the kindness of the original investigators we have had the opportunity to test many samples from e positive Negroes with apparent anti-e (not auto) in their serum. These anti-e-like antibodies are of differing specificities; two examples have been resolved by Shapiro and his colleagues[158,437], the one as anti-hr^s (plus anti-Hr) and the other as anti-hr^B, but the rest lack labels. In our last edition we gave details showing the varying reactions given by the cells of seven of these makers of anti-e-like antibody when tested with our range of anti-e, anti-e-like, anti-V and anti-VS sera.

We wondered whether these and other negro red cell samples would make a clearer story if they were studied with antibodies made in Negroes. It is perhaps of significance that both Shapiro[158] and Rosenfield[303] note that some of their

anti-e sera failed to react with the cells of Shabalala and Santi., whereas all eleven
of our routine anti-e (all from white donors) did react; furthermore, with our three
best anti-e sera the cells of Santi. gave a normal double dose effect. Our variable
reactions with anti-V and -VS sera may also be due to some of these antibodies
having been made in Whites in response to transfusion.

With more homogeneous reagents it may one day be possible to make relatively clear categories for the e of these people like those for people who have D
and have made anti-D (Table 33, page 191).

Other Rh antigens

So far we have given some details of almost all the Rh antigens defined by specific
antibodies but there are others which are less surely placed in the Rh system such
as Evans and Zd (pages 441 and 442) each of which has been found only in one
family and each of which was the cause of haemolytic disease of the newborn.

The Evans antigen occurred in an English family[379]. The propositus, his sister,
his father and his paternal grandfather have the antigen and all have an Rh complex which is like, but not identical to, $-D-$; his mother, paternal grandmother
and great-aunt do not have the Evans antigen or the $-D-$-like complex. Anti-
Evans does not react with the cells of true $-D-$ homozygotes or heterozygotes.

The Zd antigen occurred in a three-generation Czechoslovakian family[467]
travelling with cde.

SUPPRESSIONS

Under this heading are gathered very rare but theoretically very important conditions in which some or all of the expected Rh antigens are missing. In describing
the first example, in 1950, we said that a short deletion, a small piece of chromosome missing, seemed the most likely genetical background; but, for reasons to
be given, we have for some time thought that the background was very unlikely
to be as simple as this.

$-D-$

A sample of blood lacking any representation of either the C or the E series of
antigens was described by Race, Sanger and Selwyn[61,62] (1950, 1951). The
propositus was the product of a consanguineous marriage and was presumed to be
homozygous for a very rare gene complex which was given the symbol $-D-$. The
gene could be traced to a Scottish baronet born at the end of the eighteenth century, who, by two marriages, sent it on its way down two lines to the propositus.

Further examples followed: a list is given in Table 38. Notable amongst the
investigations were those of a large Canadian Indian kindred (Buchanan and
McIntyre[65-67]) and of a large inbred Nova Scotian kindred (Moore, McIntyre,
Brown, Read and Linins[284,285]). In the latter family the marriage which intro-

Table 38. Some information about the propositi and their relatives in 21 $-D-/-D-$, 1 C^wD-/C^wD-, 3 $cD-/cD-$ and 1 $(C)D^{IV}-/(C)D^{IV}-$ families

Propositus	Investigators	Race	Consanguinity of parents	Sibs of propositus		
				Hom. $-D-$	Het. $-D-$	No $-D-$
Mrs B. (O)	Race, Sanger and Selwyn[61,62], 1950	British White	half second cousins	0	0	0
Mrs V.W. (O)	Waller, Sanger and Bobbitt[63], 1953	American White	first cousins	2 (O, O)	0	1
Mrs Pep. (O)	Levine, Koch, McGee and Hill[64], 1954	American White	third cousins	0	0	0
Mrs Ca. (O)	Buchanan and McIntyre[66], 1955	American Indian	very inbred	2 (O, O)	2	1
Mrs N.† (B)	Kuniyuki and Takahara[283], 1958	Japanese	cousins	3 (O, O, B)	1	1
Mrs L.G. (O)	Moore, McIntyre, Brown and Read[284,285], 1960	Canadian White	first cousins	1 (O)	1	0
Mrs Q. (A₁)	Allen[286], 1960	American White	consanguineous	2	3	2
				0	1	0
				2 (O, A₂)	0	0
Mrs Ota* (A)	Ose and Bush[287], 1960	Japanese	first cousins	1 (A)	2	2
Mrs You. (O)	Cleghorn[154], 1961	British White	first cousins	2 (O, A₁)	0	0
Mrs G.‡ (O)	Yokoyama, Solomon, Kuniyuki and Stroup[288], 1961	Japanese	same village	1 (B)	2	2
Mrs Yos. (B)	Yokoyama, Tsuchiya, Kurata, Lodge and Dunsford[289], 1961	Japanese	not cousins same village	1 (A₁)	2	0
Mr J.M.	Ellis[311], 1961	American White	consanguineous	3 (O, B, B)	0	0
Mrs D.O. (A₂)	Chalton, Humphreys, Linins and Moore[312], 1961	Canadian White	first cousins	0	2	0
Mrs A.M.S. (A)	de Torregrosa, Rullán, Cecile, Sabater and Alberto[251], 1961	Puerto Rican White	not related	0	5	2

Table 38—continued

Propositus	Investigators	Race	Consanguinity of parents	Sibs of propositus		
				Hom. –D–	Het. –D–	No –D–
Mrs T.A. (B)	Nakajima, Misawa and Ota[252], 1965	Japanese	first cousins	2 (O, O)	0	2
Mrs M.O. (A₁,B)	Yamaguchi, Tanaka, Tsuji and Nakajima[253], 1965	Japanese	first cousins	1 (A₁,B)	3	2
II-2 (O) / Mr N. (O) / C. (O)	Unger[254], 1964 (unpublished) / Panocell donor, 1964 (unpublished) / Found at Spectra, 1965 (unpublished)	Puerto Rican / American Negro	probably related	0	0	1
Mrs M. (O)	Pope and Francis, 1966 (unpublished)	Puerto Rican				
Mrs K. (A)	Badakere and Bhatia[468], 1973	Hindu	consanguineous	0	0	0
				Hom.	Het.	No
Mrs B.G. $C^wD–/C^wD–$ (A₁)	Gunson and Donohue[261], 1957	Canadian White	second cousins	4 (O, O, A₁, A)	3	1
Mr A.L.C. $cD–/cD–$ (O)	Tate, Cunningham, McDade, Tippett and Sanger[290], 1960	American White	double first cousins	2 (A₁, A₁)	1	1
Mrs H. $cD–/cD–$ (A₁,B)	Yamaguchi, Okubo, Tomita, Yamano and Tanaka[469], 1969	Japanese	not related	0	0	0
Mme Po. $cD–/cD–$ (O)	Delmas-Marsalet, Goudemand and Tippett[470], 1969	French	first cousins	0	0	0
Mme Nou. $(C)D^{IV}–/(C)D^{IV}–$ (B)	Salmon, Gerbal, Liberge, Sy, Tippett and Sanger[380], 1969	West African	no information	0	0	1

* Pedigree also given in Silber et al.[128]
† Part of this pedigree also published by Yokoyama et al.[288]
‡ Propositus mentioned in four earlier publications.[291]
The ABO groups of the homozygotes when available have been entered in brackets, in case they are needed as donors.
See also Addenda.

duced the gene complex could be traced to that of a local woman to an English mariner shipwrecked in the Northumberland Strait and landed at Pugwash, Nova Scotia, about 1790.

No relationship has been traced between any of the propositi of Table 38. All but two of them were brought to notice because of trouble resulting from Rh antibodies they had made in response to pregnancy or transfusion. The exceptions are Mrs You., a normal blood donor, recognized by Cleghorn[154], and Mr N., a prospective candidate for the Knickerbocker (Pfizer) Panocell.

Studying, in 1960, the families of $-D-/-D-$ propositi we[292] were struck by the unexpected results of two counts: counts of the consanguinity rate of the parents of the propositi and counts of the Rh groups of the sibs of the propositi. Subsequent data have not made the consanguinity counts any less surprising.

Consanguinity of the parents of $-D-/-D-$ propositi

There is information about 18 of the 21 $-D-/-D-$ propositi of Table 38: 14 are known to be the product of consanguineous marriages and three more very likely are; this leaves only one probably not. The consanguinity rate may be as high as 80%.

The incidence of consanguinity is compared, in Table 39, with that found in the parents of propositi lacking other very common antigens, propositi who are believed to represent the homozygous state of very rare alleles and who have an incidence of probably less than one in 10,000. Such a high consanguinity rate for $-D-$ would be surprising even if the corresponding alleles were much rarer than those responsible for p, P^k, O_h, Ge— and K_0, but there is no reason for thinking that they are. Furthermore, p, P^k and O_h people, because of their regular non-immune antibodies, should announce themselves more efficiently than $-D-/-D-$ people who usually have to become immunized before they are recognized.

Table 39. Consanguinity of the parents of propositi of rare conditions thought to be recessive characters

	Consanguineous	Not related	No information
p	14	31	10
P^k	5	15	2
O_h Indians*	3	6	2
O_h Europeans	4	7	0
Ge— Europeans	2	9	4
K_0	6	7	1
$-D-/-D-$	14	4**	3
C^wD-/C^wD-	1	0	0
$cD-/cD-$	2	1	0

* Indian data collected by Bhatia and Sanghvi[255].
** Two from same village, a third probably related.

In our fourth edition we said 'The high consanguinity rate demands an explanation and the answer would probably give some insight into the organization of the Rh gene complex as a whole.' We suggested one possibility, but it was not a very good one. Several mathematico-genetical friends have bent their minds to this problem, but it still remains a puzzle. (See also Addenda.)

From Table 39 the following 2 × 2 table may be constructed:

	Not Rh	Rh
consanguinity definite	34	17
consanguinity absent or doubtful	75	5

χ^2 for 1 d.f. is 16·4 which corresponds to a probability of 1 in about 20,000.

The sibs of $-D-/-D-$ propositi

The other surprising fact that emerges from Table 38 is the high rate of sibs of $-D-/-D-$ propositi who are also $-D-/-D-$. If $-D-/-D-$ were a straightforward homozygous condition we would expect one quarter of the sibs (not, of course, counting the propositi themselves) to be $-D-/-D-$, and we find 19 out of a total of 54 sibs, which is not a significant departure. If the sibs of the two propositi, homozygous for $C^w D-$ and for $cD-$, are added to the count the excess of homozygotes does become significant ($\chi^2 = 5·41$ for 1 d.f., P = 0·02). The explanation may lie in some selection of these families that escapes us.

Serological notes

The red cells

The cells of people homozygous or heterozygous for $-D-$ have more D antigen than have ordinary DD or Dd cells: this can be shown by the ability of saline suspensions of the $-D-$ cells to be agglutinated by some incomplete anti-D sera. Most incomplete anti-D sera will agglutinate the homozygotes, $-D-/-D-$, but it is only some that will agglutinate the heterozygotes without agglutinating cDE/cDE cells (which are strong in D). But given a suitable serum it is usually easy to recognize heterozygotes within a family known to have $-D-$ if they are of the genotype $CDe/-D-$ or $cDE/-D-$: on the other hand $cDe/-D-$ and $cde/-D-$ may not show up well by this test (Lawler and Marshall[256]). We use the test as a routine in Rh grouping and have found perhaps a dozen $-D-$ heterozygotes subsequently proved by investigation of their families; but we have also found several reactors which later proved not to be $-D-$.

Though undoubtedly rare, the gene complex $-D-$, especially in the heterozygous state, is the cause of theoretical and practical difficulties in the interpretation of Rh grouping in paternity tests (see page 502).

The sera

$-D-/-D-$ people have more opportunity to become immunized than have people of pedestrian Rh genotypes for the lack all but two, D and G, of the known Rh antigens. For the same reason the antibodies they make are, not surprisingly, complex.

No evidence is yet available that the response is different to different immunizing antigens. Considering the antibodies of the first propositus, we[62] guessed that the absence of any representation of C or E antigens in the recipient, by removing some canalyzing restraint, allowed the antibody response to any C or E antigens to be somewhat hysterical and able to embrace other C or E antigens, which are presumably close relatives in structure. Anti-e was certainly present and we satisfied ourselves that separable anti-C and anti-c could, with some difficulty, be demonstrated. However, much of the antibody seemed to be directed against C and c indifferently; we were not able to demonstrate separable anti-E. Hackel[199] studied this serum and that of one of the $-D-/-D-$ American Indians who had also been immunized: using both absorption and elution methods he confirmed the earlier results and also identified anti-E and anti-ce (anti-f), and agreed that much of the antibody content appeared to be directed at various forms of C and E indifferently.

The tendency in the States is to think that these sera contain but one antibody, anti-Hr_0, directed against a single 'factor' Hr_0 produced by all the common Rh gene complexes[293]. This we would qualify by adding that separable anti-e has been a notable component of the examples we have appropriately tested.

We have tested many sera from immunized $-D-/-D-$ people: they fail to agglutinate the cells of other $-D-/-D-$ and the cells of C^wD-/C^wD-, $cD-/cD-$ and of Rh_{null} persons to be described below. The failure to agglutinate $cD-/cD-$ cells hinted at further levels of complexity, for we thought the sera contained anti-c as one component.

C^wD-

A large family with five members homozygous for this gene complex was described by Gunson and Donohue[102, 261]. Table 38 shows that the two striking peculiarities of the families of $-D-/-D-$ propositi are echoed by that of the C^wD-/C^wD- propositus: her parents are consanguineous and four of her sibs are homozygous like herself (only two would be expected to be so).

In this condition, as in $-D-$, the strength of the D antigen is exalted in both homozygotes and heterozygotes: the only other detectable Rh antigens are C^w and G.

In view of the weakness of the c antigen in $cD-/cD-$ (see below) we[318] were not surprised to find that the C^w antigen produced by C^wD- reacted much less strongly than did the C^w produced by C^wDe with all but one of our anti-C^w sera. This makes understandable the failure of C^wD-/C^wD- to react with anti-C sera (lacking anti-D) which have relatively weak anti-C^w activity.

No other example of homozygous C^wD- has been found in the 17 years since the original report: however, Mr R.R. Stapleton encountered in Sheffield a sample giving the expected reactions of C^wD-/cde (depressed C^w and elevated D). Gunson et al.[261] had noted that the original family went to Canada from an unknown locality in England early in the 19th century.

$cD-$

An inbred white family in which three members are homozygous for this gene complex was reported by Tate, Cunningham, McDade, Tippett and Sanger[290] (1960). Some details are given in Table 38.

The haploid antigens corresponding to $cD-$ could be described thus: D, more in amount than usually corresponds to one D gene; c, less than usually corresponds to one c gene and perhaps differing qualitatively (for one of many good anti-c sera failed to react at all); ce (f), less than usually corresponds to one dose. That there should be any ce antigen remains a puzzle: the cells react with the two anti-f sera from CDe/cDE persons[69,268] but they do not react with two anti-e sera, Br. and Kr., known to contain anti-f. Evidently the 'anti-f' in the two types of sera cannot be precisely the same antibody.

A Cincinatti Negro was found by Miss C. Brice to be another example of $cD-/cD-$ when the reactions of his cells paralleled those in the white family. This second propositus is not entered in Table 38 because no information about his family was available. We do not know how to classify two further homozygotes, a Negro and his mother, reported from Bethesda[392]: the D antigen was not enhanced nor was the c depressed.

In 1969, two further $cD-/cD-$ families were reported (Table 38), one French[470] and one Japanese[469]; both propositi had, like the original homozygote[290], antibody for all cells tested except those homozygous for $-D-$, $cD-$ and C^wD- and Rh_{null}. The $cD-$ complex in the French propositus produced antigens precisely like those in the original family: the Japanese propositus produced less c antigen and no f (ce), so much so that c was not detected in the mother of the propositus, who must have been $CDe/cD-$.

More recently Dr Frank Ellis sent us samples from a $CDe/cD-$ negro mother and her $cD-/cde$ daughter: on first testing the mother had appeared C+c− and the daughter C−c+.

$(C)D^{IV}-$

Salmon, Gerbal, Liberge, Sy, Tippett and Sanger[380] (1969) investigated the serum of Mme Nou (Côte d'Ivoire) whose third child had died of haemolytic disease of the newborn. The serum reacted with all cells at first tested save those of Mme Nou. herself. Elution tests suggested that Mme Nou.'s serum would not react with $-D-/-D-$ cells, and this proved correct. When the fourth baby was born, in Paris, it was successfully treated by exchange transfusion with $-D-/-D-$ blood from London.

The following is a summary of the reactions of Mme Nou.'s cells:

D not exalted, as it is in $-D-/-D-$ cells. D reactions those of Category IV (Table 33). G apparently normal. C depressed; three anti-Ce sera reacted positively and four reacted negatively, and the reactions were confirmed by elution tests. Antigen e probably absent (three of ten anti-e sera reacted weakly, but these three had not been proved free of anti-Ce); only one of the seven 'anti-e-like' antisera of page 209 did react, and that only weakly. Antigens E, c, ce, V (ce^s) and VS (e^s) all absent. With a range of anti-C sera the cells of Mme. Nou. did not give the pattern expected of $\bar{\bar{R}}^N$, nor, subsequently, did they react with anti-$\bar{\bar{R}}^N$ (page 205).

So the genotype of Mme Nou. was a 'new' one, which could be described as homozygous for $(C)D^{IV}-$. The husband of Mme Nou. is cDe/cDe or cDe/cde and the cells of their two elder children reacted weakly[380], like those of their mother, with anti-C.

The minus-minus-minus complex

This complex, which produces no Rh antigens, was first identified by Henningsen[295,296] (1958) in the heterozygous state in a Danish mother whose apparent exclusion from the parentage of her child led to a family investigation; two other heterozygous examples were disclosed, again by apparent non-maternity, in a German and a Swedish mother (Prokop and Schneider[297], 1960, Broman and Heiken[298], 1961) and we have been sent several for checking since that time. The same, or a similar, amorphic complex, in the homozygous state, is responsible for one form of Rh$_{null}$ (see page 220).

Depressed antigenic complexes

Under this heading are gathered a few gene complexes which result in weak or depressed antigens. We suspect mutant forms of C, D or E may be responsible and that these mutants may produce antigens which we cannot at present recognize for lack of the corresponding antibody. C^w will serve to illustrate what we mean: if anti-C^w had not yet been found the gene complex C^wDe, for example, would nevertheless have been distinguishable from CDe because of its weak reaction with anti-C sera (for anti-C sera usually react, relatively weakly, with cells representing C^wc).

Alternatively there may be some inhibitor site or sites incorporated in the Rh gene complex or closely linked to it. The depressing influence, whether we call it an allele of C or D or of E or an inhibitor gene, has its effect in cis: in the r^M family there is a suggestion that it may also be having some effect in trans.

Antigens corresponding to the gene complex r^G

In studying the cells of Mrs Crosby and of her family (see page 201) Allen and Tippett[279] identified only two antigens corresponding to the gene complex r^G, e (rather weak) and G. Whether it produced c was left in doubt, for no member of the family was R^1r^G. This was later settled when Levine, Rosenfield and White[299] found a representative of the extraordinarily rare genotype r^Gr^G (the product of a first cousin mating) whose cells were negative with anti-c.

Through the kindness of Dr Allen and Dr Levine we have been able to test r^Gr and r^Gr^G cells and we find them to be rather weakly positive with about one third of our anti-C sera from Rh positive donors (and so lacking anti-G). Incidentally, the r^Gr^G sample was negative with the two 'pure' anti-f sera (anti-ce) mentioned above and with anti-V (anti-ce^s) and anti-VS (anti-e^s). Some reactions of r^Gr^G cells with anti-C sera are given in Table 34 (page 201). The paper by Levine et al.[299] should be consulted: they consider r^Gr^G and r^Gr cells 'to lack C antigenic determinants, but to possess C^G, a C-like antigenic determinant.'

Three examples of negro r^Gr have been reported[300,317,258]. Dr Tippett finds that negro r^Gr cells are not easy to distinguish from r'^sr: both react with anti-VS (-e^s) sera but not with anti-V (-ce^s), but the reactions of negro r^Gr with anti-C and anti-G sera are weaker than those of r'^sr. The reactions of negro r^Gr with anti-C and anti-G are weaker than those of white r^Gr. Beattie and her colleagues[449] studied 14 such negro r^Gr and one of their families: they call the weaker G antigen G^u.

Antigens corresponding to the gene complex r^M

A sample of blood from Mrs M.R., which at first looked to be the same as that of Mrs Crosby, was described by Tippett, Sanger, Dunsford and Barber[270] but exhaustive tests showed marked differences. The antigens corresponding to the gene complex r^M are: G, depressed, some kind of C and some kind of E, both depressed.

Tippett et al.[270] noticed several hints that the complex r^M might have a trans effect: in one member of the family r^M was coupled with CD^ue, which could of course be due to chance; in two members the ce antigen produced by the trans complex was notably weak and in another the trans c antigen was very weak. Tippett et al.[270] illustrated their conclusions about r^M and compared them with r^G thus:

$$r^M \quad G \quad C \quad E$$
$$\downarrow \quad \downarrow \quad \downarrow$$
$$r^G \quad G \quad C \quad e$$
$$\downarrow \quad \downarrow$$

the arrows representing depression of the antigens. They speculated whether r^M could be a CDE or CdE gene complex which had undergone a mutation perhaps to some unknown allele of D. They also wondered whether r^G could be a mutant form of CDe or Cde. The arrows are a clear way of presenting weakness of the antigen but not convenient for type or print. On the few occasions when such gene complexes are being discussed brackets may be used in place of the arrows, for example r^Mr can be written $(C)d(E)/cde$.

Antigens corresponding to the gene complex r^L and r^t

By a succession of chances the attention of Metaxas and Metaxas-Bühler[301] (1961) was drawn to the Rh antigens of a Zürich blood donor, Mr O.L., at first, thought to be CDe/CDe. Tests on the family showed the existence of a 'new' gene complex r^L in the donor and his mother: r^L results in weak or depressed c and e antigens though in a normal f(ce) antigen. This very careful investigation may be summarized thus:

Mr O.L. $CDe/(c)d(e)$ or $CDe/(c)(D)(e)$
his mother $cD^uE/(c)d(e)$ or $cdE/(c)(D)(e)$

Two further examples and their families were reported by Heiken and Giles[264].

Tippett[169] and the late Dr Dunsford studied the family of a blood donor in which a similar gene complex was present in three generations: the gene complex, called r^t or $c^t de$, again produces depressed c antigen some e and some f, but the pattern of reactions given by anti-c sera is different in bloods representing $R^1 r^t$ from that in blood representing $R^1 r^L$. It was possible to elute anti-c from the cells of a Cc^t heterozygote after sensitization with anti-c capable of agglutinating them, but not after exposure to an anti-c serum which did not agglutinate them. Some years later[475] the cells of a white Australian $c^t de$ propositus were found to give reactions identical with those of the original $c^t de$ English donor. c^t is not the same as the c allele described by Heustis et al.[160], for Cc^t cells do not react with the majority of anti-c sera (including that of Huestis et al.).

Antigens corresponding to the gene complexes $(C)D(e)$ and $(C^w)D(e)$

Two gene complexes producing depressed C and e antigens, $\bar{\bar{R}}^N$ and $(C)D(e)$, are now known each to produce an antigen recognizable by a specific antibody (pages 204–206). At least one such complex, $(C)D(e)$, results in an elevated D antigen[264], but whether it produces a specific antigen is not yet known[465].

The frequencies in Sweden of such complexes as $(C)D(e)$ and $(c)d(e)$ were estimated by Rasmuson and Heiken[305]. Families with similar gene complexes were observed among 1,000 families tested by Chown et al.[462].

Kornstad and Larsen[471] describe a complex $(C^w)D(e)$ which produces normal D, and weak C^w, C and e: the family was informative and showed the new complex aligned in *trans* with CDe, cDE and cde.

A gene complex $(c)D(E)$ or $(c)d(E)$

Kornstad and Øyen[313] report a blood donor, Miss T.S., who is superficially CDe/cDE but whose c and E antigens are much depressed. The depressed complex, either $(c)D(E)$ or $(c)d(E)$ was traced in five other members of her family. Heiken[382] investigated two families in which a rather weak c and E were segregating together: one of them had previously been reported[58] as an example of E^u (see page 196).

Rh_{null} AND UNLINKED MODIFIERS

For a long time it seemed that the remaining interest in the Rh groups was the finer and finer subdividing of the known antigens and antibodies. Then the subject caught fire again when LW and Rh_{null} made a splendid blaze which is not yet burnt out. These two conditions are inter-related but Rh_{null} will be described first.

The Rh_{null} condition

A gust of fresh air seemed to disperse the Rh mists when Vos, Vos, Kirk and Sanger[294] (1961) reported a sample of blood with no Rh antigens at all. The propositus, an Australian aboriginal woman, Mrs E.N., a prospector for gold in the Western Desert, had, unfortunately, no close relative alive[294, 399]. According to the rules of her tribe her parents should not have been closely related, but in such a small breeding population some consanguinity seems likely, for the total population was then only about 2,000. The propositus had no Rh antibody in her serum: she was first noticed during an anthropological survey.

The condition was originally indicated thus $---/---$, but later observations made this notation quite inappropriate and the name 'Rh_{null}' was suggested by Ceppellini[334] and generally adopted.

Amongst several possible causes the first to be considered was that Mrs E.N. 'lacked a frequent gene necessary for the production of some Rh precursor substance', and this is the present view.

The next year Levine and his colleagues[320] found that the cells of Mrs E.N. reacted negatively with the 'D-like' antibody which was later to be called anti-LW (page 228).

The next step was the finding of a second example of Rh_{null}, this time in a white American patient. Mrs L.M. belonged to a large family but the Rh groups of her husband and her daughter were alone enough to throw real light on the adumbrated background of Rh_{null} (Levine, Celano, Falkowski, Chambers, Hunter and English[334–336]): inhibition was indeed responsible, just as it was for the Bombay condition. The husband of Mrs L.M. was *cde/cde* and their daughter *CDe/cde*. Therefore Mrs L.M. had certainly one and presumably two perfectly normal *Rh* gene complexes though she herself could not express them as antigens.

The third Rh_{null} propositus was, however, of a different genetic background: in the family reported by Ishimori and Hasekura[339, 385] the phenotype is clearly due not to inhibition of normal *Rh* genes but to homozygosity for a silent, or amorphic, allele at the *Rh* locus.

So there are at least two types of Rh_{null}: one, which we have come to call the regulator type, is caused by a 'regulator' gene which is *not* part of the *Rh* complex locus and the other, the amorph type, is caused by a silent or amorphic gene which *is* part of the *Rh* complex locus. The regulator type of Rh_{null} can be recognized when a parent or child of the propositus has both C and c or both E and e antigens.

The amorph type of Rh_{null} can be recognized when, for example, in the family an apparent CDe/CDe parent has an apparent cDE/cDE child. Sometimes, even when parents are available, the type of Rh_{null} is not disclosed. The pedigrees in Figure 14 represent the two types: they are abbreviated versions of as yet unpublished pedigrees. We give these two as a change from the original pedigrees of Levine et al.[336] and Ishimori and Hasekura[339, 385] which have been reproduced so many times.

We borrowed the convenient word 'regulator' from the great work of Jacob and Monod. Though the operon system of genetic control worked out in E. coli has not yet been shown to apply to mammals some think it likely to be: it has been considered for haemoglobin[486, 487] and Mäkelä and Stocker[488] (1969) wrote of ABO, Hh, Lewis and secretor in Jacob-Monod terms, and, more recently, there is the valiant attempt, to be referred to on page 241, to fit Rh into an operon scheme (Rosenfield, Allen and Rubinstein[438], 1973).

Without understanding any of the subtleties of operon activity, the bare skeleton of the loci involved given in Jacob and Monod's 1961 review[489] seems made for complex blood group systems. At its very simplest the operon consists of an operator gene and two or three structural genes closely linked to it. The operator controls the activity of these structural genes (the structural genes specify protein). A regulator locus, not closely linked to the operon, produces messenger RNA which, after uniting with certain specific metabolites in the cytoplasm, goes on to influence the activity of the operator gene. Mutation can happen at the regulator, operator and structural loci.

That the regulator locus is not part of the Rh locus is nicely demonstrated by the relatives of the Rh_{null} propositus of Guévin et al.[403]: the parents are first cousins and both CDe/cde, one Rh_{null} sib must be genetically CDe/cde (because her husband is cDE/cde, 3 children CDe/cde and 1 cDE/cde). Had the regulator been part of the Rh locus this Rh_{null} sib would, in view of the consanguinity of her parents, have to be genetically CDe/CDe or cde/cde.

The propositi and their families

Some details of all the Rh_{null} families we know about are given in Table 40.

The regulator seems to be more frequent than the amorph type. So far there is no way of distinguishing the two serologically: at first we[413] wondered whether the SsU disturbance, to be mentioned below, might be the prerogative of the regulator type, but this was ruled out when the Sea Lapp family (No. 13) was found.

The consanguinity rate of parents of propositi homozygous for a rare condition is expected to be high, but in this list it seems too high and echoes our puzzlement concerning $-D-/-D-$ (page 213); however, in this case the sib count seems just right: 8 Rh_{null} to 23 not Rh_{null}, when 7·75 to 23·25 would be expected.

In some of the families the Rh antigens of the parents or children of the propositi are markedly depressed, but in others they seem quite normal.

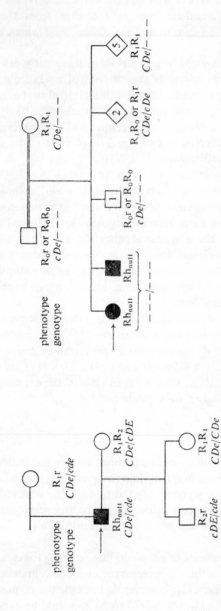

Fig. 14. Two kinds of Rh$_{null}$. The example on the left is of the 'regulator' type, controlled by an inhibitor gene unlinked to *Rh*: the family demonstrates that both alleles of the propositus are normal, though unable to express themselves as antigens. (Part of a family investigated by Hrubiško et al.[410].)

The example on the right is of the type caused by a 'silent' or amorphic allele at the *Rh* locus: the parents of the Rh$_{null}$ sibs are superficially *cc* and *CC*, with *cc* and *CC* children, thus disclosing the type of Rh$_{null}$ in the family. (Part of a family investigated by Dr. P. Oestgaard.)

Table 40. Rh$_{null}$: information collected from the literature or from our records

References	Race	Type of Rh$_{null}$	Rh antigens of relatives depressed	Sibs of propositi Rh$_{null}$:	not	Parental consanguinity
1. Vos et al.[294]	Australian aboriginal	?	Yes[399]	0	0	see text
2. Levine et al.[335,336]	USA, White	regulator	Yes	0	3	No
3. Ishimori et al.[385,400]	Japanese	amorph	none noted	0	1	Yes
4. Haber et al.[401,402]	USA, White	regulator	No	0	0	Yes
5. Guévin et al.[403]	French Canadian	regulator	Yes	2	2	Yes
6. Sturgeon[404]	USA, White	?	?	1[411]	0	not known
7. Senhauser et al.[405]	USA, White	regulator	Yes	0	0	Yes
8. Seidl et al.[406]	German	probably amorph	single dose	1	0	Yes
9. Polesky et al.[407,408]	USA, White	regulator	No	2	0	No
10. Nagel et al.[409]	German	?	somewhat	0	0	Yes
11. Hrubiško et al.[410]	Czech	regulator	No	0	1	same village
12. Stevenson et al.[411]	USA, White	regulator	No ?	1	5	Yes
13. Oestgaard[412]	Norwegian Sea Lapp	amorph	?	1	8	Yes
14. Müller[482]	Swiss	regulator	Yes	0	3	No

The *CDE* genotypes of the propositi of the regulator type appear, not surprisingly, to be random: *CDe*, *cde* and *cDE* have all been shown to be completely inhibited.

Ascertainment

The first Rh_{null} was ascertained during a population survey: of the others, four were brought to notice by antibody in their serum (Nos. 2, 4, 6, 10), three through having haemolytic anaemia (Nos. 8, 11, 12) and four were found in routine testing of blood donors, hospital or antenatal patients (Nos. 3, 5, 7, 9, 13, 14).

Antibody in Rh_{null} people

Some have made antibody presumed to be in response to transfusion or pregnancy. The antibody in some reacts with all cells tested (including $-D-/-D-$ etc.) but not with Rh_{null} (Nos. 4, 8 and the sister of 9), and this antibody has been given the number anti-Rh29 by the New York workers[401, 402]. The antibody in one Rh_{null} male donor (No. 10) arose without known stimulus: it differed from anti-Rh29 only by failing to react with $-D-/-D-$ cells, thus lacking any anti-D or anti-LW components. No. 2 had anti-e and anti-C in her serum[336, 414], while No. 6 and another sister of No. 9 had unidentified weak antibodies. Two Rh_{null} sisters of No. 5 had no Rh antibody though they had 4 and 3 children respectively.

Genetic pathway

Figure 15 is a satisfying attempt to relate the observed Rh reactions of the people with ordinary CDE antigens but no LW (to be described below) to those of the people listed in Table 40 who have neither CDE nor LW antigens. A precursor substance 1 is imagined which in the presence of the very common allele X^1 (X being unlinked to the *Rh* locus) is converted into substance 2. In Rh_{null} people of the regulator type, who are homozygous for the rare allele X^0, there is no conversion so substance 2 is absent. When, as normally happens, substance 2 is made, it is then converted by the *CDE* genes into Rh antigens some facet of which is further converted into LW antigen by *LW* which is dominant in effect. In the absence of *LW*, that is in the homozygote *lwlw*, there is no conversion to LW and the person has Rh antigens but no LW antigen. People of the amorph type of Rh_{null} presumably have substance 2 but their Rh genotype ($---/---$) is incapable of producing Rh antigens and as a consequence they are left also without LW antigen. Dr Giblett uses the symbols X^1 and X^0 for the 'aboriginal' genes which we think an improvement on the Xr^1 and Xr^0 of Levine *et al.*[334, 336].

Other antigens affected by the Rh_{null} state

The recognition that the regulator type of Rh_{null} had some defect of the cell surface fell to Schmidt, Lostumbo, English and Hunter[338], in 1967, who found that

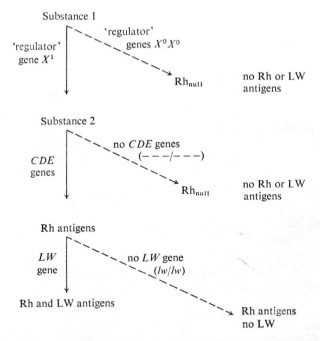

Fig. 15. Genetic pathways in the biosynthesis of Rh and LW antigens: a possible scheme taken from Tippett[415]. This is another way of putting the diagram of Giblett[416].

the cells of the propositus in Levine's family (No. 2, Table 40) gave peculiar reactions with anti-s and anti-U sera.

Other cases of Rh$_{null}$ were then and thereafter looked at from the point of view of upsets of the S, s and U antigens. In our Unit we were lucky to be given the opportunity to test for such antigenic upsets the cells of all but Nos. 2 and 3 in Table 40.

We found that S, s and U reactions known to be falsely negative were given only when the antiglobulin test was used. When saline reacting anti-S or anti-s sera were used no false negative reactions were seen, whereas when the antiglobulin test was needed about half of our anti-S, anti-s and anti-U sera gave false negative reactions. We suspect that the change to the surface of this type of Rh$_{null}$ cell may result in a less firm attachment of S, s and U to their antibody which may not always survive the rigorous washing prior to the antiglobulin test. This we suspect for two reasons: first, S+, s+Rh$_{null}$ cells are capable of absorbing anti-S and anti-s from sera with which they do not react by other tests: and second, an anti-S and an anti-s serum in our collection which react positively with Rh$_{null}$ cells in saline fail to react by the antiglobulin test, although they react well by this test with control cells.

The degree of suppression of S, s and U reactions varies in different propositi and may even vary between Rh$_{null}$ sibs. Perhaps it can vary in time: on two occasions we found the S, s and U reactions of No. 8 (Table 40) to be normal, but on a third they were slightly weakened.

In the regulator type of Rh_{null} cells we found the antigens M and N slightly enhanced but would not have thought much of this had not Dr Sturgeon and Dr Metaxas reported the same thing[404]. Another antigen we found affected by the Rh_{null} state was En^a: both of our anti-En^a sera reacted slightly, but unmistakably, more strongly with the cells of five examples of Rh_{null} than with those of ordinary $En(a+)$ people. We also found the Kidd and Dombrock antigens to be slightly enhanced.

McGinniss and her colleagues[476, 477] described IgM and, later, IgG antibodies, which they called anti-precursor, in four patients with anaemia: the sera reacted with Rh_{null} and other 'null' cells but not with 'normal' cells unless they were pre-papainized.

In Helsinki, Dr Nordling measured the electrophoretic mobility of one example of Rh_{null} of the regulator type and found it to be normal[413]. Normal also were the two Rh_{null} sibs of Seidl et al.[406].

The antigen i may be enhanced in Rh_{null} people[338] and this is presumably due to marrow stress consequent on their anaemia.

Only with the last but one Rh_{null} of Table 40 (No. 13) did it become clear that the SsU upset could occur in the amorphic as well as the regulatory type.

Rh_{null} disease

In the notable paper of 1967, in which Schmidt, Lostumbo, English and Hunter[338] recorded the finding of the SsU upset in Rh_{null} blood, is also described what later became known as Rh_{null} disease. The observation was first made on propositus No. 2 (Table 40) and repeated in the same year on propositus No. 1 (Schmidt and Vos[389]) and later found to be a general truth: the majority of Rh_{null} people have a compensated anaemia which may be severe but more often seems to be slight and may require sophisticated tests to detect. The anaemia may be shown by high reticulocyte counts, shortened survival time of their own Cr labelled blood, high foetal haemoglobin and raised i antigen strength. To these signs was later added the presence of stomatocytes (Sturgeon[404], 1970).

Now that Nicholson, Masouredis and Singer[417] have shown that the Rh antigens, probably protein, are an integral part of the red cell wall it is not surprising, as Levine[418] points out, that the Rh_{null} condition should be responsible for a defect in the structure of the wall.

Moulds[408] refers to a suggestion by Dr Rosenfield that the term 'Rh_{null} syndrome' is preferable to 'Rh_{null} disease', and we agree.

Heterogeneity of Rh_{null}

With fortunate segregation of the Rh groups in the families of Rh_{null} people two clear genetic types, the regulator and the amorphic, can be distinguished. There is, however, heterogeneity in the regulator type. Sometimes the propositus is anaemic and sometimes healthy. Sometimes his SsU antigens are depressed and sometimes normal, and in our Unit, it was noticed that the extent of the depression of these antigens is variable. Sometimes the Rh antigens of close relatives are depressed and sometimes not. Further, Stevenson et al.[411] record positive fixation-elution tests after exposure to anti-D of the cells of one Rh_{null} (sib of No. 12) but not of another (sib of No. 6). This was confirmed by Dr Tippett, using an anti-D serum which gave negative fixation-elution results with the cells of three other examples of Rh_{null}, one of which was known to have D in his genotype; she also observed that the cells of the sib of No. 12 were unlike those of other Rh_{null} samples in reacting, though weakly, with some immune sera from homozygous $-D-$, $cD-$ and C^wD- people.

We guess that the same X^0 allele is having slightly different effects in different environments.

Other unlinked modifiers

Chown, Lewis, Kaita and Lowen[419, 420] reported a fine investigation of a person whose phenotype at first appeared to be r^G but whose genotype proved to be R^1R^2. The inhibition of the relevant antigens was due to her being homozygous for a modifier gene unlinked to Rh: her parents were consanguineous like those of most Rh_{null} propositi. The patient had a condition indistinguishable from Rh_{null} disease, and her SsU antigens were rather weak.

The cells of the patient, besides reacting with anti-G, showed traces of other Rh antigens: and, unlike Rh_{null} cells, they reacted well with immune sera from homozygous $-D-$, $cD-$ and C^wD- and $\bar{R}^N$ people, and they reacted with anti-LW. The name Rh_{mod} was suggested for this phenotype[420].

In view of the heterogeneity of the regulator type of Rh_{null} one cannot help wondering whether the same X^0 allele is responsible but in this environment not being so successful in damping down the Rh and LW antigens—one of several possibilities considered by Chown and his colleagues.

A perhaps similar, but less inhibited, example is to be reported by Rosenfield et al.[421].

Earlier hints of unlinked depressors

The blood of two sisters was investigated by Dunsford and Tippett[302]; both were CDe/cde and family tests showed that they should have identical CDe gene complexes. In spite of this, one sister was found to be notably weaker than the other in the antigens D, Ce, c, ce and e, i.e. $(C)(D)(e)/(c)d(e)$, while being just as strong in the antigens M, s and k (these being the other antigens for which their genotypes were alike). The difference is a stable character for it was unchanged on retesting many months later. The parents were not consanguineous.

Another possible example of the effect of an unlinked depressor gene was reported by Giles and Bevan[330]. Two sisters, who should have been normal CDe/cDE (because their parents were normal cDE/cDE and CDe/CDe

respectively) both appeared to represent the genotype $(C)D(e)/(c)D(E)$. Furthermore, one of the sisters had a son to whom she gave a cDE gene complex which, in him, produced the expected antigens of normal strength. The parents of the two sisters were not consanguineous.

A family is reported[383] in which a child is $CDe/(c)D(E)$, the mother cDE/cde, two sibs CDe/cDE. Since the C, D and e antigens of the child are normal his two depressed antigens were attributed to mutation. Mutation is a word not to be juggled with lightly and we do not think too much weight should be given to this case. In the ABO system, for example, an unlinked inhibitor gene was found to affect the A but not the B of an AB person (see page 27).

THE LW ANTIGEN

The antibody which we now call anti-Rh_0, or anti-D, was first described by Levine and Stetson[2] in 1939 and in the next year the work on the anti-rhesus antibody, made by rabbits and guinea-pigs injected with the cells of rhesus monkeys, was published by Landsteiner and Wiener[1] (1940). The properly called anti-rhesus antibody appeared to have the same specificity as that of Levine and Stetson's patient, so the human antibody acquired the name of anti-Rh (and later anti-Rh_0).

However, it is now clear that the antigen in human blood corresponding to the true anti-rhesus antibody is not the same as the clinically important antigen called Rh_0 or D. But this realization came too late to change the name of the clinically important groups *from* Rh, for that name was in the title of perhaps a thousand papers. As a way out of this dilemma Dr Levine suggested that the name for the true rhesus antigen should be changed instead, and that it should be called LW, in honour of Landsteiner and Wiener.

The first difference between the two antibodies was observed by Fisk and Foord[155], as early as 1942, and they reported that all newborn babies, whether Rh positive or Rh negative, as defined by human anti-Rh sera, were positive with guinea-pig anti-rhesus serum. The guinea-pig antibody was, many years later, seen to be anti-LW.

In 1952 Murray and Clark[157] made one of the most surprising observations in the history of Rh when they found that heat extracts of human Rh negative red cells could stimulate the formation of apparent anti-D in guinea-pigs. Levine and his colleagues[135, 321] (1961) confirmed this and observed that the 'D-like' antibody differed from human anti-D in that it still agglutinated D cells after they had been blocked with incomplete anti-D. Again, the antibody was later to be identified as anti-LW.

In 1955, through the kindness of Dr A. Cahan and Dr J. Wallace, we were able to test two extraordinary blood samples, both of them from CDe/cde white people (Miss B. and Mrs G.) who had in their serum a rather weak but easily identifiable 'anti-D'. This 'anti-D' did not react by the antiglobulin method and, more strange, it could be absorbed by dd cells. This latter peculiarity called to mind the

Murray-Clark effect just described, a correct association as was to be seen later. These two antibodies were mutually compatible and were later realized to be the first human examples of anti-LW.

The families of LW− propositi

In 1962 Dr Wallace obtained a second sample from Mrs G. and also samples from members of her family and our Unit was again associated in the investigation. By this time Rh_{null} had been recognized and cells were available and proved negative

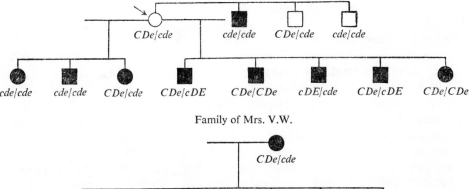

Fig. 16. Two families showing that Rh and LW are genetically independent of each other. Black = LW+: hollow = LW−. (Upper pedigree from Tippett[169]: lower from Swanson and Matson[331].)

with the serum of Mrs G. and of Miss B., and this has been true of subsequent examples of anti-LW.

The results of testing the cells of the family of Mrs G. with the two anti-LW sera, that of Mrs G. herself and that of Miss B., are shown in Figure 16. The cells of Mrs G. and of her brothers were then sent to Dr Levine's laboratory for tests with their guinea pig anti-LW of 1961 and, as expected, the results were the same as those given by the human anti-LW.

That the gene responsible for the antigen LW is not part of the Rh complex locus was first established by Tippett[169] in her thesis in the following succinct words:

'The argument is as follows. If LW were part of the Rh gene complex and its absence were a dominant character then Mrs G. should have given the absence either to the four children to whom she gave her *CDe* or to the three children to whom she gave her *cde*. If, on the other hand, LW were part of the Rh gene complex and its absence were a recessive character then Mrs G.'s youngest brother could not differ, as he does, from her in Rh genotype.'

Further details about Mrs G. were given by Levine, Celano, Wallace and Sanger[332].

An antibody in the serum of a Mrs VW. investigated by Swanson and Matson[331] gave reactions so like those of Mrs G. and Miss B. that a sample was sent to our Unit where Dr Tippett found the cells of Mrs VW. to be negative with the anti-LW of Mrs G. and Miss B. Tests on the family (Figure 16) confirmed that LW and Rh are genetically independent of each other.

All that is known of the family of Miss B. is that her two sibs, both Rh positive, were compatible with her serum[422].

We know of only two more reports of families which demonstrate the inheritance of the LW− condition. Both were brought to notice by the presence of anti-LW in the serum of the propositus. The first was described by de Veber *et al.*[423] (1971). The antibody, presumably stimulated by pregnancy, was present in the serum of a woman, Mrs Big., who had never been transfused. Mrs Big. is *CDe/cde* and LW−; she has four *CDe/cde* sibs, three of them LW+ and one LW−. The second was described by Swanson *et al.*[424] (1974). This anti-LW was present in the serum of an elderly transfused *CDe/cDE* LW− man, Mr Wald., who has a *cDE/cde* LW− sister and thus between them they confirm the genetical independence of *Rh* and *LW*. Another sister, now dead, was married to a first cousin and one of their two sons is *cDE/cde* LW−. This paper appears to be the only one giving information for or against consanguinity in the parents of LW− propositi.

Sibs of LW− propositi

The five families provide the following sib count (excluding the propositus): LW+ 10, LW− 7. This does not differ significantly from the expected 12·75 to 4·25.

Frequency of LW

LW− people are very rare: the propositi so far have selected themselves by having anti-LW in their serum. Using the more embracing anti-LW serum of Mrs Big., de Veber *et al.*[423] found all of 10,552 unselected Canadian donors to have LW: we know of no random tests with other anti-LW sera.

Other notes about LW

Using titrations of the anti-LW of Mrs VW., Swanson, Polesky and Matson[333] found the amount of LW antigen to be the same in cells representing one or two

D genes; a wide range of genotypes was included. Cells representing *dd* or *D^ud* gave much weaker reactions, but again the reactions were the same for a variety of genotypes.

Unlike the guinea-pig anti-LW, that of Mrs VW. did not react more strongly with cord than with adult cells[333]: this surprised us, for Dr Tippett had found that the anti-LW of Mrs VW., like that of Mrs G. and Miss B., did react more strongly with cord cells than with adult cells. The explanation was technical: in Minneapolis the anti-LW was titrated in serum while in London saline was used. The diluting serum for some unexplained reason masks the difference between adult and cord cells.

Klun and Muschel[384] found that red cell stroma treated with certain anti-D sera will fix complement whether the stroma be prepared from Rh positive, Rh negative or LW negative cells. They suggest that the fixation is on account of some precursor Rh substance.

In 1974, Swanson and her colleagues[424] coordinated the results, from several laboratories, of tests with 10 anti-LW sera against 10 examples of LW− cells. An impressive pattern emerged: it appears that these are two kinds of anti-LW and two kinds of 'LW−' red cells. One anti-LW is anti-LW+LW$_1$, analogous to anti-A+A$_1$ in the ABO system, an exemplar is the serum Big. whose cells are *lwlw*, corresponding to O: the other is anti-LW$_1$, corresponding to anti-A$_1$, exemplars of which are the sera VW and Wald., whose cells are LW$_2$, corresponding to A$_2$. The multitude are LW$_1$. This seems to be a useful distinction and, as Swanson *et al.*[424] point out, could on rare occasion be important in transfusion. No doubt further subdivisions will follow. These LW$_1$ and LW$_2$ symbols have to be distinguished from those suggested by Levine *et al.*[390] to represent the greater strength of the LW antigen in normal Rh positive cells compared with that in normal Rh negative cells.

Immune anti-LW in animals

It was, of course, the original immunization of rabbits and guinea pigs by rhesus monkey cells (Landsteiner and Wiener [1, 10] 1940, 1941) that began all the coil about anti-Rh and the antibody later to be called anti-LW. The extreme complexity of the immune response was demonstrated by Wiener, Moor-Jankowski and Brancato[425] in 1969.

Levine and Celano[390] (1967) succeeded in producing anti-LW in guinea pigs or rabbits by injecting them with rhesus, baboon or human red cells and subsequently absorbing the immune serum with LW− human cells.

Polesky *et al.*[426] (1968) recorded their results of immunizing guinea pigs with Rh$_{null}$, with LW− and with cord cells. Subsequent absorption with Rh$_{null}$ and LW− cells gave indications which the authors interpreted as possibly anti-substance 2. This interpretation fitted a genetical pathway scheme given in our last edition (page 217) but does not seem to fit the present and better scheme of Giblett[416] and Tippett[415] (Figure 15).

Now that human anti-LW sera are available it seems to us clearer to give more weight to the work with human anti-LW.

Auto- and transient anti-LW

Auto-anti-LW is a not uncommon compound of serum from patients with 'warm' auto-immune acquired haemolytic anaemia (Celano and Levine[386], Vos *et al.*[427]).

Transient auto-anti-LW formed in Rh negative people in the process of making anti-D is the subject of two interesting running accounts by Giles and Lundsgaard[398] and by Chown and his colleagues[428].

Perrault[429] found 10 examples of 'cold' auto-anti-LW in screening 45,000 samples with the Auto Analyzer: none of the 10 donors had haemolytic anaemia, some were pregnant and all were Rh positive.

LW as judged by auto-anti-LW looks heterogeneous and very difficult.

If we were to do justice to the papers in this section we should never finish the chapter.

The whole subject of LW is reviewed by Beck[430] (1973) and, more recently, by Giles[431].

OTHER NOTES ABOUT Rh

Quantitative aspects of the Rh antigens

The amount of an Rh antigen which we detect by serological methods depends on a number of influences which are gradually being sorted out. Those so far recognized are: (1) Dosage effects; (2) 'Position' effects due to fellow genes in *cis* (i.e. on the same chromosome); (3) 'Position' effects due to fellow genes in *trans* (i.e. on the opposite chromosome); (4) Specificity of antiserum not being what it was thought to be.

These influences, especially the first three, often operate together and the resulting picture is not obviously clear but a few comparisons can be made in which only one of the influences is to be seen at work at a time. Some quantitative work has to be reassessed now that the existence of antibodies to compound antigens has been recognized (page 199); also we now know that anti-c and anti-e often have an anti-ce component and that certain anti-C may be mainly anti-Ce.

Dosage effects

That two *M* (or *N*) genes would make more of the corresponding antigen than would one gene was recognized by the discoverers of the MN system. Dosage effects in Rh were first recognized with anti-c sera[16]: they have on occasion proved useful as a research tool. Other sera sometimes showing the effect well are anti-

C^w[28, 145], anti-E[73, 74, 197], anti-e[23] and anti-f (anti-ce)[69]. Only a slight effect could be detected[73] with anti-C. No effect has yet been recorded in using the antisera anti-V (-ce^s), anti-VS (-e^s), anti-rh$_i$ (-Ce) or anti-G.

These differences show themselves above the other influences that are presumably in action. For example $C^w De/C^w De$ reacts more strongly[28] with anti-C^w than does $C^w De/CDe$ and this comparison is one of the most straightforward, yet it is complicated by the possible effect of a C in *trans* on the amount of C^w.

Cis-*effects*

The earliest example of this effect happens to be one of the few possible uncomplicated comparisons. Lawler and Race[73] (1950) found that there was more detectable E in cdE/cde than in cDE/cde. Because the presence of D seemed to have a depressing effect on the C, E and e antigens Lawler and Race were led to guess that perhaps a common basic substance, of limited amount, was needed by all the Rh genes for their function. This guess seemed to be supported by the subsequent finding of $-D-/-D-$ red cells which have more D than any other DD cells yet found[62, 63], and would presumably be free of any competition for basic material.

Trans-*effects*

These were demonstrated by Lawler and Race[73] who observed that, for example, more detectable C antigen resulted from CDe/cde than from CDe/cDE and that more E resulted from cDE/cde than from cDE/CDe.

A *trans*-effect was beautifully demonstrated by Ceppellini, Dunn and Turri[41] (1955). When investigating the antigen D^u in 1948 we were puzzled because we encountered too many examples of the genotype CD^ue/Cde. Ceppellini and his colleagues showed that these are not true D^u but ordinary CDe whose D gene cannot express itself fully in the presence of Cde. When such an apparent CD^ue segregates, in a family, away from Cde it discloses itself as a normal CDe.

The inhibitory effect of Cde has been confirmed[76, 262, 394] and CdE has been found[260] to behave like Cde in this respect. However, Cde and CdE do not always have a depressing effect on the D antigen produced by the opposite chromosome[76, 315].

This very interesting phenomenon, which is illustrated in Figure 17, explains only the minority of D^u, and they are of the 'high grade' type.

The effect of antibodies to compound antigens

By using certain chosen anti-C and anti-E sera a difference could be demonstrated in the apparent amount of C and E antigen in the red cells of donors whose genotypes contain the same Rh genes, C, D, E, etc., but in different alignments[75] (see page 200).

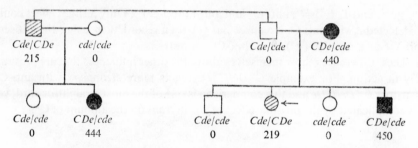

Fig. 17. The effect of *Cde* on the expression of a fellow *D* gene: simulation of D^u. (After Ceppellini, Dunn and Turri[41], 1955.) The numbers represent total scores for titrations with six anti-D sera. Black represents a normal D; hatching represents results which previously would have been interpreted as 'high grade' D^u.

Mixed effects

As already pointed out, most comparisons of antigen strength measure the effect of different types of gene interaction. Levine, Celano, Lange and Stroup[33] have pursued the competitive effect of *C* and *D* and illustrated how it works both ways in *trans* to reduce the amount of D in *CDe/CDe*: they suggest that in this genotype it may work both ways in *cis* too, which seems likely. Using selected anti-D sera they found that a dosage effect of *D* could be demonstrated in the comparison *cDE/cDE* versus *cDE/cde*, that is, when the known competitive effect of *C* on *D* is eliminated.

All these quantitative observations have been made by the use of simple titration tests; later and more sophisticated methods have confirmed them and sometimes allowed estimation of the number of antigen sites on the red cell.

By quantitative agglutination methods Silber, Gibbs, Jahn and Akeroyd (1961)[127, 128] studied the D anti-D reaction: this they measured by counts of inagglutinable cells (a method used by the Wurmsers in their work on the thermodynamics of ABO reactions). The results gave very clear confirmation that *DD* cells react more strongly than *Dd* in the comparison between *cDE/cDE* and *cDE/cde*, and in that between *cDe/cDe* and *cDe/cde*. Silber *et al.*[128] concluded that decreasing amounts of D antigen resulted from the gene complexes −D−, *cDE*, *cDe* and *CDe*, which was in accord with the general impressions (which Galton said are never to be trusted) of most blood group workers.

Gibbs and Rosenfield[341] used the same method to test with anti-D, -*C*, -c and anti-E the cells of a large family with genotypes representing the six combinations of *Cde*, *cde*, *CDe* and *cD^uE*. In contrast to assays of D, those of C, c and E suggested that there was 'more homogeneity in regard to specific binding affinities of these antiserums and antigenic determinants'.

Further recent work on the more serological aspects of Rh is to be found in the following references: 342–347, 395. A masterly review of the modern serology of blood group reactions is to be found in Chapter 5 of Mollison's 5th edition of *Blood Transfusion in Clinical Medicine*[435] (1972).

More sophisticated quantitative methods used to estimate
the number of antigen sites

By quantitative antiglobulin tests Wiener and Gordon[34] (1953) estimated that, compared with the number of D antigen sites, a red cell has about one-tenth that number of Fy[a] sites and about one-quarter that number of K sites.

By the use of I[131] labelled anti-D, Boursnell, Coombs and Rizk[60] (1953) estimated the number of D sites on *CDe/CDe* cells to be about 5,500.

By an anti-globulin fixation method Grubb[99] (1955) estimated that the minimum number of D sites on *CDe/CDe* cells was about 2,000.

By the use of I[131] labelled anti-D, Masouredis[133] confirmed that *DD* differed from *Dd* when there was no interference from *C* and estimated that one *DD* red cell (lacking *C*) had about 10,300 D antigen sites while a *Dd* cell (lacking *C*) had about 6,400. When *C* was present the values were *DD* 7,400 and *Dd* 4,600. Masouredis and Sturgeon[387] applied the same technique to the study of various D[u] samples.

By the use of ^{125}I labelled anti-γ globulin reagent, Rochna and Hughes-Jones[348] (1965) estimated the following number of sites:

Probable genotype	Range of D antigen sites per cell
CDe/cde	9,900–14,600
cDe/cde	12,000–20,000
cDE/cde	14,000–16,600
CDe/CDe	14,500–19,300
CDe/cDE	23,000–31,000
cDE/cDE	15,800–33,300

The tests involved four different examples of each of these genotypes except *CDe/CDe* of which there were three.

In 1971, Hughes-Jones, Gardner and Lincoln[445] reported further measurements using ^{125}I labelled anti-γ globulin. Four −*D*−/−*D*− samples were added to those measured for D: as expected, their number of D sites was very high, it ranged from 110,000 to 202,000.

Measurement of the c sites of three examples of *cc* and three of *Cc* gave the results *cc* average 79,000 and *Cc* average 43,000.

Measurement of the e sites of two *ee* and two *Ee* gave the results *ee* 18,200 and 24,400 and *Ee* 14,500 and 13,400.

Measurement of the E sites in a fine range of genotypes confirmed earlier results of simple titrations: *EE* scored about twice *Ee* and the E in *cdE/cde* was between a single and a double dose.

D antigen sites as seen by the electron microscope

Two fascinating papers by Nicholson, Masouredis and Singer[417] (1971) and by Singer and Nicholson [444] (1972) describe how Rh positive red cells were sensitized with ^{125}I labelled anti-D then lysed; their membranes spread flat were then picked up on an electron microscope grid and stained with a ferritin conjugated goat anti-human γ globulin preparation. The ferritin particles were distributed in discrete clusters, within a circle of about 300 Å radius, 2 to 8 particles in each, and this was interpreted as so many ferritin conjugated antiglobulin molecules bound to a single anti-D antibody molecule and corresponding to a single D site. The number of D sites thus flagged corresponded well with the amount of ^{125}I labelled anti-D molecules bound per unit area.

The D antigen sites appeared 'to be distributed in an aperiodic and essentially random two dimensional array on the erythrocyte membrane'. By the technique used the antigen sites of the outer surface alone were stained, not those of the inner surface.

The authors give the indirect evidence that the D antigen is protein and a picture is drawn of these protein molecules as not static but mobile in the lipid of the cell membrane.

Many references to work on biological membranes are to be found in those two papers. Some earlier attempts on the biochemistry of D are to be found in the following papers: 138–142, 314, 367–374, 396.

Development of the Rh antigens

The Rh antigens are well developed before birth[103–105, 134]. Chown[106] examined a foetus of about six weeks of age and of 32 mm. from crown to rump: the cord blood was *cDE/cde* and gave a direct positive antiglobulin reaction. The mother had anti-D as a result of previous pregnancies. Anti-D was also detected in the serum of the foetus.

We have found the antigens V (ce^s), f (ce), VS (e^s) and rh_i (Ce) well developed in cord cells, and so is the antigen LW (see page 228).

Rh mosaics, not mosaic for other antigens

At the time of our last edition there were six examples of this condition which had been a mystery for years:

1   Mrs Eik., Norwegian, aged 80+, fracture (Vogt and Hartmann[143]; Vogt[349]). *cDE/cde + cde/cde*, about 50:50. No relatives available.
2   Mrs de G., Scottish, aged 26, pregnancy (Cameron[350]). *CDe/cde + cde/cde*, about 18:82. Mother, brother and two children *CDe/CDe*, father and sister *CDe/cde*.Karyotype later found to be normal.
3   Polycythemia vera male patient, Swedish, aged 62 (Levan, Nichols Hall, Löw, Nilsson and Nordén[351]). *cDE/cde + cde/cde*. Brother *cDE/cde*.
4   Mrs Eng., Swedish, aged 43, gastric ulcer (Broman and Nilsson[352]). *cDe/cde + cde/cde*, roughly 30:70. Sibs: 3 *cDe/cde*, 1 *CDe/CDe*, 1 *CDe/cde* (or *CDe/cDe*). Children: *cde/cde* and *cDe/cde*.
5   Mrs Lis., Swedish, aged 33, pregnancy (Broman and Nilsson[352]). *CDe/cde + cde/cde*. Mother *CDe/CDe*, sister *CDe/cDE*.

6   Mrs Ost., Swedish, aged 79 (Broman and Nilsson[352]). *CDe/cde + cde/cde*. Sister *cDE/cde*, child *CDe/CDe*.

All the patients had been retested over periods of time and the condition was not transient.

Samples from five of the six propositi were kindly sent to us but all we could do was to confirm the original findings. The mixtures are separable and each pair of separated components is identical for all groups save Rh.

Various possible explanations could be ruled out by one or another of the families: twin and dispermic chimerism, a theoretical possible *Rh* allele comparable to A_3, a disease change associated with leukaemia, and somatic crossing-over. Somatic mutation seemed very unlikely and so, at the time, did the theoretical possibility of clones of monosomal cells in the marrow. Of course, there may be several causes.

Then, in 1970, Mannoni *et al.*[439] reported a patient with myelofibrosis who had a mixture of Rh, *CDe/cde* and *cde/———*. There was also a double population of A cells, one reacting with anti-A_1 and one not. This case echoed No. 3 above and drew the attention of Callender *et al.*[440] when they were observing the onset and progress of an Rh mixture in a man with polycythaemia vera. Originally, in 1965, he was *CDe/cDE* but five years later he had a mixture of two populations, one *CDe/cDE* and one apparently *CDe/CDe*. The patient showed clones of cytogenetically abnormal cells which were attributed to his treatment with radio phosphorus, and this led Callender and her colleagues to consider the Rh mosaicism of their case as reflecting clones of normal *CDe/cDE* cells and clones of monosomic *CDe* cells derived from a damaged Rh chromosome.

This seems a very satisfactory explanation, and the presence of monosomic clones would fit serologically all six cases listed above, and two others investigated by Stapleton[441]:

Mrs Dav., English, pregnancy. *cDE/cde + cde/cde*, about 30:70. Father *CDe/cDE*, mother *cDE/cde*, child *cDE/cde*.

Miss S.B., aged 12, English, unexplained anaemia. *CDe/cde + cde/cde*, about 25:75. Father *cde/cde*, mother *CDe/CDe*.

The only snag arose after *Rh* became known to be on autosome No. 1 and no cytogenetic abnormality of No. 1 was to be seen in Callender's case or in that of Jenkins and Marsh to be described below. On the other hand, a man with myelofibrosis reported by Marsh *et al.*[447] (1974), who had a mixture of *CDe/cde + cde/cde*, about 7:93 (father *cde/cde*, mother *CDe/CDe*), did have a cytogenetic mixture, a normal population plus a population representing an unbalanced translocation involving chromosomes 1, 4 and 7.

During the proof stage of this book the detailed investigation of two more examples was reported (Habibi *et al.*[483], 1974). Both patients had the same mixture: 30% *CDe/cde* and 70% *cde/cde*. All four No. 1 chromosomes again appeared perfectly normal. The authors thought somatic mutation the likeliest cause.

9

A similar, but perhaps distinct, phenomenon

The remarkable mosaic described by Jenkins and Marsh[353] (1965) is distinguished from the nine above. A healthy male blood donor was found to be a mosaic: 30% of his cells were *CDe/cde*, Fy(a+) and 70% *cde/cde*, Fy(a−). The father is *CDe/CDe*, Fy(a+b−) and the mother *CDe/cde*, Fy(a−b+). The explanation preferred was that a somatic mutation had happened at a locus responsible for producing some precursor substance used by both the *Rh* and *Duffy* genes. But after it became known that the *Rh* and the *Duffy* loci were both on autosome No. 1 the idea of a monosonic clone seemed to afford the obvious explanation[442, 443]. In 1973 the donor was therefore retested[443] and his antigens were just as before but his karyotype, now done for the first time, showed an absolutely normal No. 1, and the rest of his chromosomes were normal too. A small unnoticeable deletion could hardly be invoked, for *Rh* and *Fy* are known to be a long way apart on their chromosome[446].

ABO protection against Rh immunization

This now very large and important subject has been so ably dealt with by Mollison[435] (*Blood Transfusion in Clinical Medicine*, 5th edition, 1972) that we shall not attempt an account. It all began with the observation by Levine[354], in 1943, that mothers of children with haemolytic disease of the newborn due to anti-Rh were more often compatibly mated on the ABO system than were unselected women.

Prevention of Rh immunization

Nearly 20 years later, thought about this ABO protection was to lead to the beginning of the brilliant work in Liverpool and in New York and Raritan which resulted in this triumph of preventive medicine. The literature is enormous but the story is condensed in several books: in *'Prevention of Rh hemolytic disease'* by Pollack, Gorman and Freda[450] and *'Rh immunisation and its prevention'* by Woodrow[355] and in a very useful reprinting of selected papers with commentaries by Sir Cyril Clarke[356], *'Rh haemolytic disease. Original papers with commentaries'*. There is also an interesting book by a professional writer, David R. Zimmerman[451], *'Rh. The intimate history of a disease and its conquest'*, to which Dr James D. Watson wrote an introduction.

No evidence for acquired tolerance to the antigen D

Professor Rogers Brambell and Mr N.A. Mitchison independently arrived at a brilliant explanation of why so few Rh negative women are in fact immunized by their offspring. That it is not the true explanation takes only a little from the pleasure such an idea gives.

Towards the end of 1950 Professor Brambell and Mr Mitchison inquired of the present authors whether the Blood Transfusion Service had any record of the Rh groups of the maternal grandmothers of children with haemolytic disease. In the words of Professor Brambell: 'The essence of Burnet's "marker" concept seems to be that the organism cannot produce antibodies to antigens to which it is exposed sufficiently early in its development. Assuming that maternal blood-group antigens, as well as antibodies, can reach the foetus, the young should never be able to develop antibodies to either its own *or its mother's antigens*. Thus an Rh negative child of an Rh positive mother should never be able to form anti-Rh, whereas an Rh negative child of an Rh negative mother should be able to do so. Is this the explanation of the erratic reaction to Rh immunization of Rh negative people?'

There were at the time no facts to answer this question, but steps to find some were taken by Booth, Dunsford, Grant and Murray[357]. They tested 113 maternal grandmothers of children suffering from haemolytic disease due to anti-D: 46 of the grandmothers were *dd* which is exactly the number expected to be *dd* out of 113 mothers of perfectly ordinary *dd* persons.

Subsequent investigations confirmed that there was no evidence for the acquisition, *in utero*, of tolerance to the antigen D[358, 359]. In one of these investigations[360], irregularities, interpreted as evidence of tolerance, were later found[361] to have other causes. On the contrary, it is suggested[388] that an Rh positive mother may give her Rh negative daughter a first immunizing dose *in utero*.

In spite of this, we guess tolerance to Rh could be acquired: a genetically *OO* chimera twin with A cells in his circulation does not make anti-A, and it seems unlikely, as mentioned on page 527, that a genetically *dd* chimera twin, like Madame Ko. (page 523), with D positive cells in her circulation, could ever make anti-D, whatever her challenge.

A curious inhibition of D:anti-D agglutination

Freiesleben and Jensen[378] investigated a very peculiar and informative example of anti-D which could be inhibited in some of its reactions by a factor to be found in all normal sera tested. The factor was thought 'to occur with the lipoproteins.' The factor inhibits the straight agglutination and indirect antiglobulin agglutination of cells in a saline medium. Fixation of antibody and antigen was shown not to be inhibited, only the agglutination was inhibited. When papain was involved in the system the inhibition was abolished. An apparently identical anti-D was investigated by Dybkjaer[381].

Rh and acquired haemolytic anaemia

The first realization that Rh played the main part in the serology of acquired haemolytic anaemia of the 'warm' antibody type came with the observation, in 1953 by Weiner, Battey, Cleghorn, Marson and Meynell[362], that the 'non-specific' auto-antibody, common to such patients, had in fact the specificity anti-e. There-after cells of such exotic genotypes as $-D-/-D-$ and LW− were also used to distinguish various classes of warm autoantibodies. (References to the Rh aspect of this vast subject may be found in W. Weiner[363], W. Weiner and Vos[364], in Dacie[365], and in Celano and Levine[386].)

Worlledge, Carstairs and Dacie[366] showed that warm auto-antibodies induced by α-methyldopa are of Rh specificity and are not directed against the drug.

Rh antibodies in fluids other than serum

Very soon after the discovery of Rh, Witebsky, Anderson and Heide[200, 201] found that anti-Rh could be present in the milk of women whose serum contained the antibody; this was confirmed[137]. Van Bolhuis[202] found incomplete anti-D in several amniotic fluids belonging to babies suffering from haemolytic disease of the newborn. Eaton, Morton, Pickles and White[203] found anti-Yt^a in ascitic fluid, and Dr Pickles told us that, at Oxford, they also found examples of anti-A, anti-B, anti-c and anti-Le^a in this fluid. Zeitlin[204] reported a case of ascites that was a source of enormous quantities of anti-E.

The search for Rh antigens other than on the red cells is mentioned on pages 41–43.

Model making

Several attempts to make schemes that might fit the observed Rh interactions, and lull a little our bewilderment, have already been mentioned. The shortage of chemical information allows the fancy to roam and this it has done with much ingenuity. References to some theoretical papers are: Nijenhuis[248], Lauer[375], Boettcher[257], Knox[376] and Edwards[452].

The fundamental problem of how much complexity should be assigned to antigens and how much to antibodies has been bravely tackled by Hirschfeld[377] and Perrault[472].

A PRESENT VIEW OF Rh

There seems no limit to the marvellous complexity of this system of antigens and antibodies. The system can be understood at various levels, that of Rh+ and Rh−, for example, or that of the original CDE, with satisfaction and the knowledge can be applied with accuracy.

The CDE scheme has been of enormous value in describing observed relation-ships and anticipating others, but the question arises whether it has anything more to offer, whether thought about some of the latest observations is handicapped if attempts are made to fit them to the pattern.

Some believe that the time of usefulness of such committed symbols as C and c and rh′ and hr′, which denote alternatives, has passed, as far as pioneer work is

concerned. It is felt that for further advance the notation must be freed of all inter-
pretive meaning and record only reactions, plus, minus or weak, between cells and
numbered antisera. The subject was dealt with most expertly by Rosenfield,
Allen, Swisher and Kochwa[322] in 1962, who pointed out weaknesses of both the
CDE and Rh-Hr notations, and devised a numerical notation. We believe that
CDE is still the best practical way of *communicating* knowledge about Rh though
it is best *stored* for future use in the numerical form; but it has to be thawed out and
reconstituted in familiar terms, at any rate for the older generation of workers.

There is undoubtedly some underlying order: there are antigens which behave
as if controlled by simple alleles, C, c, C^w and E, e and E^w, and antigens which
correspond to compounds of these, ce, Ce, CE, for example, and we cannot ignore
this order.

Tests on families show that minute differences in the Rh antigens are most
punctiliously transmitted to the next generation, and these extraordinarily sensitive reflections of the genetic code show three series of alternative antigens. Since
a fundamental property of genes is to have alternative forms, or alleles, far and
away the most economical hypothesis was that the antigens were reflecting activity
at three sites where Mendelian substitution could go on, and this, in 1944, led
Fisher to propose three closely linked loci.

Though revolutionary at the time, parallels were soon found in other species,
notably Drosophila[340, 307, 308], phage, bacteria and moulds[309, 310], mouse[306] and,
years later, HL-A in man[473]. The arrival of the cistron[309, 310] with its many mutational sites removed the need to specify three 'genes'—one cistron could suffice.
This, together with the concept of regulators, or unlinked controller loci, and
operators, or built-in controller loci, dominated the view of Rh for many years;
but the latest sesame is 'conjugated operons'.

A very satisfying attempt to rationalize as a whole the infinite variety of Rh
reactions was made by Rosenfield, Allen and Rubinstein[438] (1973). Their paper is
an intellectual *tour de force*; it is hard going, and must be read and re-read by
anyone wanting to grasp what Rh may be like at heart.

The paper fuses Fisher's view of Rh with modern knowledge of gene structure.
Such attempts, as we have said, had been made before, but the main present
advance seems to us to be the application of the idea of conjugated operons, in
this following the description of work on the λ phage (Watson[474], 1970), and the
translation in detail of the immense variety of qualitative and quantitative Rh
interactions into terms of such a pattern of control.

The model is based on three adjacent structural genes *D*, *C* and *E* (in their old
order) interspersed with operators or promoters having a left to right direction of
control.

This important paper is written in a dogmatic style but the authors say, towards the end, disarmingly, that the model is entirely speculative. Though experts
can pick a few holes in the fabric, if half of the explanations are right this paper
may come to be looked upon as the first major achievement towards enlightenment since Fisher.

REFERENCES

1 LANDSTEINER K. and WIENER A.S (1940) An agglutinable factor in human blood recognized by immune sera for rhesus blood. *Proc. Soc. exp. Biol. N.Y.*, **43**, 223.

2 LEVINE P. and STETSON R.E. (1939) An unusual case of intragroup agglutination. *J. Amer. med. Ass.*, **113**, 126–127.

3 WIENER A.S. and PETERS H.R. (1940) Hemolytic reactions following transfusions of blood of the homologous group, with three cases in which the same agglutinogen was responsible. *Ann. Int. Med.*, **13**, 2306–2322.

4 LEVINE P., KATZIN E.M. and BURNHAM L. (1941) Isoimmunization in pregnancy, its possible bearing on the etiology of erythroblastosis fetalis. *J. Amer. med. Ass.*, **116**, 825–827.

5 LEVINE P., VOGEL P., KATZIN E.M. and BURNHAM L. (1941) Pathogenesis of erythroblastosis fetalis: statistical evidence. *Science*, **94**, 371–372.

6 LEVINE P., BURNHAM L., KATZIN E.M. and VOGEL P. (1941) The role of isoimmunization in the pathogenesis of erythroblastosis fetalis. *Am. J. Obst. Gynec.*, **42**, 925–937.

7 LINNET-JEPSEN P., GALATIUS-JENSEN F. and HAUGE M. (1958) The inheritance of the Gm serum group. *Acta genet.*, **8**, 164–196.

8 RACE R.R., SANGER RUTH, TIPPETT PATRICIA, NOADES JEAN and HAMPER JEAN (1961) Quoted in the 4th edition of this book.

9 GALATIUS-JENSEN F. (1958) On the genetics of the haptoglobins. *Acta genet.*, **8**, 232–247.

10 LANDSTEINER K. and WIENER A.S. (1941) Studies on an agglutinogen (Rh) in human blood reacting with anti-rhesus sera and with human isoantibodies. *J. exp. Med.*, **74**, 309–320.

11 WIENER A.S. (1941) Hemolytic reactions following transfusion of blood of the homologous group. II. *Arch. Path.*, **32**, 227–250.

12 LEVINE P. (1942) The pathogenesis of fetal erythroblastosis. *N.Y. State J. Med.*, **42**, 1928–1934.

13 WIENER A.S. and LANDSTEINER K. (1943) Heredity of variants of the Rh type. *Proc. Soc. exp. Biol. N.Y.*, **53**, 167–170.

14 RACE R.R. and TAYLOR G.L. (1943) A serum that discloses the genotype of some Rh positive people. *Nature, Lond.*, **152**, 300.

15 WIENER A.S. and SONN EVE B. (1943) Additional variants of the Rh type demonstrable with a special human anti-Rh serum. *J. Immunol.*, **47**, 461–465.

16 RACE R.R., TAYLOR G.L., BOORMAN KATHLEEN E. and DODD BARBARA E. (1943) Recognition of Rh genotypes in man. *Nature, Lond.*, **152**, 563.

17 RACE R.R., TAYLOR G.L., CAPPELL D.F. and MCFARLANE MARJORY N. (1944) Recognition of a further common Rh genotype in man. *Nature, Lond.*, **153**, 52–53.

18 WIENER A.S. (1943) Genetic theory of the Rh blood types. *Proc. Soc. exp. Biol. N.Y.*, **54**, 316–319.

19 RACE R.R. (1948) The Rh genotypes and Fisher's theory. *Blood*, **3**, suppl. 2, 27–42.

20 FISHER R.A., cited by RACE R.R. (1944) An 'incomplete' antibody in human serum. *Nature, Lond.*, **153**, 771–772.

21 RACE R.R., TAYLOR G.L., IKIN ELIZABETH W. and PRIOR AILEEN M. (1944) The inheritance of allelomorphs of the Rh gene in fifty-six families. *Ann. Eugen., Lond.*, **12**, 206–210.

22 MURRAY J., RACE R.R. and TAYLOR G.L. (1945) Serological reactions caused by the rare human gene Rh_z, *Nature, Lond.*, **155**, 112.

23 MOURANT A.E. (1945) A new rhesus antibody. *Nature, Lond.*, **155**, 542.

24 DIAMOND L.K. (1946) Paper read at Rh and Hematology Congress, Dallas.

25 HILL J.M. and HABERMAN S. (1948) Two examples of sera containing the anti-d agglutinin predicted by Fisher and Race. *Nature, Lond.*, **161**, 688.

26 HABERMAN S., HILL J.M., EVERIST B.W. and DAVENPORT J.W. (1948) The demonstration and characterization of the anti-d agglutinin predicted by Fisher and Race. *Blood*, **3**, 682–688.

27 Bosch Clara van den (1948) The very rare Rh genotype R_yr (CdE/cde) in a case of erythroblastosis foetalis. *Nature, Lond.*, **162**, 781.

28 Callender Sheila T. and Race R.R. (1946) A serological and genetical study of multiple antibodies formed in response to blood transfusion by a patient with lupus erythematosus diffusus. *Ann. Eugen., Lond.*, **13**, 102–117.

29 Stratton F. and Renton P.H. (1954) Haemolytic disease of the newborn caused by a new Rh antibody, anti-C^x. *Brit. med. J.*, **i**, 962–965.

30 Race R.R., Sanger Ruth and Lawler Sylvia D. (1948) Rh genes allelomoprhic to C. *Nature, Lond.*, **161**, 316.

31 Race R.R., Sanger Ruth and Lawler Sylvia D. (1948) Allelomorphs of the Rh gene C. *Heredity*, **2**, 237–250.

32 Race R.R. and Sanger Ruth (1951) The Rh antigen C^u. *Heredity*, **5**, 285–287.

33 Levine P., Celano M., Lange S. and Stroup Marjory (1959) The influence of gene interaction on dosage effects with complete anti-D sera. *Vox Sang.*, **4**, 33–39.

34 Wiener A.S. and Gordon Eve B. (1953) Quantitative test for antibody-globulin coating human blood cells and its practical applications. *Amer. J. clin. Path.*, **23**, 429–446.

35 Stratton F. (1946) A new Rh allelomorph. *Nature, Lond.*, **158**, 25.

36 Race R.R., Sanger Ruth and Lawler Sylvia D. (1948) The Rh antigen D^u. *Ann. Eugen., Lond.*, **14**, 171–184.

37 Renton P.H. and Stratton F. (1950) Rhesus type D^u. *Ann. Eugen., Lond.*, **15**, 189–209.

38 Stratton F. and Renton P.H. (1948) Rh genes allelomorphic to D. *Nature, Lond.*, **162**, 293.

39 Race R.R., Sanger Ruth and Lawler Sylvia D. (1948) Rh genes allelomorphic to D. *Nature, Lond.*, **162**, 292.

40 Ceppellini R. in Ceppellini R. and Nasso S. and Tecilazich F. (1952) *La Malattia Emolitica del Neonato*, Milano.

41 Ceppellini R., Dunn L.C. and Turri M. (1955) An interaction between alleles at the Rh locus in man which weakens the reactivity of the Rh_0 factor (D^u). *Proc. nat. Acad. Sci., Wash.*, **41**, 283–288.

42 Renton P.H. (1949) The Rhesus factor D^u. M.D. Thesis, University of Manchester.

43 Rosenfield R.E., Vogel P., Miller E.B. and Haber Gladys (1951) Weakly reacting Rh positive (D^u) bloods. *Blood*, **6**, 1123–1134.

44 Broman B. (1952) Further observations on the Rh antigen D^u. Paper read at the 4th International Congress of Hematology, Mar del Plata.

45 Darnborough J. (1957) The incidence of D^u in blood donors in Yorkshire with special reference to the ccD^uee phenotype. *Vox Sang.*, **2**, 93–99.

46 Dunsford I. (1948) A variant of the rhesus antigen D. *Ann. Eugen., Lond.*, **14**, 142–143.

47 Dunsford I. (1953) Homozygous D^u (D^u/D^u) cell in a family of rare Rhesus genotypes. *Ann. Eugen., Lond.*, **17**, 283–285.

48 Walsh R.J. (1952) Variants of the blood group gene D in two native races. *Med. J. Aust.*, **2**, 405–407.

49 Eldon K. (1950) Le facetur D^u. *Rev. Hémat.*, **5**, 294–304.

50 Shapiro M. (1951) The ABO, MN, P and Rh blood group systems in the South African Bantu. *S. Afr. med. J.*, **25**, 187–192.

51 Rosenfield R.E., Haber Gladys, Gibbel Natalie (1958) A new Rh variant. *Proc. 6th Congr. int. Soc. Blood Transf.*, 90–95.

52 Geiger J. and Wiener A.S. (1958) An Rh_0 positive mother with serum containing potent Rh antibodies, apparently of specificity anti-Rh_0, causing erythroblastosis fetalis. *Proc. 6th Congr. int. Soc. Blood Transf.*, 36–40.

53 Renton P.H. and Hancock Jeanne A. (1955) An individual of unusual Rh type. *Vox Sang.* (O.S.), **5**, 135–142.

54 Renton P.H. and Hancock Jeanne A. (1956) Variability of the Rhesus antigen D. *Brit. J. Haemat.*, **2**, 295–304.

55 Greenwalt T.J. and Sanger Ruth (1955) The Rh antigen E^w. *Brit. J. Haemat.*, **1**, 52–54.

[56] CEPPELLINI R., IKIN ELIZABETH W. and MOURANT A.E. (1950) A new allele of the Rh gene E. *Boll. Ist. Siero. Milanese*, **29**, 123–124.

[57] CEPPELLINI R. (1950) L'antigène Rh E^u. *Rev. Hémat.*, **5**, 285–293.

[58] MOURANT A.E., IKIN ELIZABETH W., HÄSSIG A., HÄSSIG ROSINA and HOLLÄNDER L. (1952) Uber das Vorkommen des Rhesusgens E^u in einer Ostschweizer Familie. *Schwiez. med. Wschr.* **82**, 1100 (6 pages in reprint).

[59] SUSSMAN L.N. (1955) The rare blood factor rh(″) or E^u. *Blood*, **10**, 1241–1245.

[60] BOURSNELL J.C., COOMBS R.R.A. and RIZK VIVIEN (1953) Studies with marked antisera. Quantitative studies with antisera marked with iodine^{131} isotope and their corresponding red-cell antigens. *Biochem. J.*, **55**, 745–758.

[61] RACE R.R., SANGER RUTH and SELWYN J.G. (1950) A probable deletion in a human Rh chromosome. *Nature, Lond.*, **166**, 520.

[62] RACE R.R., SANGER RUTH and SELWYN J.G. (1951) A possible deletion in a human Rh chromosome: a serological and genetical study. *Brit. J. exp. Path.*, **32**, 124–135.

[63] WALLER R.K., SANGER RUTH and BOBBITT O.B. (1953) Two examples of the $-D-/-D-$ genotype in an American family. *Brit. med. J.*, **i**, 198–199.

[64] LEVINE P., KOCH ELIZABETH A., MCGEE R.T. and HILL G.H. (1954) Rare human isoagglutinins and their identification. *Amer. J. clin. Path.*, **24**, 292–304.

[65] BUCHANAN D.I. and MCINTYRE J. (1955) The descendants and contemporaries of Louis L'Iroquois. *Proc. 5th Congr. int. Soc. Blood Transf.*, Paris, 133–144.

[66] BUCHANAN D.I. and MCINTYRE J. (1955) Consanguinity and two rare matings. *Brit. J. Haemat.*, **1**, 304–307.

[67] BUCHANAN D.I. (1956) Blood genotypes $-D-/-D-$ and $CDe/-D-$. Transfusion therapy and some effects of multiple pregnancy. *Amer. J. clin. Path.*, **26**, 21–28.

[68] ROSENFIELD R.E., VOGEL P., GIBBEL NATALIE, SANGER RUTH and RACE R.R. (1953) A 'new' Rh antibody, anti-f. *Brit. med. J.*, **i**, 975.

[69] SANGER RUTH, RACE R.R., ROSENFIELD R.E., VOGEL P. and GIBBEL NATALIE (1953) Anti-f and the 'new' Rh antigen it defines. *Proc. nat. Acad. Sci., Wash.*, **39**, 824–834.

[70] JONES A.R., STEINBERG A.G., ALLEN F.H., DIAMOND L.K. and KRIETE B. (1954) Observations on the new Rh agglutinin anti-f. *Blood*, **9**, 117–122.

[71] DENATALE A., CAHAN A., JACK J.A., RACE R.R. and SANGER RUTH (1955) V: a 'new' Rh antigen, common in Negroes, rare in white people. *J. Amer. med. Ass.*, **159**, 247–250.

[72] GIBLETT ELOISE R., CHASE JEANNE and MOTULSKY A.G. (1957) Studies on anti-V, a recently discovered Rh antibody. *J. Lab. clin. Med.*, **49**, 433–439.

[73] LAWLER SYLVIA D. and RACE R.R. (1950) Quantitative aspects of Rh antigens. 1950 *Proceedings of the International Society of Hematology*, 168–170.

[74] MALONE R.H. and DUNSFORD I. (1951) The Rhesus antibody anti-E in pregnancy and blood transfusion. *Blood*, **6**, 1135–1146.

[75] RACE R.R., SANGER RUTH, LEVINE P., MCGEE R.T., LOGHEM J.J. VAN, HART MIA V.D. and CAMERON C. (1954) A position effect of the Rh blood-group genes. *Nature, Lond.*, **174**, 460.

[76] CHOWN B. and LEWIS MARION (1957) Occurrence of D^u type of reaction when CDe or cDE is partnered with Cde. *Ann. hum. Genet.*, **22**, 58–64.

[77] MOURANT A.E. (1954) *The Distribution of the Human Blood Groups*, pp. 438, Blackwell Scientific Publications, Oxford.

[78] FISHER R.A. (1946) The fitting of gene frequencies to data on rhesus reactions. *Ann. Eugen., Lond.*, **13**, 150–155.

[79] FISHER R.A. (1947) Note on the calculations of the frequencies of rhesus allelomorphs. *Ann. Eugen., Lond.*, **13**, 223–224.

[80] RACE R.R., MOURANT A.E., LAWLER SYLVIA D. and SANGER RUTH (1948) The Rh chromosome frequencies in England. *Blood*, **3**, 689–695.

[81] MURRAY J. (1944) Rh antenatal testing. A suggested nomenclature. *Lancet*, **ii**, 594.

[82] MURRAY J. (1944) A nomenclature of subgroups of the Rh factor. *Nature, Lond.*, **154**, 701.

83 RACE R.R. in MOLLISON P.L., MOURANT A.E. and RACE R.R. (1954) *The Rh Blood Groups and their Clinical Effects*, Medical Research Council Memorandum No. 27, Her Majesty's Stationery Office, London.

84 RACE R.R., MOURANT A.E. and McFARLANE MARJORY N. (1946) Travaux récents sur les antigènes et anticorps Rh avec une étude particulière de la thèorie de Fisher. *Rev. Hémat.*, **1**, 9–21.

85 BOYD W.C. (1955) Maximum likelihood calculation of Rh gene frequencies in Pacific populations. *Nature, Lond.*, **176**, 648.

86 BOYD W.C. (1954) Shortened maximum likelihood estimation of Rh gene frequencies. *Amer. J. hum. Genet.*, **6**, 303–318.

87 BOYD W.C. (1955) Simple maximum likelihood methods for calculating Rh gene frequencies in Pacific populations. *Amer. J. phys. Anthrop.*, **13**, 447–453.

88 HEIKEN A. and RASMUSON MARIANNE (1966) Genetical studies on the Rh blood group system. *Hereditas Lund*, **55**, 192–212.

89 WIENER A.S. (1948) Genetic transmission of two rare blood group genes. *Nature, Lond.*, **162**, 735.

90 SUSSMAN L.N. and WALD N. (1950) The rare gene r^y (CdE). *Amer. J. hum. Genet.*, **2**, 85–90.

91 PHANSOMBOON S. and POLLAK O.J. (1950) Study of an American Negro family with the rare Rh genotype $r^y r$ (CdE/cde). *J. Immunol.*, **65**, 711–714.

92 CEPPELLINI R. (1951) Identification du chromosome r^y (CdE) dans quatre générations. *Il Sangue*, **24**, 157.

93 GROVE-RASMUSSEN M., LOGHEM J.J. VAN, MAGNÉE WILLY and SOUCHARD L. (1951) The rare gene CdE (r_y) in a Basque family. *Ann. Eugen., Lond.*, **16**, 131–133.

94 HÄSSIG A., ROSIN S. and ROTHLIN A. (1955) Über die Häufigkeit des Rhesus-Chromosoms CdE = R_y in der Schweiz. *Schweiz. med. Wschr.*, **85**, 909–912.

95 DUNSFORD I. and ASPINALL P. (1951) The Rh chromosome $C^w dE$ (Ry^w) occurring in three generations. *Nature, Lond.*, **168**, 954–955.

96 HEIDE H.M. V.D., MAGNÉE WILLY and LOGHEM J.J. VAN (1951) Blood group frequencies in the Netherlands. *Amer. J. hum. Genet.*, **3**, 344–347.

97 CHAUDHRI I.M., IKIN ELIZABETH W., MOURANT A.E. and WALBY JEAN A.E. (1952) The blood groups of the people of North-West Pakistan. *Man* (Paper No. 250, no vol. nor page number in reprint).

98 SANGER RUTH (1949) An unusual Rh chromosome combination. *Nature, Lond.*, **165**, 655.

99 GRUBB R. (1955) An estimate of the number of Rh receptors on a single red cell. *Acta genet.*, **5**, 377–380.

100 BOORMAN KATHLEEN E., DODD BARBARA E. and JOHNSTONE AVRIL (1951) A family showing the existence of the Rh gene complex $CD^u E$. *Brit. J. exp. Path.*, **32**, 49–50.

101 WIENER A.S., GORDON EVE B. and COHEN LAURA (1952) A new rare Rhesus agglutinogen. *Amer. J. hum. Genet.*, **4**, 363–372.

102 GUNSON H.H. and DONOHUE W.L. (1958) The blood genotype $C^w D-/C^w D-$. *Proc. 6th Congr. int. Soc. Blood. Transf.*, 123–126.

103 BORNSTEIN S. and ISRAEL M. (1942) Agglutinogens in fetal erythrocytes. *Proc. Soc. exp. Biol. N.Y.*, **49**, 718–720.

104 STRATTON F. (1943) Demonstration of the Rh factor in the blood of a 48 mm. embryo. *Nature, Lond.*, **152**, 449.

105 MOLLISON P.L. and CUTBUSH MARIE (1949) Personal communication.

106 CHOWN B. (1955) On a search for rhesus antibodies in very young foetuses. *Arch. Dis. Childh.*, **30**, 232–233.

107 STEINBERG A.G. (1965) Evidence for a mutation or crossing-over at the Rh locus. *Vox Sang.*, **10**, 721–724.

108 DAHR P. (1942) Untersuchungen über eine neue erbliche agglutinable Blutkörpercheneigenschaft beim Menschen. *Deutsch. med. Wochen.*, **14**, 345–347.

109 WIENER A.S. and SONN EVE B. (1943) Heredity of the Rh factor. *Genetics*, **28**, 157–161.

[110] RACE R.R., TAYLOR G.L., CAPPELL D.F. and MCFARLANE MARJORY N. (1943) The Rh factor and erythroblastosis foetalis. *Brit. med. J.* ii, 289–293.

[111] BROMAN B. (1944) The blood factor Rh in man. *Acta Paed.*, **31**, suppl. 2, 178 pp.

[112] WIENER A.S., SONN EVE B. and BELKIN R.B. (1943) Heredity and distribution of the Rh blood types. *Proc. Soc. exp. Biol. N.Y.*, **54**, 238–240.

[113] WIENER A.S. and SONN EVE B. (1946) The Rh series of genes, with special reference to nomenclature, *Ann. N.Y. Acad. Sci.*, **46**, 969–988.

[114] WIENER A.S., SONN EVE B. and POLIVKA H.R. (1946) Heredity of Rh blood types. V. Improved nomenclature; additional family studies with special reference to Hr. *Proc. Soc. exp. Biol. N.Y.*, **61**, 382–390.

[115] WIENER A.S., SONN-GORDON EVE B. and HANDMAN LILIAN (1947) Heredity of the Rh blood types. VI. Additional family studies, with special reference to the theory of multiple allelic genes. *J. Immunol.*, **57**, 203–210.

[116] WIENER A.S. (1949) Heredity of the Rh blood types. VII. Additional family studies, with special reference to the genes R^z and r^y. Proceedings of the 8th International Congress of Genetics, *Hereditas*, suppl. vol, 1949.

[117] WIENER A.S., GORDON EVE B. and HANDMAN LILLIAN (1949) Heredity of the Rh blood types *Amer. J. hum. Genet.*, **1**, 127–140.

[118] BRENDEMOEN O.J. (1952) Inheritance of the Rh antigens: C-c-D-E in 114 families. *Acta path. microbiol. scand.*, **31**, 67–70.

[119] RACE R.R., TAYLOR G.L., IKIN ELIZABETH W. and DOBSON AILEEN M. (1945) The inheritance of allelemorphos of the Rh gene: a second series of families. *Ann. Eugen., Lond.*, **12**, 261–265.

[120] STRATTON F. (1945) The inheritance of the allelomorphs of the Rh gene with special reference to the Rh' and Rh" genes. *Ann. Eugen., Lond.*, **12**, 250–260.

[121] MCFARLANE MARJORY (1946) The inheritance of allelomorphs of the Rh gene in fifty families. *Ann. Eugen., Lond.*, **13**, 15–17.

[122] CHOWN B., OKAMURA Y. and PETERSON R.F. (1946) Inheritance of allelomorphs of the Rh gene in Canadians of Japanese race: a study of 65 families. *Canad. J. Res., E.* **24**, 144–147.

[123] BESSIS M. (1947) *La maladie hémolytique du nouveau-né*, pp. 263, Masson & Cie., Paris.

[124] SANGER RUTH, RACE R.R., WALSH R.J. and MONTGOMERY CARMEL (1948) An antibody which subdivides the human MN blood groups. *Heredity*, **2**, 131–139.

[125] LAWLER SYLVIA D., BERTINSHAW DOREEN, SANGER RUTH and RACE R.R. (1950) Inheritance of the Rh blood groups: 150 families tested with anti-C-c-C^w-D-E and anti-e. *Ann. Eugen., Lond.*, **15**, 258–270.

[126] WIENER A.S. (1945) Recent advances in knowledge of the Rh blood factors, with special reference to the clinical applications. *Trans. Stud. Coll. Phyns Philad.*, **13**, 105–122.

[127] SILBER R., GIBBS MARY B., JAHN ELSA F. and AKEROYD J.H. (1961) Quantitative hemagglutination studies in the Rh blood group system. I. The assay of the anti-D (Rh_0) agglutinin. *Blood*, **17**, 282–290.

[128] SILBER R., GIBBS MARY B., JAHN ELSA F. and AKEROYD J.H. (1961) Quantitative hemagglutination studies in the Rh blood group system. II. A study of the D (Rh_0) agglutinogen. *Blood*, **17**, 291–302.

[129] KORNSTAD L., RYTTINGER L. and HÖGMAN C. (1960) Two sera containing probably naturally occurring anti-C^w, one of them also containing a naturally occurring anti-Wr^a. *Vox Sang.*, **5**, 330–334.

[130] FISHER R.A. and RACE R.R. (1946) Rh gene frequencies in Britain. *Nature, Lond.*, **157**, 48.

[131] FISHER R.A (1947) The Rhesus factor: a study in scientific method. *Am. Scien.*, **35**, 95–103.

[132] FISHER SIR RONALD (1953) Population genetics. *Proc. Roy. Soc. B.*, **141**, 510–523.

[133] MASOUREDIS S.P. (1960) Relationship between Rh_0 (D) genotype and quantity of I^{131} anti-Rh_0 (D) bound to red cells. *J. clin. Invest.*, **39**, 1450–1462.

[134] SPEISER P. (1959) Ueber die bisher jüngste menschliche Frucht (27 mm/2.2g), an der bereits

die Erbmerkmale A₁, M, N, s, Fy(a+), C, c, D, E, e, Jk(a+?) im Blut festgestellt werden konnten. *Wien klin. Wschr.*, **71**, 549–551.

135   LEVINE P., CELANO M., FENICHEL R. and SINGHER H. (1961) A 'D'-like antigen in Rhesus red blood cells and in Rh-positive and Rh-negative red cells. *Science*, **133**, 332–333.

136   ANDRESEN E. (1967) Irregular transmission of a blood-group complex in one family of pigs following irradiation. *Vox Sang.*, **12**, 25–31.

137   SPEISER P., SCHANZER A. and KARRER K. (1953) Über Immunkörper gegen erbliche Blutkörperchenantigene in der Muttermilch. *Z. Kinderheilkunde*, **72**, 509–520.

138   HACKEL E., SMOLKER R.E. and FENSKE SUE A. (1958) Inhibition of anti-Rh and anti-Lutheran sera by ribonucleic acid derivatives. *Vox Sang.*, **3**, 402–408.

139   HACKEL E. and SPOLYAR K.S. (1960) Anti-c and anti-e inhibition by ribonucleic acid derivatives. *Vox Sang.*, **5**, 517–522.

140   HACKEL E. and SMOLKER R.E. (1960) Effect of ribonuclease on erythrocyte antigens. *Nature, Lond.*, **187**, 1036–1037.

141   BOYD W.C., MCMASTER MARJORIE H. and WASZCZENKO-ZACHARSZENKO EUGENIA (1959) Specific inhibition of anti-Rh serum by 'unnatural' sugars. *Nature, Lond.*, **184**, 989–990.

142   DODD M.C., BIGLEY NANCY J. and GEYER VIRGINIA B. (1960) Specific inhibition of Rh₀ (D) antibody by sialic acids. *Science*, **132**, 1398–1399.

143   VOGT ELSA and HARTMANN O. (1962) Unpublished observations.

144   PROKOP O. (1959) Das Rh-mosaik $R_z^w R_1$ aufgefunden. *Klin. Wschr.*, **37**, 882.

145   PROKOP O. and RACKWITZ A. (1959) Eine weitere Beobachtung von R_z^w in der seltenen Kombination $R_z^w R_1^w$ mit einer Bemerkung über den Dosiseffekt von C^w, *Blut*, **5**, 279–281.

146   CLEGHORN T.E. (1960) The demonstration of the Rh chromosome C^wDE. *Vox Sang.*, **5**, 171–172.

147   RACE R.R., SANGER RUTH, LAWLER SYLVIA D. and KEETCH D.V. (1948) Blood groups of Latvians, A₁A₂BO, MN and Rh. *Ann. Eugen., Lond.*, **14**, 134–138.

148   ALLISON A.C., HARTMANN O., BRENDEMOEN O.J. and MOURANT A.E. (1952) The blood groups of the Norwegian Lapps. *Acta path. microbiol. scand.*, **31**, 334–338.

149   ALLISON A.C., BROMAN B., MOURANT A.E. and RYTTINGER L. (1956) The blood groups of the Swedish Lapps. *J. Roy. anthrop. Inst.*, **86**, 87–94.

150   KORNSTAD L. (1959) The frequency of the Rh antigen C^w in 2,750 Oslo blood donors. *Vox Sang.*, **4**, 225–230.

151   KAARSALO E., KORTEKANGAS A.E., TIPPETT PATRICIA A. and HAMPER JEAN (1962) A contribution to the blood group frequencies in Finns. *Acta path. microbiol, scand.*, **54**, 287–290.

152   RACE R.R., SANGER RUTH and LAWLER SYLVIA D. (1960) The Rh antigen called c^v, a revocation. *Vox Sang.*, **5**, 334–336.

153   PLAUT GERTRUDE, BOOTH P.B., GILES CAROLYN M. and MOURANT A.E. (1958) A new example of the Rh antibody, anti-C^x. *Brit. med. J.*, **i**, 1215–1217.

154   CLEGHORN T.E. (1961) *The Occurrence of Certain Rare Blood Group factors in Britain.* M.D. thesis, University of Sheffield.

155   FISK R.T. and FOORD A.G. (1942) Observations on the Rh agglutinogen of human blood. *Amer. J. clin. Path.*, **12**, 545.

156   SANGER RUTH, NOADES JEAN, TIPPETT PATRICIA, RACE R.R., JACK J.A. and CUNNINGHAM C.A. (1960) An Rh antibody specific for V and R'^s. *Nature, Lond.*, **186**, 171.

157   MURRAY J. and CLARK E.C. (1952) Production of anti-Rh in guinea pigs from human erythrocytes. *Nature, Lond.*, **169**, 886–887.

158   SHAPIRO M. (1960) Serology and genetics of a new blood factor: hr^s. *J. forens. Med.*, **7**, 96–105.

159   LAYRISSE M., LAYRISSE ZULAY, GARCIA ESPERANZA, WILBERT J. and PARRA R.J. (1961) New Rh phenotype Dcce^fe^f found in a Chibcha Indian tribe. *Nature, Lond.*, **191**, 503–504.

160   HUESTIS D.W., CATINO MARY LU and BUSCH SHIRLEY (1964) A 'new' Rh antibody (anti-Rh 26) which detects a factor usually accompanying hr´. *Transfusion, Philad.*, **4**, 414–418.

161 KAITA HIROKO, LEWIS MARION and CHOWN B. (1964) The Rh antigen E^w. *Transfusion, Philad.*, **4**, 118–119.

162 WINTER NANCY, MILKOVICH LUCILLE and KONUGRES ANGELYN A. (1966) A third example of the Rh antigen, E^w. *Transfusion, Philad.*, **6**, 271–272.

163 O'RIORDAN J.P., WILKINSON J.L., HUTH M.C., WILSON T.E., MOURANT A.E. and GILES C.M. (1962) The Rh gene complex cdE^u. *Vox Sang.*, **7**, 14–21.

164 VAN LOGHEM J.J. (1947) Production of Rh agglutinins anti-C and anti-E by artificial immunization of volunteer donors. *Brit. med. J.* **2**, 958–959.

165 VOS G.H. and KIRK R.L. (1962) A 'naturally-occurring' anti-E which distinguishes a variant of the E antigen in Australian aborigines. *Vox Sang.*, **7**, 22–32.

166 SANGER RUTH, WALSH R.J. and KAY M. PATRICIA (1951) Blood types of natives of Australia and New Guinea. *Amer. J. phys. Anthrop.*, **9**, 71–78.

167 NIJENHUIS L.E. (1961) *Blood Group Frequencies in the Netherlands, Curaçao, Surinam and New Guinea: a Study in Population Genetics.* Doctoral Thesis, University of Amsterdam, 106–109.

168 VAN LOGHEM J.J., BARTELS H.L.J.M. and HART M. V.D. (1949) La production d'un anticorps anti-C^w par immunisation artificielle d'un donneur bénévole. *Rev. Hémat.*, **4**, 173–176.

169 TIPPETT PATRICIA (1963) *Serological Study of the Inheritance of Unusual Rh and Other Blood Group Phenotypes.* Ph.D. Thesis. University of London.

170 GROBBELAAR B.G. and MOORES P.P. (1963) The third example of anti-hr^s. *Transfusion, Philad.*, **3**, 103–104.

171 STURGEON P. (1962) The Rh_0 variant—D^u. I. Its frequency in a mixed population. *Transfusion, Philad.*, **2**, 234–243.

172 STURGEON P. (1962) The Rh_0 variant—D^u. II. Its detection with a direct tube test. *Transfusion, Philad.*, **2**, 244–255.

173 MOLLISON P.L. and CUTBUSH MARIE (1949) La maladie hémolytique chez un enfant D^u. *Rev. Hémat.*, **4**, 608–612.

174 VOGEL P. and ROSENFIELD R.E. Unpublished observations, cited by Rosenfield R.E., Vogel P., Miller E.B. and Haber Gladys (1951) Weakly reacting Rh positive (D^u) bloods. *Blood*, **6**, 1123–1134.

175 ARGALL C.I., BALL J.M. and TRENTELMAN E. (1953) Presence of anti-D antibody in the serum of a D^u patient. *J. Lab. clin. Med.*, **41**, 895–898.

176 HOLMAN C.A. (1951) Cited in 2nd, 3rd and 4th editions of this book.

177 LARYRISSE M., LAYRISSE ZULAY, GARCIA ESPERANZA and PARRA J. (1961) Genetic studies of the new Rh chromosome Dce^lf(Rh_o^l) found in a Chibcha tribe. *Vox Sang.*, **6**, 710–719.

178 SPEISER P. (1958) Frequenz und Bedeutung seltener Rhesusmerkmale (C und E bei Rhesus-Negativen, D^u und C^w). *Blut*, **4**, 1–7.

179 SCHMIDT P.J., MORRISON ELEANOR and SHOHL JANE (1959) The antigenicity of the Rh_0 variant (D^u) in transfusion practice. *Proc. 7th Congr. int. Soc. Blood Transf.* 569–571.

180 MARSTERS R.W. and SCHLEIN F.C. (1959) The inheritance of the Rh_0 variant D^u. *Vox Sang.*, **4**, 350–366.

181 PROKOP O., HUNGER H. and DÜRWALD W. (1960) Beobachtungen über ein D-hemmendes Prinzip in einer Sippe. *Dtsch. Z. gerichtl. Med.*, **50**, 553–558.

182 WIENER A.S., GEIGER J. and GORDON EVE B. (1957) Mosaic nature of the Rh_0 factor of human blood. *Exp. Med. Surg.*, **15**, 75–82.

183 ANDERSON LOIS D., RACE G.J. and OWEN MAY (1958) Presence of anti-D antibody in an Rh (D)-positive person. *Amer. J. clin. Path.*, **30**, 228–229.

184 RACE R.R. (1944) An 'incomplete' antibody in human serum. *Nature, Lond.*, **153**, 771.

185 UNGER L.J., WIENER A.S. and WIENER L. (1959) New antibody (anti-Rh^B) resulting from blood transfusion in an Rh-positive patient. *J. Amer. med. Ass.*, **170**, 1380–1383.

186 LAWLER SYLVIA D. and LOGHEM J.J. VAN (1947) The Rhesus antigen C^w causing haemolytic disease of the newborn. *Lancet*, **ii**, 545.

THE Rh BLOOD GROUPS 249

187 BROMAN B. (1948) Paper read at the 8th International Congress of Genetics, Stockholm.
188 COLLINS J.O., SANGER RUTH, ALLEN F.H. and RACE R.R. (1950) Nine blood group antibodies in a single serum following multiple transfusions. *Brit. med. J.*, **1**, 1297–1299.
189 LOGHEM J.J. VAN, KLOMP-MAGNEE W. and BAKX C.J.A. (1953) Haemolytic disease of the
newborn due to iso-immunization by the antigens c and Cᵂ. *Vox Sang.* (O.S.), **3**, 130–
132.
190 CHOWN B. and LEWIS MARION (1954) The occurrence of an Rh haemagglutinin of specificity
anti-Cᵂ in the absence of known stimulation: suggestions as to cause. *Vox Sang.* (O.S.),
4, 41–45.
191 VOGEL P. (1954) Current problems in blood transfusion. *Bull. N. Y. Acad. med.*, **30**, 657–674.
192 WEINER W. (1956) Personal communication.
193 RACE R.R. and SANGER RUTH (1956) Unpublished observations.
194 UNGER L.J. and WIENER A.S. (1959) A 'new' antibody anti-Rhᶜ, resulting from isosensitization by pregnancy with special reference to the heredity of a new Rh-Hr agglutinogen
ℜh₂ᶜ. *J. Lab. clin. Med.*, **54**, 835–842.
195 SACKS M.S., WIENER A.S., JAHN ELSA F., SPURLING CARROLL L. and UNGER L.J. (1959)
Isosensitization to a new blood factor Rhᴰ with special reference to its clinical importance. *Ann. intern. Med.*, **51**, 740–747.
196 SIMMONS R.T. and KRIEGER VERA I. (1960) Anti-Rh₀(D) antibodies produced by iso-
immunization in an Rh positive mother of the unusual genotype ℜ¹rᵧ (CDᵘe/CdE).
Med. J. Aust., **2**, 1021–1022.
197 SCHLEYER F. (1953) Reaktionen von anti-E-Serumfraktionen mit verschiedenen E-Geno-
typen. *Zeitschr. f. Hygiene*, **137**, 48–60.
198 FRANCIS BETTY J., HATCHER D.E. and MARCUSE P.M. (1960) An Rh₀ (D) positive patient
whose serum contains anti-Rh₀ (D) antibodies. *Vox Sang.*, **5**, 324–329.
199 HACKEL E. (1957) Rh antibodies in the serum of two −D−/−D− people. *Vox Sang.*, **2**, 331–
341.
200 WITEBSKY E., ANDERSON G.W. and HEIDE ANNE (1942) Demonstration of Rh antibody in
breast milk. *Proc. Soc. exp. Biol. N.Y.*, **49**, 179–183.
201 WITEBSKY E. and HEIDE ANNE (1943) Further investigations on presence of Rh antibodies in
breast milk. *Proc. Soc. exp. Biol. N.Y.*, **52**, 280–281.
202 BOLHUIS J.H. VAN (1948) *Placenta en Rhesus Antagonisme*, J.J. Groen and Zoon N.V.,
Leiden. Pages 21, 105, 106, 139.
203 EATON B.R., MORTON J.A., PICKLES MARGARET M. and WHITE K.E. (1956) A new antibody,
anti-Ytᵃ, characterizing a blood group of high incidence. *Brit. J. Haemat.*, **2**, 333–341.
204 ZEITLIN R.A. (1957) A neglected source of blood-group antibodies. *Lancet*, **i**, 915.
205 DIAMOND L.K. (1944) Progress report to Committee on Medical Research of the Office of
Scientific Research and Development. *OEM*. cmr. 384, Jan. 1st.
206 WIENER A.S. (1944) A new test (blocking test) for Rh sensitization. *Proc. soc. exp. Biol.
N.Y.*, **56**, 173–176.
207 COCA A.F. and KELLY MARGARET F. (1921) VI. A Serological study of the bacillus of
Pfeiffer. *J. Immunol.*, **6**, 87–101.
208 PAPPENHEIMER A.M. (1940) Anti-egg albumin antibody in the horse. *J. exp. Med.*, **71**,
263–269.
209 HEIDELBERGER M., TREFFERS H.P. and MAYER M. (1940) A quantitative theory of the
precipitin reaction. VII. The egg albumin-antibody reaction in antisera from the rabbit
and horse. *J. exp. Med.*, **71**, 271–282.
210 SHIBLEY G.S. (1929) Studies in agglutination. IV. The agglutination inhibition zone.
J. exp. Med., **51**, 825–841.
211 KLECZKOWSKI A. (1941) Effect of heat on flocculating antibodies of rabbit antisera. *Brit. J.
exp. Path.*, **22**, 192–208.
212 DIAMOND L.K. and ABELSON NEVA M. (1945) The importance of Rh inhibitor substance in
anti-Rh serums. *J. clin. Investig.*, **24**, 122–126.

213 COOMBS R.R.A. and RACE R.R. (1945) Further observations on the 'incomplete' or 'blocking' Rh antibody. *Nature, Lond.*, **156**, 233.

214 MOHN J.F. (1956) Studies on the thermal inactivation of Rh antibodies. *Prog. 6th Congr. int. Soc. Blood Transf.*, 73–74.

215 BOYD W.C. (1946) Effect of photo-oxidation on isohemagglutinating antibodies. *J. exp. Med.*, **83**, 221–225.

216 BOYD W.C. (1946) The effect of high pressures on hemagglutinating antibodies. *J. exp. Med.*, **83**, 401–407.

217 BAAR H.S. (1945) The Race-Wiener test in haemolytic disease of the newborn. *Nature, Lond.*, **155**, 789.

218 DIAMOND L.K. and ABELSON NEVA M. (1945) The demonstration of anti-Rh agglutinins, an accurate and rapid slide test. *J. Lab. clin. Med.*, **30**, 204–212.

219 DIAMOND L.K. and ABELSON NEVA M. (1945) The detection of Rh sensitization: evaluations of tests for Rh antibodies. *J. Lab. clin. Med.*, **31**, 668–674.

220 DIAMOND L.K. and DENTON R.L. (1945) Rh agglutination in various media with particular reference to the value of albumin. *J. Lab. clin. Med.*, **30**, 821–830.

221 CAMERON J.W. and DIAMOND L.K. (1945) Chemical, clinical and immunological studies on the products of human plasma fractionation. XXIX. Serum albumin as a diluent for Rh typing reagents. *J. clin. Investig.*, **24**, 793–801.

222 WIENER A.S., UNGER L.J. and JACK J.A. (1960) Preuve de l'existence d'un nouveau gène allèle Rh R^{1cd}. *Rev. Hémat.*, **15**, 286–290.

223 UNGER L.J. and WIENER A.S. (1959) Some observations on the blood factor Rh^A of the Rh-Hr blood group system. *Acta Genet., Med. et Gemell.*, 2nd suppl., 13–25.

224 WIENER A.S. and UNGER L.J. (1959) Rh factors related to the Rh_0 factor as a source of clinical problems. *J. Amer. med. Ass.*, **169**, 696–699.

225 UNGER L.J. and WIENER A.S. (1959) Observations on blood factors Rh^A, Rh^α, Rh^B, and Rh^C. *Amer. J. clin. Path.*, **31**, 95–103.

226 UNGER L.J. and WIENER A.S. (1959) Some observations on blood factors Rh^A, Rh^B and Rh^C of the Rh-Hr blood group system. *Blood*, **14**, 522–534.

227 UNGER L.J., WIENER A.S. and KATZ L. (1959) Studies on blood factors Rh^A, Rh^B and Rh^C. *J. exp. Med.*, **110**, 495–510.

228 COOMBS R.R.A., MOURANT A.E. and RACE R.R. (1945) Detection of weak and 'incomplete' Rh agglutinins: a new test. *Lancet*, **ii**, 15.

229 COOMBS R.R.A., MOURANT A.E. and RACE R.R. (1945) A new test for the detection of weak and 'incomplete' Rh agglutinins. *Brit. J. exp. Path.*, **26**, 255–266.

230 COOMBS R.R.A., MOURANT A.E. and RACE R.R. (1946) In vivo isosensitization of red cells in babies with haemolytic disease. *Lancet*, **i**, 264–266.

231 MORESCHI C. (1908) Neue Tatsachen uber die Blutkörperchenagglutination. *Zbl. Bakt.*, **46**, 49–51.

232 PICKLES MARGARET M. (1946) Effects of cholera filtrate on red cells as demonstrated by incomplete Rh antibodies. *Nature, Lond.*, **158**, 880.

233 MORTON J.A. and PICKLES MARGARET M. (1947) Use of trypsin in the detection of incomplete anti-Rh antibodies. *Nature, Lond.*, **159**, 779.

234 PITTENGER R.G., McQUISTON DOROTHY and STURGEON P. (1964) The Rh_0 variant—D^u. III. A field trial of the D^u tube test in typing donor bloods. *Transfusion, Philad.*, **4**, 361–366.

235 SUSSMAN L.N. and WIENER A.S. (1964) An unusual Rh agglutinogen lacking blood factors Rh^A, Rh^B, Rh^C and Rh^D. *Transfusion, Philad.*, **4**, 50–51.

236 WIENER A.S. and UNGAR L.J. (1962) Further observations on the blood factors Rh^A, Rh^B, Rh^C and Rh^D. *Transfusion, Philad.*, **2**, 230–233.

237 WARREN JENNIFER K. (1962) The frequency of the occurrence of anti-D^B (Anti-Rh^B) in anti-D (anti-Rh) sera. *Vox Sang.*, **7**, 381–383.

238 CHOWN B., KAITA HIROKO, LEWIS MARION, ROY R.B. and WYATT LOUISE (1963) A 'D-positive' man who produced anti-D. *Vox Sang.*, **8**, 420–429.

239 MACPHERSON C.R., STEVENSON T.D. and GAYTON J. (1966) Anti-D in a D-positive man, with positive direct Coombs test and normal red cell survival. *Amer. J. clin. Path.*, **45**, 748–750.

240 CHOWN B., LEWIS MARION, KAITA HIROKO and PHILIPPS SYLVIA (1964) The Rh antigen D^w (Wiel). *Transfusion, Philad.*, **4**, 169–172.

241 LEWIS MARION, MACPHERSON C.R. and GAYTON JANICE (1965) The Rh complex R_1^{wo} (CD^{w}e). *Can. J. Genet., Cytol.*, **7**, 259–261.

242 DUNSFORD I. (1962) A new Rh antibody—anti-CE. *Proc. 8th Congr. europ. Soc. Haemat.*, Vienna 1961. Paper No. 491.

243 KEITH PRISCILLA, CORCORAN PATRICIA A., CASPERSEN KARI and ALLEN F.H. (1965) A new antibody; anti-Rh (27) (cE) in the Rh blood-group system. *Vox Sang.*, **10**, 528–535.

244 GOLD E.R., GILLESPIE E.M. and TOVEY G.H. (1961) A serum containing 8 antibodies. *Vox Sang.*, **6**, 157–163.

245 SHAPIRO M. (1964) Serology and genetics of a 'new' blood factor: hr^H. *J. forens. Med.*, **11**, 52–66.

246 ROSENFIELD R.E., HABER GLADYS V. and DEGNAN T.J. (1964) Rh alleles, $R^{-10, 20}$, and new evidence for $R^{2,4}$. *Vox Sang.*, **9**, 168–174.

247 JAKOBOWICZ RACHEL, WHITTINGHAM SENGA, BARRIE JEAN U. and SIMMONS R.T. (1962) A further investigation on polyvalent anti-C (rh′) and anti-G (rh^G) antibodies produced by iso-immunization in pregnancy. *Med. J. Aust.*, **i**, 895–896.

248 NIJENHUIS L.E. (1961) Comments on the genetical structure of the Rhesus system. *Vox Sang.*, **6**, 229–232.

249 STOUT T.D., MOORE B.P.L., ALLEN F.H. and CORCORAN PATRICIA (1963) A new phenotype —D+G— (Rh: 1, −12). *Vox Sang.*, **8**, 262–268.

250 ZAINO E.C. (1965) A new Rh phenotype, Rh$_o$rh, G-negative. *Transfusion, Philad.*, **5**, 320–321.

251 DE TORREGROSA M., RULLÁN MIMOSA M., CECILE C., SABATER AMELIA and ALBERTO C. (1961) Severe erythroblastosis in a primigravida associated with absence of Rh chromosomes. *Amer. J. Obstet. Gynec.*, **82**, 1375–1378.

252 NAKAJIMA H., MISAWA S. and OTA K. (1965) A further example of D—/D—— ($\overline{\overline{R}}^o\overline{\overline{R}}^o$) found among the Japanese. *Proc. Jap. Acad.*, **41**, 488–492.

253 YAMAGUCHI Y., TANAKA S., TSUJI Y. and NAKAJIMA H. (1965) A new example of the rare D——($\overline{\overline{R}}^o$) of Rh blood groups in Japan. *Proc. Jap. Acad.*, **41**, 493–498.

254 UNGER L.J. (1964) A family pedigree showing the transmission of rare and 'new' Rh-Hr genes. *Transfusion, Philad.*, **4**, 173–176.

255 BHATIA H.M. and SANGHVI L.D. (1962) Rare blood groups and consanguinity: 'Bombay' phenotype. *Vox Sang.*, **7**, 245–248.

256 LAWLER SYLVIA D. and MARSHALL RUTH (1962) A serological study of −D− heterozygotes in the same family. *Vox Sang.*, **7**, 305–314.

257 BOETTCHER B. (1964)The Rh 'deletion' phenotypes and the information they provide about the Rh genes. *Vox Sang.*, **9**, 641–652.

258 HUESTIS D.W. and STERN K. (1962) Immunization to Rh$_o$(D) observed in pregnancy of a woman with type rh^G(G). *Transfusion, Philad.*, **2**, 419–422.

259 BOORMAN KATHLEEN E. and LINCOLN P.J. (1962) A suggestion as to the place of r^G and r^M on the Rh system. *Ann. hum. Genet.*, **26**, 51–58.

260 MCGEE R., LEVINE P. and CELANO M. (1957) First example of genotype r^{y}r^y—a family study. *Science*, **125**, 1043.

261 GUNSON H.H. and DONOHUE W.L. (1957) Multiple examples of the blood genotype C^{w}D−/ C^{w}D− in a Canadian family. *Vox Sang.*, **2**, 320–331.

262 LEVINE P., CELANO M., MCGEE R., MUSCHEL L.H. and GRISET T.A. (1957) D^u and gene interaction in a family study. *P. H. Andresen Festskrift*, Munksgaard, Copenhagen, 144–155.

[263] WIENER A.S., OWEN R.D., STORMONT C. and WEXLER I.B. (1956) Medico-legal applications of blood-grouping tests. *J. Amer. med. Ass.*, **161**, 233–239.

[264] HEIKEN A. and GILES CAROLYN M. (1965) On the Rh gene complexes $D--$, $D(C)(e)$ and $d(c)(e)$. *Hereditas, Lund.*, **53**, 171–186.

[265] BROMAN B., HEIKEN A., TIPPETT PATRICIA A. and GILES CAROLYN M. (1963) The $D(C)(e)$ gene complex revealed in the Swedish population. *Vox Sang.*, **8**, 588–593.

[266] TIPPETT PATRICIA and SANGER RUTH (1962) Observations on subdivisions of the Rh antigen D. *Vox Sang.*, **7**, 9–13.

[267] LEVINE P., WHITE JANE, STROUP MARJORY, ZMIJEWSKI C.M. and MOHN J.F. (1960) Haemolytic disease of the newborn probably due to anti-f. *Nature, Lond.*, **185**, 188–189.

[268] GRUNDORFER J., KOPCHIK WILMA, TIPPETT PATRICIA and SANGER RUTH (1961) Anti-f in the serum of a CDe/cDE person: the second example. *Vox Sang.*, **6**, 618–619.

[269] ROSENFIELD R.E. and HABER GLADYS V. (1958) An Rh blood factor, rh_i (Ce), and its relationship to hr (ce). *Amer. J. hum Genet.*, **10**, 474–480.

[270] TIPPETT PATRICIA A., SANGER RUTH, DUNSFORD I. and BARBER MARGARET (1961) An Rh gene complex, r^M, in some ways like r^G. *Vox Sang.*, **6**, 21–33.

[271] LAYRISSE M., SANGER RUTH and RACE R.R. (1959) The inheritance of the antigen Di^a: evidence for its independence of other blood groups systems. *Amer. J. hum. Genet.*, **11**, 17–25.

[272] BARNICOT N.A., GARLICK J.P. and ROBERTS D.F. (1960) Haptoglobin and transferrin inheritance in northern Nigerians. *Ann. hum. Genet.*, **24**, 171–183.

[273] ROSENFIELD R.E., HABER GLADYS V., SCHROEDER RUTH and BALLARD RACHEL (1960) Problems in Rh typing as revealed by a single negro family. *Amer. J. hum. Genet.*, **12**, 147–159.

[274] STURGEON P., FISK R., WINTLER CONSTANCE and CHERTOCK RHODA (1959) Observations with pure anti-C on a variant of C common in Negroes. *Proc. 7th Congr. int. Soc. Blood Transf.*, 293–300.

[275] STURGEON P. (1960) Studies on the relation of anti-rh'N (C^N) to Rh blood factor rh_i (Ce). *J. forens. Sci.*, **5**, 287–293.

[276] ZOUTENDYK A. and TEODORCZUK H. (1960) The Rh factor C in South African Bantu. *Nature, Lond.*, **187**, 790–791.

[277] ZOUTENDYK A. and TEODORCZUK H. (1962) Rh factors C and G in South African Bantu. *Proc. 8th Congr. int. Soc. Blood Transf.*, 183–186.

[278] RACE R.R. and SANGER RUTH (1961) Whither Rh? Int. Symp. on Imm. and Biochem. of Human Blood, Amsterdam 1959. *Vox Sang.*, **6**, 227–228.

[279] ALLEN F.H. and TIPPETT PATRICIA A. (1958) A new Rh blood type which reveals the Rh antigen G. *Vox Sang.*, **3**, 321–330.

[280] JAKOBOWICZ RACHEL and SIMMONS R.T. (1959) Iso-immunization in a mother which demonstrates the 'new' Rh blood antigen G (rh^G) and anti-G (rh^G). *Med. J. Aust.*, **2**, 357–358.

[281] VOS G.H. (1960) The evaluation of specific anti-G (CD) eluate obtained by a double absorption and elution procedure. *Vox Sang.*, **5**, 472–478.

[282] ALLEN F.H. and TIPPETT PATRICIA A. (1961) Blocking tests with the Rh antibody anti-G. *Vox Sang.*, **6**, 429–434.

[283] KUNIYUKI M. and TAKAHARA N. (1958) Two cases of peculiar blood groups. *Blood and Transfusion*, J. Japan Soc. Blood Trans., **4**, 206–208 (in Japanese).

[284] MOORE B.P.L., McINTYRE J., BROWN FRANCES and READ H.C. (1960) Recognition of the rare Rh chromosome $D--$. *Canad. med. Ass. J.*, **82**, 187–191.

[285] READ H.C., BROWN FRANCES, LININS ILGA, McINTYRE J. and MOORE B.P.L. (1961) New examples of $D--/D--$, *Vox Sang.*, **6**, 362–365.

[286] ALLEN F.H. (1960) In *J. Pediat.*, **57**, 281–286.

[287] OSE T. and BUSH O.B. (1960) Erythroblastosis fetalis. Report of cases with one caused by gene deletion. *Prog. 8th Congr. int. Blood Transf.*, II-c-13.

288 YOKOYAMA M., SOLOMON J.M., KUNIYUKI M. and STROUP MARJORY (1961) $\overline{\overline{R}}{}^0$ (D––) in two Japanese families with a note on its genetic interpretation. *Transfusion, Philad.*, 1, 273–279.

289 YOKOYAMA M., TSUCHIYA T., KURATA M., LODGE T. and DUNSFORD I. (1961) Unpublished observations.

290 TATE HERMINE, CUNNINGHAM C., McDADE MARY G., TIPPETT PATRICIA A. and SANGER RUTH (1960) An Rh gene complex Dc–. *Vox Sang.*, 5, 398–402.

291 YOKOYAMA M. and FURUHATA T. (1957) On the discovery of rare Rh genotype. *Proc. imp. Acad. Japan*, 33, 233–235; also (1958) *Ochanomizu Medical Journal*, 6, 105–137, and *Programs* 1957, 1958 AABB meetings.

292 RACE R.R. and SANGER RUTH (1960) Consanguinity and certain rare blood groups. *Vox Sang.*, 5, 383–384.

293 WIENER A.S. (1958) Blood group nomenclature. *Science*, 128, 849–852.

294 VOS G.H., VOS DELL, KIRK R.L. and SANGER RUTH (1961) A sample of blood with no detectable Rh antigens. *Lancet*, i, 14–15.

295 HENNINGSEN K. (1958) A new 'deleted' Rh-chromosome. *Nature, Lond*, 181, 502.

296 HENNINGSEN K. (1959) A family study involving a new rare Rh-chromosome (d–– or –––), *Proc. 7th Congr. int. Soc. Blood Transf.*, 567–568.

297 PROKOP O. and SCHNEIDER W. (1960) Das Rhesusmosaik $R_1/\ldots$ *Dtsch. Z. gerlichtl. Med.*, 50, 423–428.

298 BROMAN B. and HEIKEN A. (1962) Unpublished observations.

299 LEVINE P., ROSENFIELD R.E. and WHITE JANE (1961) The first example of the Rh phenotype $r^G r^G$. *Amer. J. hum. Genet.*, 13, 299–305.

300 KEVY S.V., SCHMIDT P.J. and LEYSHON W.C. (1959) A second example of the blood type 'rh^G'. *Vox Sang.*, 4, 257–266.

301 METAXAS M.N. and METAXAS-BÜHLER MARGRIT (1961) An Rh gene complex which produces weak c and e antigens in a mother and her son. *Vox Sang.*, 6, 136–141.

302 DUNSFORD I. and TIPPETT PATRICIA (1960) Unpublished observations.

303 ROSENFIELD R.E. (1961) Exceptional inheritance of Rh phenotypes. Paper read at 2nd Int. Meeting Foren. Path. and Med. Also published in part in reference 322.

304 GIBLETT ELOISE R. and CHASE JEANNE (1959) Js^a, a 'new' red-cell antigen found in Negroes; evidence for an eleventh blood group system. *Brit. J. Haemat.*, 5, 319–326.

305 RASMUSON MARIANNE and HEIKEN A. (1966) Frequency of occurrence of the human Rh complexes $D(C)(e)$, $d(c)(e)$, D–– and –––. *Nature, Lond.*, 212, 1377–1379.

306 GORER P.A. and MIKULSKA Z.B. (1959) Some further data on the H-2 system of antigens. *Proc. roy. Soc. B.*, 151, 57–69.

307 CARLSON E.A. (1958) The bearing of a complex-locus in Drosophila on the interpretation of the Rh series. *Amer. J. hum. Genet.*, 10, 465–473.

308 CARLSON E.A. (1959) Comparative genetics of complex loci. *Quart. Rev. Biol.*, 34, 33–67.

309 BENZER S. (1955) Fine structure of a genetic region in bacteriophage. *Proc. nat. Acad. Sci., Wash.*, 41, 344–354.

310 BENZER S. (1957) The elementary units of heredity from *The Chemical Basis of Heredity*, The Johns Hopkins Press, Baltimore, 70–93.

311 ELLIS F.R. (1961) Unpublished observations.

312 CHALTON MARY, HUMPHREYS PATRICIA, LININS ILGA and MOORE B.P.L. (1963) A third Canadian family with the Rh chromosome D––. *Transfusion, Philad.*, 3, 100–102.

313 KORNSTAD L. and ØYEN R. (1967) An Rh gene complex producing weak c and E antigens. *Vox Sang.*, 13, 417–422, and *Nordisk Med.*, 77, 326.

314 SPRINGER G.F., WILLIAMSON P. and BRANDES W.C. (1961) Blood group activity of gram-negative bacteria. *J. exp. Med.*, 113, 1077–1093.

315 SIMMONS R.T. (1962) The inheritance of CdE and a 'low-grade' CD^{u}e (not due to suppression) in three generations. *Vox Sang.*, 7, 79–82.

316 METAXAS M.N., METAXAS-BÜHLER M., BÜTLER R. and ROMANSKI Y. (1964) Two examples of the Rh genotype *CdE/CdE* (RyRy) in a Swiss family. *Vox Sang.*, **9**, 698–711.

317 STERN K. and BERGER MARY (1961) Experimental immunization to rh^G. *Amer. J. clin. Path.*, **35**, 520–525.

318 TIPPETT PATRICIA, GAVIN JUNE and SANGER RUTH (1962) The antigen C^w produced by the gene complex C^w*D*–, *Vox Sang.*, **7**, 249–250.

319 CHOWN B., LEWIS MARION and KAITA HIROKO (1962) A 'new' Rh antigen and antibody. *Transfusion, Philad.*, **2**, 150–154.

320 LEVINE P., CELANO M., VOS G.H. and MORRISON J. (1962) The first human blood, –––/ –––, which lacks the 'D-like' antigen. *Nature, Lond.*, **194**, 304–305.

321 LEVINE P., CELANO M., FENICHEL R., POLLACK W. and SINGHER H. (1961) A 'D-like' antigen in rhesus monkey, human Rh positive and human Rh negative red blood cells. *J. Immunol.*, **87**, 747–752.

322 ROSENFIELD R.E., ALLEN F.H., SWISHER S.N. and KOCHWA S. (1962) A review of Rh serology and presentation of a new terminology. *Transfusion, Philad.*, **2**, 287–312.

323 MOHR J. (1954) *A Study of Linkage in Man*, pp. 119, Munksgaard, Copenhagen.

324 MÄKELÄ O., ERIKKSON A.W. and LEHTOVAARA RAIMO (1959) On the inheritance of the haptoglobin serum groups. *Acta genet.*, **9**, 149–166.

325 V.D. WEERDT CHRISTINA M. (1965) *Platelet Antigens and Iso-immunization*. Doctoral Thesis, 'Aemstelstad', Amsterdam, pp. 108.

326 MOHR J. (1966) Genetics of fourteen marker systems: associations and linkage relations. *Acta genet.*, **16**, 1–58.

327 STEINBERG A., SHWACHMAN H., ALLEN F.H. and DOOLEY R.R. (1956) Linkage studies with cystic fibrosis of the pancreas. *Amer. J. hum. Genet.*, **8**, 162–176.

328 GREUTER W., HESS M., RENAUD N., SCHMITTER M. and BÜTLER R. (1963) Beitrag zur Genetik des Gm- und Gc-Serumgruppensystems anhand von Untersuchungen an Schweizerfamilien. *Arch. Klaus-Stift. VererbForsch.*, **38**, 77–92.

329 LINNET-JEPSEN P. (1965) *Undersøgelser over Gm(a) Faktoren: Specielt i det første leveår.* M.D. Thesis, University of Aarhus, pp. 256.

330 GILES CAROLYN M. and BEVAN BERYL (1964) Possible suppression of Rh-antigens in only one generation of a family. *Vox Sang.*, **9**, 204–208.

331 SWANSON JANE and MATSON G.A. (1964) Third example of a human 'D-like' antibody or anti-LW. *Transfusion, Philad.*, **4**, 257–261.

332 LEVINE P., CELANO M.J., WALLACE J. and SANGER RUTH (1963) A human 'D-like' antibody. *Nature, Lond.*, **198**, 596–597.

333 SWANSON J., POLESKY H.F. and MATSON G.A. (1965) The LW antigen of adult and infant erythrocytes. *Vox Sang.*, **10**, 560–566.

334 LEVINE P., CHAMBERS J.W., CELANO M.J., FALKOWSKI F., HUNTER O.B. and ENGLISH C.T. (1965) A second example of –––/––– or Rh$_{null}$ blood. *Proc. 10th Congr. int. Soc. Blood Transf.*, Stockholm 1964, 350–356.

335 LEVINE P., CELANO M.J., FALKOWSKI F., CHAMBERS J., HUNTER O.B. and ENGLISH C.T. (1964) A second example of –––/––– blood, or Rh$_{null}$. *Nature, Lond.*, **204**, 892.

336 LEVINE P., CELANO M.J., FALKOWSKI F., CHAMBERS J., HUNTER O.B. and ENGLISH C.T. (1965) A second example of –––/––– or Rh$_{null}$ Blood. *Transfusion, Philad.*, **5**, 492–500.

337 RACE R.R. (1964) Latest on blood groups, presented at NATO Advanced Course on Human Population Genetics, Rome; and (1965) Modern concepts of the blood group systems. *Ann. N.Y. Acad. Sci.*, **127**, 884–891.

338 SCHMIDT P.J., LOSTUMBO MARY M., ENGLISH CAROL T. and HUNTER O.B. (1967) Aberrant U blood group accompanying Rh$_{null}$. *Transfusion, Philad.*, **7**, 33–34.

339 ISHIMORI T. and HASEKURA H. (1966) A case of a Japanese blood with no detectable Rh blood group antigen. *Proc. Jap. Acad.*, **42**, 658–660.

340 GREEN M.M. and GREEN K.C. (1949) Crossing-over between alleles at the *lozenge* locus in *Drosophila melanogaster. Proc. nat. Acad. Sci., Wash.*, **35**, 586–591.

341 GIBBS MARY B. and ROSENFIELD R.E. (1966) Immunochemical studies of the Rh system. IV. Hemagglutination assay of antigenic expression regulated by interaction between paired Rh genes. *Transfusion, Philad.*, **6**, 462–474.

342 MASOUREDIS S.P. (1962) Reaction of I^{131} anti-Rh$_0$ (D) with enzyme treated red cells. *Transfusion, Philad.*, **2**, 363–374.

343 GOODMAN H.S. and MASAITIS LILLIAN (1962) II. Analysis of the agglutination reactions characteristic of the Rh system. *Transfusion, Philad.*, **2**, 332–337.

344 BARNES A.E. and FARR R.S. (1963) The influence of race and phenotype on the erythrocyte D antigen studied by I^{131}-labelled anti-D. *Blood*, **21**, 429–446.

345 EVANS R.S., TURNER ELIZABETH and BINGHAM MARGARET (1963) Studies of I^{131} tagged Rh antibody of D specificity. *Vox Sang.*, **8**, 153–176.

346 KOCHWA S. and ROSENFIELD R.E. (1964) Immunochemical studies of the Rh system. I. Isolation and characteriziation of antibodies. *J. Immunol.*, **92**, 682–692.

347 ROSENFIELD R.E. and KOCHWA S. (1964) Immunochemical studies of the Rh system II. Capacity of antigenic sites of different phenotypes to bind and retain Rh antibodies. *J. Immunol.*, **92**, 693–701.

348 ROCHNA ERNA and HUGHES-JONES N.C. (1965) The use of purified ^{125}I-labelled anti-γ globulin in the determination of the number of D antigen sites on red cells of different phenotypes. *Vox Sang.*, **10**, 675–686.

349 VOGT ELSE (1964) Humane blod-chimaerer. *Nord. med.*, **71**, 510.

350 CAMERON C. (1963) Unpublished observations.

351 LEVAN A., NICHOLS W.W., HALL B., LÖW B., NILSSON S.-B. and NORDÉN A. (1964) Mixture of Rh positive and Rh negative erythrocytes and chromosomal abnormalities in a case of polycythemia. *Hereditas, Lund.*, **52**, 89–105.

352 BROMAN B. and NILSSON S.-B. (1964) Unpublished observations.

353 JENKINS W.J. and MARSH W.L. (1965) Somatic mutation affecting the Rhesus and Duffy blood group systems. *Transfusion, Philad.*, **5**, 6–10.

354 LEVINE P. (1943) Serological factors as possible causes in spontaneous abortions. *J. Hered.*, **34**, 71–80.

355 WOODROW J.C. (1970) Rh immunisation and its prevention. *Ser. Haematol.*, **3**, part 3, 1–151.

356 CLARKE C.A. (1974) *Rh haemolytic disease. Original papers with commentaries.* Medical and Technical Publishing Company, Newcastle.

357 BOOTH P.B., DUNSFORD I., GRANT JEAN and MURRAY SHEILAGH (1953) Letter to the Editor, *Brit. med. J.*, **ii**, 41–42.

358 WARD H.K., WALSH R.J. and KOOPTZOFF OLGA (1957) Rh antigens and immunological tolerance. *Nature, Lond.*, **179**, 1352–1353.

359 MAYEDA K. (1962) The self marker concept as applied to the Rh blood group system. *Amer. J. hum. Genet.*, **14**, 281–289.

360 OWEN R.D., WOOD H.R., FOORD A.G., STURGEON P. and BALDWIN L.G. (1954) Evidence for actively acquired tolerance to Rh antigens. *Proc. nat. Acad. Sci., Wash.*, **44**, 420–424.

361 LEVINE P. and STURGEON P. (1961) Personal communication.

362 WEINER W., BATTEY D.A., CLEGHORN T.E., MARSON F.G.W. and MEYNELL M.J. (1953) Serological findings in a case of haemolytic anaemia with some general observations on the pathogenesis of this syndrome. *Brit. med. J.*, **ii**, 125–128.

363 WEINER W. (1961) The serology of acquired haemolytic anaemia (hyperimmune type). Paper read at VIIIth Cong. Europ. Soc. Haemat., Vienna.

364 WEINER W. and VOS G.H. (1963) Serology of acquired hemolytic anemias. *Blood*, **22**, 606–613.

365 DACIE J.V. (1962) *The Haemolytic Anaemias, Congenital and Acquired*, 2nd edition. Part II. *The Auto-Immune Haemolytic Anaemias.* Churchill, London.

366 WORLLEDGE SHEILA M., CARSTAIRS K.C. and DACIE J.V. (1966) Autoimmune haemolytic anaemia associated with α-methyldopa therapy. *Lancet*, **ii**, 135–139.

[367] HACKEL E. (1964) Anti-Rh inhibition by RNA derivatives and amino acids. *Vox Sang.*, **9**, 56–59.

[368] RULE A.H. and BOYD W.C. (1964) Relationships between blood group agglutinogens: role of sialic acids. *Transfusion, Philad.*, **4**, 449–456.

[369] CHATTORAJ A. and BOYD W.C. (1965) Inhibition of hemagglutinins by amino acids. *Vox Sang.*, **10**, 700–707.

[370] JOHNSON G.A. and McCLUER R.H. (1961) Relation of sialic acid to $Rh_0(D)$ antigen. *Proc. Soc. exp. Biol. Med.*, **107**, 692–694.

[371] PRAGER M.D., HOPKINS G. and FOSTER M. (1963) The effect of phosphatases and organic phosphates on Rh reactions. *Vox Sang.*, **8**, 410–419.

[372] DODD M.C., BIGLEY NANCY J., JOHNSON G.A. and McCLUER R.H. (1964) Chemical aspects of inhibitors of $Rh_0(D)$ antibody. *Nature, Lond.*, **204**, 549–552.

[373] PRAGER M.D. and LOWRY MILDRED E. (1966) On the possible relation of sialic acid to the Rh factor. *Transfusion, Philad.*, **6**, 577–583.

[374] WATKINS WINIFRED M. (1966) Blood-group substances. *Science*, **152**, 172–181.

[375] LAUER A. (1964) Die Vererbungsweise im Rh-System. *Blut*, **10**, 99–112.

[376] KNOX E.G. (1966) A notional structure for the rhesus antigens. *Brit. J. Haemat.*, **12**, 105–113.

[377] HIRSCHFELD J. (1973) Some notes on the Rh-system—a complex-complex model. *Vox Sang.*, **24**, 21–32.

[378] FREIESLEBEN E. and JENSEN K.G. (1964) Inhibition of an anti-D by a normal serum factor. *Vox Sang.*, **9**, 65–69.

[379] WEINER W., WROBEL D.M. and GAVIN JUNE (1966 and 1968) Unpublished observations.

[380] SALMON C., GERBAL A., LIBERGE GENEVIÈVE, SY B., TIPPETT PATRICIA and SANGER RUTH (1969) Le complexe génique D^{IV} (C)–. *Rev. fr. Transf.*, **12**, 239–247.

[381] DYBKJAER E. (1966) Unpublished observations.

[382] HEIKEN A. (1967) Demonstration of the Rh gene complex $D(c)(E)$. *Vox Sang.*, **13**, 158–164.

[383] HEIKEN A. and GILES C.M. (1967) Evidence of mutation within the rhesus blood group system. *Nature, Lond.*, **213**, 699–700.

[384] KLUN MARY J. and MUSCHEL L.H. (1966) Complement fixation by the anti-Rh_0 (D) antibody. *Nature, Lond.*, **212**, 159–161.

[385] ISHIMORI T. and HASEKURA H. (1967) A Japanese with no detectable Rh blood group antigens due to silent Rh alleles or deleted chromosomes. *Transfusion, Philad.*, **7**, 84–87.

[386] CELANO M.J. and LEVINE P. (1967) Anti-LW specificity in autoimmune acquired hemolytic anemia. *Transfusion, Philad.*, **7**, 265–268.

[387] MASOUREDIS S.P. and STURGEON P. (1965) Quantitative serologic and isotopic studies on the Rh_0 variant-D^u. *Blood*, **25**, 954–975.

[388] TAYLOR JANE F. (1967) Sensitization of Rh-negative daughters by their Rh-positive mothers. *New Engl. J. Med.*, **276**, 547–551.

[389] SCHMIDT P.J. and VOS G.H. (1967) Multiple phenotypic abnormalities, associated with Rh_{null} (———/———). *Vox Sang.*, **13**, 18–20.

[390] LEVINE P. and CELANO M.J. (1967) Agglutinating specificity for LW factor in guinea pig and rabbit anti-Rh serums. *Science*, **156**, 1744–1746.

[391] MORTON N.E. and ROSENFIELD R.E. (1967) A new Rh allele, r^{yn} ($R^{-1, 2, w3, w4}$). *Transfusion, Philad.*, **7**, 117–119.

[392] LEYSHON W.C. (1967) The Rh gene complex $cD-$ segregating in a negro family. *Vox Sang.*, **13**, 354–356.

[393] HOPKINS D.F. (1967) Observations on Rh (D^u) blood donations in Scotland. *Vox Sang.*, **13**, 431–440.

[394] GUNSON H.H. and SMITH D.S. (1967) The depressant effect of the Cde(R') chromosome on the D^u antigen. *Vox Sang.*, **13**, 423–430.

[395] MASOUREDIS S.P., DUPUY MARY E. and ELLIOT MARGARET (1967) Relationship between

Rh$_0$ (D) zygosity and red cell Rh$_0$ (D) antigen content in family members. *J. clin. Invest.*, **46**, 681–694.

396 CHORPENNING F.W., TRAUL K.A., ANDERSON ANN A., COWELL D.L. and PAUL R.A. (1967) Purification and characterization of Rh-active material from erythrocytes. *Transfusion, Philad.*, **7**, 373. (Abstract.)

397 BELL C.A. and ZWICKER HELEN (1967) Donath Landsteiner hemolysin with anti-HI specificity. *Transfusion, Philad.*, **7**, 384. (Abstract.)

398 GILES CAROLYN M. and LUNDSGAARD ANNE (1967) A complex serological investigation involving LW. *Vox Sang.*, **13**, 406–416.

399 BOETTCHER B. and HASEKURA H. (1971) Rh blood groups of Australian aborigines in the tribe containing the original Rh$_{null}$ propositus. *Vox Sang.*, **21**, 200–209.

400 HASEKURA H., ISHIMORI T., FURUSAWA S., KAWAGUCHI H., KAWADA K., SHISHIDO H., KOMIYA M., FUKUOKA Y. and MIWA S. (1971) Hematological observations on the $\bar{r}$h (———/———) propositus, the homozygote of amorphic Rh blood group genes. *Proc. Jap. Acad.*, **47**, 579–583.

401 HABER G.V., BASTANI A., ARPIN P.D. and ROSENFIELD R.E. (1967) Rh$_{null}$ and pregnancy complicated by maternal anti-'total Rh'. I. Anti-Rh29 (Rh). *Transfusion, Philad.*, **7**, 389.

402 BAR-SHANY S., BASTANI A., CUTTNER J. and ROSENFIELD R.E. (1967). Rh$_{null}$ and pregnancy complicated by maternal anti-'total Rh'. II. Additional evidence of multiple anomalies associated with the Rh: −29m (rh$_m$) variety of Rh$_{null}$ red cells. *Transfusion, Philad.*, **7**, 389–390.

403 GUÉVIN R.M., TALIANO V., PARADIS D.J. and COUTURE FRANCE (1967) Personal communication.

404 STURGEON P. (1970) Hematological observations on the anaemia associated with blood type Rh$_{null}$. *Blood*, **36**, 310–320.

405 SENHAUSER D.A., MITCHELL M.W., GAULT D.B. and OWENS J.H. (1970) Another example of phenotype Rh$_{null}$. *Transfusion, Philad.*, **10**, 89–92.

406 SEIDL S., SPIELMANN W. and MARTIN H. (1972) Two siblings with Rh$_{null}$ disease. *Vox Sang.*, **23**, 182–189.

407 POLESKY H.F., MOULDS J. and HANSON MARGARET (1971) Three Rh$_{null}$ siblings: a family study. Abstracts AABB Meeting, Chicago, p. 83.

408 MOULDS J. (1973) 'Rh$_{nulls}$: amorphs and regulators' in *A Seminar on Recent Advances in Immunohematology*, AABB Meeting, Bal Harbour.

409 NAGEL V., KNEIPHOFF HILTRUT, PEKKER ST., HOPPE H.H., SANGER RUTH and TIPPETT PATRICIA (1972) Unexplained appearance of antibody in an Rh$_{null}$ donor. *Vox Sang.*, **22**, 519–523.

410 HRUBIŠKO M., FABRYOVA LIBUSA, LIPSIC T. and SANGER RUTH (1972) Another case of Rh$_{null}$ disease. Abstracts AABB and ISBT Meeting, Washington, p. 15.

411 STEVENSON M.M., ANIDO V., TANNER A.M. and SWOYER J. (1973) Rh 'null' is not always null. *Brit. Med. J.*, **1**, 417.

412 OESTGAARD P. (1973) Unpublished observations.

413 SANGER RUTH and RACE R.R. (1971) Immunogenetics of certain antigens of the red cell membrane. *Nouv. Rev. fr. Hemat.*, **11**, 878–884.

414 HOLLAND P.V., McGINNISS M.H. and SCHMIDT P.J. (1972) Rh$_{null}$ disease—further observations. Abstracts AABB and ISBT Meeting, Washington, p. 15.

415 TIPPETT PATRICIA (1972) A present view of Rh. *Pathologica*, **64**, 29–38.

416 GIBLETT ELOISE R. (1969) *Genetic Markers in Human Blood*. Blackwell Scientific Publications, Oxford, p. 308.

417 NICOLSON G.L., MASOUREDIS S.P. and SINGER S.J. (1971) Quantitative two-dimensional ultrastructural distribution of Rh$_0$(D) antigenic sites on human erythrocyte membranes. *Proc. Nat. Acad. Sci.*, **68**, 1416–1420.

418 LEVINE P. (1972) Specificity of Rh null disease. Abstracts AABB and ISBT Meeting, Washington, p. 14.

[419] CHOWN B., LEWIS MARION, KAITA HIROKO and LOWEN BONNIE (1971) A new cause of haemolytic anaemia? *Lancet*, **i**, 396.

[420] CHOWN B., LEWIS MARION, KAITA HIROKO and LOWEN BONNIE (1972) An unlinked modifier of Rh blood groups: effects when heterozygous and when homozygous. *Amer. J. Hum. Genet.*, **24**, 623–637.

[421] ROSENFIELD R.E. and McGUIRE DELORES (1973) Personal communication.

[422] LEY A.B. and HARRIS JEAN P. (1956) Personal communication.

[423] DE VEBER L.L., CLARK G.W., HUNKING M. and STROUP M. (1971) Maternal anti-LW. *Transfusion, Philad.*, **11**, 33–35.

[424] SWANSON J.L., MILLER J., AZAR M. and McCULLOUGH J.J. (1974) Evidence for heterogeneity of LW antigen revealed in family study. *Transfusion, Philad.* **14**, 470–474.

[425] WIENER A.S., MOOR-JANKQWSKI J. and BRANCATO G.J. (1969) LW factor. *Haematologia* **3**, 385–393.

[426] POLESKY H.F., SWANSON JANE and OLSON CAROL (1968) Guinea pig antibodies to ? Rh-Hr precursor. *Proc. 11th Congr. int. Soc. Blood Transf.*, Sydney 1966. Bibl. haemat., No. 29, part 1, pp. 384–387. Karger, Basel/New York, Ed. L.P. Holländer.

[427] VOS G., PETZ L., GARRATTY G. and FUDENBERG H. (1973) Autoantibodies in acquired hemolytic anemia with special reference to the LW system. *Blood*, **42**, 445–453.

[428] CHOWN B., KAITA H., LOWEN B. and LEWIS M. (1971) Transient production of anti-LW by LW-positive people. *Transfusion, Philad.*, **11**, 220–222.

[429] PERRAULT R. (1973) 'Cold' IgG autologous anti-LW. *Vox Sang.*, **24**, 150–164.

[430] BECK M.L. (1973) 'The LW system: a review and current concepts' in *A Seminar on Recent Advances in Immunohematology*, AABB Meeting, Bal Harbour.

[431] GILES CAROLYN M. (1974) In preparation.

[432] JAKOBOWICZ RACHEL, GOLDBERG BRONIA and SIMMONS R.T. (1967) The rare Rh gene $C^w dE$ (r^{yw}) found in two generations of a Caucasian family. *Med. J. Aust.*, **2**, 738.

[433] FINNEY R.D., BLUE A.M. and WILLOUGHBY M.L.N. (1973) Haemolytic disease of the newborn caused by the rare rhesus antibody anti-C^x. *Vox Sang.*, **25**, 39–42.

[434] HARRISON J. (1970) The 'naturally occurring' anti-E. *Vox Sang.*, **19**, 123–131.

[435] MOLLISON P.L. (1972) *Blood Transfusion in Clinical Medicine*, 5th ed. Blackwell Scientific Publications, Oxford, pp. 830.

[436] GROBEL R.K. and CARDY J.D. (1971) Hemolytic disease of the newborn due to anti-E^w. A fourth example of the Rh antigen, E^w. *Transfusion, Philad.*, **11**, 77–78.

[437] SHAPIRO M., LE ROUX MARJORIE and BRINK STEFANIE (1972) Serology and genetics of a new blood factor: hr^B. *Haematologia*, **6**, 121–128.

[438] ROSENFIELD R.E., ALLEN F.H. and RUBINSTEIN P. (1973) Genetic model for the Rh blood-group system. *Proc. Nat. Acad. Sci.*, **70**, 1303–1307.

[439] MANNONI P., BRACQ CHRISTINE, YVART J. and SALMON C. (1970) Anomalie de fonctionnement du locus Rh au cours d'une myelofibrose. *Nouv. Ref. fr. Hemat.*, **10**, 381–388.

[440] CALLENDER SHEILA T., KAY H.E.M., LAWLER SYLVIA D., MILLARD ROSEMARY E., SANGER RUTH and TIPPETT PATRICIA A. (1971) Two populations of Rh groups together with chromosomally abnormal cell lines in the bone marrow. *Brit. Med. J.*, **1**, 131–133.

[441] STAPLETON R.R. (1973) Personal communication.

[442] RACE R.R. (1972) Lecture to Plenary Session, *XIII Congr. Int. Soc. Blood Transfusion*, Washington.

[443] MARSH W.L. and CHAGANTI R.S.K. (1973) Blood group mosaicism involving the Rhesus and Duffy blood groups. *Transfusion, Philad.*, **13**, 314–315.

[444] SINGER S.J. and NICOLSON G.L. (1972) The fluid mosaic model of the structure of cell membranes. *Science*, **175**, 720–731.

[445] HUGHES-JONES N.C., GARDNER BRIGITTE and LINCOLN P.J. (1971) Observations of the number of available c, D and E antigen sites on red cells. *Vox Sang.*, **21**, 210–216.

[446] SANGER RUTH, TIPPETT PATRICIA, GAVIN JUNE and RACE R.R. (1973) Failure to demon-

strate linkage between the loci for the Rh and Duffy blood groups. *Ann. Hum. Genet.*, **36**, 353–354.

447 MARSH W.L., CHAGANTI R.S.K., GARDNER F.H., MAYER K., NOWELL P.C. and GERMAN J. (1974) Mapping human autosomes: evidence supporting assignment of Rhesus to the short arm of chromosome No. 1. *Science*, **183**, 966–968.

448 CASE J. (1973) Quantitative variation in the G antigen of the Rh blood group system. *Vox Sang.*, **25**, 529–539.

449 BEATTIE K.M., NEITZER G.M., ZANARDI V. and ZUELZER W.W. (1971) G^u, a variant of G. *Transfusion, Philad.*, **11**, 152–156.

450 POLLACK W., GORMAN J.G. and FREDA V.J. (1969) Prevention of Rh hemolytic disease. In *Progress in Hematology*, VI, pp. 121–147. Eds. E. Brown and C.V. Moore, Heinemann Medical Books, London.

451 ZIMMERMAN D. (1973) *Rh. The Intimate History of a Disease and its Conquest*, pp. 371, Macmillan Publishing Co., Inc., New York.

452 EDWARDS J.H. (1968) The Rhesus locus. *Vox Sang.*, **15**, 392–395.

453 WILKINSON SUSAN L., VAITHIANATHAN T. and ISSITT P.D. (1974) The high incidence of anti-HL-A antibodies in anti-D typing reagents. Illustrated by a case of Matuhasi-Ogata phenomenon mimicking a 'D with anti-D' situation. *Transfusion, Philad.*, **14**, 27–33.

454 ALTER A.A., GELB A.G. and LEE ST.L. (1964) Hemolytic disease of the newborn caused by a new antibody (anti-Go^a). *Proc. 9th Congr. int. Soc. Blood Transf.*, Mexico 1962, 341–343.

455 ALTER A.A., GELB A.G., CHOWN B., ROSENFIELD R.E. and CLEGHORN T.E. (1967) Gonzales (Go^a), a new blood group character. *Transfusion, Philad.*, **7**, 88–91.

456 LEWIS M., CHOWN B., KAITA H., HAHN D., KANGELOS M., SHEPEARD W.L. and SHACKELTON K. (1967) Blood group antigen Go^a and the Rh system. *Transfusion, Philad.*, **7**, 440–441.

457 LOVETT D.A. and CRAWFORD M.N. (1967) Js^b and Go^a screening of negro donors. *Transfusion, Philad.*, **7**, 442.

458 CHOWN B., LEWIS M., KAITA H., HAHN D., SHACKELTON K. and SHEPEARD W.L. (1968) On the antigen Go^a and the Rh system. *Vox Sang.*, **15**, 264–271.

459 LASSITER G.R., ISSITT P.D., GARRIS M.L. and WELBORN R. (1969) Further studies on the D^{Cor} (Go^a) antigen of the Rh system. *Transfusion, Philad.*, **9**, 282.

460 LEWIS MARION, KAITA HIROKO and CHOWN B. (1971) The inheritance of the Rh blood groups. I. Frequencies in 1,000 unrelated Caucasian families consisting of 2,000 parents and 2,806 children. *Vox Sang.*, **20**, 500–508.

461 MOURANT A.E., KOPEĆ ADA C. and DOMANIEWSKA-SOBCZAK KAZIMIERA (1974) *The Distribution of the Human Blood Groups and other Biochemical Polymorphisms.* 2nd edition, Oxford University Press.

462 CHOWN B., LEWIS MARION and KAITA HIROKO (1971) The inheritance of the Rh blood groups. II. Expression of the Rh antigens in random unrelated Caucasian families. *Vox Sang.*, **21**, 126–134.

463 CHOWN B., LEWIS MARION and KAITA HIROKO (1971) The Rh system. An anomaly of inheritance, probably due to mutation. *Vox Sang.*, **21**, 385–396.

464 ALLEN F.H. and ROSENFIELD R.E. (1972) Review of Rh serology. Eight new antigens in nine years. *Haematologia*, **6**, 113–120.

465 GILES CAROLYN M. and SKOV F. (1971) The *CDe* rhesus gene complex; some considerations revealed by a study of a Danish family with an antigen of the rhesus gene complex (*C*)*D*(*e*) defined by a 'new' antibody. *Vox Sang.*, **20**, 328–334.

466 GILES CAROLYN M., CROSSLAND J.D., HAGGAS W.K. and LONGSTER G. (1971) An Rh gene complex which results in a 'new' antigen detectable by a specific antibody, anti-Rh33. *Vox Sang.*, **21**, 289–301.

467 ŠVANDA M., PROCHÁZKA R., KOUT M. and GILES CAROLYN M. (1970) A case of haemolytic disease of the newborn due to a new red cells antigen, Zd. *Vox Sang.*, **18**, 366–369.

468 BADAKERE S.S. and BHATIA H.M. (1973) Haemolytic disease of the newborn in a −D−/ −D− Indian woman. *Vox Sang.*, **24**, 280–282.

[469] YAMAGUCHI H., OKUBO Y., TOMITA T., YAMANO H. and TANAKA M. (1969) A case of Rh gene complex *cD–/cD–* found in a Japanese. *Proc. Jap. Acad.*, **45**, 618–620.

[470] DELMAS-MARSALET Y., GOUDEMAND M. and TIPPETT P. (1969) Un nouvel exemple de génotype rhésus cD–/cD–. *Rev. fr. Transf.*, **12**, 233–238.

[471] KORNSTAD L. and LARSEN ANNA M.H. (1973) A possible $D(C^w)(e)$ gene complex of the Rh system. *Vox Sang.*, **25**, 385–389.

[472] PERRAULT R. (1972) Low concentration antibodies. VI. Immunogenesis of anti-f. A new look at the Rh system. *Upsala J. med. Sci.*, suppl. 12, pp. 65.

[473] DAUSSET J. (1972) Similarities between the HL-A system and other immunogenetic systems. *Vox Sang.*, **23**, 153–164.

[474] WATSON J.D. (1970) *Molecular Biology of the Gene*, 2nd edition, W.A. Benjamin, Inc., New York, pages 444–445 and 487–490.

[475] ALBREY J.A., POLLARD M., GILES CAROLYN M. and TIPPETT PATRICIA (1970) Personal communication.

[476] McGINNISS M.H., KAPLAN H.S., BOWEN A.B. and SCHMIDT P.J. (1969) Agglutinins for 'null' red blood cells. *Transfusion, Philad.*, **9**, 40–42.

[477] McGINNISS MARY H., SCHMIDT P.J. and PERRY MILDRED (1973) Auto-agglutinins to 'null' red blood cells. Abstract 26th AABB Meeting, Bal Harbour, 114.

[478] DAVIDSOHN I., STERN K., STRAUSER E.R. and SPURRIER WILMA (1953) Be, a new 'private' blood factor. *Blood*, **8**, 747–754.

[479] STERN K., DAVIDSOHN I., JENSEN F.G. and MURATORE R. (1958) Immunologic studies on the Be^a factor. *Vox Sang.*, **3**, 425–434.

[480] McCREARY J., MACILROY M., COURTENAY D.G. and OHMART D.L. (1973) The second example of anti-Be^a causing hemolytic disease of the newborn. *Transfusion, Philad.*, **13**, 428–431.

[481] DUCOS J., MARTY YVONNE, RUFFIÉ J., GAVIN JUNE, TEESDALE PHYLLIS and TIPPETT PATRICIA (1974) In preparation.

[482] MÜLLER SUZANNE (1974) Unpublished observation.

[483] HABIBI B., LOPEZ M. and SALMON C. (1974) Two new cases of Rh mosaicism. Selective study of red cell populations. *Vox Sang.*, **27**, 232–242.

[484] STURTEVANT A.H. (1925) The effects of unequal crossing over at the Bar locus in Drosophila. *Genetics*, **10**, 117–147. Also, reprinted in *Classic Papers in Genetics*, 1959, ed. Peters A.J., Prentice Hall International, Inc., London.

[485] BRIDGES C.B. (1935) Salivary chromosome maps. *J. Hered.*, **26**, 60–64.

[486] MOTULSKY A.G. (1962) Controller genes in synthesis of human haemoglobin. *Nature, Lond.*, **194**, 607–609.

[487] ZUCKERKANDL E. (1964) Controller-gene diseases: the operon model as applied to β-thalassemia, familial fetal hemoglobinemia and the normal switch from the production of fetal hemoglobin to that of adult hemoglobin. *J. Molec. Biol.*, **8**, 128–147.

[488] MÄKELÄ P. HELENA and STOCKER B.A.D. (1969) Genetics of polysaccharide biosynthesis. *Ann. Rev. Genet.*, **3**, 291–322.

[489] JACOB F. and MONOD J. (1961) Genetic regulatory mechanisms in the synthesis of proteins. *J. Molec. Biol.*, **3**, 318–356.

[490] BEVAN BERYL and GILES CAROLYN M. (1974) Personal communication.

Chapter 6
The Lutheran Blood Groups

The antibody which defines the Lutheran blood groups was briefly reported by Callender, Race and Paykoç[1a], in 1945: a fuller description was given by Callender and Race[1] in 1946. The antibody was present in the serum of a patient suffering from lupus erythematosus diffusus. This patient had been many times transfused and produced, as well as anti-c and anti-N, the first example of anti-C^w, and the only example so far found of anti-Levay.

The Lutheran antibody was undoubtedly immune in nature. It appeared after a transfusion of blood containing, as was subsequently discovered, the provocative antigen. The name of the donor was Lutheran.

The symbols L and l were originally used for the genes but as these symbols were later used also for the Lewis groups something had to be done. A few meetings of interested people[2] were held and the following notation agreed upon:

genes: Lu^a, Lu^b
phenotypes: Lu(a+), Lu(a−)
antibodies: anti-Lu^a, anti-Lu^b (should it be discovered).

This notation proved so convenient for Lutheran and for Lewis that it has been used for almost all systems discovered since the meeting.

(However, a convenient modification was suggested by Dr E.B. Ford: the first antibody and antigen of a system is given the superscript a, e.g. Lu^a, as before, but the hypothetical antithetical antibody and antigen are given no superscript, e.g. Lu, until the antibody is found. Once the antibody is found the superscript b is conferred on the antibody, antigen and gene.)

The antigen Lu^a was shown by Callender and Race[1] to be inherited as a dominant character.

Ten years later, in 1956, the expected anti-Lu^b was discovered by Cutbush and Chanarin[3], and, as so often happened, a second example was found within a few months[4]. The finding of anti-Lu^b established the positive existence of the antigen and gene Lu^b for which symbols had been used confidently for ten years.

The first indication that Lutheran, like other systems, was not as straightforward as at first appeared came with the finding of the phenotype Lu(a−b−) by Crawford, Greenwalt, Sasaki, Tippett, Sanger and Race[19] (1961) and then came the recognition of its puzzling relationship to the Auberger groups (Tippett[29],

1963). Next, an antibody anti-Lu^{a}Lu^b was found which reacted with all cells except those of the phenotype Lu(a–b–) (Darnborough, Firth, Giles, Goldsmith and Crawford[30], 1963).

Then, during the last five years, came the recognition, by Molthan, Crawford, Marsh and Allen[52] of a pair of alleles, Lu^9 and Lu^6, related to the *Lutheran* locus in the same way as, for example, *C* and *c* are related to *E* and *e* at the *Rh* complex locus. During this same period of time, a series of antibodies emerged, mostly in the U.S.A., which gave negative reactions with Lu(a–b–) cells and with the donors' own cells but positive reactions with the cells of all others tested: the nature of the relationship between the Lutheran system and most of these antibodies is yet unknown.

As a result of the work of Jan Mohr in Copenhagen in 1951, the *Lutheran* locus and the *secretor* locus had the distinction of providing the first example of autosomal linkage in man, and, incidentally, the first example of autosomal crossing-over. In 1954 Mohr adumbrated two further linkages, since confirmed, between *myotonic dystrophy* and *Lutheran*, and *myotonic dystrophy* and *secretor*. Furthermore it was the *Lutheran-secretor* linkage that gave the first hint that crossing-over in man is more frequent in the female than in the male: but these very fine contributions of the Lutheran groups to human genetics will be described in the chapter on mapping of the autosomes.

FREQUENCIES

Tests with anti-Lu^a only

As a basis for calculations we may take the first three reports[1, 5, 6] of tests on unrelated English people: in a total of 1,373 samples 105 (or 7·65%) were Lu(a+) and 1,268 (92·35%) were Lu(a–). The gene frequencies are:

$$Lu^b = \sqrt{0.9235} = 0.9610$$
$$\text{and } Lu^a = 1 - 0.9610 = 0.0390$$

and the phenotype and genotype frequencies are:

$$Lu(a-) \quad Lu^bLu^b = 0.9235$$
$$Lu(a+) \begin{cases} Lu^aLu^b = 0.0750 & \text{or } 0.9804 \\ Lu^aLu^a = 0.0015 & \text{or } 0.0196 \end{cases} \begin{matrix} \text{of all} \\ Lu(a+) \end{matrix}$$

These expectations fit very well with the Canadian series tested with anti-Lu^a and anti-Lu^b to be noted below.

Many series of tests with anti-Lu^a on people in different parts of the world have been reported: they were summarized by Mourant[7], by Gonzenback *et al.*[8] and by Hartmann *et al.*[32]

Tests with anti-Lu^b only

Though fewer series have been tested with anti-Lu^b they are large ones—they have to be if an Lu(b–) is to be found. In tests on 5,682 white people[3, 20, 21, 22, 33] five Lu(b–) were found: the expected number, according to the English frequencies based on the tests with anti-Lu^a, is 8·5. All five proved to be, as expected, Lu(a+b–) and not Lu(a–b–).

Tests with anti-Lu^a and anti-Lu^b

Substantial series of tests are those of Chown, Lewis and Kaita[34] on 1,456 Manitoban white people and of Dublin et al.[51] on 1,201 white Bostonians. The Canadian figures follow, the frequencies for Boston were almost identical:

	obs.	exp.
Lu(a+b–)	2	1·75
Lu(a+b+)	99	99·44
Lu(a–b+)	1,355	1,354·81

The agreement between the observed and expected phenotypes is extraordinarily close. The gene frequencies on which the expected numbers are based are obtained by simple counting: in the sample there are 103 Lu^a genes and 2,809 Lu^b genes, that is, in proportion, 0·0354 Lu^a to 0·9646 Lu^b. These figures are very close indeed to those for England (0·0390 to 0·9610), based on tests with anti-Lu^a alone.

Chown, Lewis and Kaita[34] tested, with both antisera, a further 600 white Manitoban women but with Mennonite names: they had nearly twice the frequency of Lu^a found in the other white Manitobans.

Tests with anti-Lu^{a}Lu^b (anti-Lu3) only

Anti-Lu^{a}Lu^b reacts with all cells save those of the phenotype Lu(a–b–). In tests on 18,069 British donors, Darnborough et al.[30] found only one Lu(a–b–).

INHERITANCE

Callender and Race[1] tested the blood of relatives of Lu(a+) propositi and concluded that the Lu^a antigen was inherited as a dominant character.

From the English genotype frequencies given above the expected frequency of the six genotypically different matings can be calculated in the usual manner together with the children expected therefrom (page 141). In Table 41 these genotypes are reduced to the more practical level of phenotype frequencies when anti-Lu^a alone is used.

Families tested with anti-Lu^a only

Table 42 summarizes published results of tests on white families: they confirmed that the antigen Lu^a was inherited in a straightforward way.

Table 41. The expected distribution of the Lutheran phenotypes, as judged by anti-Lu[a] in English parents and offspring

Matings		Proportion of children from each mating	
Type	Frequency	Lu(a+)	Lu(a−)
Lu(a+) × Lu(a+)	0·0058	0·7586	0·2414
Lu(a+) × Lu(a−)	0·1413	0·5099	0·4901
Lu(a−) × Lu(a−)	0·8529	—	1·0000
	1·0000		

In several of the series in Table 42 the families were selected for having Lu(a+) members. When the Lu(a+) propositus was an offspring he is not included in the count: very much more often the propositus was a parent and this naturally has upset the relative incidence of the three mating types. If the six unselected series[12, 18, 35−37] are counted separately the incidence of the three mating types and of the children therefrom agrees well with the calculated expectation, as may be seen in the lowest two rows of the table.

In Table 42 there appear to be two rather wide departures from the almost 50:50 Lu(a+) and Lu(a−) offspring expected of the mating Lu(a+) × Lu(a−). Mohr's[38] finding of too many Lu(a+) offspring can be, at least in part, attributed to one family with 11 children all Lu(a+): the Lu(a+) parent must have been *Lu^aLu^a*. Greenwalt[23] found, on the other hand, too many Lu(a−) offspring: this was no doubt because his series included a number of young children and, as Greenwalt and his colleagues[39] later showed, the antigen is not well developed in early life and can easily be missed. Greenwalt's families[23] were the offspring of Lu(a+) blood donors.

Mohr[9, 13] tested many large Danish families for the Lutheran groups. They were selected for size and for having at least one parent Lu(a+); 27 of them with 124 children were published in the two papers on linkage between the *Lutheran* and '*Lewis*' (later seen to be *secretor*) loci and were further selected for having Lu(a−) children. These families supported the theory of inheritance but cannot easily be subjected to the present analysis.

Families tested with anti-Lu[a] and anti-Lu[b]

The only substantial series of families tested with both antisera are those reported by Chown, Lewis and Kaita[34] which are reproduced in Table 43. The observed figures fit perfectly with those calculated from the white population of Manitoba (excluding the Mennonites). It is estimated that if a third allele of *Lu^a* and *Lu^b* exists in this population it would have to have a frequency of probably less than 0·02.

Table 42. White families tested with anti-Lu[a]

		Total number of matings	children	Lu(a+) × Lu(a+) No. of matings	Children Lu(a+)	Children Lu(a−)	Lu(a+) × Lu(a−) No. of matings	Children Lu(a+)	Children Lu(a−)	Lu(a−) × Lu(a−) No. of matings	Children Lu(a+)	Children Lu(a−)
1. Callender and Race[1] Mainwaring and Pickles[5]	British	12	21	1	3	0	11	8	10			
2. Lawler[11]	British	47	97	1	2	1	12	12	5	34	0	77
3. Our Unit[12,18]	British	379	871	3	5	1	40	44	39	336	0	782
4. Our Unit 1958–66	British	216	420	0			21	23	17	195	0	380
5. Our Unit 1958–66	N. European	92	259	0			20	35	34	72	0	190
6. van der Weerdt[35]	Dutch	13	51	0			3	9	6	10	0	36
7. Linnet-Jepsen[36]	Danish	7	20	0			3	6	3	4	0	11
8. Linnet-Jepsen et al.[37]	Danish	48	91	0			12	15	19	36	0	57
9. Mohr[38]	Norwegian	68	231	3	10	0	15	38	23	50	0	160
10. Greenwalt[23]	U.S.A.	73	334	1	4	0	72	146	184			
		955	2,395									
Families unselected for Lutheran groups (series 3, 4, 5, 6, 7, 8)		755	1,712	3	5	1	99	132	118	653	0	1,456
expected					4·6	1·4	106·7	127·5	122·5	643·9	–	1,456·0

Table 43. Five hundred Canadian families tested with anti-Lu^a and anti-Lu^b. (From Chown, Lewis and Kaita[34], 1966)

Matings			Children						
			Lu(a+b−)		Lu(a+b+)		Lu(a−b+)		
	obs.	exp.	obs.	exp.	obs.	exp.	obs.	exp.	Total
Lu(a+b−) × Lu(a+b−)	0	0·00							
Lu(a+b−) × Lu(a+b+)	0	0·10							
Lu(a+b−) × Lu(a−b+)	1	1·10	0	0	1	1	0	0	1
Lu(a+b+) × Lu(a+b+)	4	2·35	3	3.25	7	6·5	3	3·25	13
Lu(a+b+) × Lu(a−b+)	59	63·55	0	0	92	92	92	92	184
Lu(a−b+) × Lu(a−b+)	436	432·90	0	0	0	0	1,194	1,194	1,194
	500	500·00							1,392

THE PHENOTYPE Lu(a−b−)

The first example of Lu(a−b−), a phenotype now known to be extremely rare, was found by the propositus herself (Crawford et al.[19], 1961). Two kinds of Lu(a−b−) can be distinguished by pedigree evidence, one is a dominant and the other a recessive character. They may also be distinguished serologically: Stanbury and Francis[40], and Tippett[53] showed that fixation-elution tests using anti-Lu^b, anti-Lu^{a}Lu^b and, on appropriate occasion[53, 54], anti-Lu^a sera, are positive with cells of the dominant type but negative[53] with those of the recessive type of Lu(a−b−).

A summary of all the Lu(a−b−) families known to us is attempted in Table 44: the information about one of them does not disclose to which type, dominant or recessive, it belongs.

The recessive kind of Lu(a−b−)

Darnborough, Firth, Giles, Goldsmith and Crawford[30] encountered the first example of anti-Lu^{a}Lu^b in the serum of Mrs L.B., a patient whose red cells gave the reaction Lu(a−b−). No other example of Lu(a−b−) was found in the family, and from dosage tests with anti-Lu^b it was also suspected that the mode of inheritance was not of the Crawford type. That the phenotype Lu(a−b−) can be a recessive character is shown clearly by the families of Mrs Mo. and Mr Fuj. (Table 44).

The recessive Lu(a−b−) phenotype may be thought of as the reflexion of homozygosity for a rare allele Lu which is either 'silent' or making some antigen yet undetected. Lu must be rare indeed, because only three, or probably four, unrelated recessive Lu(a−b−) propositi are known (Table 44) and because there is no disturbance of distribution in the families summarized in Table 43. However, a Toronto family found by Mrs Marie Crookston and tested with many Lutheran antisera in several laboratories, including our own, is best explained by the presence in it of *Lu*. The phenotypes were: father Lu(a–b+), mother Lu(a+b+) and both children Lu(a+b–); the father must be of the genotype *Lu^{b}Lu* and the children *Lu^{a}Lu*.

The dominant kind of Lu(a–b–)

Apparently inert, or 'minus-minus', phenotypes are known in most other blood group systems and they behave like recessive characters, but Lu(a–b–) of the Crawford type does not[19]. The pedigree in Figure 18 alone was enough to show that the character is dominant, and this was supported by later families. From Table 44 the propositi are seen to have 21 sibs Lu(a–b–) and 20 *not* Lu(a–b–), and to have 21 children Lu(a–b–) and 27 children *not* Lu(a–b–), both counts close to the 50:50 expected of a dominant character.

In our last edition we wrote:

'Perhaps a reasonable guess would be that there is a locus, spatially independent of the *Lutheran* locus, which when occupied by the usual alleles, in the normal homozygous state, lets though some precursor substance needed by the Lutheran genes. Lu(a–b–) people may have at this locus a rare allele, dominant in effect, which converts the precursor substance into something unsuitable for the subsequent production of Lu^b, and we would guess, of Lu^a also.'

That Lu^a is also suppressed was made very likely by a Dutch family reported by Tippett[53] (1971) and made certain by the Canadian family, Lar., reported by Taliano, Guévin and Tippett[54] (1973). Furthermore, part of a Canadian family, reproduced in Figure 19, showed that the dominant inhibition of Lu^b and of Lu^a is not controlled from the *Lutheran* locus. The argument is as follows: I-2 transmitted the inhibitor to II-7 with her *Lu^a* allele, but II-7 in turn gave it to III-8 with his *Lu^b* allele; there has been recombination between the inhibitor locus and the *Lutheran* locus.

The need for a symbol for this inhibitor system therefore arose, and Taliano and his colleagues[54] suggested *In(Lu)* for the locus and also for the rare allele responsible for the inhibition, and *in(Lu)* for the very common 'normal' allele. Later, as will be seen below, *In(Lu)* was found to control the expression of other loci.

Other notes about the inhibitor *In(Lu)*

The Auberger groups are described in Chapter 14. About 18% of white people are Au(a–) and the rest Au(a+). In 1963 Tippett[29, 44] found that in the Crawford family (Figure 18) the 7 Lu(a–b–) members were Au(a–) while the 6 members who were not Lu(a–b–) were all Au(a+). The association between Lu(a–b–) of the dominant type and Au^a negativeness was soon established (see page 384) but only recently has the nature of the relationship become clearer: Crawford, Tippett and Sanger[66] (1974) found that *In(Lu)* inhibits not only the Lutheran antigens and the Au^a antigen but also the antigens P$_1$ and i (see pages 147 and 453 respectively).

Table 44. The families of Lu(a−b) propositi (+ + = Lu(a+b+), − + = Lu(a−b+), − − = Lu(a−b−))

Propositus and some relatives	Sibs −+	Sibs −−	Spouse	Children ++	Children −+	Children −−	Father	Mother	Tests with anti-Au^a (Tippett[29,50])
DOMINANT TYPE									
1. Crawford et al.[19,29] U.S.A.									
Dr M.N. Cr.									
(Fig. 18) III-1	0	2		0	2	0	− −	− +	all 7 − − members are Au (a−)
(Fig. 18) III-2			− +	0	2	1			6 − + members tested and all are Au(a+)
(Fig. 18) III-4	2	0							
(Fig. 18) II-1	0	1							
(Fig. 18) III-10									
2. Darnborough et al.[30] England									
Mrs S.H.	1	1	− +	0	0	0	− −	− +	all 3 − − members tested are Au(a−) all 3 − + members tested are Au(a+)
3. Stanbury and Francis[40] U.S.A.									
Mr McKel.	0	2	− +	0	0	2	− +		3 − − tested: 2 Au(a−) 1 Au(a+) 1 − + tested: Au(a+)
4. Wright and Moore[41] Canada									
Mr A.W. and his half sibs	0	2	− +	0	1	2	− −	d / − +	2 − − tested: Au(a−) 1 − + tested: Au(a+)
father's sibs									
— sister	0	2		0	2	2			
— sister	2	1		0	2	1			
— pat. uncle	1			0	2	0			
— pat. aunt				0	1	2			
— pat. cous.	1	1		0	0	1			
— pat. cous.				0	3	2			
5. Brice and Hoxworth[43] U.S.A. (Negro)									
Mr M.T.	1	2	− +	0	1	0	− +		all 4 − − are Au(a−) father Au(a+) no others tested
6. Tippett[53] Netherlands									
Mrs Di.	2	1	− +	2	1	0			
7. Taliano et al.[54] Canada									
Mr Lar. and his	2	1	+ +	0	1	1	− +		6 − − tested: 4 Au(a−) 2 Au(aw) 1 − + tested: Au(a−)
— mother				0	1	1			
— brother				0	2	2			
8. Gellerman[67] U.S.A. (Malayan)									
Mrs Deg.	0	2						− −	

Table 44—*continued*

Propositus and some relatives	Sibs −+	Sibs −−	Spouse	Children ++	Children −+	Children −−	Father	Mother	Tests with anti-Au^a (Tippett[29,50])
9. Gellerman[67] U.S.A.									
Miss R.L. and her	1	0					−	−	
— mother	1	0						−+	
10. Gellerman[67] U.S.A.									
Mrs Pec.	2	0							
11. Salmon[68] France									
Mons F.E. and his							−+		4 −− tested all Au(a−)
									7 −+ tested: 4 Au(a+)
									3 Au(a−)
— mother	1	1							
— mat. aunt			−+	0	1	1			
— mat. cous.			−+	0	2	1			
12. Tippett[70] Sardinia									
Mr Spa.	2	0					−+		
13. Contreras and Tippett[71,70] Sardinia									
Mr Pin. and his	2	2					−+		6 −− tested all Au(a−)
									7 −+ tested: 4 Au(a+)
									3 Au(a−)
— mother	1	1					−+	−	
— mat. aunt			−+	0	1	1			
	== 20	== 21		== 2	== 25	== 21			
RECESSIVE TYPE									
a. Darnborough et al.[30] England									
Mrs L.B.			++	0	2	0	−+	d	
b. Brown et al.[42,55] Canada									
Mrs G. Mo. and her			−+	0	2	0	−+	−+	1 −− tested: Au(a+)
									no others tested
— cous. VI-2	1	0	++	1	1	0			
— cous. VI-9	1	0							
c. Myhre et al.[69] U.S.A. (Japanese)									
Mr Fuj.	3	1	−+	0	5	0	−+	−+	
TYPE NOT GENETICALLY DISCLOSED									
d. Melonas and Noto[48] U.S.A. (Negro)									
Mrs H.H.	2	0						−+	propositus Au(a+)
									no others tested

Ascertainment: The propositi in all the families of the dominant type were recognized in routine tests with anti-Lu^a and anti-Lu^b or with anti-Lu^aLu^b (anti-Lu3). The propositi of families *a* to *d* brought themselves to notice by having anti-Lu^aLu^b (anti-Lu3) in their serum.

Consanguinity: There was no known consanguinity in any of the parents of propositi excepting the much inbred family b, and the Japanese family c.

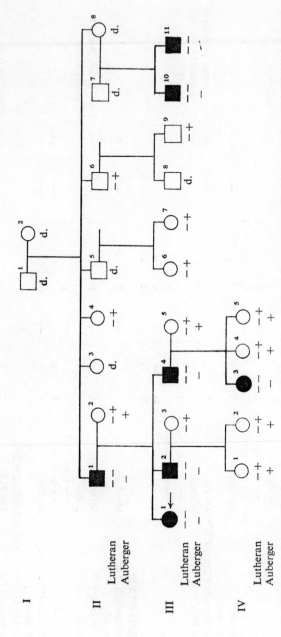

Fig. 18. The inheritance of Lu(a−b−) in the family Cr. (From Crawford, Greenwalt, Sasaki, Tippett, Sanger and Race[19], 1961, with a few later additions.) The minus or plus signs of the upper rows represent the reactions with anti-Lu[a] and Lu[b], those of the lower rows with anti-Au[a] (Tippett,[29] 1963).

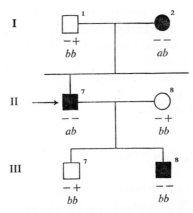

Fig. 19. Part of the pedigree of the Lar. family showing that the gene responsible for the dominant type of Lu(a–b–) is not part of the *Lutheran* locus (Taliano, Guévin and Tippett[54], 1973). –– = Lu(a–b–) (black), –+ = Lu(a–b+); the *Lutheran* genotypes, *ab* or *bb*, of the three Lu(a–b–) members were determined by fixation-elution tests. For argument see text.

This new finding has, of course, made the notation *In(Lu)* less appropriate, and no doubt in time someone will think of a better.

For many years it seemed possible that the *Auberger* locus was part of the *Lutheran* complex locus, but in 1974 Dr Salmon and his colleagues found the long hoped for informative type of family which showed the two loci to be separate and unlikely even to be linked.

In considering the way the inhibitor might work Crawford *et al.*[66] wrote:

'The question arises whether *In(Lu)* causes some surface change which makes difficult the attachment of certain antibodies, or whether it causes alteration to a substance needed in the building of certain antigens, but to this we have no answer. If Lu(a–b–) does reflect some change to the cell surface it is presumably an innocuous change, for the senior author knows of no anaemia in the seven Lu(a–b–) members of her family.

'Incidentally, the fact that *In(Lu)* is capable of depressing, often out of recognition, antigens of genetically independent systems, P_1 for example, calls for further caution in attributing to the Lutheran system the series of "public" antibodies having the common property of failing to react with Lu(a–b–) cells, at any rate if judged only by tests with samples of the dominant type.'

Linkage relations of In(Lu)

As we have said, the family reported by Tippett[53] and that by Taliano *et al.*[54] combined to show that *In(Lu)* is not part of the *Lutheran* locus, and the family described by Contreras and Tippett[71] showed it not to be part of the *P* locus. There is no information about its genetical relationship to the *Auberger* or the *Ii* loci.

Incidentally, *In(Lu)* has also been shown not to be sited at any of the following structural loci[53, 54, 71]: *ABO*, *MNSs*, *Rh*, *Kell*, *Duffy*, *Kidd* and *Yt*, nor is it carried on the X or on the Y.

In our Unit Dr Patricia Tippett has on occasion found samples sent as Lu(a–b–) to react with anti-Lu^{a}Lu^b (anti-Lu3): further investigation showed them to be either Lu(a–bw) or Lu(awbw). Similar samples have been noted in other laboratories[56] and called the Lu(w) phenotype. From our limited family studies the depressed Lu^a and Lu^b antigens appear to be the result of modifying genes apparently echoing somewhat faintly the more powerful gene behind the dominant Lu(a–b–) phenotype.

THE EXPANDING LUTHERAN SYSTEM

In 1971 the first of what was to become a series of antibodies related in some way to the Lutheran system was reported from the United States. As successive antibodies disclosed themselves they were given numbers anti-Lu4, -Lu5 etc. and at the time of writing the number approaches Lu:20, though not all have been published. Most of these antibodies had earlier appeared to be antibodies to unknown 'public' antigens until the observation that they reacted negatively with Lu(a–b–) cells gave the clue that they were related to the Lutheran system. That the antibodies were not all the same was evident because, while reacting negatively with Lu(a–b–) and with their owner's cells, they were positive with the cells of other owners. Much of this expansion was due to the wide distribution by Dr Mary Crawford of her own Lu(a–b–) cells. A summary of the reactions is given in Table 46 (page 275); not all the crop of new antibodies were of the 'public' type.

In the description to follow we have singled out the antigens Lu9 and Lu6 because family evidence has shown the manner of their relationship to the *Lutheran* locus. The rest we have gathered under the heading of 'para-Lutheran' antigens, from which they could be promoted as their inheritance becomes clearer.

With the promise of a second series of alleles, *Lu*^{6} and *Lu*^{9}, Lutheran looks very much like joining Rh, MNSs and Kell as a complex system; so a reference here to phylogeny (page 181) and to the operon pattern of inheritance (pages 221 and 241) may be appropriate.

Notation. The notation adopted for the recently recognized antigens in the Lutheran system, Lu9 and Lu6, and for the para-Lutheran antigens about to be described, is that proposed by Rosenfield et al.[58] (1962) for the Rh system; it is succinctly stated by Molthan et al.[52] in relation to Lu9: 'The antibody: anti-Lu9; the antigen: Lu9; the gene: *Lu*^{9}; phenotypes: Lu:9 and Lu:–9.'

The antigens Lu9 and Lu6

An expansion of the Lutheran system, comparable to that of the Kell system when Kp^a and Kp^b were recognized (page 286), followed the finding in Philadelphia of an antibody in the serum of Mrs Mull. Mrs Mull lacked the corresponding rare antigen but her husband and a number of his relatives and all three of their children had it. Mrs Mull was Lu(a–b+) and fortunately Lu^a and Lu^b were segregating in the family, and in their excellent account Molthan, Crawford, Marsh and Allen[52] (1973) give the fine pedigree reproduced in Figure 20. It shows that the antigen Lu9 is a dominant character and that the gene Lu^9 is linked to the *Lutheran* locus (lod score at θ 0·0 = 6·3) with no recombination on 14 occasions when it could have been observed. It was clear that Lu^9 is part of the *Lutheran* complex locus. It cannot be an allele at the Lu^aLu^b mutational site because Lu(a+b+) can be Lu:9. Presumably the relationship of Lu9 to Lutheran is like that of C to D or E in Rh, or of K to Kp or Js in Kell.

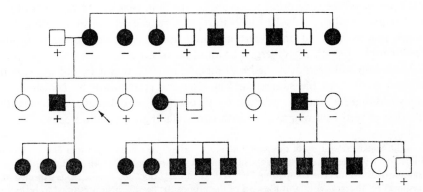

Fig. 20. Lu9 and Lu[a] types in the Mull family. All members of the family are Lu(b+). The first child of the proposita died in infancy, was not tested for Lu9 or Lu[a], and was omitted from the pedigree. Black = Lu:9; white = Lu:−9; + = Lu(a+); − = Lu(a−). (From Molthan, Crawford, Marsh and Allen[52], 1973.)

Frequency of Lu:9

This is shown in Table 45 which is taken from the original paper. In a random sample of 521 there were 9, or 1·7%, Lu:9. The significantly higher proportion of Lu:9 in Lu(a+b+) than in Lu(a−b+) samples was interpreted as evidence of a

Table 45. Tests with anti-Lu9 on persons of four Lutheran phenotypes. (From Molthan, Crawford, Marsh and Allen[52], 1973.)

Sample	Lutheran phenotype	Number tested	Number Lu:9	Number Lu:−9
Random	Lu(a−b+)	474	4	470
Random	Lu(a+b+)	47	5	42
Selected	Lu(a+b−)	13	0	13
Selected	Lu(a−b−)	8	0	8

Among the 512 random samples, there is an excess of Lu:9 bloods among those that are Lu(a+b+); no more than one would be expected. The probability of such a discrepancy occurring by chance is small (p = 0·000465 by Fisher's exact method).

'linkage disequilibrium' and as further support for Lu^9 belonging to the *Lutheran* complex locus (just as *C* is aligned with *e* more often than with *E* at the *Rh* complex locus). According to our calculations the frequency of the gene complexes are: Lu^aLu^9 0·005, Lu^aLu^{-9} 0·040, Lu^bLu^9 0·004 and Lu^bLu^{-9} 0·951.

Relationship of Lu9 to Lu6

Evidence that Lu^6 belongs to the *Lutheran* complex locus came when two unrelated people of the very rare Lu:−6 phenotype, and two Lu:−6 relatives of one of them, were all found to be Lu:9. Furthermore, the cells of these four Lu:−6 people reacted more strongly with anti-Lu9 than did the cells of heterozygous Lu:9 people. Lu^6 clearly emerged as an allele of Lu^9.

Anti-Lu6 had been described by Marsh[56], in 1972, and a second example by Wrobel *et al.*[57], in the same year but after the recognition by Molthan and Crawford that Lu^9 and Lu^6 were alleles. Wrobel and her colleagues noted that the reaction of anti-Lu6 was weaker with cord cells than with adult cells.

The elegant simplicity of this Lu9:Lu6 story was a little ruffled when in a Danish family, studied by Dybkjaer *et al.*[61], the propositus was Lu:−6 and had in her serum the third known example of anti-Lu6. The compatible Lu:−6 sister of the propositus was Lu:9, as expected of a presumed Lu^9 homozygote. But the cells of the propositus herself, also presumed to be homozygous for Lu^9, reacted only very weakly with anti-Lu9, and this remains to be explained. Furthermore, the newborn babies of the propositus and of her sister were Lu:w6, −9, though this would be explained if Lu9 should prove not to be developed by the time of birth.

Para-Lutheran antigens

We are using this name to cover the series of antigens which are certainly related to the Lutheran system, but in a way not yet understood. As mentioned above the antibodies corresponding to these 'public' antigens are all alike in that they fail to react with Lu(a−b−) cells of the dominant or recessive type or with their own cells, or perhaps with the cells of some of their sibs: all are different in that they react with each other's cells. Their reactions are summarized in Table 46.

Table 46 includes only those para-Lutheran antigens which have been published at the time of writing, and one other (Anton.) tested in our Unit. All these antibodies have been tested against cells of both the dominant and recessive types of Lu(a−b−): all, like anti-Lu^{a}Lu^b (Lu3) and anti-Lu6, react only weakly with Lu(awbw) and Lu(a−bw) samples mentioned on page 272.

We do not intend to give details of all the para-Lutheran antibodies: references may be found in the legend to Table 46. Lu:10 (Sing.) lacks a reference but is mentioned on occasion in the other papers quoted; the antibody is weak and its rumoured antithetical relationship to Lu:5 (Dr F.H. Allen, personal communication) will sort itself out in time.

The antibody anti-Lu4 may be taken as typical of the series. The Much. antigen

Table 46. Antibodies and phenotypes in the Lutheran and para-Lutheran series

Phenotype	Anti- Lu^a 1	Lu^b 2	Lu^aLu^b 3	Bar. 4	Be. 5	Jan. 6	Ga. 7	M.T. 8	Mull 9	Sing. 10	Re. 11	Much. 12	Anton.
Lu(a−b+)	−	+	+	+	+	+	+	+	−*	−*	+	+	+
Lu(a+b+)	+	+	+	+	+	+	+	+	−*	−*	+	+	+
Lu(a+b−)	+	−	+	+	+	+	+	+	−*	−*	+	+	+
Lu(a−b−)	−	−	−	−	−	−	−	−	−	−	−	−	−
Lu:−4	−	+	+	−	+	+	+	+	−	−	+	+	+
Lu:−5	−	+	+	+	−	+	+	+	−	+	+	+	
Lu:−6	−	+	+	+	+	−	+	+	−	−	+	+	+
Lu:−7	−	+	+	+	+	+	−	+	+	−	+	+	
Lu:−8	−	+	+	+	+	+	+	−	−	−	+	+	
Lu:−11	−	+	+	w	w	w	w	+	−	−	−	+	+
Lu:−12	−	w	w	+	+	+	+	w	−	−	+	−	−
Anton.	−	+	+										
References				a	bc	bd	b	e	f		i	g	h

* about 2% Lu:10. No frequencies available for Lu:10.
a Bove, Allen, Chiewsilp, Marsh and Cleghorn[59] (1971).
b Marsh[56] (1972).
c Bowen, Haist, Talley, Reid and Marsh[60] (1972).
d Wrobel, Moore, Cornwall, Wray, Øyen and Marsh[57] (1972); Dybkjaer, Lylloff and Tippett[61] (1973).
e MacIlroy, McCreary and Stroup[62] (1972).
f Molthan, Crawford, Marsh and Allen[52] (1973).
g Sinclair, Buchanan, Tippett and Sanger[63] (1973).
h Boorman and Tippett[64] (1972).
i Gralnick, Goldfinger, Hatfield, Reid and Marsh[72] (1974).

(Lu12) will also be described separately for it has been shown probably not to be controlled from the *Lutheran* locus.

The antigen Lu4

In 1971, Bove, Allen, Chiewsilp, Marsh and Cleghorn[59] found an antibody which reacted with all cells tested except the patient's own, those of two of her five sibs and all Lu(a−b−) samples tested, whether of the dominant or recessive type. The patient had been twice pregnant and had been transfused, so presumably her antibody was immune; it was not anti-Lu^{a}Lu^b because she and her two negative sibs were both normal Lu(a−b+). The family gave no clue whether the new antigen thus defined, and named Lu4, belonged to the *Lutheran* complex locus or not. The investigators favoured rather the explanation proposed in the last edition of this book for the dominant form of Lu(a−b−) and its relation to the Auberger antigen —that a dominant gene prevents the formation of a precursor substance needed for the proper expression of the *Lutheran* and *Au* genes and to these they added the *Lu^4* gene. In passing, they suggested that since nothing is known about anti-Lu^{a}Lu^b, except that it fails to react with either kind of Lu(a−b−) samples, a more suitable notation would be anti-Lu3 and this seems a good point.

The Much. antigen, Lu12

This antigen stands out from its fellows because it is known probably not to be controlled from the *Lutheran* locus, which is more than is yet known of Lu4, 5, 7, 8, 11, and Anton.

The antibody called Much. (or anti-Lu12) was described by Sinclair, Buchanan, Tippett and Sanger[63] in 1973. Like other antibodies in this series it did not react with Lu(a−b−) cells or with the cells of the maker of the antibody. Unlike the makers of anti-Lu4 to 11 and Anton, Mrs Much. was not of the phenotype Lu(a−b+) but was Lu(a−bw): her Lu^b antigen was weaker than that of heterozygous Lu(a+b+) people whereas the makers of anti-Lu4, 5, 6 and 7 are recorded as having a double dose of Lu^b. The investigators called the antibody 'Much.': they were a little doubtful about 'anti-Lu12', its place in the queue, because the corresponding antigen, alone of all the para-Lutheran antigens, could be shown probably not to be controlled by the *Lutheran* locus. Certainly the antigen was phenotypically related to the Lutheran antigens, but to call the antibody anti-Lu12 seemed like calling anti-U, which belongs to the MNSs system, anti-Rh100 because it may fail to react with Rh$_{null}$ cells. But anti-Lu12 is convenient for reference and the notation for the para-Lutheran series of antibodies will presumably be straightened out in time.

The evidence that the Much. antigen is not controlled by the *Lutheran* locus is indirect but quite impressive: in the Much. family the *Lutheran* genes were not segregating, but the *secretor* genes were, and it was clear that the locus responsible for the Much. antigen was not close to the *secretor* locus which is close to the *Lutheran* locus.

The antigen Lu5

One family (Bowen *et al.*[60]) gives a hint that *Lu⁵* may prove to be controlled from the *Lutheran* locus and eventually promoted from this 'para' section. Two of the three Lu:−5 propositi are negro, in contrast to the Lu:−4, −6, −7, −8, −12 and Anton propositi who are white.

LUTHERAN ANTIBODIES

Anti-Luᵃ (anti-Lu1)

This is not a common antibody. The second example was reported by Mainwaring and Pickles[5], in 1948. Other examples soon followed[4, 8, 10, 14–17].

Greenwalt and Sasaki[4] pointed out that anti-Luᵃ is probably not as rare as the paucity of the recorded examples would imply: they found three in testing the serum of 18,613 blood donors. In a later paper[39] with Steane they gave details of a further nine anti-Luᵃ.

The antibody may be 'naturally occurring'[4, 8, 14] or immune[1, 5, 16]. All examples so far published have been of the complete type with the exception of one reported by Francis and Hatcher[28], which behaved *in vitro* like an incomplete antibody and caused a positive direct antiglobulin reaction of the cells of two Lu(a+) babies of the propositus—though it did not cause haemolytic disease. Greendyke and Chorpenning[45] report the normal survival of Lu(a+) cells in a patient with anti-Luᵃ in her serum.

Saline agglutination tests seem to suit the majority of anti-Luᵃ: although some examples react at 37°C. the optimum temperature is usually 12°–18°C.

The appearance of the agglutination of Lu(a+) cells by anti-Luᵃ is unlike that of most other blood group reactions. Callender and Race[1] noted that the agglutinates were large but that many unagglutinated cells were constantly present, and this has been the general experience since.

Hackel and his colleagues, Smolker and Fenske[25, 26], found that anti-Luᵃ and anti-Luᵇ are partially inhibited by certain derivatives of ribonucleic acid, in this behaving like Rh antibodies but unlike other antibodies tested (anti-A, -B, -M, -N, -He, -P₁, -I).

Anti-Luᵇ (anti-Lu2)

Cutbush and Chanarin[3] found the first example in the serum of a woman who had never been transfused and who had had three healthy children. The antibody was a saline agglutinin reacting more strongly at 20°C. than at 37°C. Unagglutinated cells were recorded, but in our experience with this antibody the picture is not as striking as that given by anti-Luᵃ.

Though ten years passed between the recognition of anti-Luᵃ and the finding of the first anti-Luᵇ, other anti-Luᵇ soon followed[4, 20, 21]: many examples are now

10*

known, although only 0·15 per cent of Europeans are Lu^aLu^a and so candidates for making anti-Lu^b. The trouble the antibody causes in cross-matching tests and the necessity of its identification no doubt contribute to its apparent frequency: anti-Lu^a, on the other hand, need not be identified, for compatible donors are so easily found. Greenwalt and his colleagues[39] gave details of 32 examples tested in their laboratory.

Tests with anti-Lu^b may not be easy. Most anti-Lu^b sera do react with cells suspended in saline but give more reliable results by the antiglobulin method: for example, we found that one of them[21], though particularly good at agglutinating fresh cells in saline, gave reliable results with travelled cells only if an antiglobulin test was done.

Anti-Lu^b evidently causes more trouble than anti-Lu^a, perhaps because of its proclivity towards the incomplete. Anti-Lu^b has caused cross-matching difficulty[3, 20, 33, 39, 46], has eliminated transfused cells[27, 20], has caused a mild transfusion reaction[4, 46] and has been blamed for mild haemolytic disease of the newborn[21, 47].

As a result of serological, immunochemical and ultrafiltration studies Greenwalt and his colleagues[39] concluded that anti-Lu^b is mainly in the IgA fraction.

Anti-Lu^aLu^b (anti-Lu3)

This antibody can be made by Lu(a–b–) people. The first example was described by Darnborough and his colleagues[30], in 1963; it was almost certainly immune. A second example was reported by Melonas and Noto[48], a third by Brown and her colleagues[42] and a fourth by Myhre[69]. All four examples reacted more strongly by antiglobulin than by saline tests.

Anti-Lu9 and anti-Lu6

These are properly called Lutheran antibodies, for reasons given above. So far only one example of anti-Lu9 has been reported (Molthan *et al.*[52], 1973). It was presumably immune in origin and in our hands works best by the antiglobulin method. It reacts positively with about 2% of samples.

Of anti-Lu6 three examples are known at the time of writing[56, 57, 61]: they were all presumably immune. Negative reactors are extremely rare.

Para-Lutheran antibodies

Anti-Lu4, 5, 7, 8 and 11 *et seq.* present themselves as antibodies to 'public' antigens: negative reactors are very rare. References are to be found under Table 46. Anti-Lu10 is said to be of the 'private' type; the antibody is weak and has not yet been described in print.

OTHER NOTES ABOUT THE SYSTEM

Variations in strength of the antigens

The antigen Lu[a] varies greatly in strength in different heterozygous people[5, 49] but is of about the same strength within families[5]. Greenwalt, Sasaki and Steane[39], in testing the families of seven Lu(a+b−) propositi, demonstrated a clear dosage difference in strength of Lu[a] between homozygotes and heterozygotes.

The antigen Lu[b] also shows a dosage effect[3, 4, 20, 21, 39] but, again, the strength varies in different heterozygous people[3, 20, 39].

Beyond the weak end of the normal curve of Lu[b] and Lu[a] antigen strength are to be found occasional samples which can at first be mistaken (see page 272) for Lu(a−b−).

Development of the antigens

We tested the blood of a '12 weeks' foetus and found it to be Lu(a+). The father was subsequently found to be Lu(a+) and the mother Lu(a−); this is mentioned to show that the foetal Lu(a+) reaction could not have been due to any contamination with maternal blood. However, Greenwalt and his colleagues[39] find that in the heterozygote the Lu[a] antigen is only weakly expressed at birth and that its strength increases until about the age of 15.

The Lu[b] antigen of Lu(a−b+) cord cells is weaker than that of adults[21, 39]: it is weaker still in Lu(a+b+) infants[39]. Toivanen and Hirvonen[65] tested 72 foetuses of varying ages with anti-Lu[b]: the four aged between 7 and 9 weeks were all negative, as was one aged 10–12 weeks and one aged 16–20 weeks; about half the rest were weaker than adult samples.

Racial differences

The antigen Lu[a] can be present in Negroes as well as in Whites: it has not been found, as far as we know, in Asians, Eskimos or Australian aborigines.

Lutheran and Sw[a] (Swann)

Sw[a], one of the best investigated of the 'private' antigens, has in several publications been associated with Lutheran and has a right to be noted in this chapter. The story of the suggestive evidence of linkage between *Lu* and *Sw* and how it appeared to be shattered by one family is told in Chapter 20, page 440, where references will be found.

Though it distinguishes only 7 or 8 % of white people the Lutheran system has made an outstanding contribution to human genetics in providing, with the secretor system, the first example in man of autosomal linkage and the first example of autosomal crossing-over, and in demonstrating for the first time that crossing-over in man can be more common in the female than in the male. The system also provided the only example, so far, of a 'minus-minus' condition which is dominant—a condition eventually found to be due to an unlinked inhibitor locus capable of inhibiting antigens belonging to several genetically independent systems.

REFERENCES

[1] CALLENDER SHEILA T. and RACE R.R. (1946) A serological and genetical study of multiple antibodies formed in response to blood transfusion by a patient with lupus erythematosus diffusus. *Ann. Eugen., Lond.*, **13**, 102–117.

[1a] CALLENDER SHEILA, RACE R.R. and PAYKOC Z.V. (1945) Hypersensitivity to transfused blood. *Brit. med. J.*, **ii**, 83.

[2] A notation for the Lewis and Lutheran blood group systems (1949). A leading article. *Nature, Lond.*, **163**, 580.

[3] CUTBUSH MARIE and CHANARIN I. (1956) The expected blood-group antibody, anti-Lu^b. *Nature, Lond.*, **178**, 855–856.

[4] GREENWALT T.J. and SASAKI T. (1957) The Lutheran blood groups: a second example of anti-Lu^b and three further examples of anti-Lu^a. *Blood*, **12**, 998–1003.

[5] MAINWARING U.R. and PICKLES MARGARET M. (1948) A further case of anti-Lutheran immunization with some studies on its capacity for human sensitization. *J. clin. Path.*, **1**, 292–294.

[6] BERTINSHAW DOREEN, LAWLER SYLVIA D., HOLT HELENE A., KIRMAN B.H. and RACE R.R. (1950). The combination of blood groups in a sample of 475 people in a London hospital. *Ann. Eugen., Lond.*, **15**, 234–242.

[7] MOURANT A.E. (1954) *The Distribution of the Human Blood Group*, pp. 438, Blackwell Scientific Publications, Oxford.

[8] GONZENBACH R., HÄSSIG A. and ROSIN S. (1955) Über posttransfusionelle Bildung von Anti-Lutheran-Antikörpern. Die Häufigkeit des Lutheran-Antigens Lu^a in de Bevölkerung Nord-, West- und Mitteleuropas. *Blut*, **1**, 272–274.

[9] MOHR J. (1951) A search for linkage between the Lutheran blood group and other hereditary characters. *Acta path. microbiol. scand.*, **28**, 207–210.

[10] HEIDE H.M. V.D. and LOGHEM J.J. VAN (1951) Repartition des groupes sanguins en Hollande. *Proc. 4th Congr. int. Soc. Blood Transf.*, 383–388.

[11] LAWLER SYLVIA D. (1950) The inheritance of the Lutheran blood groups in 47 English families. *Ann. Eugen., Lond.*, **15**, 255–257.

[12] RACE R.R., SANGER RUTH and THOMPSON JOAN S. (1953) Quoted in 2nd, 3rd and 4th editions of this book but not elsewhere published.

[13] MOHR J. (1951) Estimation of linkage between the Lutheran and the Lewis blood groups. *Acta path. microbiol. scand.*, **29**, 339–344.

[14] SHAW S., MOURANT A.E. and IKIN ELIZABETH W. (1954) Hypersplenism with anti-Lutheran antibody following transfusion. *Lancet*, **ii**, 170–171.

[15] WALKER C.B.V., CAMERON C., IKIN ELIZABETH W. and MOURANT A.E. (1949) Personal communication.

[16] HOLLÄNDER L. (1955) Das Lutheran-Blutgruppensystem. Die Häufigkeit des Lutheran-Antigens in der Bevölkerung Basels. *Schweiz. med. Wschr.*, **85**, 10–11.

[17] VOGEL P. (1954) Current problems in blood transfusion. *Bull. N.Y. Acad. Med.*, **30**, 657–674.

[18] RACE R.R., SANGER RUTH and MOORES PHYLLIS (1957) Quoted in 3rd and 4th edition of this book but not elsewhere published.

[19] CRAWFORD MARY N., GREENWALT T.J., SASAKI T., TIPPETT PATRICIA, SANGER RUTH and RACE R.R. (1961) The phenotype Lu(a−b−) together with unconventional Kidd groups in one family. *Transfusion, Philad.*, **1**, 228–232.

20 METAXAS M.N., METAXAS-BÜHLER MARGRIT, DUNSFORD I. and HOLLÄNDER L. (1959) A further example of anti-Lu^b together with data in support of the Lutheran-secretor linkage in Man. *Vox Sang.*, **4**, 298–307.

21 KISSMEYER-NIELSEN F. (1960) A further example of anti-Lu^b as a cause of a mild haemolytic disease of the newborn. *Vox Sang.*, **5**, 532–537.

22 GREENWALT T.J. and SASAKI T. (1961) Unpublished observations.

23 GREENWALT T.J. (1961) Confirmation of linkage between the Lutheran and secretor genes. *Amer. J. hum. Genet.*, **13**, 69–88.

24 SANGER RUTH and RACE R.R. (1958) The Lutheran-secretor linkage in Man: support for Mohr's findings. *Hereditiy*, **12**, 513–520.

25 HACKEL E., SMOLKER R.E. and FENSKE SUE A. (1958) Inhibition of anti-Rh and anti-Lutheran sera by ribonucleic acid derivatives. *Vox Sang.*, **3**, 402–408.

26 HACKEL E. and SMOLKER R.E. (1960) Effect of ribonuclease on erythrocyte antigens. *Nature, Lond.*, **187**, 1036–1037.

27 MOLLISON P.L. (1956) *Blood Transfusion in Clinical Medicine*, 2nd edition, p. 232, Blackwell Scientific Publications, Oxford.

28 FRANCIS BETTY J. and HATCHER D.E. (1961) Hemolytic disease of the newborn apparently caused by anti-Lu^a. *Transfusion, Philad.*, **1**, 248–250.

29 TIPPETT PATRICIA (1963) *Serological Study of the Inheritance of Unusual Rh and Other Blood Group Phenotypes*. Ph.D. Thesis, University of London.

30 DARNBOROUGH J., FIRTH R., GILES CAROLYN M., GOLDSMITH K.L.G. and CRAWFORD MARY N. (1963) A 'new' antibody anti-Lu^{a}Lu^b and two further examples of the genotype Lu(a–b–). *Nature Lond.*, **198**, 796. And unpublished observations.

31 COOK P.J.L. (1965) The Lutheran-secretor recombination fraction in man: a possible sex difference. *Ann. hum. Genet.*, **28**, 393–401.

32 HARTMANN O., HEIER A.M., KORNSTAD L., WEISERT O. and ÖRJASAETER H. (1965) The frequency of the Lutheran blood group antigens, as defined by anti-Lu^a, in the Oslo population. *Vox Sang.*, **10**, 234–238.

33 CROUCHER BETTY E.E., SCOTT J.G. and CROOKSTON J.H. (1962) A further example of anti-Lu^b. *Vox Sang.*, **7**, 492–495.

34 CHOWN B., LEWIS MARION and KAITA HIROKO (1966) The Lutheran blood groups in two Caucasian population samples. *Vox Sang.*, **11**, 108–110.

35 V.D. WEERDT CHRISTINA M. (1965) *Platelet Antigens and Iso-immunization*. Doctoral Thesis, 'Aemstelstad', Amsterdam, pp. 108.

36 LINNET-JEPSEN P. (1965) *Undersøgelsen over Gm(a) faktoren. Specielt i det første leveår.* M.D. Thesis, Aarhus Universitet, pp. 256.

37 LINNET-JEPSEN P., GALATIUS-JENSEN F. and HAUGE M. (1958) On the inheritance of the Gm serum group. *Acta genet.*, **8**, 164–196.

38 MOHR J. (1966) Genetics of fourteen marker systems: associations and linkage relations. *Acta genet.*, **16**, 1–58.

39 GREENWALT T.J., SASAKI T. and STEANE E.A. (1967) The Lutheran blood groups: a progress report with observations on the development of the antigens and characteristics of the antibodies. *Transfusion, Philad.*, **7**, 189–200.

40 STANBURY ARDEN and FRANCIS BETTY (1967) The Lu(a–b–) phenotype: an additional example. *Vox Sang.*, **13**, 441–443. And personal communication.

41 WRIGHT J. and MOORE B.P.L. (1968) A family with 17 Lu(a–b–) members. *Vox Sang.*, **14**, 133–136.

42 BROWN FRANCES N.H., SIMPSON SHIRLEY L. and READ H.C. (1967) Personal communication.

43 BRICE CHARMAINE L. and HOXWORTH P.I. (1965) Some unusual observations in the search for rare donors. Paper read at A.A.B.B. Miami, and unpublished observations.

44 *Lister Institute, Report of the Governing Body* (1964) Page 35.

45 GREENDYKE R.M. and CHORPENNING F.W. (1962) Normal survival of incompatible red cells in the presence of anti-Lu^a. *Transfusion, Philad.*, **2**, 52–57.

46 MOLTHAN LYNDALL and CRAWFORD MARY C. (1966) Three examples of anti-Lu[b] and related data. *Transfusion, Philad.*, **6**, 584–589.

47 SCHEFFER HELENA and TAMAKI H.T. (1966) Anti-Lu[b] and mild hemolytic disease of the newborn. *Transfusion, Philad.*, **6**, 497–498.

48 MELONAS K. and NOTO T.A. (1965) Anti-Lu[a]Lu[b] imitating a panagglutinin. *Transfusion, Philad.*, **5**, 370. (Abstract.) And unpublished observations.

49 RACE R.R. and SANGER RUTH (1962) *Blood Groups in Man*, p. 210, 4th edition, Blackwell Scientific Publications, Oxford.

50 TIPPETT PATRICIA (1966) Unpublished observations.

51 DUBLIN T.D., BERNANKE A.D., PITT ELAINE L., MASSELL B.F., ALLEN F.H. and AMEZCUA F. (1964) Red blood cell groups and ABH secretor system as genetic indicators of susceptibility to rheumatic fever and rheumatic heart disease. *Brit. med. J.*, **ii**, 775–779.

52 MOLTHAN LYNDALL, CRAWFORD MARY N., MARSH W.L. and ALLEN F.H. (1973) Lu9, another new antigen of the Lutheran blood-group system. *Vox Sang.*, **24**, 468–471.

53 TIPPETT PATRICIA (1971) A case of suppressed Lu[a] and Lu[b] antigens. *Vox Sang.*, **20**, 378–380.

54 TALIANO V., GUÉVIN R.-M. and TIPPETT PATRICIA (1973) The genetics of a dominant inhibitor of the Lutheran antigens. *Vox Sang.*, **24**, 42–47.

55 BROWN FRANCES, SIMPSON SHIRLEY, CORNWALL SHEILA, MOORE B.P.L., ØYEN RAGNHILD and MARSH W.L. (1973) The recessive Lu(a−b−) phenotype: a family study. *Vox Sang.*, **26**, 259–264.

56 MARSH W.L. (1972) Anti-Lu5, anti-Lu6 and anti-Lu7. Three antibodies defining high frequency antigens related to the Lutheran blood group system. *Transfusion, Philad.*, **12**, 27–34.

57 WROBEL D.M., MOORE B.P.L., CORNWALL SHEILA, WRAY ELIZABETH, ØYEN RAGNHILD and MARSH W.L. (1972) A second example of Lu(−6) in the Lutheran system. *Vox Sang.*, **23**, 205–207.

58 ROSENFIELD R.E., ALLEN F.H., SWISHER S.N. and KOCHWA S. (1962) A review of Rh serology and presentation of a new terminology. *Transfusion, Philad.*, **2**, 287–312.

59 BOVE J.R., ALLEN F.H., CHIEWSILP P., MARSH W.L. and CLEGHORN T.E. (1971) Anti-Lu4: a new antibody related to the Lutheran blood group system. *Vox Sang.*, **21**, 302–310.

60 BOWEN ANN B., HAIST ANNA L., TALLEY LINDA L., REID MARION E. and MARSH W.L. (1972) Further examples of the Lutheran Lu(−5) blood type. *Vox Sang.*, **23**, 201–204.

61 DYBKJAER E., LYLLOFF K. and TIPPETT PATRICIA (1974) Weak Lu9 antigen in one Lu:−6 member of a family. *Vox Sang.*, **26**, 94–96.

62 MACILROY MIJA, McCREARY JOAN and STROUP MARJORY (1972) Anti-Lu8, an antibody recognizing another Lutheran-related antigen. *Vox Sang.*, **23**, 455–457.

63 SINCLAIR MARGARET, BUCHANAN D.I., TIPPETT PATRICIA and SANGER RUTH (1973) Another antibody related to the Lutheran blood group system (Much.). *Vox Sang.*, **25**, 156–161.

64 BOORMAN KATHLEEN E. and TIPPETT PATRICIA (1972) Unpublished observations.

65 TOIVANEN P. and HIRVONEN T. (1973) Antigens Duffy, Kell, Kidd, Lutheran and Xg[a] on fetal red cells. *Vox Sang.*, **24**, 372–376.

66 CRAWFORD MARY N., TIPPETT PATRICIA and SANGER RUTH (1974) The antigens Au[a], i and P₁ of cells of the dominant type of Lu(a−b−). *Vox Sang.*, **26**, 283–287.

67 GELLERMAN MIJA M. (1974) Unpublished observations.

68 SALMON C. (1974) Unpublished observations.

69 MYHRE B., THOMPSON MARGARET, ANSON CLAIRE, FISHKIN B. and CARTER K. (1974) A further example of the recessive Lu(a−b−) phenotype. *Vox Sang.* In the press.

70 TIPPETT PATRICIA (1973) Unpublished observations.

71 CONTRERAS MARCELA and TIPPETT PATRICIA (1934) The Lu(a−b−) syndrome and an apparent upset of P₁ inheritance. *Vox Sang.*, **27**, 369–371.

72 GRALNICK MARY A., GOLDFINGER D., HATFIELD PATRICIA A., REID MARION E. and MARSH W.L. (1974) Anti-Lu 11: another antibody defining a high frequency antigen related to the Lutheran blood group system. *Vox Sang.*, **27**, 52–56.

Chapter 7
The Kell Blood Groups

Within a few weeks of its first trial the antiglobulin test disclosed the existence of the system called Kell. The red cells of a child thought to be suffering from haemolytic disease of the newborn gave a positive direct reaction which could not be explained by Rh. In the serum of the mother, Mrs Kell., there was an antibody which sensitized the cells of her husband. and her elder child (Coombs, Mourant and Race[1], 1946) and about 7% of random blood samples[2].

The antigen appeared to be inherited as a dominant Mendelian character and this was supported by Mourant[3] who tested the blood of both parents of five K+ persons and found that in each family one or the other parent was also K+.

In 1947 a second example of anti-K was found by Wiener and Sonn-Gordon[4]. The antibody was not at first recognized as being the same as anti-K and was named Si. Other examples of anti-K soon followed and then they came thick and fast.

The expected antithetical antibody, anti-k, was found in 1949 (Levine, Backer, Wigod and Ponder[5]) and many examples have since disclosed themselves.

The age of simplicity of the Kell system was unusually long: it ended in 1957 with the finding of anti-Kp^a and the antithetical anti-Kp^b by Allen and Lewis[16]. In the same year rare people apparently devoid of all Kell antigens, K_0, were recognized (Chown, Kaita and Lewis[17]).

Up to this stage the Kell groups had made no very useful genetic distinction among Negroes, unlike the Sutter groups (Giblett[8, 10], 1958) which make a useful distinction only among Negroes. When, therefore, the Sutter groups were found to belong to the Kell system (Stroup, MacIlroy, Walker and Aydelotte[11], 1965) the interest and field of usefulness of the Kell system was greatly extended.

Further advances were the recognition that the primarily Finnish antigen Ul^a belongs to the Kell complex (Furuhjelm et al.[88, 89], 1968, 1969) and so does the recently reported antigen Wk^a (Strange et al.[90], 1974). Neither can be assigned to the K, Kp or Js departments; indeed Wk^a appears to represent a fourth series of alleles.

As is happening in the Lutheran system so in the Kell system is emerging a series of 'public' antigens associated in some way with the $-/-$ phenotype, in this case K_0. Until their genetical relationship to the Kell system is understood we refer to these antigens as para-Kell.

Of considerable interest, clinical as well as serological, is the observation, by Giblett et al.[98], 1971, that some sufferers from chronic granulomatous disease have markedly depressed Kell antigens and may make antibody to the almost universal antigen, KL, of van der Hart et al.[80], 1968.

Ignoring for the present the antigen Ul[a] and Wk[a], the Kell system of blood groups is defined by three pairs of antithetical antibodies, anti-K and anti-k, anti-Kp[a] and Kp[b], anti-Js[a] and anti-Js[b], and in the first place we shall describe the reactions of the three pairs separately.

K AND k

As far as white people are concerned the groups are still most usefully analysed for practical purposes on the basis of the K : k difference. The advances to be described in a later section add about as much to the discriminating power of the system as did the recognition of C[w] to that of Rh: the main importance of Kp[a] and Kp[b] is to the fundamental appreciation of the complexity of the system. In Negroes, on the other hand, the K : k distinction is of little practical use, for the antigen K has a frequency of less than 2%[11]; but, as will be seen, in these people Js[a] and Js[b] make such a distinction that the Kell system reaches its height of usefulness, these antigens being twice as informative in Negroes as are K and k in Whites.

Frequencies

The existence of the antigens Kp[a], Kp[b], Js[a] and Js[b] do not affect the following calculations.

Tests with anti-K

In the last edition we based our calculations on the results of antiglobulin tests on 1,018 random English donors. The tests were done some time ago in our Unit[6, 7]. A much larger series tested by Cleghorn[28] gave almost identical results:

	Our Unit	Cleghorn
K+	99 or 0·0894	792 or 0·0903
K−	1,009 or 0·9106	7,975 or 0·9097
	1,108	8,767

Since the agreement is so close there seemed no point in doing all those sums again. The gene frequencies may be calculated in the usual way:

$$k = \sqrt{0·9106} = 0·9543$$
$$\text{and } K = 1 - 0·9543 = 0·0457$$

The English genotype frequencies are:

$$\left.\begin{array}{ll} KK & 0{\cdot}0021 \text{ or } 0{\cdot}0235 \\ Kk & 0{\cdot}0872 \text{ or } 0{\cdot}9765 \end{array}\right\} \text{ of all K+}$$
$$kk \quad 0{\cdot}9107$$

The gene frequencies vary within and between European people, this is shown very clearly by two Scandinavian compilations[13, 39].

Tests with anti-k

Levine et al.[5] tested 2,500 samples with anti-k and 5, or 0·2%, were not agglutinated—which agreed perfectly with the frequency of KK given above based on the reactions of anti-K. Shapiro[14] tested 3,200 samples from South African Whites and found 5, or 0·16%, to be k−, which again agreed well with expectation.

Tests with anti-K and anti-k

Anti-k is usually conserved for tests on K+ samples, or for problems involving the Kell system. The only substantial series we know of in which anti-K and anti-k were used routinely on samples from unrelated white people are the three from Dr Bruce Chown's laboratory[9, 40, 91]. These tests on white Manitobans gave frequencies close to the English. Anti-Kp^a and anti-Kp^b were also used. It is of interest that no sample of K−k− was found in the three series (numbering 2,872, 1,277 and 1,800). The tests of Levine and his colleagues would also have detected this phenotype, so we may add their 2,500 and say that 8,449 samples of white blood were tested without any evidence of the existence of the phenotype K−k−. Nevertheless, such people do exist and, rare as they are, they cause a great practical and theoretical hullabaloo, as will be noted below.

In 14,541 Japanese, Hamilton and Nakahara[92] did however find one K−k−. The tests were on people of Hiroshima and Nagasaki but neither the K−k− nor any of his relatives had been exposed to bomb radiation; one of four sibs of the propositus was also K−k−.

Inheritance

From the genotype frequencies given above the expected frequency of the six genotypically different matings can be calculated, together with the children expected therefrom. Since anti-k is often not used, at any rate in tests on series of families, the figures in Table 47 are reduced to phenotypes when anti-K alone has been used.

In our last edition we gave details of the testing with anti-K of 2,059 European families with 4,597 children. The mating types and proportion of offspring fitted well with expectation whether this was based on the English gene frequencies ($K = 0{\cdot}0457$) or on the frequencies calculated from the $2 \times 2,059$ parents

Table 47. The expected distribution of the Kell groups in English
parents and offspring

Phenotypes

| Matings | | Proportion of children from each mating | |
Type	Frequency	K+	K−
K+ × K+	0·0080	0·7625	0·2375
K+ × K−	0·1626	0·5117	0·4883
K− × K−	0·8294	—	1·0000
	1·0000		

($K = 0·0433$). In case the references should be needed they are: 6, 7, 21, 24, 25, 42–46.

Since 1949, when Levine *et al.*[12] tested the first family with both anti-K and anti-k, many individual families thus tested are to be found in the literature, but not series of families. The only notable exceptions are the 900 white Manitoban families[91] with 2,599 children and the 130 Eskimo families[48] with 416 children, both series tested by Lewis and her colleagues.

All these families, by fitting well with expectation based on two alleles, K and k, served to consolidate the fundamental correctness of the original view of the inheritance of the two antigens K and k. The many families reported from the Rh Laboratory in Winnipeg were tested also for Kp^a and Kp^b, antigens whose place in the Kell system we shall now wrestle with.

Kp^a AND Kp^b

From the time of the discovery of anti-k in 1949 little of interest was heard of the Kell system until 1956 when Allen gave a preliminary report[15] of some fine work going on at Boston that greatly widened our view.

More detailed accounts of the work were given by Allen and Lewis[16] and by Allen, Lewis and Fudenberg[26]. Two new antibodies, anti-Kp^a and anti-Kp^b, were found and brilliantly recognized to belong to the Kell system.

The antigen Kp^a

The original anti-Kp^a sensitized the red cells of about 2% of random unrelated Whites in Boston (Table 48). The corresponding antigen was shown, by a 2 × 2 table, to be associated with the Kell system. Twelve families with Kp^a showed that the antigen was a dominant character, and all subsequent families have supported this.

Table 48 shows the incidence of Kp^a in four cities. Since practically all the 431 Kp(a+) persons will be heterozygous Kp^aKp^b the gene frequency of Kp^a may

Table 48. The frequency of the antigen Kp^a in white people

		Number tested	Kp(a+) random samples	Proportion Kp(a+)
Allen and Lewis[16]	Boston	2,363	51	0·0216
Cleghorn[28]	London	1,021	25	0·0245
Salmon[20]	Paris	3,034	49	0·0162
Chown et al.[40]	Winnipeg	1,277	32	0·0251
Dichupa et al.[87]	Winnipeg	11,239	274	0·0244
		18,934	431	0·0228

			K+ samples only	
Allen et al.[26]	Boston	255	2	0·0078
Lewis et al.[27]	Winnipeg	1,221	22	0·0181
Cleghorn[28]	London	1,379	11	0·0080
Chown et al.[40]	Winnipeg	124	1	0·0081
		2,979	36	0·0121

be taken as half the phenotype frequency, i.e. 0·0114. Table 48 also shows that the incidence of Kp^a in K+ people is only about half that in the general population. This suggested that a gene complex capable of producing both the antigen K and the antigen Kp^a might not exist, and prompted a very gallant search by Lewis, Kaita, Duncan and Chown[27]. First, 14,611 random samples were tested with anti-K; the 1,221 K+ were further tested and yielded 22 which were also Kp(a+): 17 of the families of these donors (plus one found later) were then tested. In all 18 families the K and Kp^a were seen to be segregating separately. (There is a misprint in family 16: the grandmother should be K−k+ Kp(a+b+).) Five further such families were reported and showed the separate segregation (Allen and Lewis[16], Cleghorn[28], Wright et al.[49]).

The Winnipeg group (Dichupa et al.[87]) returned to the problem by a different approach: this time they began with anti-Kp^a and then tested the Kp(a+) with anti-K. Of 11,239 random samples 274 were Kp(a+); 11 of the 274 were K+ and 9 of their families were tested. All but one of these families were informative and showed, again, that K and Kp^a were in trans.

Thus, if the gene complex KKp^a exist it probably will not be found for a long time: after all, it took five years to find the anticipated r^y when Rh groups were being done on an infinitely greater scale than are Kp groups.

The antigen k is weaker than usual (as judged by certain anti-k sera) when it is produced by the gene complex which also produces Kp^a: in other words, Kk

Kp(a+) cells may react only weakly with anti-k. This caused an extra difficulty in the pioneer work[16].

The antigen Kp^a has not, as far as we know, been found in Negroes.

The antigen Kp^b

The antithetical antigen recognized by anti-Kp^b is present in all samples so far tested except (1) those homozygous for Kp^a, (2) those heterozygous for Kp^a and heterozygous for the negative condition to be described below, and (3) those homozygous for this negative condition. All three have actually been observed, as proven by family investigations following on the finding of Kp(b−) random people.

Tests with anti-Kp^b on large numbers of random samples were done with the original serum (Rautenberg) which also contains anti-K. In tests on 5,500 Whites Allen et al.[26] found two negative (one subsequently proved to be homozygous for Kp^a and the other heterozygous for Kp^a and the negative condition). In tests on 7,251 white people Cleghorn[28], also using Rautenberg, found one negative (it was subsequently proved to be homozygous for the negative condition for it gave the reaction K−k−Kp(a−b−)). In tests on a further 6,830 Bostonians Walker et al.[38] found no negative. Chown and his colleagues[40], again using Rautenberg but checking some K+ samples with an anti-Kp^b thought not to contain anti-K, found no Kp(b−) in testing 1,277 white Manitobans; however, the 274 Kp(a+) Manitobans[87] of Table 48 provided 5 examples of Kp(a+b−).

Js^a AND Js^b

The antigen Js^a, discovered by Giblett[8] in 1958, looked like the herald of a new system. The antibody, anti-Js^a, was made by a white patient, Mr Sutter, who had been transfused. His serum sensitized the cells of about 20 % of negro donors but did not sensitize the cells of any of 240 white donors originally tested. This obviously important negro antigen was shown to be a dominant character.

Frequency of Js^a in Negroes

The three substantial series of tests on American Negroes are shown in Table 49. The heterogeneity is just significant ($\chi^2 = 6.7$ for 2 d.f.) and probably reflects differences of white admixture. Nevertheless, if the three series are pooled they give the following gene frequencies, $Js^a = 0.0828$, $Js^b = 0.9172$, which agree quite well with the frequencies calculated from the pooled results of tests with anti-Js^b also shown in Table 49, $Js^a = 0.0949$, $Js^b = 0.9051$.

The antigen Js^a was not found in Asians[10], in Eskimos[56], in North American Indians[56], in unmixed West Venezuelan Indians[57]. Giblett and Chase[10] ultimately tested nearly 500 Whites without finding a single Js(a+). (Curiously, we found one in the first 50 Whites we tested, but have not found another in many hundreds of tests since.)

Table 49. Frequency of Js^a and Js^b in Negroes

		Number tested	Js(a+)	Proportion Js(a+)
United States				
Giblett and Chase[10]	Seattle	440	86	0·1955
Stroup et al.[11]	Memphis	614	86	0·1400
Jarkowski et al.[52]	Detroit	244	34	0·1393
Congo				
Fraser et al.[53]	various tribes	660	106	0·1606
Fraser et al.[53]	Pygmies	126	6	0·0476

		Number tested	Js(b−)	Proportion Js(b−)
United States				
Walker et al.[54]	Memphis	1,001	12	0·0120
Walker et al.[54]	Milwaukee	268	1	0·0037
Huestis et al.[55]	Chicago	460	3	0·0065
Crawford[85]	Philadelphia	2,049	18	0·0088

Inheritance of Js^a

Since the original report[10] relatively few families have been published[58-63, 11]. The first four papers made clear that the Js^a antigen was genetically independent of all the established systems except P, Lutheran and Kell, for which there was, at that time, no information.

The antigen Js^b

The existence of the antigen Js^b, antithetical to Js^a, was established by Walker, Argall, Steane, Greenwalt, Sasaki and Can[63, 54, 64] when they found an antibody in the serum of a Js(a+) negro woman who had four Js(a+) children, and was therefore probably homozygous Js^{a}Js^a. The antibody failed to react with the cells of two donors who were sisters and presumed to be Js^{a}Js^a because their pooled ten children were all Js(a+). The specificity was consolidated when the serum was tested against the cells of 1,269 Negroes of whom 13 were negative and of these negatives 12 could be tested with anti-Js^a and all were found positive. Frequencies are given in Table 49.

One of the families tested by Walker et al.[54] showed the Js locus to be genetically independent of P: this left only Lutheran and Kell to be excluded before Js could be considered a new marker on the human chromosomes, a distinction which, as shown by its inclusion in this chapter, it never achieved. However, anti-Js^a and anti-Js^b make twice as useful a distinction between negro people as do anti-K, anti-k, anti-Kp^a and anti-Kp^b among white people.

Js joins the Kell system

That the 'allelic' antigens Js[a] and Js[b] belong to the Kell system was first realized by Stroup, MacIlroy, Walker and Aydelotte[11] in 1965. The primary and illuminating observation was that the cells of Mrs Peltz and Mrs Kan., the two K–k–Kp(a–b–) people described below, were Js(a–b–). Considering the rarity of Js(a–b–) this association could not possibly be a coincidence. Subsequently, five more examples of K–k–Kp(a–b–) were tested and found to be Js(a–b–).

Finally, Stroup and her colleagues embarked on a most arduous and successful genetical investigation which showed that the *Js* locus of Giblett was indeed closely, if not absolutely, linked to the *Kell* locus. First, they had to find K+ Negroes, and in testing 4,079 they found 61 (K+ incidence 0·015) and a further 14 K+ were already known to them. Of these 75 K+ Negroes six were Js(a+) and the families of five of them were tested. Three were of three generations and two were of two generations. The three-generation families gave very solid evidence of linkage between *Kell* and *Js* by including five non-recombinants; the linkage was not absolute because of one child who was apparently a recombinant, but possibly extra-marital. That this child probably was extra-marital was made more likely by the further evidence of the two two-generation families and by four two-generation families reported by Morton, Krieger, Steinberg and Rosenfield[62].

THE ANTIGEN Ul[a]

In Helsinki in 1967 a 'new' antibody, called anti-Ul[a], was found in the serum of a transfused man (Furuhjelm, Nevanlinna, Nurkka, Gavin, Tippett, Gooch and Sanger[88], 1968). Of 2,620 Helsinki blood donors 2·6% were Ul(a+); but the frequency was higher in certain Finnish isolates—up to 5%. Only one Ul(a+) was found among 501 Swedish people and none in 140 Lapps, 314 non-Scandinavian Whites, 66 Negroes, or in 5,000 Oxford[118] donors.

Tests on about 350 members of the families of 18 propositi showed that Ul[a], as expected, is a dominant character. Segregation in the families excluded *Ul[a]* from belonging to the loci for most of the blood group systems, but there was no information about Kell, because K+ is rather rare in Finland. So what proved to be a long search for K+Ul(a+) was begun: in the end three informative families were found[89] and they showed that *Ul[a]* belongs to the *Kell* complex locus, the lod score at $\theta = 0·00$ being 3·311. As Furuhjelm *et al.*[89] pointed out, this could be an indication of very close linkage rather than membership of the complex locus but they conclude 'On the other hand, and this cannot be expressed in figures, when it is known that a blood group locus is near to *Kell*, which has taken into its grasp so many antigens, the chance must be high that Ul[a] will be claimed by this complex'. 'It may therefore be assumed that the antigen Ul[a] is controlled from the *Kell* locus but there is yet no hint about the part of the locus responsible: Ul(a+) K+ k+ and Ul(a+) Kp(a+b+) samples gave no unusual reactions that might have tied *Ul[a]* to the *K* or the *Kp* series. The relationship of *Ul[a]* to the *Js* mutational site or sites will be very difficult to explore, for Js^a is almost confined to Negroes and Ul^a to Finns. If anti-Ul^b were to be found, then Ul would add a fourth series of alleles to K, Kp and Js.'

THE ANTIGENS Wk^a (WEEKS) AND CÔTÉ (K11)

The admirable investigation of an antibody to an antigen of low frequency, Wk^a, was described by Strange, Kenworthy, Webb and Giles[90] in 1974. The patient's antibody had been stimulated, about 10 years earlier, by transfusion of blood from a donor, Mr Weeks.

Frequency of the antigen Wk^a

In testing the patient's serum against 11,076 samples from blood donors in Bristol and Oxford 32 were found to be Wk(a+), a frequency of 0·3 %. It was observed that none of the 32 was K+. K+ k+ cells were then focused on and in testing 6,956 only 7 Wk(a+), or 0·1 %, were found, a significant difference from the unselected samples. In testing approximately 1,000 Kp(a+) Oxford donors none was found to be Wk(a+).

Family tests

These showed Wk^a to be a dominant character and to rule out close linkage of Wk^a with the loci for ABO, MNSs, Rh, Lutheran, Kidd and secretor. The families of 5 K+k+Wk(a+) propositi were tested and showed beautifully that Wk^a is part of the Kell system: there was no recombination on any of 13 occasions when it might have happened, and the alignment was, in each family, k with Wk^a.

Relationship of Wk^a to the antigen Côté (K11)

In 1971, Guévin, Taliano and Waldmann[100] described an antibody, anti-Côté, which had reacted with all cells tested save K_0, the maker's own cells and those of two of her eight sibs. The new antigen defined by this antibody (later given the number anti-K11) was in the limbo of what we are now calling para-Kell antigens and had been contrasted with two others there by Heistø et al.[101] (1973). Other examples of the rare Côté negative, K:−11, cells and of the antibody were subsequently found[103, 117].

But when the two unrelated Côté negative (K:−11) samples available to Strange et al.[90] were found to be strongly Wk(a+) it became clear that Wk^a and Côté (K11) were antithetical antigens. Their genetical background may be represented thus:

	Wk^a	anti-Côté (K11)
$Wk^a Wk^a$	+	−
$Wk^a Wk$	+	+
$Wk Wk$	−	+

The allelic relationship was confirmed by tests with anti-Wk^a on further unrelated K:−11 people and on the family of one of them (Stroup[117], 1974). In old fashioned terms *Wk* would be called *Wk^b*.

So Wk promotes the Côté (K11) antigen from its once para-Kell standing into the structural Kell system proper, and so adds a fourth allelic pair to *Kk*, *Kp^{a}Kp^b* and *Js^{a}Js^b*.

K$_0$, THE PHENOTYPE K−k− Kp(a−b−) Js(a−b−)

Chown, Lewis and Kaita[17] (1957) uncovered a new phenotype, K−k− Kp(a−b−), named K$_0$ for short, in two Canadian sisters of Polish extraction whose parents were second cousins: the propositus (Peltz) was brought to notice because of an antibody, named anti-Ku, in her serum which reacted with all K+ or k+ samples.

Kaita, Lewis, Chown and Gard[29] later found another example (Kan.) in a family of Finnish descent whose parents were first cousins. This second example was found as the result of a deliberate search in which 10,838 samples were tested with the anti-Ku serum of the first propositus. The pedigrees of both families were given in a later communication[37]. The third example was that found by Cleghorn and mentioned in the section on 'The antigen Kp^b', above: here too the parents were first cousins.

The observation that the cells of two K$_0$ propositi (Peltz and Kan.) were also Js (a−b−) was the prime step in placing the Js groups in the Kell system (page 290).

We now know of 14 K$_0$ propositi about whom there is family information: some details of these people and their relatives are to be found in Table 50. As Chown and his colleagues[17,29] originally supposed, the phenotype is clearly a recessive character: the sib count is very close to the expected 1:3 ratio and the consanguinity rate of the parents of the propositi is high. Incidentally, the parents and children of the propositi do not disclose themselves as heterozygotes by any dosage effects with anti-k or anti-Kp^b sera[29,50,92], though it seems they may do with anti-Kx, an eluate to be described in the antibody section below.

It was assumed that the gene responsible for the K$_0$ phenotype was an allele at the *Kell* complex locus (rather than an independent suppressor gene) because several families had been found which could only be interpreted by the postulation of such an allele, in the heterozygous state, producing no K, k, Kp^a or Kp^b antigen[16,26,30,31]. This was confirmed by the family in Table 50 reported by Nunn, Giles and Dormandy[50] in which the parents of a K$_0$ propositus were K−k+ and K+k−, and, further, a sib was K+k−. And again it was confirmed by the family reported by Lombardo, Britton, Hannon and Terry[94] in which the propositus was K$_0$, her husband K+k+ and one child K+k− and two others K−k+. We think that these two families alone provide solid evidence that K$_0$ is controlled from the *Kell* complex.

We tend to think of *K^0* as a rare allele at an operator site which switches off all activity at the *Kell* structural loci.

Table 50. The families of K_0 propositi

	Propositus	Ascertainment	Sibs (--)	Sibs (others)	Spouse	Children	Father	Mother	Consanguinity
Chown et al.[17,37]	Mrs Peltz, Canadian (Polish), her K_0 sister	anti-Ku in serum	1	2 (-+)	-+	2 (-+)	-+	-+	2nd cousins
Kaita et al.[29,37]	Mrs Kan. Canadian (Finnish), her K_0 brother	negative with Peltz serum	1	4 (-+)	-+ / -+	2 (-+) / 3 (-+)	d	-+	1st cousins
Cleghorn[28]	Miss Lim. English	negative with anti-Kp^b	0	0	-+	2 (-+)	d	d	1st cousins
Humphreys et al.[51]	David Sc. (aet. 4) Canadian Indian	anti-Ku in serum	0	0			-+	-+	uncertain
Kenny and Menichino[78]	Mrs Quat. American (Italian)	anti-Ku in serum	3	0	-+	2 (-+)	-+	+-	no
Nunn et al.[50]	Mrs Co. English	anti-Ku in serum	0	1 (++) / 1 (+-)	-+	3 (-+)	-+	-+	no
v.d. Hart[67]	Mr v.d. Laa. Dutch	anti-Ku in serum	1	4 (-+)			-+	-+	no
v.d. Hart[67]	Mr Dink. Dutch	anti-Ku in serum	0	3 (-+)			-+	-+	no
Kout[79]	Mrs J.D. Czechoslovak	anti-Ku in serum	0	1 (-+)	-+	2 (-+)	-+	d	no
Kuze and Scott[82]	Baby John M. Canadian (Sicilian)	anti-Kp^b in serum	0	1 (-+)			-+	-+	no
Garris[83]	Mr Sul. American (Russian)	anti-Ku in serum							
Simmons and Young[93]	Female Australian	anti-Ku in serum	1	3 (-+)					1st cousins
Hamilton and Nakahara[92]	Male Japanese	routine grouping	1	3 (-+)	-+	3 (-+)	d	d	possible
Lombardo et al.[94]	Female American (Italian) her K_0 brother	anti-Ku in serum	1	6 (-+)	++ / -+	1 (+-) / 2 (-+) / 6 (-+)	d	d	probable
			9	29					
		expected (1:3)	9.5	28.5					

-- = K-k-Kp(a-b-) and, when tested, Js(a-b-); -+ = K-k+Kp(a-b+); ++ = K+k+Kp(a-b+); +- = K+k-Kp(a-b+).

All but three of the propositi in Table 50 were brought to notice because they had an antibody in their serum: ten had anti-Ku (the name given to the antibody which reacts with all cells except K_0), and one had anti-Kp^b.

We have seen no suggestion that the phenotype K_0 is associated, as Rh_{null} is, with a defect of the red cell surface.

Frequency of the phenotype K_0

By 1963 Chown and his colleagues[40] had tested, with the anti-Ku serum of Mrs Peltz, 16,518 samples of red cells from random white people and had found only the one negative (Mrs Kan. of Table 50). This indicated that the phenotype frequency in Whites was of the order of 0·00006 and the gene frequency about 0·008.

Further tests, capable of detecting K_0, on 24,953 white people can be extracted from the literature[28, 26, 9, 5, 38]: only one K_0 was found, which corresponds to a frequency of 0·00004 and a gene frequency of about 0·006.

In testing 14,541 Japanese, Hamilton and Nakahara[92] found one K_0, an incidence of 0·00007 corresponding to a gene frequency of about 0·008.

EVIDENCE OF FURTHER COMPLEXITY

The fairly straightforward facts about the Kell complex dealt with so far in this chapter are summarized in Table 51. Some rare complications, included in Table 52, must now be faced.

Depressed Kell antigens

McLeod

In 1961, Allen, Krabbe and Corcoran[65] encountered a new phenotype: the cells of the propositus, McLeod, failed to react with a reagent prepared from the Peltz serum and were found to react outstandingly weakly with anti-k and anti-Kp^b; they did not react with anti-K or anti-Kp^a. McLeod's cells did react, very weakly, with the native Peltz serum[66, 11] and with another anti-Ku serum[50]. After Js was seen to belong to Kell[11], McLeod's cells were found to give an unusually weak reaction also with anti-Js^b. So the McLeod phenotype (Table 52) may be written

$$K-kw \; Kp(a-bw) \; Js(a-bw)$$

but we do not know of any convincing evidence that the phenotype is controlled from the *Kell* cistron rather than from some separate inhibitor or regulator locus or, indeed, whether it is genetic rather than environmental. The propositus however is a normal healthy person.

The parents of McLeod are not consanguineous, are of the most frequent Kell phenotype, K−k+ Kp(a−b+), and gave no clue to the genetic background of the McLeod phenotype.

Table 51. Notations for the *Kell* genes and their corresponding antigens. (Based on a table by Allen and Rosenfield[36], 1961)

Symbols as used in this chapter	Genes Short symbols (a)	(b)	Catalogue notation	Antigens produced K / K1	k / K2	Kp^a / K3	Kp^b / K4	Ku / K5	Js^a / K6	Js^b / K7	Approximate gene frequency in American Whites	Negroes
K Kp^b Js^b	K	K^b	K$^{1,-2,-3,4,5,-6,7}$	+	−	−	+	+	−	+	0·05	<0·01
k Kp^b Js^b	k	k^b	K$^{-1,2,-3,4,5,-6,7}$	−	+	−	+	+	−	+	0·94	0·91
k Kp^a Js^b	k	k^a	K$^{-1,2,3,-4,5,-6,7}$	−	+	+	−	+	−	+	0·01	
k Kp^b Js^a	k	k^s	K$^{-1,2,-3,4,5,6,-7}$	−	+	−	+	+	+	−	v. rare	0·09
K^0 (amorph)		k^0	K^0 K$^{-1,-2,-3,-4,-5,-6,-7}$	−	−	−	−	−	−	−	<0·01	

+ = antigen produced, − = no antigen.
(a) As used by Morton et al.[62]
(b) As suggested by Chown and Lewis and introduced by Allen et al.[26]

Table 52. The reactions of Kell and para-Kell antibodies, to which are added those of anti-Ge[a]

Cell samples	\	\	\	\	Antibodies (and their allotted K numbers)										
	K 1	k 2	Kp^a 3	Kp^b 4	Ku 5	Js^a 6	Js^b 7	Ul^a 10	Wk^a 17	Côté 11	KL 9	Bøc 12	San 14	Sgro 13	Ge^a
The vast majority*	− or +	+ or −	− or +	+ or −	+	− or +	+ or −	− or +	− or +	+	+	+	+	+	+
K₀	−	−	−	−	−	−	−	−	−	−	+	−	−	−	+
McLeod	−	w or −	−	w	w or −	−	w	−	−	−	−	w	−	w	+
Some CGD patients	−	w or −	−	w or −	w or −	−	w or −	−	−	−	−	w		w	+
Elsie J. et al.	−	w	$+^{**}$	−	w	−	w	−	−	w or −	+	w	−	w	+
Côté	−	+	−	+	+	−	+	−	+	−	+	+	+	+	+
Bøc	−	+	−	+	+	−	+	−	−	+	+	−	+	+	+
San	−	$+^{w}$	−	$+^{w}$	$+^{w}$	−	+	−	−	+	+	+	−	−	+
Sgro	−	$+^{w}$	−	$+^{w}$	$+^{w}$	−	$+^{w}$	−	−	+	+	+	+	−	+
Some Ge(a−)	w	w	−	w	w	−	w	−	−	+	w	+	+	+	−

* More frequent reaction given first
** Weaker than expected of $Kp^{a}Kp^{a}$

Claas

In 1968, van der Hart, Szaloky and van Loghem[80] recorded the investigation, in 1965, of the blood of a boy, Claas, in whose serum was an antibody which did not react with his own cells but which did react with all other cells at first tested, including K_0. The boy's Kell phenotype was, like that of McLeod (Table 52),

K−kw Kp(a−bw) Js(a−bw)

A sample of McLeod's cells was sent from New York and proved to be negative with the boy's serum, unlike the cells of 6,150 Dutch donors and the cells of a select panel of Kell phenotypes including K+k− and Kp(a+b−) and Js(a+b−) and four examples of K_0.

The antibody is usually referred to as anti-KL. Absorption and elution tests suggested that anti-KL is directed mainly at the whole Kell complex of antigens in general: however, some aspects of the antibody may be more specific, for van der Hart and her colleagues[80] prepared, by absorption or elution, one fraction which reacted more strongly with K−k+ cells than with K_0 cells and another fraction which gave the converse reactions. These elution tests with the Claas serum were later repeated by Marsh et al.[95] (1974) who achieved a more useful eluate of the anti-K_0 component (see anti-Kx below).

The parents of Claas are second cousins, and, like his two sibs, are of the most frequent phenotype, K−k+ Kp(a−b+) Js(a−b+). The boy suffered from 'recurrent coccal infections' and, in the light of later events, this was suspected to have been due to chronic granulomatous disease.

Further examples of anti-KL have been found[96, 97, 112].

The corresponding antigen, KL, could be classed as a para-Kell antigen (see below). Anti-KL reacts positively with K_0 cells, believed to lack all Kell antigens: its association with Kell is only in its negative reaction with the McLeod type. That McLeod type of cells react weakly with Kell antisera should not be taken to mean that McLeod's peculiarity is associated with the *Kell* locus, because, as will be seen below, some Ge(a−) samples also react weakly with Kell antisera, and the structural loci for *Kell* and *Gerbich* are genetically separate.

Chronic granulomatous disease

In 1971, Dr Eloise Giblett and her colleagues[98] made the most circumspect observation that amongst sufferers from this disease (CGD) too many have the phenotype either K_0 or McLeod.

The question is, are these people genetically K_0 or McLeod or are their Kell antigens oppressed by the process of the disease like, for example, the A antigen in leukaemia? A question which will probably be answered by the time this book comes out. At present the only evidence that sufferers may be genetically of the McLeod type is the finding by Swanson et al.[97], that both mothers of two affected cousins have notably weak k and Kp^b antigens, and so had their maternal grandmother.

Certainly not all patients with CGD have a rare Kell phenotype but the proportion that does have it should soon be known because all of them should be fully tested for the Kell groups, since the K_0 or the McLeod phenotypes are candidates for making anti-Ku or anti-KL or anti-Kp[b], any of which would cause the greatest difficulty in the finding of donors.

Experts do not agree about the manner of inheritance of CGD. For some years it was accepted as an X-borne recessive character[113], but in 1969 a sex-modified autosomal recessive way of inheritance was suggested[114]—a view which stimulated a number of letters to the *Lancet*[115].

It would be a good mark for blood grouping if the Kell abnormality happened to be an indicator of heterogeneity in the genetical background of CGD. In the families we know about via Kell abnormality all the sufferers are boys.

Acquired haemolytic anaemia

In 1972, Seyfried *et al.*[99] reported the prolonged investigation of a boy with autoimmune haemolytic anaemia. During the disease his Kell antigens were depressed and gave the McLeod picture and anti-Kp[b] was found in his serum: after his recovery his Kell antigens were perfectly normal.

Another depressed Kell phenotype

The Kell groups of a healthy Sheffield donor, Mrs Elsie J., have been studied since 1959, by the late Dr Dunsford, Dr Darnborough and by our Unit. Her phenotype (Table 52) is

$$K-kw \; Kp(a+b-) \; Js(a-bw) \; Ul(a-) \; Ku(w)$$

Apart from a difference in the Kp phenotype her cells differ from those of the McLeod and Claas type only in that they react positively with anti-KL (with which the cells of McLeod and Claas do not react). As judged by limited tests, a sister of Mrs Elsie J. appeared to be of the same phenotype.

The cells of a maker of anti-Kp[b], Mr v. Dev., sent to us from Durban by Miss Phyllis Moores gave almost identical reactions, though the weakness of the antigens was not quite so marked in a repeat sample.

Dr Brocteur kindly allowed us to join in the investigation of a family in which the propositus, Mr L.G., was again of the same phenotype as Mrs Elsie J. This family was informative: the cells of all but the propositus gave reactions of normal strength with the range of Kell antisera but their Kp reactions, using 4 examples of anti-Kp[a] and 5 of anti-Kp[b], were instructive:

	Kp[a]	Kp[b]	genotype
Mr L.G., propositus	+	−	Kp^a/K^0
his wife	−	+	Kp^b/Kp^b
his daughter	+	+	Kp^a/Kp^b
three of his sons	−	+	Kp^b/K^0
one of his sons	+	+	Kp^a/Kp^b
his brother	+	+	Kp^a/Kp^b

The most likely interpretation seems to be that Mr L.G. and 3 of his sons are heterozygous for K^0. If this be correct, then K^0 appears to be having a depressing effect on the activity of the *Kell* genes in *trans* but only when Kp^a is numbered amongst them and not when Kp^b is.

Gerbich and Kell

In 1971 Dr André-Liardet sent us a sample of blood from a Ge(a−) white person. In the routine grouping we disagreed about the Kell groups, in France the cells were found to be K+ but we made them K−. This led to further tests and the Ge(a−) person and her Ge(a−) brother were then found to react weakly with anti-K, anti-k, anti-Kp^b and anti-Js^b (Table 52). Then Dr J. Brocteur found another white family with Ge(a−) members and they too had weak Kell antigens. Other examples are now being found, though not all Ge(a−) people have depressed Kell antigens: the problem is being investigated in several laboratories.

It should be said that *Ge* is not part of the *Kell* complex locus: the evidence depends on one of the three original families (page 418). To our comfort, Dr Carolyn Giles has recently confirmed the Kell groups of the two key people in this pedigree.

No doubt there are many causes of depressed Kell antigens. For example, we found the cells of a 12-year-old boy with a deleted short arm of chromosome 18 (18p−) to react very weakly with anti-k, -Kp^b, -Ku and -KL but normally with anti-Js^b: however, their reactions were very weak also with some antibodies outside the Kell system. A sample taken six weeks later gave the same weak reactions. The cells of another 18p− person reacted normally with all antisera.

Para-Kell antigens

As in the Lutheran system, we are using 'para' to cover a series of antigens which are certainly related to the Kell system but in a way not yet understood. The antigen KL has been dealt with above. This section deals with antibodies to 'public' antigens, antibodies which are alike in that they fail to react with K$_0$ cells, with the donor's own cells and perhaps with the cells of some of the donor's sibs, and in that they react only weakly with cells of the depressed Kell phenotypes of the McLeod, Elsie J. and chronic granulomatous disease types: they react positively with all other cells tested, including the Kell defective type of Ge(a−).

The antibodies of this kind, at the time of writing, fall into three specificities distinguished by positive reactions with the cells of the donors of the other two, as may be seen in Table 52: in 1974 Côté (K11) departed from this class of antigens when it was proved to belong to the Kell system, being produced by an allele of *Wk^a*. None of the propositi was known to have consanguineous parents. The histories make it seem likely that all the antibodies were immune. In only the last of the three classes were the Kell groups of the propositi unusual (Table 52). All the propositi are Ul(a−) so none of the antibodies could be the hypothetical anti-Ul^b.

Bøc antibody

Sometimes called[102] anti-K12, the antibody was found by Heistø and his colleagues[101] in an Oslo woman who had been transfused. Her sister's cells and those of her two children were positive with her serum. A second example[102] of the antibody was found in a negro donor, Mr Spe.: his antibody reacted positively with the cells of his mother and of his three sibs. So there is, as yet, no evidence that the corresponding antigen is an inherited character.

San antibody

This antibody, reported by Heistø and his colleagues[101] at the same time as Bøc, has, we believe, recently been named anti-K14. It was found in a white woman in South Carolina. No other member of her family was tested: so evidence is lacking that the antigen is an inherited character.

Sgro antibody, anti-K13

Found by Marsh and his colleagues[104] in a male patient of Italian parentage. The Kell phenotypes of the patient and of his one compatible sib out of five were the same as those of the other people in this section but with the difference that titration tests showed all the Kell antigens to be weaker than normal, though not so very weak as McLeod. A fine family investigation led the authors to consider that the propositus and his K:−13 sib are not homozygous for a K^{-13} allele but are heterozygous $K^{-13} K^0$: this was based on tests with anti-Kx, the antibody separated from anti-KL serum (page 297). The authors conclude that the antigen K13 probably is controlled from the *Kell* complex locus: were this to be established K13 should be removed from this para-Kell section.

THE GENETIC BACKGROUND OF THE KELL SYSTEM

So far we have treated the four allelic pairs separately, and in their application to human genetics the series are quite separate: useful distinctions are made by the *K* alleles in Whites but not in Negroes, by the *Kp* alleles occasionally in Whites and by the *Js* alleles only in Negroes. The *Wk* alleles, and Ul^a make a few useful distinctions.

The complex locus controlling the four series of 'allelic' antigens appears to echo the Rh theme. Ignoring the rare K_0 phenotype and the antigens Ul^a and Wk^a, there are eight theoretically possible gene complexes in the system and these can be paired in (8/2) (8+1) or 36 different ways. These 36 possible genotypes make 27 phenotypes which would be distinguishable with the six antisera.

Of the eight possible gene complexes only four have been isolated (see Table 51, page 295) and of the 27 possible phenotypes only nine have been found. Whether the missing pieces will ever be found is questionable, for the definitive antigens (K and Kp^a on the one hand and Js^a on the other) are almost mutually exclusive in Whites and Negroes, whose interbreeding is presumably confined to recent centuries, which would give little time for recombination to produce the informative coupling alignment of genes—K with Js^a or Kp^a with Js^a.

Allen and Lewis[16], in the original paper on Kp^a and Kp^b, said 'the weight of evidence to date indicates that K and k are alleles, and that Penney [Kp^a] and Rautenberg [Kp^b] are alleles related to K and k as E and e in the Rh family are related to C and c' and this is how we think of them now though, as we have pointed out in previous editions, there was another possible interpretation which had not, and still has not, been ruled out.

The alternative possibility was that Kp^a was to K and k as C^w is to c and C and that anti-Kp^b could be thought of as anti-Kk and the antibody made by K–k–Kp(a–b–) people as anti-KkKp^a. But, with the arrival of Js^a and Js^b in the system, this attempt at economy has rather been thrown to the winds; nevertheless the possibility should, perhaps, be kept in mind until certain alignments are found which would dispose of it (for example, K and Kp^a inherited together from one parent).

If, by any chance, K, Kp^a and k were alleles, and Js^a and Js^b were separate alleles, then we would expect six gene complexes to be possible but two of them recognizable only after many years of racial admixture. On the other hand, if, after a good long time, no Js^a has been detected in coupling with K or Kp^a and should it emerge that Js^a is an allele of K, Kp^a and k (in which case anti-k, anti-Kp^b and anti-Js^b would have to be complex antibodies) then we would expect only four gene complexes at the Kell locus all of which have already been found.

Ul^a must be considered an allele at the Kell complex, but no evidence was found[89] to tie it to the K, Kp or Js series, and the same may be said[90] of Wk^a and its allele.

K^0 may be thought of as an amorph at the Kell structural locus which produces no Kell antigens, or, if preferred, as a rare allele at the Kell operator site which has switched off all activity at its neighbouring K, Kp and Js sites. That the phenotype K$_0$ can indeed be due to homozygosity at the Kell complex rather than homozygosity at an unattached regulator locus (the background of most Rh$_{null}$ phenotypes, see page 220) is shown by two informative families[50, 94]. However, K$_0$ may eventually be seen to have, like Rh$_{null}$, more than one genetical background.

A few notes on the phylogeny of complex systems are on page 181 in the Rh chapter, they apply also to Kell. Applicable also to Kell are notes about the possible fitting of Rh to a Jacob–Monod operon pattern (pages 221 and 241).

The fitting of the antigens of Table 52 which are associated with the Kell groups but not yet shown to be controlled by the Kell locus into some general pattern is a guessing game. Without chemical support any scheme is very unlikely to be true yet may be a help to remembering the facts and a stimulus to the search for objections to it.

In our last edition we proposed a scheme 'ripe for toppling' in which an antigenic substance detected by anti-KL was given an important part. We supposed KL to be controlled by a locus X separate from Kell. The scheme has not yet

11

been demolished but it needs some bolstering in face of the insurgence of chronic granulomatous disease, the para-Kell myrmidons and the Gerbich blood group system. So we felt we should try to think of some kind of pattern that might satisfy these complexities now settling on the Kell system, and here is one attempt. Just suppose: some precursor substance, XY, is needed if the *Kell* and the unlinked *Gerbich* loci are to express themselves properly. The *Kell* alleles alter the X portion of XY into X^1 plus Kell antigens, and the allele Ge^a alters the Y portion into Y^1 plus Ge^a antigen. In some CGD sufferers the X substance is grossly altered.

Such a scheme though unlikely to be correct does accommodate some of the curious reactions given in Table 52. The McLeod phenotype may result from a defective X portion of the precursor, not necessarily the same defect as that in the CGD sufferers. The somewhat depressed Kell antigens of some Ge(a–) and some people lacking the para-Kell antigens may mean that the *Kell* alleles need precursor substance unimpaired if they are to express themselves properly.

OTHER NOTES ABOUT THE KELL SYSTEM

Kell antibodies

Anti-K (anti-K1)

Innumerable examples have been found. The vast majority are frankly immune in origin and most of them the cause of cross-matching difficulty, of reaction to transfusion or of haemolytic disease of the newborn. Three convincing examples of 'naturally occurring' anti-K are known[68, 84].

Dr Levine told us long ago that anti-K, like anti-D, is more often the cause of haemolytic disease when the father's blood is compatible with the mother's on the ABO system than when it is incompatible.

Anti-K almost always works best by the indirect antiglobulin method.

A transfusion reaction with an unusual background is reported by Zettner and Bove[69]: recipient K–; first donor compatible (but later found to have anti-K in his serum); second donor compatible, but K+; second transfusion, given a few hours after the first, followed by reaction. The patient had played the part of a test tube in a blood group determination. Another such unlucky coincidence is reported by Franciosi and his colleagues[86].

Anti-k (anti-K2)

Considering that only about two in a thousand white people are of the genotype *KK* and are candidates for making anti-k, it is not surprising that the antibody is relatively rare. We know of many examples, only some of which have been published[5, 18, 14, 19, 32–34, 70, 105–107].

It seems that the antibody is usually immune in origin: no 'naturally occurring' example has yet been reported. Like anti-K, anti-k almost always works best by the antiglobulin test: one example is recorded[71] which reacts well in saline but not at all by the antiglobulin method.

Anti-Kp^a (anti-K3)

Three examples were found in Boston[16]: the first, in the serum of Mrs Penney, appeared to be 'naturally occurring' though it reacted best by the antiglobulin test. Many examples followed. Jensen[72] reported an anti-Kp^a which caused very mild haemolytic disease of the newborn: reference was made to another, this one the result of a single transfusion.

The antibody may be less rare than it appears to be because it discloses itself only if a potential donor happens to be Kp(a+), that is, about one white donor in 50.

Anti-Kp^b (anti-K4)

The original example[26] (Rautenberg) contained anti-K as well as anti-Kp^b and so did the second[23]. Absorption of these two sera by K+k− cells removed all antibody: absorption by K−k+ cells left anti-K. At the time of the last edition we had 11 examples of anti-Kp^b in our collection; some of them were absorbed with K−k+ cells without leaving any trace of anti-K and presumably they never had it. Two others lacking anti-K were the cause of mild haemolytic disease of the newborn[30, 49]. Another two[73, 74] appeared to be 'naturally occurring' and did not work by the antiglobulin method; yet another[82] was found in a seven-month-old K_0 baby (Table 50).

A transient autoimmune[99] anti-Kp^b is noted on page 298.

Considering the rarity of Kp^aKp^a candidates for making anti-Kp^b, it is surprising how many examples have been found; perhaps this is because anti-Kp^b presents a pressing cross-matching problem: it is so easy to find blood compatible with anti-Kp^a but so hard to find blood compatible with anti-Kp^b.

Anti-Ku (anti-K5)

This is the antibody present in the serum of K−k− Kp(a−b−) Js(a−b−), or K_0, people who have been immunized. The first example was found by Chown and his colleagues[17, 35]. The antibody was presumably the result of a transfusion and it later caused haemolytic disease of the newborn. Other examples are listed in Table 50: only four of these are published[50, 92−94].

Anti-Js^a (anti-K6)

The first three examples[8, 10, 75] were found in much transfused white American males and the next two[52, 76] in much transfused American females. All five examples reacted best by the antiglobulin test and the same can be said of a further three which we have been sent for confirmation. The antibody has caused haemolytic disease of the newborn[108].

Anti-Js^b (anti-K7)

Like the first example[63, 54], the next two[55, 81] presented themselves as cross-matching problems. Fourth and fifth examples were noted by Stroup *et al.*[11] in the paper in which they show Js to be part of the Kell system. Again, all the examples react best by the antiglobulin test. As would be expected, all the patients were Negroes (the genotype *Js^{a}Js^a* must scarcely exist in Whites). We know of two further examples[47, 109], one of which[109] caused haemolytic disease of the newborn.

Anti-K^w (anti-K8)

The corresponding antigen has not, as far as we know, been shown to belong to the Kell system[41]. Issitt[116] gives a short summary of K^w and notes that further work on the K^w antigen has 'foundered somewhat on the unreliability of new examples of the antibody'.

Anti-KL (anti-K9)

The powerful antibody[80] in the serum of Claas is discussed on page 297. Several examples have now been found, all of them in patients with chronic granulomatous disease[96-98, 112], or with symptoms suggestive of it.

Anti-Ul^a (anti-K10)

This antibody does belong to the Kell system[88, 89]: it was stimulated by transfusion. A second example, again Finnish, was found six years later[110] in a much transfused sufferer from lupus erythematosus diffusus: separable anti-K was also present.

Anti-Ul^a has not yet been blamed for haemolytic disease of the newborn, nor was it found in the serum of 19 Ul(a−) mothers with Ul(a+) children[88].

Anti-Côté (anti-K11) and anti-Wk^a (anti-K17)

These two antithetical antibodies are described on page 291. Both are immune: several examples of the former[100, 103, 117] have been identified, but only one of the latter[90].

Para-Kell antibodies

These antibodies, Bøc (anti-K12), San (anti-K14) and Sgro (anti-K13) are dealt with on page 300.

Anti-Kx (anti-K15)

This is a component separated from anti-KL serum, adumbrated by van der Hart et al.[80] which Marsh et al.[95, 104] named anti-Kx. The full description[95] has not yet appeared but to quote from an earlier paper[104], 'Anti-Kx reacts strongly with K_0 red cells, gives trace reactions with cells of common Kell type and reacts with clearly recognizable intermediate strength against known heterozygous K^0 samples'.

Dosage

From various publications, or from our own records, it seems that the strength of the reactions of most antisera belonging to the Kell system reflect some dosage effect of the alleles K, k, Kp^a, Kp^b, Js^a and Js^b. However, the analysis of dosage in the Kell system will no doubt prove as difficult as it is in Rh, where the alignment of the genes, both in cis and in trans, complicates the problem: a first hint was given by the observation that the k antigen is weak when the genes k and Kp^a are together in cis[16] (though this weak reaction is said to become of normal strength if the auto-analyser is used[62]). Also, the rare depressed antigens queer dosage distinctions.

Anti-Kx has been used[95] to detect heterozygosity for K_0.

Development

The K and k antigens are developed at birth. Since anti-K is such a potent cause of haemolytic disease it was not surprising that the antigen K was found well developed in a foetus of only 10 weeks, and in 6 others, of less than 16 weeks(Toivanen and Hirvonen[111], 1973). The antigen k was well developed in all of 50 foetuses tested, the youngest being 6–7 weeks[111]. Kp^a was well developed at birth[28], and in a foetus of 16 weeks[111]. Kp^b is well developed at birth, as are Js^a and Js^b[10, 55]. Js^a has been found in a 19 week negro foetus[28].

The simple distinction between K+ and K− remains clinically the most important division between white people to be made within any blood group system except ABO and Rh. At the serological and genetical level Kell is now seen to rival in complexity the ABO, MNSs, P, Rh and Lutheran systems.

REFERENCES

[1] COOMBS R.R.A., MOURANT A.E. and RACE R.R. (1946) In-vivo isosensitization of red cells in babies with haemolytic disease. Lancet, i, 264–266.
[2] RACE R.R. (1946) A summary of present knowledge of human blood groups with special reference to serological incompatibility as a cause of congenital disease. Brit. Med. Bull., 4, 188–193.

3   MOURANT A.E. Unpublished observations.
4   WIENER A.S. and SONN-GORDON EVE B. (1947) Réaction transfusionnelle hémolytique
    intra-group due a un hémagglutinogène jusqu'ici non décrit. *Rev. Hémat.*, **2**, 1–10.
5   LEVINE P., BACKER MAY, WIGOD M. and PONDER RUTH (1949) A new human hereditary
    blood property (Cellano) present in 99·8% of all bloods. *Science*, **109**, 464–466.
6   SANGER RUTH, BERTINSHAW DOREEN, LAWLER SYLVIA D. and RACE R.R. (1949) Les groupes
    sanguins humains Kell: fréquences géniques et recherche génétiques. *Rev. Hémat.*, **4**,
    32–35.
7   RACE R.R., SANGER RUTH and THOMPSON JOAN S. (1953) Quoted in 2nd edition of this
    book but not elsewhere published.
8   GIBLETT ELOISE R. (1958) Js, a 'new' blood group antigen found in Negroes. *Nature, Lond.*,
    181, 1221–1222.
9   LEWIS MARION, CHOWN B. and PETERSON R.F. (1955) On the Kell-Cellano (K-k) blood
    group: the distribution of its genes in the white population of Manitoba. *Amer. J. phys.
    Anthrop.*, **13**, 323–330.
10 GIBLETT ELOISE R. and CHASE JEANNE (1959) Js^a, a 'new' red cell antigen found in Negroes;
    evidence for an eleventh blood group system. *Brit. J. Haemat.*, **5**, 319–326.
11 STROUP MARJORY, MACILROY MIJA, WALKER R. and AYDELOTTE JANE V. (1965) Evidence
    that Sutter belongs to the Kell blood group system. *Transfusion, Philad.*, **5**, 309–314.
12 LEVINE P., WIGOD M., BACKER A. MAY and PONDER RUTH (1949) The Kell-Cellano (K-k)
    genetic system of human blood factors, *Blood*, **4**, 869–872.
13 HEIKEN A. (1962) Distribution of the Kell blood group factor K in the Swedish population,
    Acta genet., **12**, 352–358.
14 SHAPIRO M. (1952) Observations on the Kell-Cellano (K-k) blood group system with ex-
    amples of anti-K and anti-k. *S. Afr. med. J.*, **26**, 951–955.
15 ALLEN F.H. (1958) A new antigen in the Kell blood group system. *Proc. 6th Congr. int. Soc.
    Blood Transf.* 106–109.
16 ALLEN F.H. and LEWIS SHEILA J. (1957) Kp^a (Penney), a new antigen in the Kell blood group
    system, *Vox Sang.*, **2**, 81–87.
17 CHOWN B., LEWIS MARION and KAITA HIROKO (1957) A 'new' Kell blood group phenotype,
    Nature, Lond., **180**, 711.
18 LEVINE P., KUCHMICHEL A.B. and WIGOD M. (1952) A second example of anti-Cellano
    (anti-k). *Blood*, **7**, 251–254.
19 CRAWFORD HAL. (1953) A third example of the blood group antibody anti-k. *J. clin. Path.*,
    6, 52–53.
20 SALMON C. (1961) Unpublished observations.
21 RACE R.R., SANGER RUTH and MOORES PHYLLIS (1957) Quoted in 3rd and 4th editions of
    this book but not elsewhere published.
22 MOHR J. (1956) To what extent has linkage between various human blood group systems
    been excluded? *Acta genet.*, **6**, 24–34.
23 SCUDDER J., SARGENT MARY, CAHAN A., SANGER RUTH and RACE R.R. (1957) Unpublished
    observation.
24 LINNET-JEPSEN P., GALATIUS-JENSEN F. and HAUGE M. (1958) The inheritance of the Gm
    serum groups. *Acta genet.*, **8**, 164–196.
25 GALATIUS-JENSEN F. (1958) On the genetics of the haptoglobins. *Acta genet.*, **8**, 232–247.
26 ALLEN F.H., LEWIS SHEILA J. and FUDENBERG H. (1958) Studies of anti-Kp^b, a new antibody
    in the Kell blood group system. *Vox Sang.*, **3**, 1–13.
27 LEWIS MARION, KAITA HIROKO, DUNCAN DAWNA and CHOWN B. (1960) Failure to find
    hypothetic K^a (KKp^a) of the Kell blood group system. *Vox Sang.*, **5**, 565–567.
28 CLEGHORN T.E. (1961) Unpublished observations.
29 KAITA HIROKO, LEWIS MARION, CHOWN B. and GARD EILEEN (1959) A further example of
    the Kell blood group phenotype K–, k–, Kp(a–b–). *Nature, Lond.*, **183**, 1586.
30 ANDERSON LOIS, WHITE J.B., LILES BOBBIE, CAHAN A., SEPSON R. and JACK J.A. (1958) A

case of hemolytic disease of the newborn due to pure anti-Kp[b]. *Program.*, Amer. Ass. Blood Banks. There is no page number.

31 DUNSFORD I., BARBER MARGARET, HUTH MARGARET C. and WILSON T.E. (1959) A blood lacking the expected k antigen. *Vox Sang.*, 4, 148–152.

32 HEISTÖ H., VOGT ELSE and HEIER ANNA M. (1957) A case of anti-Cellano, P.H. Andresen Papers in dedication of his sixtieth birthday. Munksgaard, Copenhagen, 80–81.

33 INNELLA FILOMENA P., BOYD C.R. and STANSELL G.B. (1956) A case of anti-Cellano. *Blood,* 11, 641–647.

34 LANG B.G. and LODGE T.W. (1961) Anti-K[b] (Cellano) detected on routine ABO and D typing of donor bloods. *Vox Sang.*, 6, 353–356.

35 CORCORAN PATRICIA A., ALLEN F.H., LEWIS MARION and CHOWN B. (1961) A new antibody, anti-Ku (anti-Peltz), in the Kell blood group system. *Transfusion, Philad.*, 1, 181–183.

36 ALLEN F.H. and ROSENFIELD R.E. (1961) Notation for the Kell blood group system. *Transfusion, Philad.*, 1, 305–307.

37 CHOWN B., LEWIS MARION, KAITA HIROKO, NEVANLINNA H.R. and SOLTAN H.C. (1961) The pedigrees of two people already reported as of phenotype K–, k–, Kp(a–b–). *Vox Sang.*, 6, 620–623.

38 WALKER MARY E. and sixteen others (1961) Tests with some rare blood group antibodies. *Vox Sang.*, 6, 357.

39 KORNSTAD L., HALVORSEN K., JUEL E., WEISERT O., ØRJASAETER H. and ØSTGÅRD P. (1966) The frequency of the blood group antigen K in the Norwegian population. *Acta genet.*, 16, 231–238.

40 CHOWN B., LEWIS MARION, KAITA HIROKO and PHILIPPS SYLVIA (1963) Some blood group frequencies in a Caucasian population. *Vox Sang.*, 8, 378–381.

41 BOVE J.R., JOHNSON M., FRANCIS B.J., HATCHER D.E. and GELB A.G. (1965) Anti-K[w] defining a new antigenic determinant. Program AABB 18th Ann. Meeting, Florida, p. 60.

42 HEIKEN A. (1965) On the inheritance of the Kell blood group system. *Acta path microbiol. scand.*, 65, 255–258.

43 LINNET-JEPSEN P. (1965) *Undersogelser over Gm(a) faktoren. Specielt i det forste levear.* M.D. Thesis, Aarhus Universitet, pp. 256.

44 MOHR J. (1966) Genetics of fourteen marker systems: associations and linkage relations. *Acta genet.*, 16, 1–58.

45 V.D. WEERDT CHRISTINA M. (1965) *Platelet Antigens and Iso-immunization.* Doctoral Thesis, 'Aemstelstad', Amsterdam, pp. 108.

46 GREUTER W., HESS M., RENAUD N., SCHMITTER M. and BÜTLER R. (1963) Beitrag zur Genetik des Gm- und Gc-Serumgruppensystems anhand von Untersuchungen an Schweizerfamilien. *Arch. Klaus-Stift. VererbForsch.* 38, 77–92.

47 MARSHALL G. (1968) Another example of anti-Js[b]. *Vox Sang.*, 14, 304–306.

48 LEWIS MARION, CHOWN B. and KAITA HIROKO (1963) Inheritance of blood group antigens in a largely Eskimo population sample. *Amer. J. hum. Genet.*, 15, 203–208.

49 WRIGHT J., CORNWALL SHEILA M. and MATSINA EDA (1965) A second example of hemolytic disease of the newborn due to anti-Kp[b]. *Vox Sang.*, 10, 218–221.

50 NUNN HILARY D., GILES CAROLYN M. and DORMANDY KATHARINE M. (1966) A second example of anti-Ku in a patient who has the rare Kell phenotype, K[o]. *Vox Sang.*, 11, 611–619.

51 HUMPHREYS PATRICIA A., MOORE B.P.L. and CHOWN B. (1963) Unpublished observations.

52 JARKOWSKI T.L., HINSHAW C.P., BEATTIE K.M. and SILBERBERG B. (1962) Another example of anti-Js[a]. *Transfusion, Philad.*, 2, 423–424.

53 FRASER G.R., GIBLETT E.R. and MOTULSKY A.G. (1966) Population genetic studies in the Congo. III. Blood groups (ABO, MNSs, Rh, Js[a]). *Amer. J. hum. Genet.*, 18, 546–552.

54 WALKER R.H., ARGALL C.I., STEANE E.A., SASAKI T.T. and GREENWALT T.J. (1963) Js[b] of the Sutter blood group system. *Transfusion, Philad.*, 3, 94–99.

[55] HUESTIS D.W., BUSCH SHIRLEY, HANSON MARY LU and GURNEY C.W. (1963) A second example of the antibody anti-Js^b of the Sutter blood group system. *Transfusion, Philad.*, **3**, 260–262.

[56] CORCORAN PATRICIA A., ALLEN F.H., ALLISON A.C. and BLUMBERG B.S. (1959) Blood groups of Alaskan Eskimos and Indians. *Amer. J. phys. Anthrop.*, **17**, 187–193.

[57] LAYRISSE M. and LAYRISSE ZULAY (1959) Frequency of the new blood group antigen Js^a among South American Indians. *Nature, Lond.*, **184**, 640.

[58] LAYRISSE M., SANGER RUTH and RACE R.R. (1959) The inheritance of the antigen Di^a: evidence for its independence of other blood group systems. *Amer. J. hum. Genet.*, **11**, 17–25.

[59] BARNICOT N.A., GARLICK J.P. and ROBERTS D.F. (1960) Haptoglobin and transferrin inheritance in northern Nigerians. *Ann. hum. Genet.*, **24**, 171–183.

[60] ROSENFIELD R.E., HABER GLADYS V., SCHROEDER RUTH and BALLARD RACHEL (1960) Problems in Rh typing as revealed by a single Negro family. *Amer. J. hum. Genet.*, **12**, 147–159.

[61] ROSENFIELD R.E., HABER GLADYS V., SCHROEDER RUTH and BALLARD RACHEL (1960) A Negro family revealing Hunter-Henshaw information, and independence of the genes for Js and Lewis. *Amer. J. hum. Genet.*, **12**, 143–146.

[62] MORTON N.E., KRIEGER H., STEINBERG A.G. and ROSENFIELD R.E. (1965) Genetic evidence confirming the localization of Sutter in the Kell blood-group system. *Vox Sang.*, 10, 608–613.

[63] WALKER R.H., ARGALL C.I., STEANE E.A., SASAKI T.T. and GREENWALT T.J. (1963) Anti-Js^b, the expected antithetical antibody of the Sutter blood group system. *Nature, Lond.*, **197**, 295–296.

[64] GREENWALT T.J., WALKER R.H., ARGALL C.I., STEANE E.A., CAN R.T and SASAKI T.T. (1964) Js^b of the Sutter blood group system. *Proc. 9th Congr. int. Soc. Blood Transf.*, Mexico 1962, 235–237.

[65] ALLEN F.H., KRABBE SISSEL M.R. and CORCORAN PATRICIA A. (1961) A new phenotype (McLeod) in the Kell blood-group system. *Vox Sang.*, **6**, 555–560.

[66] LEWIS MARION (1966). Personal communication.

[67] VAN DER HART MIA (1965) Unpublished observation.

[68] MORGAN P. and BOSSOM EDITH L. (1963) 'Naturally occurring' anti-Kell (K1): two examples. *Transfusion, Philad.*, **3**, 397–398.

[69] ZETTNER A. and BOVE J.R. (1963) Hemolytic transfusion reaction due to inter-donor incompatibility. *Transfusion, Philad.*, **3**, 48–51.

[70] SCHMIDT P.J., MCGINNISS MARY H., LEYSHON W.C. and KEVY S.V. (1958) An anti-k (anti-Cellano) serum with the properties of a complete saline agglutinin. *Vox Sang.*, **3**, 438–441.

[71] THOMAS MARTHA J. and KONUGRES ANGELYN A. (1966) An anti-K2 (Cellano) serum with unusual properties. *Vox Sang.*, **11**, 227–229.

[72] JENSEN K.G. (1962) Haemolytic disease of the newborn caused by anti-Kp^a. *Vox Sang.*, **7**, 476–478.

[73] DARNBOROUGH J. and DUNSFORD I. (1959) Personal communication.

[74] MCNEIL C. and NEWMAN MARY (1966) Personal communication.

[75] MUIRHEAD E.E. (1961) Unpublished observations.

[76] GERARD MARIAN (1965) Another example of anti-Js^a. *Transfusion, Philad.*, **5**, 359.

[77] RACE R.R. and SANGER RUTH (1962) *Blood Groups in Man*, 4th edition, p. 223, Blackwell Scientific Publications, Oxford.

[78] KENNY J.J. and MENICHINO R.H. (1964) Unpublished observations.

[79] KOUT M. (1966) Personal communication.

[80] HART MIA V.D., SZALOKY AGNES and VAN LOGHEM J.J. (1968) A 'new' antibody associated with the Kell blood group system. *Vox Sang.*, **15**, 456–458.

[81] CAHAN A. (1963) Personal communication.

[82] KUZE MARTA and SCOTT MARION (1967) Unpublished observations.

83 GARRIS MARY LOU (1967) Unpublished observations on sample referred by South Nassau Hospital, Oceanside, N.Y.

84 TEGOLI J., SAUSAIS LAIMA and ISSITT P.D. (1967) Another example of a 'naturally occurring' anti-K1. *Vox Sang.*, **12**, 305–309.

85 CRAWFORD MARY N. (1967) Personal communication.

86 FRANCIOSI R.A., AWER ERICA and SANTANA M. (1967) Interdonor incompatibility resulting in anuria. *Transfusion, Philad.*, **7**, 297–298.

87 DICHUPA P.J., ANDERSON CATHERINE and CHOWN B. (1969) A further search for hypothetic K^p of the Kell system. *Vox Sang.*, **17**, 1–4.

88 FURUHJELM U., NEVANLINNA H.R., NURKKA RIITTA, GAVIN JUNE, TIPPETT PATRICIA, GOOCH ANN and SANGER RUTH (1968) The blood group antigen Ul^a (Karhula). *Vox Sang.*, **15**, 118–124.

89 FURUHJELM U., NEVANLINNA H.R., NURKKA RIITTA, GAVIN JUNE and SANGER RUTH (1969) Evidence that the antigen Ul^a is controlled from the Kell complex locus. *Vox Sang.*, **16**, 496–499.

90 STRANGE J.J., KENWORTHY R.J., WEBB A.J. and GILES C.M. (1974) Wk^a (Weeks), a new antigen in the Kell blood group system. *Vox Sang.*, **27**, 81–86.

91 LEWIS MARION, KAITA H. and CHOWN B. (1969) The inheritance of the Kell blood groups in a Caucasian population sample. *Vox Sang.*, **17**, 221–223.

92 HAMILTON H.B. and NAKAHARA Y. (1971) The rare Kell blood group phenotype K$_0$ in a Japanese family. *Vox Sang.*, **20**, 24–28.

93 SIMMONS R.T. and YOUNG N.A.F. (1968) The rare Kell blood group K–k– Kp(a–b–) or K$_0$ with anti-Ku antibody found in an Australian woman. *Med. J. Aust.*, **2**, 1040–1041.

94 LOMBARDO JOSEPHINE M., BRITTON SUSAN J., HANNON GISELLA and TERRY DOLORES (1972) K$_0$ in a sister and brother, a family study. Abstracts AABB and ISH Meeting, Washington p. 59.

95 MARSH W.L., ØYEN RAGNHILD and ALLEN F.H. (1974) Kx; a leukocyte and red cell antigen associated with the Kell system. In preparation.

96 STROUP MARJORY (1968) Personal communication.

97 SWANSON J., PARK B. and McCULLOUGH J. (1972) Kell phenotypes in families of patients with X-linked chronic granulomatous disease. Abstracts AABB and ISH Meeting, Washington, p. 26.

98 GIBLETT ELOISE R., KLEBANOFF S.J., PINCUS STEPHANIE H., SWANSON JANE, PARK B.H. and McCULLOUGH J. (1971) Kell phenotypes in chronic granulomatous disease: a potential transfusion hazard. *Lancet* i, 1235–1236.

99 SEYFRIED HALINA, GÓRSKA BARBARA, MAJ S., SYLWESTROWICZ T., GILES CAROLYN M. and GOLDSMITH K.L.G. (1972) Apparent depression of antigens of the Kell blood group system associated with autoimmune acquired haemolytic anaemia. *Vox Sang.*, **23**, 528–536.

100 GUÉVIN R.M., TALIANO V. and WALDMANN OTILIA (1971) The Côté serum, an antibody defining a new variant in the Kell system. Amer. Ass. Blood Banks, Program, 24th Annual Meeting, p. 100.

101 HEISTØ H., GUÉVIN R.-M., TALIANO V., MANN JULIA, MACILROY MIJA, MARSH W.L., TIPPETT PATRICIA and GAVIN JUNE (1973) Three further antigen-antibody specificities associated with the Kell blood group system. *Vox Sang.*, **24**, 179–180.

102 MARSH W.L., STROUP MARJORY, MACILROY MIJA, ØYEN RAGNHILD, REID MARION E. and HEISTØ H. (1973) A new antibody, anti-K12, associated with the Kell blood group system. *Vox Sang.*, **24**, 200–205.

103 MOORTHY ARA (1973) Personal communication.

104 MARSH W.L., JENSEN LEILA, ØYEN RAGNHILD, STROUP MARJORY, GELLERMAN MIJA, McMAHON F.J. and TSITSERA HELEN (1974) Anti-K13 and the K:–13 phenotype: a blood-group variant related to the Kell system. *Vox Sang.*, **26**, 34–40.

11*

[105] HOPKINS D.F. (1970) Saline agglutinating anti-K and anti-k in the apparent absence of IgM antibody. *Brit. J. Haemat.*, **19**, 749–753.

[106] KLUGE A. and JUNGFER H. (1970) Anti-K2 (Cellano) blood group antibodies. *Blut*, **21**, 357–365.

[107] CHOJNACKA-JACHIMIAK IRMINA, SEYFRIED HALINA and KOZIOLOWA HALINA (1971) An unusual case of isoimmunization by D, Cellano (k) and Duffy (Fy^b) antigens. *Arch. Immunol. Ther. Exp.*, **19**, 585–591.

[108] DONOVAN L.M., TRIPP K.L., ZUCKERMAN J.E. and KONUGRES A.A. (1973) Hemolytic disease of the newborn due to anti-Js^a. *Transfusion, Philad.*, **13**, 153.

[109] WAKE E.J., ISSITT P.D., REIHART J.K., FELDMAN R. and LUHBY A.L. (1969) Hemolytic disease of the newborn due to anti-Js^b. *Transfusion, Philad.*, **9**, 217–218.

[110] FURUHJELM U. (1973) Personal communication.

[111] TOIVANEN P. and HIRVONEN T. (1973) Antigens Duffy, Kell, Kidd, Lutheran and Xg^a on fetal red cells. *Vox Sang.*, **24**, 372–376.

[112] POOLE JOYCE (1972) A new example of anti-KL. *Med. Lab. Tech.*, **29**, 62–65.

[113] WINDHORST DOROTHY B., HOLMES BEULAH and GOOD R.A. (1967) A newly defined X-linked trait in man with demonstration of the Lyon effect in carrier females. *Lancet*, **i**, 737–739.

[114] CHANDRA R.K., COPE W.A. and SOOTHILL J.F. (1969) Chronic granulomatous disease. Evidence for an autosomal mode of inheritance. *Lancet*, **ii**, 71–74.

[115] EDWARDS J.H. (1969) Inheritance of chronic granulomatous disease. *Lancet*, **ii**, 850–851.

[116] ISSITT P.D. (1970) Applied Blood Group Serology. Published by Spectra Biologicals, p. 78.

[117] STROUP MARJORY (1974) Personal communication.

[118] BOWELL P.J. and STRANGE J.J. (1974) Personal communication.

Chapter 8
Secretors and Non-secretors

It was some time after the discovery of the ABO groups before it was realized that the antigens were not confined to the red cells but were widely distributed throughout the body. In 1910 Moss[1] demonstrated their presence in serum, though he misinterpreted the phenomenon, which was later shown by Schiff[2] to be due to the presence of antigen, and not anti-antibody, as Moss had thought.

Yamakami[30], in 1926, noted that the antigens A and B were present in saliva; but not till 1930 was it realized, by Lehrs[3] and Putkonen[4], that the character was dimorphic and that there were non-secretors as well as secretors. The ability to secrete the A, B or O antigen in the saliva was shown by Schiff and Sasaki[5] to be inherited as a Mendelian dominant character. The genes responsible are not linked to the *ABO* genes.

Friedenreich and G. Hartmann[6, 7], who studied the problem deeply, concluded that there were two distinct forms of the antigens: (1) A water soluble form not present in the red cells or serum but present in most of the body fluids and organs of a secretor. The presence of this water soluble antigen is determined by the secretor gene; (2) An alcohol soluble form of the antigen, present in all the tissues (except the brain) and in the red cells, but not present in the secretions. The alcohol soluble form is not influenced by the secretor gene.

Grubb[10] showed that the secretor phenomenon is very closely associated with the Lewis blood groups; but this aspect will be dealt with in Chapter 9.

The few subsequent facts discovered about secretion appear to conform with the views of Friedenreich and Hartmann. These facts include the *Xx* genes of Levine *et al.*[11] now usually referred to as *Hh* genes (page 22) and the *Yy* genes of Weiner *et al.*[12] (page 27). The role of the *Yy* genes is not so firmly established as that of the *Hh* genes, being based on a few families only: in the very rare genotype *yy* it appears that A is inhibited on the red cells but that the amount of A in the saliva is only slightly reduced. Chimeras (Chapter 26) have contributed also.

To be a secretor of A, for example, a person must have grown from a zygote containing:

1   At least one *A* gene. Zygotes of the genetic constitution *OO* have later acquired, by grafting (see twin chimeras, page 520), plenty of *A* genes in the marrow and perhaps elsewhere, and group A red cells in the circulation but do not secrete A.

2   At least one *Se* gene. To secrete more than traces of A a person must have started life as a zygote containing at least one *A* gene and at least one *Se* gene. A twin chimera which began life as a zygote containing an *A* gene and two *se* genes has later acquired plenty of *Se* genes in his marrow but he does not secrete A.

3   At least one *H* gene. There is, so far, information only about B people who, to be secretors, must have started life as zygotes containing at least one *H* gene. A person of the 'Bombay' type (see page 21) was of the genotype *BO, Sese*, yet she secreted no B because she lacked an *H* gene. (Unfortunately none of the families which has so far showed the inhibitory effect of *hh* on A in the red cells is capable of proving that the action of *Se* on A is, as expected, also inhibited.)

4   What is more, the *A* gene, the *Se* gene and, presumably the *H* gene must all be in the same cell. The dispermic chimera from Detroit[56, 57] (page 538) first made the present authors appreciate this point. Previously we had casually supposed that given an *Se* gene any ABH antigen around (which was not a mere graft, as in chimera twins) would be secreted: we had not pictured the interaction between the two genetically independent loci going on at the cellular level. Later, other dispermic chimeras (page 538) demonstrated this point equally clearly.

A very satisfying scheme suggesting the order in which these genes act will be found in the chapter on Lewis (Figure 22, page 342).

It seems that it should be possible to wring some information about the sphere of action of the secretor genes from a remarkable case of partial triploidy[52]: a girl whose red cells were group O and whose saliva contained B and H substance (page 540).

FREQUENCIES

In our second edition we showed that the distinction between secretors and non-secretors could be difficult to make: the then published figures for Europe varied with different workers[5, 7, 13–16] and varied with different ABO groups for the same workers. This had previously been realized by Formaggio[14] and by Andersen[15]. The main difficulty had been the classifying of group O saliva because good anti-H sera were hard to find. This was overcome by the observation of Cazal and Lalaurie[18] that saline extracts of the seeds of *Ulex europaeus* (gorse) contain a powerful anti-H; Boyd and Shapleigh[19] showed that the extract is excellent for classifying group O salivas: it can also be used (with certain reservations, see page 315) for classifying salivas of other groups.

A fine example of random people classified for ABH secretion is to be found in the controls of the Liverpool peptic ulcer investigations. These controls were unselected for ABO groups: *Ulex* was used and all samples found to be non-secretor, if from people of group A_1, A_1B, or B, were checked with anti-A or anti-B. The results were reported at succeeding totals[31, 50] but a later total was kindly given to us by Dr R.B. McConnell and this is used in Table 53.

Table 53. Secretor tests on the saliva of 1,118 random 'control' persons in Liverpool. (Data provided by Dr R.B. McConnell)

	Male	Female	Total	
		secretors		
O	211	219	430	
A	180	150	330	864 or 0·7728
B	48	35	83	
AB	12	9	21	
		non-secretors		
O	59	62	121	
A	51	48	99	254 or 0·2272
B	13	16	29	
AB	3	2	5	

Using the figures given in Table 57 the gene frequencies are:

$$se = \sqrt{0 \cdot 2272} = 0 \cdot 4767$$
$$Se = 1 - 0 \cdot 4767 = 0 \cdot 5233$$

and the genotype frequencies are:

$$Se\ Se = Se^2 = 0 \cdot 2739 \text{ or } 35 \cdot 4\%$$
$$Se\ se = 2 \times Se \times se = 0 \cdot 4989 \text{ or } 64 \cdot 6\% \text{ of all secretors}$$
$$se\ se = se^2 = 0 \cdot 2272$$

The frequencies are very close to those calculated by Glynn, Glynn and Holborrow[55] on the basis of tests with *Ulex* on the saliva of 669 Middlesex schoolchildren ($se = 0 \cdot 4783$, $Se = 0 \cdot 5217$). Nor did Lincoln and Dodd's[54] English series differ significantly, but they did find a significantly higher incidence of nonsecretors in Scotland and Ireland (they used anti-A, anti-B and *Ulex* in all tests). In a series of 3,144 University of Washington students tested by van Arsdel[32], using *Ulex* only, the proportion of non-secretors was 0·2411. The saliva of very many people in very many parts of the world has been tested for anthropological purposes and the reader is referred to Mourant *et al*[70]. The differences are very wide: we have seen accounts of non-secretors being 1% or less in Amerindians and 40% in Negroes.

INHERITANCE

The ability to secrete the ABH antigens in the saliva is a straightforward dominant character. In previous editions we gave tables showing the proportion of children expected from the various genotype and phenotype matings but this no longer seems necessary. Nor does it seem necessary to repeat the family data which went to proving the manner of inheritance though perhaps the references may be useful; they are: 15, 17, 21–23, 33–37, 51, 58, 59. The families tested since the discovery of *Ulex* must be the more reliable because of the easier classification of group O people. However, in both earlier and later series the results combine to show that secretor is a dominant character as Schiff and Sasaki[5] said in 1932. For example, for our last edition we collected from the literature 66 non-sec. × non-sec. matings with 194 children all of whom were non-secretors.

The amount of A, B or H antigen secreted is, in part, under genetic control: this is mentioned below.

Linkage relations of the *secretor* locus

The *secretor* locus is on the same chromosome as the *Lutheran* locus and they are close together. This was the first reward of a long search for autosomal linkage in man; these two linked loci were later joined by a third, that for myotonic dystrophy. The subject is returned to in Chapter 27. Linkage of marker characters with inherited diseases had long been thought of as a future tool in prognosis, but this had particular implication in that the secretor state of a young foetus can be determined from the amniotic fluid[71].

The brilliant contention of Grubb[27] (1951) that the secretor and Lewis genes though so intimately associated are nevertheless independent genetically was established by Ceppellini[24–26] and others[38, 37].

OTHER NOTES ABOUT ABH SECRETION

Development

The A, B and H antigens are well developed in the saliva of newborn babies[28, 29, 53]. Indeed, of foetuses of 35–40 mm, i.e. about 9 weeks old, Szulman writes[60] 'The primitive salivary gland cords acquire lumens in which there are blebs of secretion rich in antigen': in non-secretors there was no antigen.

As noted above the presence or absence of ABH antigens, in the proportion expected for secretors and non-secretors, can be determined in the amniotic fluid of early foetuses: Harper *et al.*[71] tested 68 samples from foetuses ranging from 9 to 24 weeks with a mean age of 17 weeks.

Secretor tests

The method we use is simple, and we claim no originality for it. From an adult we like to have 0·5 c.c. or more of saliva. A very small cotton wool swab held in Spencer-Wells forceps can conveniently be used to absorb saliva from a baby's mouth. The wet swab is then squeezed, by the forceps, and drops expressed into a small tube. If the swab is too large the squeezing simply forces the saliva into another part of the swab. With patience, neat saliva can often be collected; if this is not achieved the wet swab is squeezed in 0·5 c.c. of saline. The samples of saliva are heated in a boiling water bath for ten minutes, centrifuged hard, and the almost clear supernatant fluid removed and kept at −20°C. until it is to be tested.

This cotton wool method of collecting saliva from infants seems all right for ABH secretor tests but there is a strong hint that it is no good for Le^a secretion tests (see footnote to Table 58, page 333).

When the testing is a matter of routine, rather than the investigation of a secretion problem, we add to three tubes containing a volume of the saliva, diluted 1 in 2 in saline, a volume of anti-A, anti-B and anti-H (*Ulex*): after a few minutes a volume of A$_2$, B and O cells (about 2% suspension) is added to the appropriate tubes and we read the results any time after an hour at room temperature: absence of agglutination shows that the saliva is from a secretor. Known secretor and non-secretor salivas are tested in parallel, as controls.

The dilution of anti-A, anti-B or *Ulex* used is the one before the last to give good macroscopic agglutination in titrations with A$_2$, B or O cells respectively. We are careful to use anti-A and anti-B from donors whose antibody has not been 'boosted' by injections of blood group substance. (As far as we know most routine American anti-A and anti-B are 'boosted' while most British are not.)

We use A$_2$ cells for testing for inhibition of anti-A; in common with other workers we have found them to be a more sensitive index of inhibition than A$_1$ cells.

If *Ulex* extract alone is used to classify saliva from people of all groups it is wise to check the A$_1$, A$_1$B and B non-secretors with anti-A or anti-B.

When the problem is one of secretion we titrate the saliva and add a constant amount of antibody to each tube: the inhibition titre gives some idea of the amount of antigen secreted. A more sensitive method, which shows that non-secretors have a little of their blood group substance in their saliva, is to titrate the antiserum and add to each tube a constant amount of saliva. The subject is treated in detail by Wiener[21]. The more sensitive method is useful when looking for antigen in small amounts, as, for example, in urine.

On page 56 we referred to the varied sources of anti-H reagents; several of them have been used in secretor investigations: *Ulex europaeus*[31−34, 36, 37, 46, 55], human[35], eel[39], fowl[47, 48], *Lotus tetragonolobus*[43−45], *Cytisus sessilifolius*[46] and *Laburnum watereri*[49]. Grundbacher[88] records work on the H substance of saliva and of serum with precipitating anti-H lectins from various seeds and using Ouchterlony plates. Prokop and Geserick[90] describe a precipitin test for A and B in saliva, using *Helix pomatia* and *Evonymus europaea* respectively.

The amounts of A, B and H in the saliva of secretors

Whether the amount of A antigen in the saliva of A secretors differs according to their subgroup has, surprisingly, proved a difficult question. The answer probably depends on the kind of anti-A used for the inhibition test:

i   No or very little difference: Wiener and Kosofsky[8], using human immune anti-A and rabbit immune anti-A. Baer, Kloepfer and Rasmussen[61], using immune chicken anti-A precipitin. Hakim and Bhatia[62], using Lima bean and human anti-A (eluate from A_2 cells). Holburn and Masters[89] by radio-immunoassay.

ii   More in A_1, than in A_2 saliva: Gammelgaard[9], using human anti-A; the order of strength fell through A_1, A_2 and A_3. Boettcher[63], using human anti-A selected 'for no suggestion of "boosting"' by pregnancy or by injection. Boettcher[68, 69] using *Dolichos* as well. Hakim and Bhatia[62] using *Dolichos*. Randeria and Bhatia[72] using human anti-A. Sturgeon *et al.*[73] using commercial anti-A in an automated system.

In an important paper Clarke, McConnell and Sheppard[33] describe the results of measuring the amount of A, B and H antigen in secretors and in their secretor sibs. The following is a transcript of their summary:

'1   The sib pair data suggest that the amount of A, B or H antigen secreted by an individual is in part inherited.

2   Most of the inherited component of the variance in antigen secreted appears to be polygenic.

3   The data confirm that group O people secrete more H substance than do group A people who, in turn, secrete more than group B people, and that group AB people secrete least of all. This suggests that there may be a difference between homozygotes and heterozygotes of groups A and B with regard to the amount of H secreted.

4   The ratio of A:H secreted appears to be in part controlled genetically.

5   The distribution of the ratio of A:H substance in group A secretors indicates that many of the so-called aberrant secretors are really the arbitrarily chosen extremes of a continuous and unimodal distribution of ratios. If this be so, aberrant secretors should be defined as individuals whose A:H or B:H ratio falls more than a given number of standard deviations from the mean of the control group. Such a definition would allow people in different places, using different antisera, to compare their results.'

They considered that their method of titration distinguished two phenotype groups, secretor and non-secretor, which behaved as if controlled by a single pair of genes: that is to say, the traditional view of the genetic background was supported. They suggested that the doubts on this score raised by Morganti and his fellow workers[39–42] were due to the use of a titration method which was not capable of making a clear distinction between the two phenotypes.

The 'aberrant secretors' referred to in the summary quoted above had been described by McNeil and his co-workers[43–45] who, using *Lotus tetragonolobus* extract as anti-H, found that 'there is a respectable number of human beings of blood group A and B who secrete H, but not A or B and sometimes *vice versa*. We have yet to find a secretor of H who does not secrete an expected A or B when using *Ulex* and non-immune anti-A and anti-B. It seems that much of the aberrant trouble is due to the particular anti-H reagent used: how variable are the reactions of the different seed extracts was well demonstrated by Randeria and Bhatia[72,74].

Boettcher[69] agreed with Clarke *et al.*[33] that aberrant secretors are people with very different rates of production of antigens controlled by the *H* and the *ABO* locus.

Plato and Gershowitz[46] used *Ulex europaeus* and *Cytisus sessilifolius* in parallel to measure the amount of H in saliva. Both extracts agreed that O secretor saliva contains the most H, followed by A_2, A_1, B and AB. However, O and A_2 secretors gave a much higher titre of H when measured by *Ulex* than when measured by *Cytisus*, while B and AB secretors gave a higher titre with *Cytisus* than with *Ulex*: A_1 secretors gave about the same titre with both fluids. In a later paper[64] these quantitative tests for H are applied to families: the statistical analysis of the measurements led the authors to conclude, as Clarke, McConnell and Sheppard[33] had done, that the *amount* of antigen was under genetic control and influenced by genes other than those at the secretor locus. This also was the conclusion of Giusti *et al.*[75].

Boettcher[69], Randeria and Bhatia[72] and Sturgeon *et al.*[73] all agreed with Plato and Gershowitz[46] that the amount of H, as measured by *Ulex*, in secretor saliva descended in the order O, A_2, A_1, B. Boettcher[69] pointed out that this order differs from that given by red cells when measured for agglutination by *Ulex*, O, A_2, B, A_1.

Wolf and Taylor[66] found the amount of blood group substance to be greater in saliva from the sublingual than from the submandibular or parotid glands, and Milne and Dawes agreed[87].

A Japanese family is recorded in which several members are Le(a+) *and* secretors; furthermore they secrete A but not H. The condition has also been observed in Thais (see page 326).

A Negro of group AB was found during the course of his osteogenic sarcoma to have a much diminished A on his red cells and to have B and H but not A substance in his saliva[67].

Homozygous and heterozygous secretors

We know of two attempts to make a serological distinction between saliva from homozygous and heterozygous secretors: neither has been completely successful. Matsunaga[47] thought that *SeSe* saliva was more effective than *Sese* at inhibiting a fowl anti-H serum. We did not understand how the difference in ABO groups could be allowed for; it may be that the investigation was confined to group O salivas: the paper is in Japanese but with an English summary.

Kaklamanis, Holborow and Glynn[65] based their method on the ratio of Le^a to H substance in the saliva of group O secretors. The Le^a: H ratio was low in *SeSe Lele* and high in *Sese LeLe*; thus in these two groups (representing about 50% of all secretors) the homozygous secretors could be distinguished from the heterozygous. Medium ratios, about 1:1, were given by *SeSe LeLe* and *Sese Lele* so in these two groups the secretor zygosity could not be determined serologically.

However, Chung *et al.*[76] and Kelso[77] could not make the partial distinction between homozygotes and heterozygotes claimed by Kaklamanis *et al.*[65].

Secretor and disease

A great deal of work has established an association between secretor and three conditions:

1 Duodenal ulcer, too many group O non-secretors (Clarke *et al.*[31]).

2 Rheumatic carditis, too many non-secretors (Glynn *et al.*[85, 55], 1956, 1959; Clarke *et al.*[81], 1960; Glynn and Holborow[82], 1969).

3 Alcoholism, too many non-secretors (Camps and Dodd[83], 1967; Camps *et al.*[84], 1969). This remarkable association is not yet quite so firmly established as that with the two previous complaints; it is being actively investigated.

Immunoglobulins and secretor

Grundbacher and Shreffler[78] (1970) detected higher levels of IgG immunoglobulin and of haemolytic anti-B in the serum of secretors compared with non-secretors. The Lewis groups came into it, as expected, and the difference between secretors and non-secretors was more pronounced in Le(a—b—) people.

On the other hand, Trentleman[79] (1968) had found that Le(a+) people (non-secretors) after immunization achieved higher titres of anti-A than did Le(a—) people (mostly secretors).

In tests on 202 white people Grundbacher[86] (1972) found IgA concentrations to be significantly lower in non-secretors than in secretors.

Other blood group antigens in saliva

The antigens Le^a and Le^b are present in appropriate saliva (Chapter 9) and so is the antigen Sd^a (Chapter 17) but there is no evidence of the presence of any of the other blood group antigens. The terms secretor and non-secretor apply only to the antigens A, B and H.

The *secretor* locus

The *secretor* locus can be thought of as a 'regulator' locus which controls the expression of *H* at the site of synthesis of the glycoproteins in the secretions and hence the expression of *A* and of *B*.

We used to think that the secretor genes had no direct effect on red cells, until Gardas and Koscielak[80] (1971) found A and B antigens in both glycolipid and glycoprotein extracts of stroma from secretors but only in the glycolipid extracts from non-secretors.

Though its relation to the *ABO*, *Hh* and *Lewis* genes is complicated, the secretor:non-secretor distinction is a clear genetic marker and it shares with the Lutheran antigens the credit of providing the first example in man of autosomal linkage and of autosomal crossing-over.

REFERENCES

1   Moss W.L. (1910) *Folia Serol.*, **5**, 267. (Quoted from Wiener[21].)
2   Schiff F. (1924) Uber gruppenspezifische Serumpräcipitine. *Klin. Woch.*, **3** (16) 679–680.
3   Lehrs H. (1930) Uber gruppenspezifische Eigenschaften des menslichen Speichels. *Z. ImmunForsch.*, **66**, 175–192. (See ref. 20.)
4   Putkonen T. (1930) Uber die gruppenspezifischen Eigenschaften verschiedener Korperflussigkeiten. *Acta Soc. Med. fenn.*, '*Duodecim*', A, **14**, No. 12, 113 pages. (See ref. 20.)
5   Schiff F. and Sasaki H. (1932) Der Ausscheidungstypus, ein auf serologischem Wege nachweisbares mendelndes Merkmal. *Klin. Woch.*, **11**, 1426–1429. (See ref. 20.)
6   Friedenreich V. and Hartmann Grethe (1938) Uber die Verteilung der Gruppenantigene im Organismus der sogenannten 'Ausscheider' und 'Nichtausscheider'. *Z. ImmunForsch.*, **92**, 141–151. (See ref. 20.)
7   Hartmann Grethe (1941) *Group Antigens in Human Organs*, Munksgaard, Copenhagen. (See ref. 20.)
8   Wiener A.S. and Kosofsky I. (1941) Quantitative studies on the group-specific substances in human blood and saliva. II. Group specific substance A, with special reference to the subgroups. *J. Immunol.*, **42**, 381–393.
9   Gammelgaard A. (1942) *Om Sjaeldne, Svage A-Receptorer* (A_3, A_4, A_5 og A_x) *Hos Mennesket*, Arnold Busck, Kjøbenhavn. (See ref. 20.)
10 Grubb R. (1948) Correlation between Lewis blood group and secretor character in man. *Nature, Lond.*, **162**, 933.
11 Levine P., Robinson Elizabeth, Celano M., Briggs Olive and Falkinburg L. (1955) Gene interaction resulting in suppression of blood group substance B. *Blood*, **10**, 1100–1108.
12 Weiner W., Lewis H.B.M., Moores Phyllis, Sanger Ruth and Race R.R. (1957) A gene, *y*, modifying the blood group antigen A. *Vox Sang.* **2**, 25–37.
13 Simmons R.T., Semple N.M. and Graydon J.J. (1951) The Lewis (Le^a) blood group and secretor types. A review: their correlation in the blood and saliva of white Australians. *Med. J. Aust.*, **1**, 105–110.
14 Formaggio T.G. (1951) Ricerche sullo sviluppo e l'eliminazione delle proprietà gruppali. Nota III—Diversita di distribuzione del tipo 'secretore' nei gruppi sanguigni A.B.O. *Minerva Medicolegale*, **71**, pages 1–20 (in reprint).
15 Andersen A. (1952) Investigations in the inheritance of the characters secretor and non-secretor. *Acta path. microbiol. scand.*, **31**, 448–461.
16 Thompson Joan S. (1953) Unpublished data.
17 Moharram I. (1943) The group properties in the saliva of the Egyptian population. *Laboratory and Medical Progress*, **4**, 1–13.
18 Cazal P. and Lalaurie M. (1952) Recherches sur quelques phyto-agglutinines spécifiques des groupes sanguins ABO. *Acta haemat.*, **8**, 73–70.
19 Boyd W.C. and Shapleigh Elizabeth (1954) Separation of individuals of any blood group into secretors and non-secretors by use of a plant agglutinin (lectin). *Blood*, **9**, 1195–1198.
20 Translations of these papers have been published by the Blood Bank Center, U.S. Army Medical Research Laboratory, Fort Knox, Kentucky, 40121.
21 Wiener A.S. (1943) *Blood Groups and Transfusion*, 3rd edition, Thomas, Springfield.
22 Race R.R., Sanger Ruth, Lawler Sylvia D. and Bertinshaw Doreen (1949) The Lewis blood groups of 79 families. *Brit. J. exp. Path.*, **30**, 73–83.
23 Chown B. and Lewis Marion (1955) The inheritance of the blood group and secretor genes in the Blood Indians of Alberta, Canada. *Amer. J. phys. Anthrop.* **13**, 473–478.
24 Ceppellini R. and Siniscalco M. (1955) Una nuova ipotesi genetica per il sistema Lewis-Secretore e suoi riflessi nei riguardi di alcune evidenze di linkage con altri loci. *Revista dell'Istituto Sieroterapico Italiano*, **30**, 431–445. (See ref. 20.)

25 CEPPELLINI R. (1955) Nuova interpretazione sulla genetica dei caratteri Lewis eritrocita e salivari derivante dall'analisi di 87 famiglie. Supplement to: *La Ricerca Scientifica*.

26 CEPPELLINI R. (1955) On the genetics of secretor and Lewis characters: a family study. *Proc. 5th Congr. int. Soc. Blood Transf.* Paris, 207–211.

27 GRUBB R. (1951) Observations on the human group system Lewis. *Acta path. microbiol. scand.*, **28**, 61–81.

28 WIENER A.S. and BELKIN RUTH B. (1943) Group-specific substances in the saliva of the new born. *J. Immunol.* **47**, 467–470.

29 FORMAGGIO T.G. (1951) Development and secretion of the blood group factor O in the newborn. *Proc. Soc. exp. Biol., N.Y.*, **76**, 554–556.

30 YAMAKAMI K. (1926) The individuality of semen, with reference to its property of inhibiting specifically isohemoagglutination. *J. Immunol.*, **12**, 185–189.

31 CLARKE C.A., EVANS D.A.P., McCONNELL R.B. and SHEPPARD P.M. (1959) Secretion of blood group antigens and peptic ulcer. *Brit. med. J.*, **i**, 603–607.

32 ARSDEL P.P. VAN (1958) The usefulness of the plant-lectin, *Ulex europaeus*, in a large-scale blood group study. *Vox Sang.*, **3**, 448–455.

33 CLARKE C.A., McCONNELL R.B. and SHEPPARD P.M. (1960) A genetical study of the variation in ABH secretion. *Ann. hum. Genet.*, **24**, 295–307.

34 CEPPELLINI R., DUNN L.C. and INNELLA FILOMENA (1959) Immunogenetica II. Analisi genetica formale dei caratteri Lewis con particolare riguardo alla natura epistatica dell specificita serologica Le^b. *Folia hered. path.*, **8**, 261–296.

35 SNEATH JOAN S. and SNEATH P.H.A. (1959) Adsorption of blood group substances from serum on to red cells. *Brit. med. Bull*, **15**, 154–157.

36 BIANCO IDA, SILVESTRONI E., LAWLER SYLVIA D., MARSHALL RUTH and SINISCALCO M. (1960) Further contributions to the study of Lewis and secretor characters. *Vox Sang.*, **5**, 337–348.

37 GREENWALT T.J. (1961) Confirmation of linkage between the Lutheran and secretor genes. *Amer. J. hum. Genet.*, **13**, 69–88.

38 SANGER RUTH and RACE R.R. (1958) The Lutheran-secretor linkage in Man: support for Mohr's findings. *Heredity*, **12**, 513–520.

39 MORGANTI G., CRESSERI A., SERRA A., BEOLCHINI P.E., BARBAINI S. and GIANOTTI G.A. (1959) Comparative studies on the A, B, O (H) blood substances in the saliva and the milk. *Vox Sang.*, **4**, 267–277.

40 MORGANTI G. (1959) La 'secrezione paradossa' quale causa di errore nelle determinazioni di gruppo sanguigno ABO effettuate su secreti e su sangue disseccato. Rivista di Medicina Legale e Legislazione Sanitaria, **1**, 242–248.

41 MORGANTI G. (1960) Reazioni paradossali dei sieri agglutinanti anti-A ed anti-B. *La Tranfusione del Sangue*, **5**, 83–95.

42 MORGANTI G. (1960) Recenti acquisizioni sulla secrezione delle sostanze gruppospecifiche A, B, H (O). *Rivista di Emoterapia ed Immunoematologia*, **7**, 1–42.

43 McNEIL C., TRENTELMAN E.F., KREUTZER VIRGINIA O. and FULLMER C.D. (1957) Aberrant secretion of salivary A, B, and H group substances in human beings. *Amer. J. clin. Path.* **28**, 145–151.

44 McNEIL C., TRENTELMAN E.F., FULLMER C.D., KREUTZER VIRGINIA O. and ORLOB RUTH B. (1957) The significance of blood group conflicts and aberrant salivary secretion in spontaneous abortion. *Amer. J. clin. Path.*, **28**, 469–480.

45 McNEIL C., TRENTELMAN E.F., HELMICK WILLA MAE, ORLOB RUTH and HASKELL J.G. (1960) Family blood group and secretion studies. *Vox Sang.*, **5**, 164–170.

46 PLATO C.C. and GERSHOWITZ H. (1961) Specific differences in the inhibition titers of the anti-H lectins from Cytisus sessilofolius and Ulex europaeus. *Vox Sang.*, **6**, 336–347.

47 MATSUNAGA E. (1959) Incomplete dominance of the gene for secretion of the blood group antigens in human saliva. *Jap. J. hum. Genet.*, **4**, 173–179.

48 MATSUNAGA E. and SUZUKI T. (1958) Beitrag zur Unterscheidung von Ausscheidern und Nichtausscheidern mittels Agglutinationshemmungsversuches unter besonderer Berücksichtigung der Vererbung. *Jap. J. hum. Genet.*, **3**, 1–8.

49 SPEISER P., BAUMGARTEN K. and KASERER O. (1954) Untersuchungen über die Sekretion von Blutgruppensubstanzen im Speichel und in Tumorflüssigkeiten. *Z. ImmunForsch.*, **111**, 168–176.

50 MCCONNELL R.B. (1960) The mechanism by which blood group antigens influence gastrointestinal disorders. *Proc. int. Cong. Gastroenterologv*, 41–45.

51 LAWLER SYLVIA D., MARSHALL RUTH and ROBERTS D.F. (1960) The Lewis and secretor characters in the Fulani and Habe. *Ann. hum. Genet.*, **24**, 271–282.

52 ELLIS J.R., MARSHALL RUTH, NORMAND I.C.S. and PENROSE L.S. (1963) A girl with triploid cells. *Nature, Lond.*, **198**, 411.

53 LAWLER SYLVIA D. and MARSHALL RUTH (1961) Lewis and secretor characters in infancy. *Vox Sang.*, **6**, 541–554.

54 LINCOLN P.J. and DODD BARBARA E. (1972) Variation in secretor and Lewis type frequencies within the British Isles. *J. Med. Genet.*, **9**, 43–45.

55 GLYNN A.A., GLYNN L.E. and HOLBOROW E.J. (1959) Secretion of blood-group substances in rheumatic fever. A genetic requirement for susceptibility? *Brit. med. J.*, **ii**, 266–270.

56 BEATTIE KATHRYN M., ZUELZER W.W., MCGUIRE DELORES A. and COHEN FLOSSIE (1964) Blood group chimerism as a clue to generalized tissue mosaicism. *Transfusion, Philad.*, **4**, 77–86.

57 ZUELZER W.W., BEATTIE KATHRYN M. and REISMAN L.E. (1964) Generalized unbalanced mosaicism attributable to dispermy and probable fertilization of a polar body. *Amer. J. hum. Genet.*, **16**, 38–51.

58 PRICE EVANS D.A., DONOHOE W.T.A., BANNERMAN R.M., MOHN J.F. and LAMBERT R.M. (1966) Blood groups gene localization through a study of mongolism. *Ann. hum. Genet.*, **30**, 49–67.

59 KERDE C. (1961) Cited by PROKOP O., and UHLENBRUCK G. (1963) *Lehrbuch der menschlichne Blut-und Serumgruppen.* Thieme, Leipzig.

60 SZULMAN A.E. (1965) The ABH antigens in human tissues and secretions during embryonal development. *J. Histochem. Cytochem.*, **13**, 752–754.

61 BAER H., KLOEPFER H.W. and RASMUSSEN URSULA (1961) Immunochemistry and genetics of blood group O. II. A study of the secretion of blood group A, B and O (H) substances in the saliva of family groups using precipitating antibody prepared in chickens. *J. Immunol.*, **87**, 342–350.

62 HAKIM S.A. and BHATIA H.M. (1965) Serological specificity of anti-A on the basis of inhibition reactions. *Ind. Jour. med. Res.*, **53**, 291–297.

63 BOETTCHER B. (1964) Inhibition of a human anti-A serum by salivas from A_1 and A_2 persons. *Aust. J. exp. Biol. med. Sci.*, **42**, 703–706.

64 PLATO C.C. and GERSHOWITZ H. (1962) Differences between families in the amount of salivary H substances. *Ann. hum. Genet., Lond.*, **26**, 47–50.

65 KAKLAMANIS EVANGELIA, HOLBOROW E.J. and GLYNN L.E. (1964) A method for differentiating homozygous from heterozygous secretors of ABH blood-group substances. Its application to the study of secretor status in rheumatic fever. *Lancet*, **i**, 788–790.

66 WOLF R.O. and TAYLOR L.L. (1964) The concentration of blood-group substance in the parotid, sublingual, and submaxillary salivas. *J. dent. Res.*, **43**, 272–275.

67 TEGOLI J., SANDERS C.W., HARRIS J.P. and ISSITT P.D. (1967) Unusual suppression of secretion of blood group substance A. *Vox Sang.*, **13**, 285–287.

68 BOETTCHER B. (1967) Precipitation of a substance in salivas from A_1 and A_2 secretors. *Aust. J. exp. Biol. med. Sci.*, **45**, 425–493.

69 BOETTCHER B. (1967) Correlations between inhibition titres of blood group substances in salivas from A_1, A_2 and B secretors. *Aust. J. exp. Biol. med. Sci.*, **45**, 495–506.

[70] MOURANT A.E., KOPEĆ ADA C. and DOMANIEWSKA-SOBCZAK KAZIMIERA (1974) *The Distribution of the Human Blood Groups and Other Biochemical Polymorphisms*, 2nd edition, Oxford University Press.

[71] HARPER P., BIAS WILMA B., HUTCHINSON JUDITH R. and McKUSICK V.A. (1971) ABH secretor status of the fetus: a genetic marker identifiable by amniocentesis. *J. Med. Genet.*, **8**, 438–440.

[72] RANDERIA K.J. and BHATIA H.M. (1971) Quantitative inhibition studies on the ABH and Lewis antigens in saliva. *Indian J. med. Res.*, **59**, 1737–1753.

[73] STURGEON P., McQUISTON DOROTHY and CAMP S. VAN (1973) Quantitative studies on salivary blood group substances. II. Normal values. *Vox Sang.*, **24**, 114–125.

[74] BHATIA H.M. and RANDERIA K.J. (1970) Studies on blood group antigens in saliva: incidence and type of aberrant secretors. *Indian J. med. Res.*, **58**, 194–201.

[75] GIUSTI G.V., PANARI G. and FLORIS M.T. (1972) Population and family studies on the amount of salivary ABH blood group substances. *Vox Sang.*, **22**, 54–63.

[76] CHUNG C.S., PITT E.L. and DUBLIN T.D. (1965) Heterozygous ABH secretor and susceptibility to rheumatic fever. *Amer. J. Hum. Genet.*, **17**, 352–358.

[77] KELSO J. (1968) Quantitative aspects of Lewis-secretor interaction in saliva. *Vox Sang.*, **14**, 282–288.

[78] GRUNDBACHER F.J. and SHREFFLER D.C. (1970) Effects of secretor, blood, and serum groups on isoantibody and immunoglobulin levels. *Amer. J. Hum. Genet.*, **22**, 194–202.

[79] TRENTELMAN E.F. (1968) A relationship between Lewis type and immunologic responsiveness to blood group specific substances. *Transfusion, Philad.*, **8**, 172–173.

[80] GARDAS A. and KOŚCIELAK J. (1971) A, B and H blood group specificities in glycoprotein and glycolipid fractions of human erythrocyte membrane. Absence of blood group active glycoproteins in the membranes of non-secretors. *Vox Sang.*, **20**, 137–149.

[81] CLARKE C.A., McCONNELL R.B. and SHEPPARD P.M. (1960) ABO blood groups and secretor character in rheumatic carditis. *Brit. Med. J.*, **i**, 21–23.

[82] GLYNN L.E. and HOLBOROW E.J. (1969) Blood groups and their secretion in rheumatic fever. *Rheumatology*, **2**, 113–130.

[83] CAMPS F.E. and DODD BARBARA E. (1967) Increase in the incidence of non-secretors of ABH blood group substances among alcoholic patients. *Brit. Med. J.*, **i**, 30–31.

[84] CAMPS F.E., DODD BARBARA E. and LINCOLN P.J. (1969) Frequencies of secretors and non-secretors of ABH group substances among 1,000 alcoholic patients. *Brit. Med. J.*, **4**, 457–459.

[85] GLYNN A.A., GLYNN L.E. and HOLBOROW E.J. (1956) The secretor status of rheumatic-fever patients. *Lancet*, **ii**, 759–762.

[86] GRUNDBACHER F.J. (1972) Immunoglobulins, secretor status, and the incidence of rheumatic fever and rheumatic heart disease. *Hum. Hered.*, **22**, 399–404.

[87] MILNE R.W. and DAWES C. (1973) The relative contributions of different salivary glands to the blood group activity of whole saliva in humans. *Vox Sang.*, **25**, 298–307.

[88] GRUNDBACHER F.J. (1973) Lectins in precipitin reactions with soluble H substance of human saliva and serum. *Science*, **181**, 461–463.

[89] HOLBURN A.M. and MASTERS CAROLE A. (1974) The radioimmunoassay of serum and salivary blood group A and Le^a glycoprotein. *Brit. J. Haemat.*, **28**, 157–167.

[90] PROKOP O. and GESERICK G. (1972). An 'anti-secretor'-reagent for the direct estimation of the Se-status by precipitation. *Haematologia* **6**, 135–137.

Chapter 9
The Lewis Groups

The antibody, anti-Le^a, which agglutinates the red cells of about 22% of Europeans, was described by Mourant[1], in 1946. Subsequent work has revealed a remarkable complex of interaction between the Lewis, the secretor and the ABO systems. At first the red cell antigen Le^a appeared to be a recessive character[4] but it is no longer so interpreted.

In 1948 Andresen[9] described the almost antithetical antibody anti-Le^b. Then, later in 1948, Grubb[16] made the surprising observation that persons whose red cells were Le(a+) were ABH non-secretors—a rule sometimes broken in the Orient.

Grubb[16, 10] and Brendemoen[18] independently found that the saliva of Le(a+) people strongly inhibited anti-Le^a and that the saliva of the majority of Le(a–) people also inhibited anti-Le^a but did so less strongly. Brendemoen[18] also found Le^a substance in the serum of Le(a+) persons.

In 1951 Grubb[10] proposed a general theory of the Lewis groups based on the presence or absence of the antigens of the saliva rather than of the red cells. The remarkably far-seeing ideas of Grubb were strongly supported by the very fine work of Ceppellini[8, 19, 28]. It is in the light of the theory of Grubb and Ceppellini that we now see the Lewis system.

In 1955 Sneath and Sneath[20] made the important observation that red cells lacking Le^a or Le^b will take up these antigens from plasma containing them.

The chemistry of the Lewis antigens was studied by Morgan and Watkins from the time their presence in saliva was first recognized, and this work led to the beautiful concept of the genetical pathways leading to the presence of the ABH and Lewis antigens of the red cells and saliva, a concept reached also by Ceppellini as a result of his genetical studies.

It is now clear that the antigen Le^a was in fact identified in non-secretor saliva by Japanese workers in 1939 (Ueyama[47, 51], Furuhata and Ueyama[52]) by means of a precipitin reaction with certain normal chicken sera. The antigen and antibody were called 'T' and anti-'T'. No doubt due to the war and to language difficulties the work was overlooked in the West. In the 1950s a great deal of work was done in Japan on the 'T': anti-'T' reaction and on the distribution of the 'T' antigen in the body and in body fluids. Abstracts of 13 papers were published in the Nagasaki Igakkai Zassi alone, mostly by Kitashima or by Isii. ('T' and anti-'T' must be distinguished from Friedenreich's 1930 antigen T and its antibody.)

Before looking at the Lewis and related systems as a whole it seems necessary to describe separate contributions to knowledge, some of which have led to or followed and supported the general views of Grubb and Ceppellini.

THE RED CELL ANTIGEN Le^a

Innumerable examples of anti-Le^a have now been found and the frequency of Le(a+) red cells has been determined in many races. In England[2] the frequency of Le(a+) is 22·38 % (based on a total of 1,796 tests of which 402 were positive). In almost every country of Europe the frequency has proved to be about the same[2, 3]. The incidence of Le(a+) is quite independent of the ABO groups[2].

Mourant[1] established that the Le(a+) character of red cells was inherited. Andresen[4] observed that the parents of Le(a+) persons could both be Le(a–) and therefore proposed the theory that Le(a+) was a recessive Mendelian character. (Andresen found that this was not generally true for children under the age of about eighteen months.) The theory was applied to English families tested in our Unit (those in Table 54) and the close agreement between observed and expected seemed to be overwhelmingly strong support for the theory of recessive inheritance of the red cell antigen Le^a: nevertheless, though superficially correct the recessive theory was shown to be fundamentally wrong by the brilliant work of Grubb to be described below. A consequence of Grubb's interpretation was that the mating Le(a+) × Le(a+) should produce an occasional Le(a–) child, which would have been incompatible with the recessive theory: such families were eventually found (Ceppellini and Siniscalco[28]; Ceppellini, Dunn and Innella[62]; two are to be seen in Table 54; one is recorded by Lamm et al.[130] and one was found in our Unit).

THE RED CELL ANTIGEN Le^b

Andresen[9], in 1948, described the first example of the antibody anti-Le^b which appeared to be identifying an antigen 'allelic' to Le^a. Very many examples of the antibody have now been found and most of them, like the original, give good positive reactions only if the cells being tested are group O or group A$_2$.

When tests are confined to group O and group A$_2$ samples there is general agreement[6, 10–14] that the frequencies of European phenotypes are about: Le(a+b–) 22 % and Le(a–b–) 6 % or less. In Negroes the incidence of the phenotype Le(a–b–) is considerably higher[11, 15, 62, 65, 66]—from 16 to 22%.

Anti-Le^b sera exist, as first reported by Brendemoen[21], well able to detect Le^b in the red cells of A$_1$ people. More will be said below about these two kinds of anti-Le^b.

Presumably because of the A$_1$ difficulty few genetical investigations involving red cell tests with anti-Le^b have been reported: 44 of the families of Andresen et al.[7] were tested with anti-Le^b, and so were 279 of our 464 families. Series were also tested by Jordal[67] and by Greenwalt[60].

Table 54. The antigen Le^a: tests on the red cells of white families

		Total number of matings	children	Le(a+) × Le(a+) No. of matings	Children Le(a+)	Le(a−)	Le(a+) × Le(a−) No. of matings	Children Le(a+)	Le(a−)	Le(a−) × Le(a−) No. of matings	Children Le(a+)	Le(a−)
1. Our Unit 1949–59	English	464	1,025	18	39	0	167	130	229	279	72	555
2. Andresen et al.[7], 1950	Danish	71	170	4	14	0	28	20	49	39	13	74
3. Mohr[55], 1954	Danish	75	299	3	12	0	18	28	39	54	31	189
4. Steinberg et al.[38], 1956	U.S.A.	35	106	5	15	0	14	14	33	16	5	39
5. Jordal[54], 1957	Danish	188	482	8	24	0	63	40	106	117	34	278
6. Galatius-Jensen et al.[58,59], 1958	Danish	184	431	10	26	0	58	38	99	116	24	244
7. Greenwalt[60], 1961	U.S.A.	73	340	1	5	0	21	42	52	51	30	211
8. Linnet-Jepsen[56], 1965	Danish	19	48	1	3	1	6	2	14	12	3	25
9. Mohr[105], 1966	Norwegian	127	457	3	12	0	39	50	81	85	32	282
10. Price-Evans et al.[106], 1966	English	66	132	3	6	0	26	12	40	37	5	69
		1,302	3,490	56	156	1	440	376	742	806	249	1,966
Andersen[61], 1959	Danish			7	22	1						
				63	178	2						
				exp.*	*175·7*	*4·3*						

* Expected, according to the theory of Grubb and to the frequencies of McConnell (Table 57).

Judged by the red cells only, the inheritance of Le^b was obscure: matings Le(b+) × Le(b+) produced Le(b+) and Le(b−) children, but so did matings Le(b−) × Le(b−), even when all members were group O[68, 62]. The subject is returned to on page 332.

THE RED CELL ANTIGENS Le^a AND Le^b AND ABH SECRETION

In the autumn of 1948 Dr Grubb of Lund, working at the Lister Institute, made the observation[16], which greatly added to the interest of these groups, that practically all, if not all, persons whose red cells were Le(a+) were also salivary non-secretors of A, B and H substance. All subsequent investigations on adults have confirmed this, with the exceptions to be noted below; these apart there is general agreement that in adults:

Le(a+b−) red cells belong to non-secretors
Le(a−b+) red cells belong to secretors
Le(a−b−) red cells usually, but not always, belong to secretors.

The unqualified words secretor and non-secretor refer to secretion of the antigens A, B and H.

Exceptions

That the cells of O and A$_2$ adults in certain circumstances react as Le(a+b+) was first noted by Cutbush, Giblett and Mollison[24]: their reaction with anti-Le^a was, however, feeble compared with that of Le(a+b−) cells. Other, more dramatic, exceptions are:
1 Dispermic chimeras can be secretors yet have Le(a+b−) red cells: this will be explained on pages 538 and 539.
2 In races other than white, Le(a+b+) or Le(a+b−) giving strong reactions with anti-Le^a may be secretors.

A Japanese family was reported by Lewis, Kaita and Chown[63]. Since the publication the family was retested and the Winnipeg workers kindly shared the samples with our Unit. The results from the two laboratories were in complete agreement: father, mother and eldest child A$_1$ Le(a+b+) secretors of A but not of H, Le^a in saliva (in amount about equal to that in Le(a+b−) controls and more than that in Le(a−b+) controls), Le^b in saliva; two other children A$_1$ Le(a−b−) secretors of A but not of H, no Le^a or Le^b in saliva. (For the secretor tests human and snail anti-A were used and *Ulex* and human 'Bombay' anti-H.)

Similarly in Thais Chandanayingyong et al.[116] found 11 of 34 Le(a+b−) to be secretors of A or B but not of H. Again, in two large Japanese families Sturgeon and Arcilla [126] found Le(a+b+) members who were secretors, and Boettcher and Kenny[131] found about 10% of Australian aborigines to be Le(a+b+) and secretors.

These exceptions in non-Europeans should not be allowed to upset the general scheme for the background of the Lewis antigens to be given below: they might be explained by competition between the *Le*, *Se* and *H* alleles, or variants thereof, for precursor substance just as Sturgeon and Arcilla[126], for example, invoked an allele at the *secretor* locus to explain their two Japanese families.

THE ANTIGENS Le^a AND Le^b IN SALIVA AND PLASMA

It was observed independently by Grubb[16, 10] and by Brendemoen[18] that the saliva of all persons tested whose red cells were Le(a+) strongly inhibited anti-Le^a serum. The saliva of the majority of Le(a−) persons also inhibited anti-Le^a, but did so more weakly. Grubb[10] found that the saliva of 90·2% of people contained Le^a substance. He tested 1,000 South Swedish salivas—500 from men and 500 from women.

Grubb's observation[16] that the antigen Le^a was very often present in the saliva of people whose red cells lacked it led him to think of the antigens as belonging primarily to certain body fluids rather than to red cells. In 1950 Grubb wrote[23]: 'Pour nous, le système de groupe Lewis n'est pas principalement un système de groupe *sanguin*, mais un système sérologique de mucoïds hydrosolubles.' He pointed out[10] that the concept was supported by the evidence that the Le^a antigen can be washed off Le(a+) red cells[18, 17]. (Some workers[2, 24] have not been able to confirm this—perhaps it all depends on the anti-Le^a serum used to detect the removal.)

Brendemoen[18] found that the serum from persons whose red cells are Le(a+) contains Le^a substance, while serum from Le(a−) people does not. The same observation was made, independently, by Grubb and Morgan[17] and has since been confirmed[15, 69, 70].

So far, then, it seems clear that: (1) In saliva, Le^a substance is present in more than 90% of Europeans—in greater amount in people whose red cells are Le(a+b−); those people who lack Le^a substance have Le(a−b−) red cells. (2) In serum of adults, Le^a substance is easily detectable in people whose red cells are Le(a+b−); a trace of the substance has been reported[20] in people whose red cells are Le(a−b+).

Brown, Glynn and Holborow[71] found that the antigen Le^a exists in two forms, one which is readily precipitated by rabbit anti-Le^a and one which is not; the former is found in the saliva of Le(a+b−) people and the latter in the saliva of Le(a−b+) people. The same observation was made, using chicken anti-Le^a, by Baer, Naylor, Gibbel and Rosenfield[72].

The amount of Le^a in saliva in various ABO and Lewis phenotypes has been intensively studied (Kaklamanis *et al.*[107], Kelso[132], Sturgeon *et al.*[126, 133], Boettcher and Kenny[131], Randeira and Bhatia[134]).

The puzzling fact that some Le^a substance is present in the saliva of Le(a−b−) non-secretors has recently been recorded by Gunson and Latham[125], by

Andresen[135] and by Sturgeon et al.[126]. How this is related to the type of ant-Le^a serum used as indicator, or to the Le^c antigen (page 336) is yet to be unravelled.

Less clear is the distribution of Le^b substance: there seems no doubt that it can be present both in saliva and in serum[10, 21, 15, 8, 20, 22]. Contradictory results in the literature are undoubtedly due to there being at least two kinds of anti-Le^b (see page 339). Both types of sera agree in showing that Le^b substance is present in the saliva of people whose red cells are Le(a−b+).

Other sites of Le^a

Lawler[73] found that the milk is a richer source of the Le^a substance than is the saliva in recently delivered women who have an *Le* gene.

McConnell[74] found that Le^a substance is present in gastric juice, reflecting in amount that in the saliva. More surprisingly, he found urine to be a rich source of Le^a substance.

McConnell found Le^a substance in seminal fluid and so did Lodge and Usher[108]: this is in sharp disagreement with Grubb[10] who detected no Le^a in the seminal fluid of five Le(a+) men.

None of these findings would have been surprising had the Japanese work of the 1950s, referred to early in this chapter, been accessible: the 'T' substance had there been found in saliva, serum, milk, urine, seminal fluid, amniotic fluid, meconium, gum arabic, etc. Interest in the presence of Le^a-like substance in gum arabic has recently been reawakened by Matsuzawa[122].

TRANSFORMATION OF THE LEWIS GROUPS OF RED CELLS

Sneath and Sneath[20] (1955) made the important observation that if red cells lacking Le^a and Le^b are suspended in plasma containing Le^a or Le^b they will take these antigens on board. In this respect the Lewis antigens behave like the J antigen of cattle (Ferguson, Stormont and Irwin[25, 26]), and the R antigen of sheep (Rendel, Sorensen and Irwin[101, 102]).

The phenomenon was first observed *in vivo* when blood from an Le(a+b−) donor was given to an Le(a−b+) patient. From a post-transfusion sample of the patient's blood the donor cells were recovered (by differential Rh agglutination) and they were found to have become Le(a+b+). The effect could be reproduced *in vitro* (Table 55).

So we must think of the Lewis antigens of the red cells not as being directly genetically predetermined (as are all the other known human red cell antigens) but as being passively acquired from antigens of the plasma.

The experiment of Sneath and Sneath had, in fact, been performed by Nature some 45 years before when she established the vascular anastomoses between the chimera twins later investigated by Nicholas, Jenkins and Marsh[27] (1957): from

Table 55. Reactions of red blood cells with Lewis antisera after incubation in plasma from different donors for 24 hours. (From Sneath and Sneath[20], 1955)

Plasma from persons of Lewis phenotype	Lewis substances in the plasma		Red cells of Lewis group					
			Le(a+b−)		Le(a−b+)		Le(a−b−)	
			reactions with anti-					
	Le^a	Le^b	Le^a	Le^b	Le^a	Le^b	Le^a	Le^b
Le(a+b−)	+	−	+	−	+	+	+	−
Le(a−b+)	trace	+	+	+	−	+	−	+
Le(a−b−)	−	−	+*	−	−	+*	−	−

* After three days, these reactions were extremely weak, whereas the other agglutination eactions were almost as strong as those given by fresh cells.

the published pedigree it can be seen that red cells destined, had they stayed at home, to be Le(a+b−) have grown up Le(a−b+) after emigration into a twin of that constitution; and, similarly, cells destined to be Le(a−b+) have grown up Le(a+b−).

Mäkelä and Mäkelä[22] repeated the Le^b part of the experiments of Sneath and Sneath and confirmed the results. They record some further very interesting observations: saliva from people whose red cells were Le(b+) strongly inhibited the available anti-Le^b serum (a good one) but serum from the same people would not inhibit. The transforming power, on the other hand, was the reverse of what might have been expected: the saliva would not transofrm Le(b−) cells though the serum did.

The Mäkeläs did another very ingenious experiment. They incubated the red cells of five A$_1$ Le(b−) secretors of Le^b with the plasma of a person whose red cells were A$_2$ Le(b+). All five samples of A$_1$ cells readily became Le(b+). The plasma of these five would not transform O Le(b−) cells into Le(b+). In this way they seem to have demonstrated beyond doubt that the absence or weakness of the Le^b reaction of the red cells of A$_1$ people is due to shortage of Le^b substance in their plasma rather than to reluctance of their cells to receive it. The same was shown to apply to cord blood. (This brilliant demonstration is in terms of the kind of Le^b recognized by the serum used. It may not apply to the kind of Le^b recognized by other anti-Le^b sera—such as those, first reported by Brendemoen[21], which work quite well with the red cells of A$_1$ secretors of Le^b.)

Mäkelä, Mäkelä and Kortekangas[123] studied the mechanism of adsorption of Le^a and Le^b on to red cells lacking these antigens and concluded that there was no evidence 'that enzymatic synthesis was part of the process'.

THE THEORY OF GRUBB AND OF CEPPELLINI

In 1951 Grubb[10] proposed a general theory of the Lewis groups which seemed at the time too complicated to believe, and it lacked the support of family investigations. However, in 1955, Ceppellini's family studies[8, 19, 28] were published and appeared to confirm with only minor modification the extraordinarily far-seeing ideas of Grubb (Table 56).

Grubb's fundamental observation[10] was that the Lewis groups when judged by the presence of Le^a in the saliva are independent of the presence there of the ABH antigens. Previously this true lack of association had been hidden from ordinary eyes by the rigid association of Le(a+) red cells with non-secretor saliva.

Ceppellini[8] confirmed this lack of association between the Lewis and secretor systems and so have later workers: in Table 57 it can be seen that about the same proportion of secretors have Le^a in their saliva (Les) as have non-secretors.

Ceppellini tested the saliva and red cells of 84 Ferrarese families with 262 children and showed, as had been postulated by Grubb, that the presence of Le^a in the saliva was controlled by a gene dominant in effect and independent of the secretor genes. Ceppellini called the genes L and l but he and later workers have changed to Le and le.

The essence of the theory is shown in Table 56. Although the Se se and Le le genes segregate independently (for which the evidence will be given below) they interact in some of their phenotypic effects; the interaction is needed to explain why, when Le is present, non-secretors of ABH secrete more Le^a than do secretors. Interaction is also needed to explain Le^b.

Table 56. The Lewis and ABH secretor system according to the theory of Grubb and Ceppellini

Genotypes	Antigens				
	ABH	of saliva			of red cells
		Le^a	Le^{bL}	Le^{bH}	
SeSe LeLe SeSe Lele Sese LeLe Sese Lele	+	+	+	+	Le(a−b+)
sese LeLe sese Lele	−	+	−	−	Le(a+b−)
SeSe lele Sese lele	+	−	−	+	Le(a−b−)
sese lele	−	−	−	−	Le(a−b−)

A previous discrepancy between the observations of Grubb and of Ceppellini can be attributed to their having used different kinds of anti-Le^b sera—see text.

One consequence of the theory of the Lewis groups is that an occasional Le(a+) × Le(a+) mating should produce an Le(a−) child, the mating being of the genotype $sese$ $Lele$ × $sese$ $Lele$ from which a quarter of the children should be $sese$ $lele$. Several such families have been encountered, as noted earlier in the section on Le^a in the red cells.

Table 57. The antigens Le^a and ABH in the saliva of random people

Population	Investigators	Total tested	Sec. Les	Non-sec. Les	Sec. nL	Non-sec. nL	Gene frequencies Le	le
Swedish	Grubb[10], 1951	1,000	715	187	83	15	0·6870	0·3130
			0·7150	0·1870	0·0830	0·0150		
Ferrarese	Ceppellini[8], 1955	518	374	83	50	11	0·6569	0·3431
			0·7220	0·1602	0·0965	0·0212		
Ferrarese	Bianco et al.[64], 1960	132	94	24	12	2	0·6743	0·3257
			0·7121	0·1818	0·0909	0·0152		
West Africans	Barnicot and Lawler[65], 1953	125	43	24	35	23	0·3188	0·6812
			0·3440	0·1920	0·2800	0·1840		
Charleston Negroes	Ceppellini et al.[62], 1959	236	138	44	40	14	0·5217	0·4783
			0·5847	0·1864	0·1695	0·0593		
Northern Nigerians (Fulani + Habe)	Lawler et al.[66], 1960	145	94	12	29	10	0·4813	0·5187
			0·6483	0·0828	0·2000	0·0690		
English	McConnell[74], 1961	1,000	735	231	28	6	0·8156	0·1844
			0·7350	0·2310	0·0280	0·0060		

Les = Le^a present; nL = Le^a absent.

The place of Le^b in the system is less certain and this is probably the cause of the alternative theories of the Lewis groups to be mentioned below. However, it is now generally agreed that anti-Le^b sera give two patterns of reaction in inhibition tests (see Table 56, and page 339) while behaving alike in their reactions with red cells, at any rate of group O and A_2. Grubb[10] was using anti-Le^{bH} and naturally assumed Le^b to be a direct product of the gene Se. Ceppellini[8] used anti-Le^{bL} and considered Le^b a product of the action of the genes Se and Le.

A consequence of Ceppellini's theory of Le^b is that Le(a+b−) × Le(a−b−) matings should produce some Le(a−b+) children and this indeed they do. Because of difficulty of testing A_1 cells with anti-Le^b only families with all Le(a−) members O or A_2 should be countenanced. Many such families must now have been found, the first two were:

> Father O Le(a−b−) sec. nL, mother A_1 Le(a+b−) non-sec. Les; one child O Le(a+b−) non-sec. Les, one child O Le(a−b+) sec. Les. (Sanger and Race[68]).
> Parents O Le(a+b−) non-sec. Les and O Le(a−b−) sec. nL; 3 children O Le(a−b+) sec. Les and 2 children O Le(a−b−) sec. nL (Ceppellini, Dunn and Innella[62]).

The Le^b antigen on the red cells of all these four Le(a−b+) children whose parents lack Le^b on the red cells could be due to their having received an Se gene from one parent and an Le gene from the other.

The fact that an O_h person has been proved to have Se and Le genes yet found to lack the antigen Le^b we interpreted[120] as meaning that the very common gene H is required as well as Se and Le in the production of Le^b.

However, the last word on Le^b rests with Morgan and Watkins and their colleagues. Inhibition tests led them to think of Le^b as a result of interaction between the genes Le and H (Figure 4, page 60) and not between Le and Se as Ceppellini had supposed; and this was triumphantly confirmed at the chemical level (Marr, Donald, Watkins and Morgan[121], 1967).

Frequencies and inheritance of the saliva phenotypes
Les and nL

The frequencies are given in Table 57. Various symbols have been used for the phenotypes: in this account Les = Le^a substance present in the saliva and nL = no Le^a substance present.

The results of family tests are given in Table 58. Several of the series have been analysed by the investigators and found to be in reasonable agreement with expectation. In the outstanding paper of Ceppellini, Dunn and Innella[62] the families are classified and analysed in the ten phenotypically different matings involving both the secretor and Lewis systems.

The expected frequencies in England of the various matings and the proportion of issue are to be found in Table 59: the calculations were based on the sample of

1,000 random people tested by McConnell[74] (Table 57). According to Table 59 only nL children are to be expected from matings nL × nL: this agrees with observation, for in Table 58 there are six such matings with 14 nL children and a further mating has been recorded by Marshall[75] with all three children nL.

Table 58. Inheritance of the antigen Le[a] of the saliva
(Les = Le[a] present: nL = Le[a] absent)

	Matings								
	Les × Les			Les × nL			nL × nL		
		Children			Children			Children	
	No.	Les	nL	No.	Les	nL	No.	Les	nL
Ceppellini[8], 1955, Ferrara, 84 families with 262 children	67	184	14	17	40	24	0	0	0
Bianco et al.[64], 1960, Ferrara, 66 families with 180 children	53	142	5	12	24	8	1	0	1
Ceppellini et al.[62], 1959, Charleston Negroes, 38 families with 161 children	24	86	14	10	30	20	4	0	11
Lawler et al.[66], 1960, Nigerians (Habe), 28 families with 61 children	16	27	5	11	17	10	1	0	2
Sneath and Sneath[57], 1959, English, 52 families with 109 children	39	73	3	13	22	11	0	0	0
McConnell[74], 1961, English, 113 families with 434 children	109	415	6	4	10	3	0	0	0
Greenwalt[60], 1961, Milwaukee, 72 families with 287 children*	60	225	13	12	37	12	0	0	0

* After subtraction of salivas taken from children by a swab: such samples are recorded by Greenwalt[60] and show a significant excess of nL—a timely warning.

Table 59. The expected distribution of the Le[a] antigen in the saliva of English parents and offspring

| | Matings | | Proportion of children from each mating | |
Type	Frequency	Les	nL
Les × Les	0·9332	0·9758	0·0242
Les × nL	0·0657	0·8440	0·1560
nL × nL	0·0012	—	1·0000

Genetical independence of the *Lele* and *Sese* loci

Three families have been reported which show clearly independent segregation of the Lewis and secretor genes and so prove that the two loci are at any rate not closely linked. The families are: 348 C of Ceppellini and Siniscalco[28], No. 13 of

12

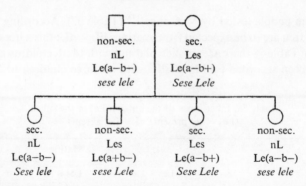

Fig. 21. Family illustrating the independent inheritance of the secretor and Lewis genes (after Sneath and Sneath[57]): the *Se* gene of the mother has gone with her *le* gene to the first child but with her *Le* gene to the third child; the mother's *se* gene has gone with her *Le* to the second child and with her *le* to the fourth child.

Sanger and Race[68] and a family of Sneath and Sneath[57] shown in Figure 21. If the two loci were on the same chromosome they must be too far apart for the intervening distance to be directly measured, for of 13 informative children at least six would have to be recombinants.

Evidence is accumulating[28, 68, 60] to show that the Lewis genes are not at any rate closely linked to the Lutheran genes (which are quite closely linked to the secretor genes—see Chapter 27).

An investigation in Paris made linkage between Lewis and red cell acid phosphatase seem a possibility, but this was not supported by work at Yale (see Chapter 27).

OTHER NOTES ABOUT THE LEWIS SYSTEM

Other Lewis antigens

Antigens of Le(a–b–) red cells

In 1957 Iseki, Masaki and Shibasaki[86] described the production of an antibody, named anti-Le^c, by injecting a rabbit with Le(a–b–) secretor saliva and absorbing the immune serum with enzyme treated Le(a+b–) and Le(a–b+) cells. The result of testing the cells of 485 Japanese persons with anti-Le^a, anti-Le^b and anti-Le^c were

+ – –	– + –	– – +
107	369	9
22·06%	76·08%	1·86%

The anti-Le^c was incomplete, rather weak, and reacted only in the cold: Le(a–b–) cells alone reacted positively, 8 of the 9 tested were from secretors and 1 was from a non-secretor.

In a second paper, Iseki et al.[93] recorded the testing of 5 families with the three antisera and in seeking for an explanation of the results had to postulate a system in which Le^c is dominant in effect over Le^b and Le^a, and Le^b dominant over Le^a, as far as the red cell antigens were concerned.

Because this anti-Le^c of the Gunma University workers reacted with the cells of Le(a–b–) secretors *and* non-secretors it now seems, in the light of investigations in Moscow and Lancaster about to be described, that perhaps the antibody could be thought of as anti-Le^c+Le^d.

Lodge, Andersen and Gold[112] in a very complicated analysis of five Lewis antisera (which will have to be consulted in the original) also found evidence of an antigen present in Le(a–b–) cells when an antiglobulin test on papainized cells was used. The results of inhibition and absorption tests are complicated and the authors themselves consider that more work should be done on other sera before trying to include these reactions, and those of anti-Le^c, in general theories about Lewis.

Magard

Andersen[92] (1958) investigated the serum of an A_2 Le(a–b+) patient suffering from cancer of the stomach (from whom no saliva was available). An antibody was present with the baffling property of agglutinating preferentially the cells of A_1 Le(a–b–) secretors and, rather less strongly, those of A_2 Le(a–b–) secretors. Absorption tests showed that A substance and not B, H, Le^a or Le^b would inhibit the antibody.

Andersen's interpretation was that the gene *Se* in the absence of *Le* alters the character of the A antigen of the red cells and that this alteration is recognized by the serum Magard. This view is not incompatible with the scheme of Figure 22.

Le^d

In 1970, Potapov[124] described two antibodies made by injecting a goat with saliva from an O Le (a–b+) secretor person: the immune serum after absorption with

Table 60. Addition to Table 56 required by Potapov's[124] (1970) finding of anti-Le^d and his postulation of anti-Le^c (later found by Gunson and Latham[125], 1972)

Saliva		Red cells			
		reactions with anti-			
		Le^a	Le^b	Le^c	Le^d
Sec.	Les	–	+	–	–*
Non-sec.	Les	+	–	–	–
Sec.	nL	–	–	–	+
Non-sec.	nL	–	–	+	–

* reaction not yet confirmed in practice.

trypsinized Le(a+b−) cells contained a strong anti-Le^b and a less strong antibody which failed to react with Le(a+b−) cells and with Le(a−b−) cells from non-secretors but did react with Le(a−b−) cells from secretors. This antibody Potapov called anti-Le^d, leaving 'anti-Le^c' free for a then hypothetical antibody expected to react only with cells from Le(a−b−) non-secretors.

Anticipating the finding of anti-Le^c, Potapov made additions to the scheme for Lewis and secretor which we have summarized in Table 60.

Le^c

In the serum of an Le(a−b+) secretor patient who had once been transfused and four times pregnant, Gunson and Latham[125] (1972) found a cold agglutinin which reacted only with the cells of Le(a−b−) non-secretor people and so established the existence of the anti-Le^c adumbrated by Potapov[124]. The Le^c: anti-Le^c reaction was inhibited strongly by saliva from Le(a−b−) non-secretors, less strongly by that from Le(a−b−) secretors and Le(a+b−) non-secretors, and hardly at all by that from Le(a−b+) secretors. The reaction was inhibited by three purified glycoproteins isolated from ovarian cysts of Le(a−b−) non-secretors and by the trisaccharide 3 fucosyllactose. A number of other sugars failed to inhibit the reaction. The inhibitions were just as expected by Professor Watkins who contributes some explanatory paragraphs to the paper which must be read as a whole.

Dr Potapov (personal communication, 1973) successfully induced anti-Le^c in one of four goats by injecting 210 ml of boiled saliva from two Le(a−b−) non-secretors. The immune serum, diluted 1 part in 15 parts of saline, was absorbed with trypsinized Le(a+) or Le(d+) or Le(b+) red cells. The resulting preparations could be used for distinguishing between O Le(c+) and O Le(d+) cells, the cells being trypsinized (or papainized) beforehand.

Through the kindness of Dr Potapov we were able in our Unit to test the goat reagent in parallel with the human anti-Le^c of Gunson and Latham[125] with completely concordant results: Le(a−b−) cells from non-secretors were agglutinated, while Le(a−b−) cells from secretors were not.

It is comforting to note that in extending the Lewis system from two to four antigens no new alleles need be invoked, and with this Dr Potapov concurs[148]. From the work of Morgan and Watkins the Le^a and Le^b structures have long been seen to be derived from Type 1 precursor chains (see Figure 4, page 60), and Watkins suggests that Le^c and Le^d are derived from Type 2 precursor chains.

Le^x

In 1949 Andresen and Jordal[40] described anti-X, later[45, 67] called anti-Le^x, which was considered by many workers to be anti-Le^a plus anti-Le^b, not necessarily in separable state. However, the Danish workers have never thought of anti-Le^x as anti-Le^a plus anti-Le^b and Jordal[45] showed that anti-Le^x reacts with approximately the same proportion of cord samples as of adult samples, which is quite unlike the behaviour of anti-Le^a and anti-Le^b (see below). Anti-Le^x reacts equally well with O, A$_2$ and A$_1$ cells. Andersen[104] describes and discusses the heterogeneity of two sera both of which reacted only with Le(a+b−) and Le(a−b+) cells: both were inhibitable by salivas containing Le^a substance. Andersen concluded that anti-Le^x might be detecting on the red cells a product of the gene *Le^a* (which we now call *Le*). Andresen[94] is more definite, he says:

'Consequently, *anti-Le^x must be considered as a specific agglutinin*, which has a corresponding specific receptor X closely related to the Le^a substance. The presence of receptor X in the blood cells is always accompanied by the presence of Le^a substance in the secretions. The presence of the X receptor is entirely independent of the subject's secretor/non-secretor status. There is no correlation between the X receptor and Le^b substance.'

Sturgeon and Arcilla[126] (1970) agreed that anti-Le^x reacts as strongly with cells of the commonest infants' phenotype Le(a−b−x+) as with adult Le(a+b−) or Le(a−b+) cells. They included anti-Le^x in their 'semiquantitative' work on the red cells and saliva of families of the rare Le(a+b+) people, and in a study of the development of the Lewis antigens. They, in line with Andresen[94], consider Le^x to be a product of the *Le* gene which is not affected by the *Sese* or *Hh* genes.

However, Andresen[135] did find some Le^x substance in the saliva of Le(a−b−) non-secretors (though not in that of Le(a−b−) secretors). This presence of Le^x awaits explanation, as does the presence of some Le^a substance in the saliva of Le(a−b−) non-secretors[125, 135, 126] (page 327). Further discussion of the background of Le^x is to be found in a recent paper by Arcilla and Sturgeon[150].

A$_1$Le^b

In 1968, Seaman, Chalmers and Franks[127], found a 'new' antibody, anti-A$_1$Le^b, when cross-matching the serum of a patient named Siedler. The patient had never been transfused and his serum reacted with red cells having both A$_1$ and Le^b antigens but did not react with cells having only one or neither of these two antigens. The antigen was shown to be present in the saliva of people whose red cells had A$_1$ and Le^b. The secretor state of the person was not recorded.

A second example of the antibody was found in very unusual circumstances and faced Crookston, Tilley and Crookston[128] (1970) with a problem which they solved in a brilliant investigation. In short, the female of a twin chimera pair (Chapter 26) was genetically group O but half her red cells were A$_1$, grafted from her brother. Her serum contained anti-A$_1$Le^b, and this agglutinated the A$_1$Le(b+) cells of her twin brother (then aged 35) but did not agglutinate those A$_1$ cells of her brother treasured in her own circulation. As a solution to this puzzle the authors deduced that the ability to make the antigen A$_1$Le^b cannot be grafted but requires the presence of at least one A_1, *Se* and *Le* gene in the true genetic constitution and, further, that the antigen is made at some unknown site and secondarily taken up by the red cells. The female twin cannot make A$_1$Le^b because she lacks a constitutional A_1 gene, so her brother's cells in her circulation have to go without A$_1$Le^b. Her brother on the other hand does make A$_1$Le^b, which is taken up by his cells.

The deduction was beautifully confirmed by experiments *in vitro*[128] and *in vivo*[129]: it was observed that O Le(a−b−) and O Le(a+b−) cells took up A_1Le^b from plasma containing it. And see Tilley *et al.*[151], 1975.

A third example of an antibody which reacted with red cells only if they carried both A_1 and Le^b was investigated by Gundolf[149]. The antibody was found in the serum of an A_1 person who was unusual in secreting in her saliva some A but no H substance, and whose red cells were also deficient in H. This anti-A_1Le^b was, like that of Crookston *et al.*[128] (and personal communication), inhibited by saliva from all A secretors whether from Les or nL people but, unlike the Canadian example, it was also inhibited by the saliva of O Les people.

Lewis antisera

Anti-Le^a in human serum

Since Mourant first tested the serum of Mrs Lewis many hundred examples of anti-Le^a have been found. The majority are too weak to be useful; most of them 'occur naturally' and react best at temperatures lower than 37°C. Occasionally the antibody appears to be immune in origin and on rare occasions it has been blamed for haemolytic reactions to transfusion[30-36]. Not infrequently anti-Le^a sera will haemolyse Le(a+) cells in the presence of complement.

Most, if not all, anti-Le^a sera contain some weak anti-Le^b and come from people of the phenotype Le(a−b−); we have not ourselves encountered an example of anti-Le^a from a person of the phenotype Le(a−b+), nor had Miller *et al.*[15] who further observed that the saliva of donors of anti-Le^a sera contains A, B and H substance but lacks both Le^a and Le^b substances. Pettenkofer and Hoffbauer[37], on the other hand, did find anti-Le^a in Le(a−b+) donors, which is difficult to understand if Table 56 be correct and all Le(a−b+) people have Le^a antigen in their body.

Anti-Le^a sera have been used in complement binding studies[82,83].

Powerful anti-Le^a sera are few and far between and unless the cells are in good condition it is easy to get the wrong answer—this applies also to anti-Le^b. The use of papain improves the reaction of many examples of Lewis antisera.

A lymphocytotoxic serum with unknown non-HL-A specificity was found by Dorf *et al.*[136] to detect Le^a antigen on the lymphocytes of Le(a+) people: further, four out of five anti-Le^a sera were found to have lymphocytotoxic anti-Le^a properties.

Anti-Le^a in animal sera

As mentioned at the beginning of this chapter a precipitin for saliva of non-secretors was described in 1939 by Japanese workers (Ueyama[47,51], Furuhata and Ueyama[52]). The antibody was found in the serum of certain normal chickens and in the serum of a chicken injected with group O non-secretor saliva.

Anti-Le^a sera, either of the precipitating or agglutinating type, have since been produced in chickens[72], rabbits[84, 85, 86, 71, 87] and in goats[88, 89, 117, 118] by the injection of non-secretor saliva[84, 89], of substances isolated from ovarian cysts of non-secretors[84, 85, 86, 71, 72] and of tanned rabbit red cells coated with Le^a substance[87].

Anti-Le^b

Anti-Le^b, like anti-Le^a, is usually found in the serum of Le(a−b−) persons, but they are non-secretors of ABH and of Le^a and Le^b substances[10, 15, 39]. However, examples of anti-Le^b in A_1 or A_1B, Le(a+b−), non-sec, Les people have been reported[21, 109, 137] and we have heard of others[138]: all these antibodies were of the anti-Le^{bH} type mentioned below. Useful anti-Le^b with agglutinating and precipitating properties has been made in goats[117, 118].

Anti-Le^b sera often contain some anti-H and indeed they have properties in common with anti-H: they react most strongly with O and A_2 cells, and salivas that inhibit anti-Le^b inhibit anti-H and, furthermore, most anti-Le^b are found in A_1 or A_1B persons. We have, however, tested two anti-Le^b sera from group O donors sent by Dr Mary Crawford and Dr Cleghorn and several from group B people. The ABO groups of a series of over 500 makers of Lewis antibodies are recorded by Kissmeyer-Nielsen[119].

Some, perhaps most, anti-Le^b sera, like the original example of Andresen[9], react specifically only with O and A_2 cells: others, like that first described by Brendemoen[21], react specifically with A_1 cells as well.

It is now generally agreed that inhibition studies show that there are two kinds of anti-Le^b sera:

1 Anti-Le^{bH} (anti-Le$_1^b$) which is inhibited by the saliva of all ABH secretors, whether they be from Le(a−b+) or Le(a−b−) persons.

2 Anti-Le^{bL} (anti-Le$_2^b$) which is inhibited by saliva from ABH secretors who have Le^a in the saliva but not by those secretors who lack Le^a, that is Le(a−b−) sec. people.

We have used the notation of Ceppellini, Dunn and Innella[62] followed, in brackets, by that of Sneath and Sneath[57]. Ceppellini[80] says that these two types of anti-Le^b 'give an identical pattern of reactions against red cells': Sneath and Sneath[57] suggest that anti-Le^{bH} sera are those that react strongly only with O and A_2 cells while anti-Le^{bL} sera are those whose specificity is but little affected by the presence of A_1.

Bird[90, 110] suggests that anti-H may be thought of as anti-H+H$_1$, by analogy with anti-A+A$_1$, and that anti-Le^b may be anti-H$_1$. Kissmeyer-Nielsen[91] sent us two powerful anti-H sera from Le(a+b−) persons which at least do not contradict this idea, for they react more strongly with Le(b+) than with Le(b−) cells and all antibody is removed by absorption with O Le(a−b−) and O Le(a+b−) cells. Bird's suggestion would be compatible with Figure 22; the anti-H$_1$ presumably corresponds to anti-Le^{bH} in the subdivision of Le^b sera above. Wiener, Gordon and Moor-Jankowski[111] also take this view.

When Kornstad[137] used A_1 and O cells of different Lewis phenotypes in parallel absorptions of anti-Le^b sera, from 2 Le (a+b−) and from 4 Le(a−b−) donors, he found the antisera from the Le(a+b−) persons had a greater affinity for H than for Le^b, while antisera from the Le(a−b−) donors had greater affinity for Le^b than for H. While being cautious about the small number of sera tested Kornstad was left favouring the idea that there exists 'a wide spectrum of antibodies ranging from a pure anti-H via anti-H (Le^b) and anti-Le^b (H) to a pure anti-Le^b'.

Other Lewis antibodies

Anti-Le^x, anti-Le^c, anti-Le^d, the Magard antibody and anti-A_1Le^b have been dealt with in the sections concerning their corresponding antigens (pages 334–338). Jeannet et al.[139] reported two non-HL-A cytotoxic antisera of the specificity anti-A_1Le^b: they reacted only with lymphocytes of people whose red cells had A_1 and Le^b.

Development of the Lewis antigens

Andresen first observed that the distribution of the Lewis phenotypes were different during the first few months of life[4]. Rosenfield and Ohno[46] found that cord blood gave the reaction Le(a−b−). Jordal[45] tested 50 foetuses of 3–6 months of age and all of them were Le(a−b−), as were 152 cord samples. Jordal also found that anti-Le^x reacts with about the same proportion of cord cell samples as of adult samples. Cutbush, Giblett and Mollison[24] found that 13 out of 22 samples of cord blood gave a positive antiglobulin reaction with their anti-Le^a serum. Bronnikova[140], using goat immune antisera, was able to detect Le^a and Le^b in enzyme treated foetal and newborn cells.

Extensive studies on the Lewis groups of the blood of children are to be found in four Scandinavian papers[4,48,45,96]. Soon after birth the antigens appear and by three months over 80 % of children give the reaction Le(a+); this soon falls and by about two years of age the adult level of 20 %, or so, is reached. Le(b+), on the other hand, is rarer in young children than in adults: the adult frequency of around 70 % is reached only at about six years of age[45]. Le^x, on the other hand, is well developed at birth[45,126].

Lawler and Marshall[69,70] found Le^a and Le^b to be present at birth in saliva and serum though absent from the red cells. Babies who are to become Le(a+b−) have Le^a but not Le^b in their serum and saliva; babies who are to become Le(a−b+) have Le^a and Le^b in both serum and saliva—the Le^a in the serum is detectable only during the phase when the red cells are Le(a+b+); babies who are to become Le(a−b−) have neither Le^a nor Le^b in their serum or saliva.

At another stage in life the antigens may vary: in the words of Brendemoen[49] 'the agglutinability of cells for anti-Le^a and anti-Le^b sera are considerably reduced during pregnancy for reasons unknown'. A striking example of Le^a disappearing from the red cells during pregnancy and returning thereafter is recorded[97], and the same phenomenon has been reported[141] from Bombay in women of the O_h type.

Other theories about Lewis

In this chapter we have given great prominence to the theory of Grubb and Ceppellini, but it is not inconceivable that it will founder on yet uncharted facts and that one of the other theories, which at present seem less hopeful, may have to come to the rescue.

The theory of Andresen, Andersen, Jordal and Henningsen[7, 40, 41] was designed to explain the reactions of anti-Le^x. The theory applies to red cell antigens: according to it there are two alleles of the Lewis gene, Le^a and Le^b, Le^a is recessive in its effect and Le^b is dominant (at any rate in group O adults), but these genes cannot express themselves in the absence of an independent gene X. X produces the antigen X recognized by anti-Le^x. Though it does not seem possible to dispute the theory arguing only from red cells, it does not appear to accommodate the facts about saliva: for example, it does not allow for the probably invariable presence of Le^a substance in the saliva of Le(a−b+) people of whom about one-third, according to the theory, should be Le^bLe^b. However, Andresen[94] has extended the theory to include secretions and the two kinds of anti-Le^b and the 'Magard' antibody.

Pettenkofer's theory[42, 43] (1953) required three Lewis alleles, Le^a, Le^b and Le^c: it was criticized by Grubb[44] and supported by Iseki, Masaki and Shibasaki[93] who interpret the red cell phenotypes defined by the use of anti-Le^a, anti-Le^b and their anti-Le^c sera as follows: Le(a+b−c−) = Le^aLe^a, Le(a−b+c−) = Le^aLe^b and Le^bLe^b, Le(a−b−c+) = Le^aLe^c, Le^bLe^c and Le^cLe^c. However, this theory would not allow Le(a+) × Le(a+) matings to produce Le(a−) children—which they occasionally do (see page 324).

In 1958 Wiener and Wexler[95] put forward a theory which we could not distinguish from that of Pettenkofer. Wiener, Gordon and Moor-Jankowski[111] no longer take this view: their present theory does not, as far as we can see, differ from that of Grubb and Ceppellini except in that Le^b is considered to be part of H, as first suggested by Bird[90, 110]. They make the comfortable proposal that if Le^b is really part of H it should be ignored in the Lewis notation, as it is in the ABO notation. But their proposed red cell phenotype notation does not cope with the common situation in which only anti-Le^a is available.

Chemistry of the Lewis substances

In 1951 Annison and Morgan[50, 103] isolated Le^a substance from pseudomucinous ovarian cysts and this was followed by a great deal of work by Professor Morgan and Dr Winifred Watkins[98, 77, 78, 99, 100, 113, 114]. This was one of the steps towards the triumphant synthesis quoted in the next section.

In 1967, Marr, Donald, Watkins and Morgan[121], described the chemical analysis of Le^b substance which fitted beautifully into the general pattern.

12*

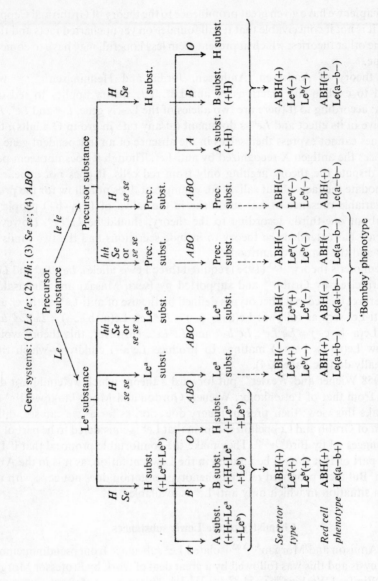

Gene systems: (1) *Le le*; (2) *Hh*; (3) *Se se*; (4) *ABO*

Fig. 22. Possible genetical pathways for the bio-synthesis of A, B, H and Le^a substances. (From Watkins[113], 1965.)

The postulated fucosyltransferase responsible for Le activity was identified in 1969 (Grollman, Kobata and Ginsburg[142]; Chester and Watkins[143]).

It is beyond our powers to comment usefully on the advanced chemical work on the Lewis antigens. We feel all we can do is to give some recent references from which the reader may find what he wants: for example Watkins[144]; Marcus and Cass[145]; Grollman, Kobata and Ginsburg[142]; Marcus[146, 147].

GENETICAL PATHWAYS TOWARDS BLOOD GROUP GLYCOPROTEINS IN SALIVA

It would be surprising if Figure 22 tells the whole story but it rationalizes in a most satisfying way the very complicated interactions known to exist between the *ABO*, the *secretor*, the *Hh* and the *Lewis* genes. The figure is taken from Watkins[113]; it is based on the brilliant work of Morgan and Watkins[76-78] and of Ceppellini[79, 80]. There is biochemical and genetical evidence for the order in which the genes play their part: first the *Lewis* genes, then the *Hh* genes[81, 29] and the *secretor* genes and finally the *ABO* genes. The genes *le, h, se* and *O* are thought of as amorphs, or at least to have no effect that yet can be detected.

When first put forward this scheme predicted the existence of the rare O_h Le(a−b−) red cell phenotype which was duly found[115] (and see page 23) and the scheme has very comfortably accommodated the recently recognized antigens Le^d and Le^c.

A diagram of the chemical differences between the substances involved in the progress is given on page 60. The subject seems to us to be the scientific high water mark of blood group enquiry.

REFERENCES

[1] MOURANT A.E. (1946) A 'new' human blood group antigen of frequent occurrence. *Nature, Lond.*, **158**, 237.

[2] RACE R.R. and SANGER RUTH (1954) *Blood Groups in Man*, 2nd edition, pp. 400, Blackwell Scientific Publications, Oxford.

[3] MOURANT A.E. (1954) *The Distribution of the Human Blood Groups*, pp. 438, Blackwell Scientific Publications, Oxford.

[4] ANDRESEN P.H. (1948) Blood group with characteristic phenotypical aspects. *Acta path. microbiol. scand.*, **24**, 616–618.

[5] RACE R.R., SANGER RUTH, LAWLER SYLVIA D. and BERTINSHAW DOREEN (1949) The Lewis blood groups of 79 families. *Brit. J. exp. Path.*, **30**, 73–83.

[6] THOMPSON JOAN S. (1953) Quoted in 2nd edition of this book.

[7] ANDRESEN P.H., ANDERSEN A., JORDAL K. and HENNINGSEN K. (1950) Corrélation entre le système Lewis et le système sécréteur-non-sécréteur. (Recherches sur 71 familles.) *Rev. Hémat.*, **5**, 305–314.

[8] CEPPELLINI R. (1955) On the genetics of secretor and Lewis characters: a family study. *Proc. 5th Congr. int. Soc. Blood Transf.*, Paris, 207–211.

[9] ANDRESEN P.H. (1948) The blood group system L. A new blood group L_2. A case of epistasy within the blood groups. *Acta path. microbiol. scand.*, **25**, 728–731.

10 GRUBB R. (1951) Observations on the human group system Lewis. *Acta path. microbiol. scand.*, **28**, 61–81.

11 MILLER E.B., ROSENFIELD R.E. and VOGEL P. (1951) On the incidence of some of the new blood agglutinogens in Chinese and Negroes. *Amer. J. phys. Anthrop.*, **9**, 115–126.

12 BRENDEMOEN O.J. (1953) Personal communication.

13 SALMON C. and MALASSENET R. (1953) Considérations sur les anticorps anti-Lewis et pourcentage des différents phénotypes Lewis chez les donneurs de sang de Paris. *Rev. Hémat.*, **8**, 183–188.

14 IKIN ELIZABETH W. (1953) Cited by Mourant, A.E.[3]

15 MILLER E.B., ROSENFIELD R.E., VOGEL P., HABER GLADYS and GIBBEL NATALIE (1954) The Lewis blood factors in American Negroes. *Amer. J. Phys. Anthrop.*, **12**, 427–444.

16 GRUBB R. (1948) Correlation between Lewis blood group and secretor character in man. *Nature, Lond.*, **162**, 933.

17 GRUBB R. and MORGAN W.T.J. (1949) The 'Lewis' blood group characters of erythrocytes and body fluids. *Brit. J. exp. Path.*, **30**, 198–208.

18 BRENDEMOEN O.J. (1949) Studies of agglutination and inhibition in two Lewis antibodies. *J. Lab. clin. Med.*, **34**, 538–542.

19 CEPPELLINI R. (1955) Nuova interpretazione sulla genetica dei carratteri Lewis eritrocitari e salivari derivante dall'analisi di 87 famiglie. Supplement to *Ric. sci. Mem.*, **25**, 3–9 (in offprint).

20 SNEATH JOAN S. and SNEATH P.H.A. (1955) Transformation of the Lewis groups of human red cells. *Nature, Lond.*, **176**, 172.

21 BRENDEMOEN O.J. (1950) Further studies of agglutination and inhibition in the Le^a-Le^b system. *J. Lab. clin. Med.*, **36**, 335–341.

22 MÄKELÄ O. and MÄKELÄ PIRJO (1956) Le^b antigen. Studies on its occurrence in red cells, plasma and saliva. *Ann. Med. exp. Fenn.*, **34**, 157–162.

23 GRUBB R. (1950) Quelques aspects de la complexité des groupes ABO. *Rev. Hémat.*, **5**, 268–275.

24 CUTBUSH MARIE, GIBLETT ELOISE R. and MOLLISON P.L. (1956) Demonstration of the phenotype Le(a+b+) in infants and in adults. *Brit. J. Haemat.*, **2**, 210–220.

25 FERGUSON L.C., STORMONT C. and IRWIN M.R. (1942) On additional antigens in the erythrocytes of cattle. *J. Immunol.*, **44**, 147–164.

26 STORMONT C. (1949) Acquisition of the J substance by the bovine erythrocyte. *Proc. nat. Acad. Sci., Wash.*, **35**, 232–237.

27 NICHOLAS J.W., JENKINS W.J. and MARSH W.L. (1957) Human blood chimeras: a study of surviving twins. *Brit. med. J.*, i, 1458–1460.

28 CEPPELLINI R. and SINISCALCO M. (1955) Una nuova ipotesi genetica per il sistema Lewis secretore e suoi riflessi nei riguardi di alcune evidence di linkage con altri loci. *Revista dell'Istituto Sieroterapico Italiano*, **30**, 431–445.

29 LEVINE P., ROBINSON ELIZABETH, CELANO M., BRIGGS OLIVE and FALKINBURG L. (1955) Gene interaction resulting in suppression of blood group substance B. *Blood*. **10**, 1100–1108.

30 KRIEGER VERA I. and SIMMONS R.T. (1949) The second example of anti-Lewis serum found in Australia. *Med. J. Aust.*, **1**, 85–86.

31 VRIES S.I. DE and SMITSKAMP H.S. (1951) Haemolytic transfusion reaction due to an anti-Lewis^a agglutinin. *Brit. med. J.*, i, 280–281.

32 BRENDEMOEN O.J. and AAS K. (1952) Hemolytic transfusion reaction probably caused by anti-Le^a. *Acta med. scand.*, **141**, 458–460.

33 MATSON G.A., COE J. and SWANSON JANE (1955) Hemolytic transfusion reaction due to anti-Le^a agglutinin. *Blood*, **10**, 1236–1240.

34 LAUER A., CLAUSS J. and HOPPE H.H. (1954) Die Lewis-Blutgruppen als Ursache von Transfusionzwischenfällen. *Dtsch. med. Wschr.*, **79**, 1869. (Not seen.)

35 MERRILD-HANSEN B. and MUNK-ANDERSEN G. (1957) Haemolytic transfusion reaction caused by anti-Le^a. *Vox Sang.*, **2**, 109–113.

36 PETERSON E.T. and CHISHOLM R. (1958) A hemolytic transfusion reaction due to anti-Le^a. *Proc. 6th Congr. int. Soc. Blood Transf.*, 59–62.

37 PETTENKOFER H.J. and HOFFBAUER H. (1954) Über die Bedeutung des Lewis-Blutgruppensystems für die Entstehung eines Morbus haemolyticus neonatorum. *Zbl. Gynäk*, **76**, 576–583.

38 STEINBERG A., SHWACHMAN H., ALLEN F.H. and DOOLEY R.R. (1956) Linkage studies with cystic fibrosis of the pancreas. *Amer. J. hum. Genet.*, **8**, 162–176.

39 GRUBB R. (1955) A note on anti-Le^b and reagents predominantly reacting with group O cells. *Amer. J. phys. Anthrop.*, **13**, 663–665.

40 ANDRESEN P.H. and JORDAL K. (1949) An incomplete agglutinin related to the L-(Lewis) system. *Acta path. microbiol. scand.*, **26**, 636–638.

41 ANDRESEN P.H. and HENNINGSEN K. (1951) The Lewis blood group system and the X-system in 5 Tables. *Acta haemat.*, **5**, 123–127.

42 PETTENKOFER H.J. (1953) Serologie und Vererbung des Lewis-Blutgruppensystems. *Z. ImmunForsch.*, **110**, 217–227.

43 PETTENKOFER H.J. (1953) Zur Genetik des Lewis-Blutgruppensystems. *Naturwissenschaften* **40**, 321–322.

44 GRUBB R. (1953) Zur Genetik des Lewis-Systems. *Naturwissenschaften*, **40**, 560–561.

45 JORDAL K. (1956) The Lewis blood groups in children. *Acta path. microbiol. scand.*, **39**, 399–406.

46 ROSENFIELD R.E. and OHNO G. (1953) Unpublished observations cited by Miller *et al.*[15]

47 UEYAMA R. (1939) Ueber das neue Antigen 'T' entdeckt im menschlichen Speichel des Nicht-ausscheiders. *Hanzaigaku-Zasshi*, **13**, 51–64 (in Japanese).

48 JORDAL K. and LYNDRUP S. (1952) The distribution of C-D and Le^a in 1,000 mother-child combinations. *Acta path. microbiol. scand.*, **31**, 476–480.

49 BRENDEMOEN O.J. (1952) Some factors influencing Rh immunization during pregnancy. *Acta path. microbiol. scand.*, **31**, 579–583.

50 ANNISON E.F. and MORGAN W.T.J. (1951) The 'Lewis' (Le^a) human blood-group substance. *Biochem. J.*, **49**, 24.

51 UEYAMA R. (1940) Studien über die neuen Typensubstanzen in Sekreten. *Jap. J. med. Sci. VII Social Med. Hyg.*, **3**, 23–25 (not seen).

52 FURUHATA T. and UEYAMA R. (1939) On the new antigen-antibody 'T and anti-T preci-pitin'. *Tokyo Izisinsi*, **3120**, 271–273. (In Japanese, not seen.)

53 RACE R.R., SANGER RUTH and MOORES PHYLLIS (1957) Quoted in 3rd edition of this book, but not elsewhere published.

54 JORDAL K. (1957) The Lewis blood group Le^a in adults. *Danish med. Bull.*, **4**, 210–217.

55 MOHR J. (1954) *A Study of Linkage in Man*, pp. 119, Munksgaard, Copenhagen.

56 LINNET-JEPSEN P. (1965) *Undersøgelser over Gm(a) faktoren. Specielt i det første leveår.* M.D. thesis, Aarhus Universitet, pp. 256.

57 SNEATH JOAN S. and SNEATH P.H.A. (1959) Adsorption of blood-group substances from serum on to red cells. *Brit. med. Bull.*, **15**, 154–157.

58 LINNET-JEPSEN P., GALATIUS-JENSEN F. and HAUGE M. (1958) The inheritance of the Gm serum groups. *Acta genet.*, **8**, 164–196.

59 GALATIUS-JENSEN F. (1958) On the genetics of the haptoglobins. *Acta genet.*, **8**, 232–247.

60 GREENWALT T.J. (1961) Confirmation of linkage between the Lutheran and secretor genes. *Amer. J. hum. Genet.*, **13**, 69–88.

61 ANDERSEN J. (1959) On the genetics of the Lewis system. *Acta path. microbiol. scand.*, **47**, 445–448.

62 CEPPELLINI R., DUNN L.C. and INNELLA FILOMENA (1959) Immunogenetica II. Annalisi genetica formale de caratteri Lewis con particolare riguardo alla natura epistatica della specificita' serologica Le^b. *Fol. hered. path.*, **8**, 261–296.

63 LEWIS MARION, KAITA HIROKO and CHOWN B. (1957) The blood groups of a Japanese population. *Amer. J. hum. Genet.*, **9**, 274–283.

64 BIANCO IDA, SILVERSTRONI E., LAWLER SYLVIA D., MARSHALL RUTH and SINISCALCO M. (1960) Further contributions to the study of Lewis and secretor characters. *Vox Sang.*, **5**, 337–348.

65 BARNICOT N.A. and LAWLER SYLVIA D. (1953) A study of the Lewis, Kell, Lutheran and P blood group systems and the ABH secretion in West African Negroes. *Amer. J. phys. Anthrop.*, **11**, 83–90.

66 LAWLER SYLVIA D., MARSHALL RUTH and ROBERTS D.F. (1960) The Lewis and secretor characters in the Fulani and Habe. *Ann. hum. Genet.*, **24**, 271–282.

67 JORDAL K. (1958) The Lewis factors Le^b and Le^{x}and a family series tested by anti-Le^a, anti-Le^b, and anti-Le^x. *Acta path. microbiol. scand.*, **42**, 269–284.

68 SANGER RUTH and RACE R.R. (1958) The Lutheran-secretor linkage in Man: support for Mohr's findings. *Heredity*, **12**, 513–520.

69 LAWLER SYLVIA D. and MARSHALL RUTH (1961) Significance of the presence of Lewis substances in serum during infancy. *Nature, Lond.*, **190**, 1020.

70 LAWLER SYLVIA D. and MARSHALL RUTH (1961) Lewis and secretor characters in infancy. *Vox Sang.*, **6**, 541–554.

71 BROWN PATRICIA C., GLYNN L.E. and HOLBOROW E.J. (1959) Lewis^a substance in saliva. A qualitative difference between secretors and non-secretors. *Vox Sang.*, **4**, 1–12.

72 BAER H., NAYLOR I., GIBBEL NATALIE and ROSENFIELD R.E. (1959) The production of precipitating antibody in chickens to a substance present in the fluids of non-secretors of blood groups A, B and O. *J. Immunol.*, **82**, 183–189.

73 LAWLER SYLVIA D. (1960) Blood group substances in human milk. *Proc. 7th Congr. europ. Soc. Haemat.*, London 1959, part II, 1219–1222.

74 McCONNELL R.B. (1961) Lewis blood group substances in body fluids. Paper read at the 2nd International Conference of Human Genetics.

75 MARSHALL RUTH (1690) ABH-secretor and Lewis characters in three population samples. *Proc. 7th Congr. europ. Soc. Haemat.*, London 1959, part II, 1227–1231.

76 WATKINS WINIFRED M. and MORGAN W.T.J. (1959) Possible genetical pathways for the biosynthesis of blood group mucopolysaccharides. *Vox Sang.*, **4**, 97–119.

77 MORGAN W.T.J. (1959) Some immunological aspects of the products of the human blood group genes. *Ciba Foundation Symposium on Biochemistry of Human Genetics*, 194–216, Churchill, London.

78 WATKINS WINIFRED M. (1959) Some genetical aspects of the biosynthesis of human blood group substances. *Ciba Foundation Svmposium on Biochemistry of Human Genetics*, 217–238, Churchill, London.

79 CEPPELLINI R. (1959) Immunogenetica I^o—Analisi fenotypica al livello submolecolare: le specificita' serologiche multiple dei mucoidi gruppospecifici salivari. *Folia hered. path.*, **8**, 201–226.

80 CEPPELLINI R. (1959) Physiological genetics of human factors. *Ciba Foundation Symposium on Biochemistry of Human Genetics*, 242–261, Churchill, London.

81 WATKINS WINIFRED M. and MORGAN W.T.J. (1955) Some observations on the O and H characters of human blood and secretions. *Vox Sang.* (O.S.), **5**, 1–14.

82 POLLEY MARGARET J. and MOLLISON P.L. (1961) The role of complement in the detection of blood group antibodies: special reference to the antiglobulin test. *Transfusion, Philad.*, **1**, 9–22.

83 STRATTON F. (1961) Complement-fixing blood group antibodies with special reference to the nature of anti-Le^a. *Nature, Lond.*, **190**, 240–241.

84 TOYAMA S. (1956) Studies on S-T blood typing system. 1. On the incomplete immune cold T agglutinin. *Jap. J. leg. Med.*, **10**, 105–122. (In Japanese, not seen.)

85 GLYNN A.A., GLYNN L.E. and HOLBOROW E.J. (1956) The secretor status of rheumatic-fever patients. *Lancet*, **ii**, 759–762.

86 ISEKI S., MASAKI S. and SHIBASAKI K. (1957) Studies on Lewis blood group system. I. Le^c blood group factor. *Proc. imp. Acad. Japan*, **33**, 492–497.

87 LEVINE P. and CELANO M. (1960) The antigenicity of Lewis (Le^a) substance in saliva coated on to tanned red cells. *Vox Sang.*, **5**, 53–61.

88 TSUGANEZAWA M. (1956) On the anti-T antibody in the goat anti-T immune serum, especially on the incomplete anti-T agglutinin. *Jap. J. leg. Med.*, **10**, 545–552. (In Japanese, not seen.)

89 KERDE C., BRUNK R., FÜNFHAUSEN G. and PROKOP O. (1960) Über die Herstellung von Anti-Lewis-Seren an Capra hircus L. *Z. ImmunForsch.*, **119**, 462–468.

90 BIRD G.W.G. (1958) *Erythrocyte Agglutinins from Plants.* Ph.D. Thesis, London.

91 KISSMEYER-NIELSEN F. (1961) Unpublished observations.

92 ANDERSEN J. (1958) Modifying influence of the secretor gene on the development of the ABH substance. A contribution to the conception of the Lewis group system. *Vox Sang.*, **3**, 251–261.

93 ISEKI S., MASAKI S. and SHIBASAKI K. (1957) Studies on Lewis blood group system. II. Distribution and heredity of Le^c blood group factor. *Proc. imp. Acad., Japan* **33**, 686–691.

94 ANDRESEN P.H. (1961) Relations between the ABO, secretor/non-secretor, and Lewis systems with particular reference to the Lewis system. *Amer. J. hum. Genet.*, **13**, 396–412.

95 WIENER A.S. and WEXLER I.B. (1958) *Heredity of the Blood Groups.* Grune and Stratton, New York and London, 31–38.

96 BRENDEMOEN O.J. (1961) Development of the Lewis blood group in the newborn. *Acta path. microbiol. scand.*, **52**, 55–58.

97 ROSENFIELD R.E., HABER GLADYS V., KISSMEYER-NIELSEN F., JACK J.A., SANGER RUTH and RACE R.R. (1960) Ge, a very common red-cell antigen. *Brit. J. Haemat.*, **6**, 344–349.

98 WATKINS WINIFRED M. and MORGAN W.T.J. (1957) Specific inhibition studies relating to the Lewis blood group system. *Nature, Lond.*, **180**, 1038–1040.

99 MORGAN W.T.J. and WATKINS WINIFRED M. (1959) Some aspects of the biochemistry of the human blood group substances. *Brit. med. Bull.*, **15**, 109–113.

100 MORGAN W.T.J. (1960) A contribution to human biochemical genetics; the chemical basis of blood group specificity. *Proc. roy. Soc.*, B, **151**, 308–347.

101 RENDEL J., SORENSEN A.N. and IRWIN M.R. (1954) Evidence for epistatic action of genes for antigenic substances in sheep. *Genetics*, **39**, 396–408.

102 RENDEL J. (1957) Further studies on some antigenic characters of sheep blood determined by epistatic action of genes. *Acta agric. Scand.*, **7**, 224–259.

103 ANNISON E.F. and MORGAN W.T.J. (1952) Studies in immunochemistry. 10. The isolation and properties of Lewis (Le^a) human blood group substances. *Biochem. J.*, **50**, 460–472

104 ANDERSEN J. (1960) Serological studies on two Lewis sera (so-called anti-X sera), with a note on the 'X' character. *Acta path. microbiol. scand.*, **48**, 374–384.

105 MOHR J. (1966) Genetics of fourteen marker systems: associations and linkage relations. *Acta genet.*, **16**, 1–58.

106 PRICE EVANS D.A., DONOHOE W.T.A., BANNERMAN R.M., MOHN J.F. and LAMBERT R.M. (1966) Blood group gene localization through a study of mongolism. *Ann. hum. Genet.*, **30**, 49–67.

107 KAKLAMANIS EVANGELIA, HOLBOROW E.J. and GLYNN L.E. (1964) A method for differentiating homozygous from heterozygous secretors of ABH blood-group substances. *Lancet*, i, 788–790.

108 LODGE T.W. and USHER A. (1962) Lewis blood group substances in seminal fluid. *Vox Sang.*, **7**, 329–333.

109 GARRATTY G. and KLEINSCHMIDT GILLIAN (1965) Two examples of anti-Le^b detected in the sera of patients with the Lewis phenotype Le(a+b−). *Vox Sang.*, **10**, 567–571.

110 BIRD G.W.G. (1959) Haemagglutinins in seeds. *Brit. med. Bull.*, **15**, 165–168.

111 WIENER A.S., GORDON EVE B. and MOOR-JANKOWSKI J. (1964) The Lewis blood groups in man. A review with supporting data on non-human primates. *J. forens. Med.*, **11**, 67–83.

[112] LODGE T.W., ANDERSEN J. and GOLD E.R. (1965) Observations on antibodies reacting with adult and cord Le(a–b–) cells, with O_h Le(a–b–) cells and a soluble antigen present in certain salivas. *Vox Sang.*, **10**, 73–81.

[113] WATKINS WINIFRED M. (1965) Relationship between structure, specificity and genes within the ABO and Lewis blood-group systems. *Proc. 10th Congr. int. Soc. Blood Transf.*, Stockholm 1964, 443–452.

[114] WATKINS WINIFRED M. (1966) Blood-group substances. *Science*, **152**, 172–181.

[115] GILES CAROLYN M., MOURANT A.E. and ATABUDDIN A.-H. (1963) A Lewis-negative 'Bombay' blood. *Vox Sang.*, **8**, 269–272.

[116] CHANDANAYINGYONG D., SASAKI T.T. and GREENWALT T.J. (1967) Blood groups of the Thais. *Transfusion, Philad.*, **7**, 269–276.

[117] MARCUS D.M. and GROLLMAN A.P. (1966) Studies of blood group substances. I. Caprine precipitating antisera to human Le^a and Le^b blood group substances. *J. Immunol.*, **97**, 867–875.

[118] MARCUS D.M., BASTANI A., ROSENFIELD R.E. and GROLLMAN A.P. (1967) Studies of blood group substances. II. Hemagglutinating properties of caprine antisera to human Le^a and Le^b blood group substances. *Transfusion, Philad.*, **7**, 277–280.

[119] KISSMEYER-NIELSEN F. (1965) Irregular blood group antibodies in 200,000 individuals. *Scand. J. Haemat.*, **2**, 331–342.

[120] RACE R.R. and SANGER RUTH (1958 and 1962) *Blood Groups in Man*, 3rd edition p. 210, and 4th edition p. 248. Blackwell Scientific Publications, Oxford.

[121] MARR ANNE M.S., DONALD A.S.R., WATKINS WINIFRED M. and MORGAN W.T.J. (1967) Molecular and genetic aspects of human blood-group Le^b specificity. *Nature, Lond.*, **215**, 1345–1349.

[122] MATSUZAWA S. (1967) Two incomplete agglutinins associated with anti-Le^a in rabbit antisera against gum arabic. *Vox Sang.*, **13**, 218–224.

[123] MÄKELÄ O., MÄKELÄ P. HELENA and KORTEKANGAS A. (1967) In vitro transformation of the Lewis blood groups of erythrocytes. *Ann. Med. exp. Fenn.*, **45**, 159–164.

[124] POTAPOV M.I. (1970) Detection of the antigen of the Lewis system, characteristic of the erythrocytes of the secretory group Le(a–b–). *Probl. Haemathol.* (Moscow), no. 11, 45–49. (In Russian, with summary in English.)

[125] GUNSON H.H. and LATHAM VALERIE (1972) An agglutinin in human serum reacting with cells from Le(a–b–) non-secretor individuals. *Vox Sang.*, **22**, 344–353.

[126] STURGEON P. and ARCILLA M.B. (1970) Studies on the secretion of blood group substances. I. Observations on the red cell phenotype Le(a+b+x+). *Vox Sang.*, **18**, 301–322.

[127] SEAMAN MURIEL J., CHALMERS D.G. and FRANKS D. (1968) Siedler: an antibody which reacts with A_1Le(a–b+) red cells. *Vox Sang.*, **15**, 25–30.

[128] CROOKSTON MARIE C., TILLEY CHRISTINE A. and CROOKSTON J.H. (1970) Human blood chimaera with seeming breakdown of immune tolerance. *Lancet*, **ii**, 1110–1112.

[129] SWANSON JANE, CROOKSTON MARIE C., YUNIS E., AZAR M., GATTI R.A. and GOOD R.A. (1971) Lewis substances in a human marrow-transplantation chimaera. *Lancet*, **i**, 396.

[130] LAMM L.U., KISSMEYER-NIELSEN F. and HENNINGSEN K. (1970) Linkage and association studies of two phosphoglucomutase loci (PGM_1 and PGM_3) to eighteen other markers. Analysis of the segregation at the marker loci. *Human Heredity*, **20**, 305–318.

[131] BOETTCHER B. and KENNY R. (1971) A quantitative study of Le^a, A and H antigens in salivas of Australian Caucasians and Aborigines. *Human Heredity*, **21**, 334–345.

[132] KELSO J. (1968) Quantitative aspects of Lewis-secretor interaction in saliva. *Vox Sang.*, **14**, 282–288.

[133] STURGEON P., McQUISTON DOROTHY and CAMP S. VAN (1973) Quantitative studies on salivary blood group substances. II. Normal values. *Vox Sang.*, **24**, 114–125.

[134] RANDERIA K.J. and BHATIA H.M. (1971) Quantitative inhibition studies on the ABH and Lewis antigens in saliva. *Indian J. Med. Res.*, **59**, 1737–1753.

135 ANDRESEN P.H. (1972) Demonstration of Le^x substance in the saliva of ABH non-secretors. *Vox Sang.*, **23**, 262–269.

136 DORF M.E., EGURO S.Y., CABRERA G., YUNIS E.J., SWANSON J. and AMOS D.B. (1972) Detection of cytotoxic non-HL-A antisera. I. Relationship to anti-Le^a. *Vox Sang.*, **22** 447–456.

137 KORNSTAD L. (1969) Anti-Le^b in the serum of Le(a+b−) and Le(a−b−) persons: absorption studies with erythrocytes of different ABO and Lewis phenotypes. *Vox Sang.*, **16**, 124–129.

138 RACE R.R. and SANGER RUTH (1968) *Blood Groups in Man*, 5th edition, Blackwell Scientific Publications, Oxford, p. 319.

139 JEANNET M., BODMER J.G., BODMER W.F. and SCHAPIRA M. (1972) Lymphocytotoxic sera associated with the ABO and Lewis red cell blood groups. In *Histocompatability Testing*, Munksgaard, Copenhagen, pp. 493–499.

140 BRONNIKOVA M.A. (1971) Les singularités de transformation du système Lewis avec l'age. *Proc. 12th Congr. int. Soc. Blood Transf.*, Moscow, 1969, 83–86. Karger, Basel.

141 CAMOENS HAZEL, SATHE MALTHI, JOSHI V.B., BHATIA H.M. and SHARMA R.S. (1971) Variations in the Le^a in O_h (Bombay) phenotype during pregnancy. *Indian J. Med. Sci.*, **25**, 313–314.

142 GROLLMAN EVELYN F., KOBATA A. and GINSBURG V. (1969) An enzymatic basis for Lewis blood types in man. *J. clin. Invest.*, **48**, 1489.

143 CHESTER M.A. and WATKINS WINIFRED M. (1969) α-L-fucosyltransferases in human submaxillary gland and stomach tissues associated with the H, Le^a and Le^b blood group characters and ABH secretor status. *Biochem. biophys. Res. Commun.*, **34**, 835.

144 WATKINS WINIFRED M. (1972) The biochemical basis of human blood group ABO and Lewis polymorphism. Review article in Annual Report, The Lister Institute of Preventive Medicine, 12–29.

145 MARCUS D.M. and CASS LOUISE E. (1969) Glycosphingolipids with Lewis blood group activity: uptake by human erythrocytes. *Science*, **164**, 553–555.

146 MARCUS D.M. (1969) The ABO and Lewis blood-group system. Immunochemistry, genetics and relation to human disease. *New Engl. J. Med.*, **280**, 994–1006.

147 MARCUS D.M. (1970) Discussion: The nature of the Le^a and Le^b antigens in human plasma. *Ann. N.Y. Acad. Sci.*, **169**, 161–163.

148 POTAPOV M.I. (1973) Genetic aspects of the secretion in saliva of antigens of the Lewis system. *Genetika (U.S.S.R.)*, **5**, 138–143. (In Russian, with summary in English.)

149 GUNDOLF F. (1973) Anti-A_1Le^b in serum of a person of a blood group A_1h. *Vox Sang.*, **25**, 411–419.

150 ARCILLA MINERVA B. and STURGEON P. (1974) Le^x, the spurned antigen of the Lewis blood group system. *Vox Sang.*, **26**, 425–438.

151 TILLEY C.A., CROOKSTON N.C., BROWN B.L. and WHERRETT J.R. (1975) A and B and A_1Le^b substances in glycosphingolipid fractions of human serum. *Vox Sang.*, **28**, 25–33.

Chapter 10
The Duffy Blood Groups

The discovery of the Duffy system was briefly reported by Cutbush, Mollison and Parkin[1] early in 1950; a fuller account was given by Cutbush and Mollison[2] later in that year.

The antibody, anti-Fy^a, was found in the serum of Mr Duffy who suffered from haemophilia and who had been transfused several times during the previous 20 years. The corresponding antigen, Fy^a, was present in the cells of about two thirds of English people and was inherited as a dominant character.

Further examples of anti-Fy^a were found almost immediately. The first example of the antithetical antibody, anti-Fy^b, was found in 1951 by Ikin, Mourant, Pettenkofer and Blumenthal[3, 4], and it gave all the reactions expected of it.

In 1955 Sanger, Race and Jack[5] found, to their surprise, that the majority of Negroes were of the phenotype Fy(a−b−) not found in Whites: the symbol *Fy* was used for the gene or genes responsible for this condition. In the years that followed, tests with anti-Fy^a and anti-Fy^b on families made us realize[14] that heterozygotes for the Fy(a−b−) condition must exist as a rarity in Whites and it seemed reasonable to suppose that the genetical background was the same as that responsible for the Fy(a−b−) so common in Negroes. However, Chown and his colleagues[37, 45] have since established that these rare white heterozygotes are usually not heterozygous for *Fy* but for a gene *Fy^x* which makes a small amount of Fy^b antigen, detectable with appropriate anti-Fy^b sera, and that *Fy* is an extreme rarity in Whites.

Since the last edition of this book three new Duffy antibodies, anti-Fy3, -Fy4 and -Fy5, have been identified. These antibodies are of considerable theoretical interest but for one reason or another have contributed relatively little to the usefulness of a system already having great powers of genetic discrimination.

In 1963 the *Duffy* locus was found to be linked to the locus for a congenital cataract, and when, in 1968, it was found to be linked to an inherited visible abnormality of chromosome No. 1 it had the great distinction of being the first locus in man to be assigned to a particular autosome (page 564).

FREQUENCIES AND INHERITANCE IN WHITES

Innumerable unrelated people and thousands of families must now have been tested with anti-Fy^a. Five early series of tests[2, 6–8, 25, 26] on random English people,

1,944 in all, provided these frequencies[14]:

Fy(a+)	Fy(a−)
66·51%	33·49%

which agree well with subsequent results for Northern Europeans in general. (Details of over a thousand white families tested with anti-Fy^a were given in our last edition: they are not repeated here but the references are kept and are: 6–8, 24, 26, 39, 11, 28, 29, 40–43).

The first English series tested with both anti-Fy^a and anti-Fy^b was from our Unit[25] and from Dr Cleghorn's laboratory[26]; 909 donors were distributed as follows:

Fy(a+b−)	Fy(a+b+)	Fy(a−b+)	Fy(a−b−)
178	435	296	0
19·58%	47·86%	32·56%	

In 1962 we recorded[14] how certain families had made us aware that hetero-zygotes of an Fy(a−b−) condition must be present in white people and an example of such a family is given in Figure 23. At the time it seemed reasonable to suppose that the genetical background was the same as that of the Fy(a−b−) so common in Negroes and we estimated that the gene responsible, then called Fy, might have a frequency as high as 0·03. From the work of Chown, Lewis and Kaita[37, 45] it has become clear that 0·02 is nearer the mark and, furthermore, that the condition has two causes, much the commoner of which is a gene Fy^x that makes a weak Fy^b antigen, detected only by selected anti-Fy^b sera: the less common cause is a gene indistinguishable from that behind the Fy(a−b−) of Negroes.

The weak Fy^b reaction corresponding to the gene Fy^x can easily be missed, as indeed it must have been in most of the rare families, like that in Figure 23, and also in the 909 unrelated English series above, but it makes little practical dif-ference if it is classified as due to Fy.

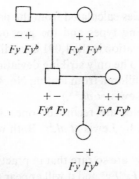

Fig. 23. An English family illustrating the inheritance of the allele Fy. Were the existence of Fy in white people not known both the father and his daughter would have appeared to be extra-marital. The family was tested before Fy could be distinguished from Fy^x (see text). (Samples sent by Professor Paul Polani.)

The best Duffy tests are the two series of Manitoba families reported by Chown, Lewis and Kaita[37, 45]. The gene, genotype and phenotype frequencies, calculated from 2,182 parents of 1,091 families are given in Table 61 and may be taken as gospel for white people. (Incidentally, the gene frequencies fit perfectly the English series if Fy^x and Fy are pooled.)

Table 61. Duffy frequencies in Whites
(After Chown, Lewis and Kaita[37, 45], 1965, 1972)

	Genes	
Fy^a		0·425
Fy^b		0·557
Fy^x		0·016
Fy		0·002

Genotypes		Phenotypes	
Fy^aFy^a	0·1806	Fy(a+b−)	0·1823
Fy^aFy	0·0017		
Fy^aFy^x	0·0136	Fy(a+b±)	0·0136
Fy^aFy^b	0·4735	Fy(a+b+)	0·4735
Fy^bFy^b	0·3102	Fy(a−b+)	0·3302
Fy^bFy^x	0·0178		
Fy^bFy	0·0022		
Fy^xFy^x	0·0003	Fy(a−b±)	0·0004
Fy^xFy	0·0001		
$FyFy$	0·0000	Fy(a−b−)	0·0000
	1·0000		1·0000

Fy(b±) represents weak + reaction with some anti-Fy^b sera and − with others

When the gene frequencies calculated from the parents are used to derive the expected incidence of mating types and the proportions of children expected therefrom, the fit with observation in the 1,091 Canadian families is almost perfect, as may be seen in Table 62. The only striking deviation is the unexpected finding of as many as 7 Fy(a+b−) children from mating No. 4. (Details of the three families involved are given by Lewis et al.[45].)

Two Fy^xFy^x homozygotes are recorded: one, Swedish, by Cedergren and Giles[27] and one, Canadian, by Lewis et al.[45]. Both were supported by extensive family tests.

The homozygotes Fy^xFy^x are so rare that in practice the antigen Fy^x will only be detected in the genotype Fy^aFy^x and it will appear as the phenotype Fy(a+b±). But it will probably be missed unless suitable anti-Fy^b and suitable antiglobulin sera are to hand. But the antigen Fy^x does exist and its presence can be confirmed by absorption and fixation-elution tests[37, 27] with anti-Fy^b. The product of Fy^x

Table 62. Unselected Canadian white families tested with anti-Fy^a and anti-Fy^b (After Chown, Lewis and Kaita[37,45], 1965, 1972)

	Matings		obs.	exp.	χ²	Children					
						Total	Fy(a+b−)	Fy(a+b±)	Fy(a+b+)	Fy(a−b+)	Fy(a−b±)
1.	Fy(a+b−) × Fy(a+b−)		37	*36·2*	0·02	101	101 / *101·00*				
2.	+−	++	189	*188·3*	0·00	489	257 / *244·50*		232 / *243·52*	0 / *0·98*	
3.	++	++	12	*14·1*	0·31	31	4 / *7·75*	8 / *7·75*	7 / *7·75*	12 / *7·75*	
4.	+−	−+	118	*131·4*	1·37	296	7 / *0·89*	5 / *7·99*	284 / *285·64*	0 / *1·48*	
5.	+−	++	9	*9·8*	0·07	38	0 / *0·12*	0 / *0·53*	20 / *18·35*	18 / *18·35*	0 / *0·65*
6.	++	++	261	*244·6*	1·10	750	179 / *187·50*		374 / *375·00*	197 / *187·50*	
7.	−+	++	335	*341·3*	0·12	948	5 / *1·90*	19 / *12·32*	449 / *459·78*	475 / *474·00*	
8.	−+	−+	128	*118·9*	0·70	339				339 / *338·66*	0 / *0·34*
9.	+−	+±	1	*5·4*	⎫	2	0 / *1·00*	2 / *1·00*			
10.	+−	−±	1	*0·0*	⎬ 3·03	6		6 / *6·00*			
11.	others		0	*1·0*	⎭	0					
			1,091	*1,091·0*	6·72	3,000					
					8 d.f.						
					P = 0·55						

is distinguished from that of Fy^b so far only quantitatively. This very weak Fy^b does seem to be the product of a separate allele and not merely the extreme weak end of a normal distribution curve of Fy^b antigen strength, for had this been so there should have been a lot of intervening doubtful reactions with anti-Fy^b sera, but this has not been the case.

The first white person found[14] to be Fy(a–b–) may in retrospect have been of the genotype Fy^xFy or Fy^xFy^x. The second white person found to be Fy(a–b–) and known to be of the genotype $FyFy$ was reported by Albrey et al.[46] and will be described in the section below dealing with Fy3.

Other series of unselected non-negro families[12, 26] tested with anti-Fy^a and anti-Fy^b were noted in our last two editions.

FREQUENCIES AND INHERITANCE IN NEGROES

The finding of the second example of anti-Fy^b, by Levine, Sneath, Robinson and Huntington[10], came at a time when we were testing, for another purpose, a series of blood samples from negro donors to the Knickerbocker Blood Bank, and the opportunity was taken to test them with anti-Fy^a and with the new anti-Fy^b, kindly provided by Dr Philip Levine.

The results were astonishing[5]: nearly 70 % of the samples did not react with either antibody—contrary to all previous experience in testing white people.

Our interpretation was that in Negroes there was a third allele, Fy, for which Fy(a–b–) people were assumed to be homozygous.

Should an antibody turn up which reacted with the product of the new allele, our intention was to call it anti-Fy^c and to promote Fy to Fy^c: but when, after 16 years, some such antibody was found the tide had turned in favour of numbers and it was christened anti-Fy4 and will be described below. However, until the reactions of this antibody become clearer we shall continue to use the symbol Fy.

In all, we have tested 448 samples from unselected Negroes, 304 from New York and 144 from West Indians living in England. The results are shown in Table 63. On the assumption that Fy is an allele of Fy^a and Fy^b the gene frequencies may be calculated thus:

$$Fy = \sqrt{0{\cdot}6763} \qquad\qquad\qquad = 0{\cdot}8224$$

$$Fy^b = \frac{-2Fy + \sqrt{\{(2Fy)^2 + (4 \times 0{\cdot}1987)\}}}{2} = 0{\cdot}1130$$

$$Fy^a = 1 - (Fy^b + Fy) \qquad\qquad = 0{\cdot}0646$$

In Table 63 these gene frequencies are reapplied to the 448 samples from which they were derived, and the fit between observed and expected is very close in all but the phenotype Fy(a+b+). We are not too disturbed about this small class because all the excess of observed Fy(a+b+) was in one of the four distinct series of tests that went to make up the total 448.

Table 63. The Duffy groups of 448 negro samples, 304 from New York and 144 from West Indians living in England

Anti-Fy^a	Anti-Fy^b	Observed in 448	Observed propor-tion	Interpretation	Expected proportion		Expected in 448	χ_1^2
+	−	44	0·0982	Fy^aFy^a Fy^aFy	0·0042 0·1062	0·1104	49·5	0·61
+	+	12	0·0268	Fy^aFy^b		0·0146	6·5	4·65
−	+	89	0·1987	Fy^bFy^b Fy^bFy	0·0128 0·1859	0·1987	89·0	0·00
−	−	303	0·6763	$FyFy$		0·6763	303·0	0·00
		448				1·0000	448·0	5·26

In 1955 we[5] tested 37 unselected, unrelated, West Africans from Lagos and from Accra. The results were Fy(a+b−) 0, Fy(a+b+) 0, Fy(a−b+) 4 and Fy(a−b−) 33. Though these numbers were small they strongly suggested (P = about 1 in 100) that the frequency of Fy(a−b−) is still higher amongst the West Africans than it is amongst the Negroes of New York and the West Indies. This is to be expected on the assumption that the latter people since leaving Africa have received a good many European genes.

By now many African peoples must have been tested with anti-Fy^a and anti-Fy^b, and this is one of many reasons for looking forward to the appearance of the second edition of Dr Mourant's book[38].

We do not know of any report of a series of negro families tested with anti-Fy^a and anti-Fy^b. From our own records, which include 11 West African families[5], the count is:

Fy(a−b−) × Fy(a−b−) matings 41, all 91 children Fy (a−b−)
Fy(a−b−) × Fy(a+b−) matings 4, children Fy(a−b−) 14, Fy(a+b−) 8
Fy(a−b−) × Fy(a−b+) matings 7, children Fy(a−b−) 9, Fy(a−b+) 8
Fy(a+b−) × Fy(a−b+) matings 1, children Fy(a+b−) 2, Fy(a+b+) 1

So we think that homozygosity for a third allele, Fy, is still the best guess at the genetical nature of the negro Fy(a−b−). Results of tests on random people and on families are compatible with this view. There is also some serological support[5]: in Europeans the phenotype Fy(a+b−) nearly always represents the genotype Fy^aFy^a and such samples gave a double dose reaction with an exceptionally good 'dosing' anti-Fy^a serum 'Pri'. Negro samples of the phenotype Fy(a+b−), on the other hand, gave only a single dose reaction—so here was some direct serological evidence that the phenotype Fy(a+b−) could represent a genotype with but a single Fy^a allele.

In our original paper[5] we considered also the possibility that a modifying gene might be inhibiting ordinary Fy^a or Fy^b genes. The family evidence given above shows that such a modifying gene would have to be very closely linked to, or built into, the *Duffy* locus and this, from a practical point of view, comes to the same thing as a third allele, though it does make a difference to our mental picture of the locus. In our last edition we wrote 'The finding of "anti-Fy^c" would make a straightforward third allele the most likely explanation but, though sought for in many centres for more than ten years, not a glimmer of its existence has been sighted.' But, now that anti-Fy4 seems to be emerging as the expected anti-Fy^c we are not so sure that it does contribute much evidence in favour of *Fy* being a third allele: as will be seen in the next section, it seems rather to raise fresh problems.

EXPANSION OF THE DUFFY SYSTEM

For six years after the descriptions of the rare allele *Fy^x* the system remained undisturbed by new facts, but in 1971 this phase ended with the finding of the first of three new antibodies associated with the system. Only the second of these antibodies looks like adding to the 'usefulness' of the system and this is practically confined to Negroes and further limited by shortage of the serum and weakness of the antibody in it: but all three are bound to contribute to a broader understanding of the system.

The numerical notation used for the newer Lutheran antibodies and antigens (page 272) has also been used for these recent additions to the Duffy system.

The antigen Fy3

The antibody which recognized this antigen was found in the serum of a white Fy(a−b−) Queensland woman, Mrs A.Z., who had previously been once transfused and was pregnant for the third time (Albrey, Vincent, Hutchinson, Marsh, Allen, Gavin and Sanger[46], 1971). Mrs A.Z. is the second white Fy(a−b−) person to be found, and her cells do not give the reaction of Fy^x. The parents of Mrs A.Z. are not consanguineous: the father could not be tested; the mother gave the reaction Fy(a−b+) and her genotype was confirmed to be *Fy^{b}Fy* by the offspring of a second marriage.

A.Z.'s antibody, called anti-Fy3, reacted equally strongly with all Fy(a+b−), Fy(a+b+) and Fy(a−b+) cells tested, whether from Negroes or Whites; it reacted with the two available Fy(a−b±), that is *Fy^{x}Fy^x*, samples. It did not react with her own cells or with any Fy(a−b−) cells from Negroes (247 Fy (a−b−) samples are noted in the paper and many more have since been tested); it did not react with the cells of the maker of the second example of anti-Fy3.

The specificity of the antibody could be thought of as anti-Fy^{a}Fy^b were it not that anti-Fy3 reacts strongly with cells treated with enzymes. Treatment of Fy(a+) or Fy(b+) cells with papain abolishes their reaction with anti-Fy^a or anti-Fy^b sera but enhances their reaction with Mrs A.Z.'s anti-Fy3, and with the second example of anti-Fy3 to be noted below.

The antigen Fy3 could reflect a precursor substance necessary for the production of Fy^a or Fy^b, in the way that H is a precursor of A and B. But there is a difference, because *H* is not linked to *ABO* while Fy^3 would have to be built into the *Duffy* locus; otherwise Fy(a–b–) people should be found who have transmitted an Fy^a or Fy^b gene to an offspring who had received a normal precursor gene from the other parent. No such offspring has been found in any family we have tested.

A second example of anti-Fy3 was found by Buchanan and Sinclair[47] in the serum of an Fy(a–b–) Cree Indian woman, Mrs Ye., who had been eight times pregnant but there was no record of her having been transfused. Dr Buchanan and Miss Sinclair pursued the family of Mrs Ye to an isolated area on Trout Lake, north of the Lesser Slave Lake, and kindly shared the results of their adventures with our Unit.

Their findings together with those of Miss Gavin and Miss Teesdale may be summarized:

Red cells: Mrs Ye., Fy(a–b–3–). Her 2nd husband Fy(a+bw3+). 3 children (and 1 from 1st husband) Fy(a+b–3+). 2 children Fy(a–bw3w). Mrs Ye.'s cells were Fy4+, with the reservation that this test could not be properly controlled.

Serum of Mrs Ye. The reactions of her anti-Fy3 are, like the original example, enhanced by papain and ficin. Titration scores showed Fy^aFy^a, Fy^aFy^b, Fy^bFy^b, Fy^aFy and Fy^aFy^x samples to react equally strongly, Fy^xFy^x a little less strongly and $FyFy^x$ (the two children of the Ye. family) were the weakest reactors. The antibody had no separable anti-Fy^a or anti-Fy^b component. It reacted strongly with Rh_{null} cells.

It is very striking that two non-negro Fy(a–b–) persons should make anti-Fy3 when tens of thousands of negro Fy(a–b–) people have failed to do so. This suggests that *FyFy* covers more than one genotype, and that the negro version confers an impediment to immunization by Fy(a+) or Fy(b+) cells.

The antigen Fy4

The antibody defining the antigen called Fy4 was studied in Chicago, London and New York (Behzad, Lee, Gavin and Marsh[48], 1973). A 12-year-old Fy(a+b+) negro girl with sickle cell anaemia who had had a number of transfusions, was found by Miss Susan Demistroulas in Gary, Indiana, to have in her serum, besides anti-K, an additional antibody. The problem of this second antibody was referred to Chicago: it was not a strong one but in general it gave the reactions of the anti-Fy^c sought for 18 years: it was called anti-Fy4 and was positive with all Fy(a–b–) and with the majority of negro Fy(a+b–) and Fy(a–b+) as would be expected of anti-Fy^c. But there was a surprise: like anti-Fy3, anti-Fy4 reacted with cells treated with papain, and this led the authors[48] to wonder whether the gene Fy^4 were perhaps an allele, not of Fy^a and Fy^b, but of Fy^3.

And there, in uncertainty, the genetical background of Fy4 rests: considering the frailty of the one donor, progress will probably have to await the finding of other examples of anti-Fy4. But, whatever the precise genetical background of

Fy4, we have found this small sample of anti-Fy4 effective in dividing Fy(a+b−) members of an unusually informative negro family into Fy^aFy and Fy^aFy^a.

The antigen Fy5

The first and, so far, only example of anti-Fy5 was found in the serum of a negro boy shortly before his death from leukaemia. In the course of his treatment he had had transfusions of blood and platelet concentrates. Blood for investigation was inevitably limited, but was put to very good use by Colledge, Pezzulich and Marsh[49] (1973).

The boy was of the commonest negro phenotype, Fy(a−b−) and Fy:−3. His antibody, called anti-Fy5, worked well by the antiglobulin and papain tests and at first appeared to be another example of anti-Fy3 for it reacted with all cells having the antigens Fy^a or Fy^b and failed to react with Fy(a−b−) cells. But anti-Fy3 seemed to be excluded by the observation that the boy's serum reacted positively with the cells of Mrs A.Z., the white Fy(a−b−) maker of anti-Fy3: further, it differed from Mrs A.Z.'s anti-Fy3 by reacting negatively with Rh_{null} cells of the usual Duffy phenotypes and weakly with $−D−/−D−$ cells.

It is to be hoped that further examples of anti-Fy5 will soon turn up, for it looks as if this antibody may provide the only way of distinguishing non-negro Fy(a−b−) from negro Fy(a−b−) by reacting positively with the former cells and negatively with the latter. If this prove to be so it will be interesting to know how the Fy(a−b−) of Yemenite Jews react (see 'Anthropological differences', below).

The failure of anti-Fy5 to react with Rh_{null} cells was perhaps not surprising in that anti-U and some anti-S and anti-s sera fail to react with their corresponding antigen in Rh_{null} cells, which on serological grounds we presume to be due to the failure of these antibodies to stay attached to a faulty cell membrane (see Rh chapter page 225). However, Colledge and her co-authors[49] noted that $−D−/−D−$ cells reacted more weakly than control cells with anti-Fy5, while behaving normally with other Duffy antisera. They suggested 'that the Fy5 determinant is formed by the interaction of Rhesus and Duffy gene products' and recalled the curious accident to both Rhesus and Duffy antigens reported in one of the puzzling examples of Rh mosaicism referred to on page 238.

DUFFY ANTIBODIES

Anti-Fy^a

The identification of other examples of anti-Fy^a followed quickly on the finding of the original Duffy serum[15−22]. Innumerable examples must now have been found: most of them have been immune and the cause of cross-matching difficulty or haemolytic transfusion reaction (two of them fatal[20,50]). Anti-Fy^a is not a common cause of haemolytic disease of the newborn: about a dozen cases have been reported[23,30−32].

Usually the antibody is in the incomplete form and reacts well only by the antiglobulin method. A few examples agglutinated Fy(a+) cells suspended in saline or albumin[22, 24]. Trypsin, and particularly papain, inhibit the agglutination reactions. On the other hand, the trypsin antiglobulin test shows up the anti-Fy^a:Fy(a+) reaction quite well whereas the papain anti-globulin test has been completely negative with all the anti-Fy^a sera we have tried. (We pointed out[13], some time ago, that this inhibition by papain can be useful in sorting out other antibodies in a serum which also contains anti-Fy^a or anti-Fy^b.) Anti-Fy^a is usually[51] IgG.

Anti-Fy^b

The first example of anti-Fy^b was found in 1951 during routine postnatal examination of the serum of a Berlin woman following the birth of her third child; none of the three children had haemolytic disease and the mother 'gave no history of blood transfusion' (Ikin, Mourant, Pettenkofer and Blumenthal[3, 4]). Very few tests could be done with this serum for samples taken later proved to be inert.

It was not till 1955 that the second example was found[10]. Since then we have had the opportunity of testing many further examples of anti-Fy^b: such sera often contain other antibodies.

Like anti-Fy^a, anti-Fy^b usually reacts best by the antiglobulin test and is inactivated by papain. The antibody has caused a fatal transfusion reaction[52].

Anti-Fy3, 4 and 5

The reactions of these antibodies are described earlier in the chapter.

OTHER NOTES ABOUT THE DUFFY GROUPS

Dosage and other quantitative aspects

Two doses of the gene Fy^a result in more Fy^a antigen on the red cells than does one dose. Some anti-Fy^a sera show the effect more clearly than others; particularly discriminating were the saline agglutinating anti-Fy^a (Pri.), investigated by Race, Sanger and Lehane[22] in 1953, and another such serum (Lett.) studied by Chown, Lewis and Kaita[44].

The serum Pri. besides distinguishing the cells of most heterozygotes from those of most homozygotes showed that heterozygotes have a variable amount of detectable Fy^a antigen; the tests, if repeated on second samples, showed the amount to be characteristic of the person, and not merely a reflection of experimental error. The age of the donor was shown to be one factor influencing the amount.

This variable amount of Fy^a antigen was, of course, expressed in terms of the saline agglutinin in the serum Pri.: even the lowest scoring heterozygotes gave splendid reactions with Pri. and other anti-Fy^a sera when the indirect antiglobulin test was used.

It is noted above that the serum Pri. was used to show that the cells of Fy(a+b−) people of the genotype Fy^aFy have but a single dose of the antigen Fy^a.

Cells of the phenotype Fy(a+b±) are of the genotype Fy^aFy^x. The normal single dose of Fy^a antigen of such cells with the serum Pri.[53] supports the view that Fy^x is an allele at the *Duffy* locus and does not reflect a general Duffy depression.

The first example of anti-Fy^b gave a stronger reaction with Fy^bFy^b than with Fy^aFy^b red cells[3]. The second example, on the other hand, gave only a hint of a dosage difference[10].

As judged by the first two examples, anti-Fy3 does not give a dosage effect.

Development of the antigens

Cutbush and Mollison[2] showed that the antigen Fy^a is well developed at birth; we found it in a foetus of '17 weeks', and Speiser[35] capped this by finding it in one of '40–50 days'.

Cleghorn (personal communication), using anti-Fy^a and anti-Fy^b, grouped without trouble 19 foetuses aged between 17 and 28 weeks (the details were given in our last two editions). More recently Toivanen and Hirvonen[54, 55], in comprehensive studies of foetal red cell antigens, tested samples from 39 foetuses aged from 6 weeks onwards and found both Fy^a and Fy^b to be well developed, even at the 6 to 7 week stage. The 'newer' antigens Fy3 andFy5 are developed at birth[46, 49], but we can find no note of this aspect of Fy4.

Anthropological differences

The differences between Negroes and Whites have already been dealt with at length. Of all known blood group genes *Fy* surely makes the greatest distinction between Negroes and Whites—with a frequency of probably over 90% in West Africans to about 0·1% in Whites.

The phenotype Fy(a−b−) is evidently common in Yemenite Jews. Samples from families belonging to various communities were sent to us from Israel by Dr A. Adam for Xg linkage work. We tested six families with anti-Fy^a and anti-Fy^b: each of four Yemenite families contained Fy(a−b−) members and one of two Iraqi families contained an *Fy* heterozygote. At the other end of the scale the antigen Fy^a was found in all but one of 145 Japanese[33], in all but one of 394 Koreans[34], and in all but one of 1,341 Melanesians[56]. But we are trespassing into a field the vastness of which can only be appreciated by consulting the second edition of 'The Distribution of the Human Blood Groups and other Biochemical Polymorphisms' by Mourant, Kopeć and Domaniewska-Sobczak[38], which will probably be published before this present book appears.

The Duffy system of blood groups is a powerful genetic tool, and its locus had the great distinction of being the first in man to be assigned to a particular autosome.

REFERENCES

1   CUTBUSH MARIE, MOLLISON P.L. and PARKIN DOROTHY M. (1950) A new human blood group. *Nature, Lond.*, **165**, 188.
2   CUTBUSH MARIE and MOLLISON P.L. (1950) The Duffy blood group. *Heredity*, **4**, 383–389.
3   IKIN ELIZABETH W., MOURANT A.E., PETTENKOFER H.J. and BLUMENTHAL G. (1951) Discovery of the expected haemagglutinin, anti-Fy^b. *Nature, Lond.*, **168**, 1077.
4   BLUMENTHAL G. and PETTENKOFER H.J. (1952) Über das neuentdeckte anti-Duffy^b (Fy^b). *Z. ImmunForsch.*, **109**, 267–273.
5   SANGER RUTH, RACE R.R. and JACK J. (1955) The Duffy blood groups of New York Negroes: the phenotype Fy(a–b–). *Brit. J. Haemat.*, **1**, 370–374.
6   RACE R.R., HOLT HELENE A. and THOMPSON JOAN S. (1951) The inheritance and distribution of the Duffy blood groups. *Heredity*, **5**, 103–110.
7   RACE R.R. and SANGER RUTH (1952) The inheritance of the Duffy blood groups: an analysis of 110 English families. *Heredity*, **6**, 111–119.
8   RACE R.R., SANGER RUTH and THOMPSON JOAN S. (1953) Quoted in 2nd edition of this book but not elsewhere published.
9   MOURANT A.E. (1954) *The Distribution of the Human Blood Groups*, pp. 438, Blackwell Scientific Publications, Oxford.
10 LEVINE P., SNEATH JOAN S., ROBINSON ELIZABETH A. and HUNTINGTON P.W. (1955) A second example of anti-Fy^b. *Blood*, **10**, 941–944.
11 MOHR J. (1954) Note on the inheritance of the Duffy blood group system and its possible interaction with the Rhesus groups. *Ann. Eugen., Lond.*, **18**, 318–324.
12 LEWIS MARION, CHOWN B. and KAITA HIROKO (1963) Inheritance of blood group antigens in a largely Eskimo population sample. *Amer. J. hum. Genet.*, **15**, 203–208.
13 RACE R.R. and SANGER RUTH (1958) *Blood Groups in Man*, 3rd edition, Blackwell Scientific Publications, Oxford, p. 271.
14 RACE R.R. and SANGER RUTH (1962) *Blood Groups in Man*, 4th edition, Blackwell Scientific Publications, Oxford, pp. 261–268.
15 IKIN ELIZABETH W., MOURANT A.E. and PLAUT GERTRUDE (1950) A second example of the Duffy antibody. *Brit. med. J.*, i, 584–585.
16 LOGHEM J.J. VAN and HART M. V.D. (1950) Een nieuwe bloedgroep. *Nederl. Tijdschr. v. Geneesk*, **94**, 748–749.
17 ROSENFIELD R.E., VOGEL P. and RACE R.R. (1950) Un nouvel exemplaire d'anti-Fy^a dans un sérum humain. *Rev. Hémat.*, **5**, 315–317.
18 ALLEN F.H. (1950) Personal communication.
19 JAMES J.D. and PLAUT GERTRUDE (1951) The Duffy antibody and haemophilia. *Lancet*, i, 150.
20 FREIESLEBEN E. (1951) Fatal hemolytic transfusion reaction due to anti-Fy^a (Duffy). *Acta path. microbiol. scand.*, **29**, 283–286.
21 HUTCHESON J.B., HABER JANE M. and KELLNER A. (1952) A hazard of repeated blood transfusions. Hemolytic reaction due to antibodies to the Duffy (Fy^a) factor' *J. Amer. med. Ass.*, **149**, 274–275.
22 RACE R.R., SANGER RUTH and LEHANE D. (1953) Quantitative aspects of the blood-group antigen Fy^a. *Ann. Eugen., Lond.*, **17**, 255–266.
23 BAKER J.B., GREWAR D., LEWIS MARION, AYUKAWA H. and CHOWN B. (1956) Haemolytic disease of the newborn due to anti-Duffy (Fy^a). *Arch. Dis. Childh.*, **31**, 298–299.

[24] RACE R.R., SANGER RUTH and MOORES PHYLLIS (1957) Quoted in 3rd ed. of this book but not elsewhere published.

[25] RACE R.R. and SANGER RUTH (1958, 1962 and 1968) *Blood Groups in Man*, 3rd, 4th and 5th editions, Blackwell Scientific Publications, Oxford.

[26] CLEGHORN T.E. (1961) Unpublished observations.

[27] CEDERGREN B. and GILES C.M. (1973) An Fy^xFy^x individual found in Northern Sweden. *Vox Sang.*, **24**, 264–266.

[28] LINNET-JEPSEN P., GALATIUS-JENSEN F. and HAUGE M. (1958) The inheritance of the Gm serum groups. *Acta genet.*, **8**, 164–196.

[29] GALATIUS-JENSEN F. (1958) On the genetics of the haptoglobins. *Acta genet.*, **8**, 232–247.

[30] GREENWALT T.J., SASAKI T. and GAJEWSKI M. (1959) Further examples of haemolytic disease of the newborn due to anti-Duffy (anti-Fy^a). *Vox Sang.*, **4**, 138–143.

[31] BEVAN BERYL (1959) Haemolytic disease of the newborn caused by anti-Duffy (Fy^a). *Lancet*, i, 914–915.

[32] GECZY A. (1960) A case history of a haemolytic disease of the newborn due to anti-Fy^a. *Vox Sang.*, **5**, 551–553.

[33] LEWIS MARION, KAITA HIROKO and CHOWN B. (1957) The blood groups of a Japanese population. *Amer. J. hum. Genet.*, **9**, 274–283.

[34] WON C.D., SHIN H.S., KIM S.W., SWANSON JANE and MATSON G.A. (1960) Distribution of hereditary blood factors among Koreans residing in Seoul, Korea. *Amer. J. phys. Anthrop.*, **18**, 115–124.

[35] SPEISER P. (1959) Ueber die bisher jüngste menschliche Frucht (27mm/2.2g), an der bereits die Erbmerkmale A_1, M, N, s, Fy(a+), C, c, D, E, e, Jk(a+?) im Blut festgestellt werden konnten. *Wien klin. Wschr.*, **71**, 549–551.

[36] RENWICK J.H. and LAWLER SYLVIA D. (1963) Probable linkage between a congenital cataract locus and the Duffy blood group locus. *Ann. hum. Genet.*, **27**, 67–84.

[37] CHOWN B., LEWIS MARION and KAITA HIROKO (1965) The Duffy blood group system in Caucasians: evidence for a new allele. *Amer. J. hum. Genet.*, **17**, 384–389.

[38] MOURANT A.E., KOPEĆ ADA C. and DOMANIEWSKA-SOBCZAK KAZIMIERA (1974) *The Distribution of the Human Blood Groups and other Biochemical Polymorphisms*, 2nd edition, Oxford University Press.

[39] PRICE EVANS D.A., DONOHOE W.T.A., BANNERMAN R.M., MOHN J.F. and LAMBERT R.M. (1966) Blood-group gene localization through a study of mongolism. *Ann. hum. Genet.* **30**, 49–67.

[40] MOHR J. (1966) Genetics of fourteen marker systems: associations and linkage relations. *Acta genet.*, **16**, 1–58.

[41] GREUTER W., HESS M., RENAUD N., SCHMITTER M. and BÜTLER R. (1963) Beitrag zur Genetik des Gm- und Gc-Serumgruppensystems anhand von Untersuchungen an Schweizerfamilien. *Arch. Klaus-Stift. VererbForsch.*, **38**, 77–92.

[42] V.D. WEERDT CHRISTINA M. (1965) *Platelet Antigens and Iso-immunization*. Doctoral Thesis, 'Aemstelstad', Amsterdam, pp. 108.

[43] STEINBERG A., SHWACHMAN H., ALLEN F.H. and DOOLEY R.R. (1956) Linkage studies with cystic fibrosis of the pancreas. *Amer. J. hum. Genet.*, **8**, 162–176.

[44] CHOWN B., LEWIS MARION and KATIA HIROKO (1962) Atypical Duffy inheritance in three Caucasian families: a possible relationship to mongolism. *Amer. J. hum. Genet.*, **14**, 301–308. (From the mongol point of view, see also CHOWN B., LEWIS MARION, KAITA HIROKO (1965.) Atypical Fy^b in some families with a mongol child: a revocation. *Amer. J. hum. Genet.*, **17**, 188.)

[45] LEWIS MARION, KAITA H. and CHOWN B. (1972) The Duffy blood group system in Caucasians. A further population sample. *Vox Sang.*, **23**, 523–527.

[46] ALBREY J.A., VINCENT E.E.R., HUTCHINSON J., MARSH W.L., ALLEN F.H., GAVIN JUNE and SANGER RUTH (1971) A new antibody, anti-Fy3, in the Duffy blood group system. *Vox Sang.*, **20**, 29–35.

47 BUCHANAN D.I. and SINCLAIR MARGARET (1972) Unpublished observations.
48 BEHZAD O., LEE C.L., GAVIN J. and MARSH W.L. (1973) A new anti-erythrocyte antibody in
    the Duffy system: anti-Fy4. *Vox Sang.*, **24**, 337–342.
49 COLLEDGE KATHARINE I., PEZZULICH MARISA and MARSH W.L. (1973) Anti-Fy5, an antibody
    disclosing a probable association between the Rhesus and Duffy blood group genes.
    Vox Sang., **24**, 193–199,
50 BADAKERE S.S. and BHATIA H.M. (1970) A fatal transfusion reaction due to anti-Duffy (Fy^a).
    Indian J. med. Sci., **24**, 562–564.
51 MOLLISON P.L. (1972) *Blood Transfusion in Clinical Medicine.* 5th edition, Blackwell Scien-
    tific Publications, pp. 830.
52 BADAKERE S.S., BHATIA H.M., SHARMA R.S. and BHARUCHA Z. (1970) Anti-Fy^b (Duffy) as a
    cause of transfusion reaction. *Indian J. med. Sci.*, **24**, 565–567.
53 GILES CAROLYN M. (1973) Personal communication.
54 TOIVANEN P. and HIRVONEN T. (1969) Fetal development of red cell antigens K, k, Lu^a, Lu^b,
    Fy^a, Fy^b, Vel and Xg^a. *Scand. J. Haemat.*, **6**, 49–55.
55 TOIVANEN P. and HIRVONEN T. (1973) Antigens Duffy, Kell, Kidd, Lutheran and Xg^a on
    fetal red cells. *Vox Sang.*, **24**, 372–376.
56 SIMMONS R.T., GAJDUSEK D.C., GORMAN J.G., KIDSON C. and HORNABROOK R.W. (1967)
    Presence of the Duffy blood group gene *Fy^b* demonstrated in Melanesians. *Nature, Lond.*,
    213, 1148–1149.

Chapter 11
The Kidd Blood Groups

The Kidd blood group system was discovered by Allen, Diamond and Niedziela[1] in 1951.

The 'new' antibody was found in the serum of a mother, Mrs Kidd, whose child suffered from haemolytic disease of the newborn as a result. The mother's serum also contained anti-K but this was not responsible for the disease because the child was later found to be K−. The 'new' antigen, called Jk[a], was shown to be serologically independent of the other blood groups and to be present in the blood of about 77% of white Bostonians. As expected, it was found to be inherited by means of a gene capable of expressing itself in single or double dose (Race, Sanger, Allen, Diamond and Niedziela[2], 1951).

Other examples of anti-Jk[a] were soon found and, in 1953, the awaited antibody, anti-Jk[b], disclosed itself (Plaut, Ikin, Mourant, Sanger and Race[3]) and, again, further examples quickly followed.

The phenotype Jk(a−b−) was first found in a Filipina of some Spanish and Chinese ancestry (Pinkerton, Mermod, Liles, Jack and Noades[19], 1959). Other examples followed, mostly from the Pacific area. Such people were presumed to be homozygous for a third and yet silent allele, Jk. Several Jk(a−b−) persons have an antibody which gives the reactions of anti-Jk[a]Jk[b] but its real specificity may not be as simple as this.

Europeans heterozygous for a silent allele indistinguishable from Jk were early realized to exist[24], but whether the genetic background is the same as that of the eastern Jk is not known.

FREQUENCIES

Six early series of tests with anti-Jk[a] established the frequency of the antigen in Europeans[1, 2, 4−7]. In total, 4,275 people were distributed as follows:

Jk(a+)	Jk(a−)
3,266	1,009
76·40%	23·60%

From which figures the gene $Jk^b = \sqrt{0.2360} = 0.4858$
and the gene $Jk^a = 1 - 0.4858 = 0.5142$

and the genotype frequencies are

$$\left.\begin{array}{l} Jk^aJk^a \ 0.2644 \text{ or } 0.3461 \\ Jk^aJk^b \ 0.4996 \text{ or } 0.6539 \end{array}\right\} \text{ of all Jk(a+)}$$
$$Jk^bJk^b \ 0.2360$$

Gene frequencies counted from the 2,102 parents of 1,051 Canadian families tested by Chown, Lewis and Kaita[35, 46] with both anti-Jk^a and anti-Jk^b are almost identical:

$$Jk^b = 0.4838 \qquad Jk^a = 0.5162$$

As will be seen below, the gene Jk must exist in Europeans though in practice family tests are needed to show its presence: in theory it might be detected by infinitely laborious titrations with good dosing anti-Jk^a or anti-Jk^b sera with unrelated samples. We estimate that Jk may have a frequency in Europeans of 0.01 or less.

INHERITANCE

In our last edition we analysed 9 series of white families tested with anti-Jk^a (refs. 2, 9, 22, 20, 6, 35–37): in all there were 1,197 families and 3,116 children and the incidence of children fitted well enough the incidence calculated on the two allele hypothesis.

Chown, Lewis and Kaita[35, 46] have tested over a thousand families with anti-Jk^a and anti-Jk^b: the results of their two series are combined in Table 64. The expected incidence of the various mating types, calculated from the gene frequencies obtained from the 2,102 parents, is close to the observed incidence. The distribution of children from the various matings is very close to the expected mendelian ratios, based on two alleles Jk^a and Jk^b. Though Jk does exist in white people[24], its frequency is too low to upset the good fit based on two alleles. No doubt the three Jk(a−b+) children with a Jk(a+b−) parent reflect the presence of Jk in the family, for there was no reason to doubt the parentage of any of the three.

In our own tests with anti-Jk^a and anti-Jk^b on unrelated people and on families we have been troubled by an excess of Jk^aJk^b heterozygotes. In previous editions we wrote:

'Perhaps the simplest explanation is that anti-Jk^a is recognizing a single antigen and anti-Jk^b is not: the anti-Jk^b sera probably contain another antibody. As different anti-Jk^b sera were used in the two investigations we guess that the extra antibody belongs to the Kidd system. Perhaps anti-Jk^b corresponds to, say, anti-c + anti-E in the Rh system: it is only to be expected that the Kidd antigens will prove more complicated than they have appeared up to now'.

13

While we are still having the same old trouble, it is rather irksome that Chown, Lewis and Kaita[35] have so triumphantly avoided it, as may be seen in Table 64.

Table 64. 1051 Canadian families tested with anti-Jk^a and anti-Jk^b (From Chown, Lewis and Kaita[35,46], 1965, 1973)

Type	Matings Number obs.	exp.	Total	Children Jk(a+b−) obs.	exp.	Jk(a+b+) obs.	exp.	Jk(a−b+) obs.	exp.
Jk(a+b−) × Jk(a+b−)	76	74·62	203	203	203	0	0	0	0
Jk(a+b−) × Jk(a+b+)	263	279·67	714	367	357	346	357	1	0
Jk(a+b−) × Jk(a−b+)	127	131·06	357	0	0	355	357	2	0
Jk(a+b+) × Jk(a+b+)	287	262·22	756	179	189	386	378	191	189
Jk(a+b+) × Jk(a−b+)	249	245·83	736	0	0	367	368	369	368
Jk(a−b+) × Jk(a−b+)	49	57·60	132	0	0	0	0	132	132
	1,051	1,051·00	2,898						
	$\chi^2_5 = 4\cdot8$								

THE PHENOTYPE Jk(a−b−)

When the cells of a Filipina, with some Spanish and Chinese ancestry, were found to be Jk(a−b−) it was assumed that either a third allele, *Jk*, must exist or that the condition reflected the presence of a modifying gene (Pinkerton, Mermod, Liles, Jack and Noades[19], 1959).

The patient was brought to notice because of antibody in her serum which reacted with all cells at first tested except her own. The antibody was called anti-Jk^{a}Jk^b.

Many Jk(a−b−) people are now known: at least a dozen selected themselves by having anti-Jk^{a}Jk^b in their serum and a few of these have been reported[39,40,47]; random Jk(a−b−) people have been found in searches for compatible donors. In general, Jk(a−b−) has been found among Filipino-Spanish[19], Hawaian-Chinese[19,40], Chinese[39], Polynesians, particularly Samoans and Maoris, Thais, Mato Grosso Indians[23] but, one example was found in a North African. (Personal communications from Dr J.M. Staveley, Mr J.A. Albrey, Dr L.E. Mermod, Dr Dasnayanee Chandanayingyong and Dr C. Salmon.)

The question of the genetic background of the Jk(a−b−) phenotype, whether it be due to an allele at the *Kidd* locus or to an inhibitory gene, remains unanswered: in either case the background is presumably a homozygous one, and what family evidence there is supports this[39,40,47].

The gene *Jk* in Europeans

Crawford and her colleagues[24] reported a family in which a gene indistinguishable, so far, from the Pacific *Jk* is present in three generations. Illegitimacy could not be entertained, for the key members had proved themselves legitimate by inheriting the extremely rare Lu(a–b–) phenotype. By 1967, we had tested two other families, one Finnish and the other English, in which *Jk* was presumably present: in both a Jk(a+b–) father has a Jk(a–b+) child: although paternity could not be proved in either family, the other groups gave no evidence that the children were extramarital. We have encountered other examples more recently.

The gene *Jk* must however be infrequent in Europeans: were it not, the results of Chown and his colleagues[35, 46] using anti-Jk^a and anti-Jk^b (Table 64) would hardly have fitted so well with the expectations based on a two allele calculation.

KIDD ANTIBODIES

When first discovered, the original anti-Jk^a would agglutinate cells suspended in saline but it later 'went off' *in vivo* and an indirect antiglobulin test had to be used. Apparent 'going off', both *in vivo* and *in vitro*, seems a common trouble with Kidd antisera. The trypsin antiglobulin test[10] can be very helpful in making an anti-Jk^a or anti-Jk^b serum work, and so may the addition of complement[11, 25]. We prefer an antiglobulin test on papainized cells. Antibodies of the Kidd system are usually[26] of the IgG type but may be IgM.

Anti-Jk^a

The discovery[1] of anti-Jk^a was quickly followed by the identification of other examples[5, 12–14]: hundreds of examples must have been found since but not many of them reported[15, 21, 27–31, 41, 48].

Anti-Jk^a has been the rare cause of haemolytic disease of the newborn[1, 15, 30, 42] and of reaction to transfusion[21, 28, 31, 43].

Anti-Jk^b

The first example was found, together with anti-Fy^a, in the serum of a woman who had had a reaction to her second transfusion[3]. Within six months two more examples were recognized[16, 17], both accompanied by several other antibodies. Many examples have now been found though few reported[18, 32, 33, 45, 48]. Anti-Jk^b has caused haemolytic disease of the newborn[32, 33, 44].

As mentioned earlier in this chapter, there is a hint that some anti-Jk^b sera may contain more than one Kidd antibody.

Anti-Jk^{a}Jk^b (anti-Jk3)

This was the name given to the antibody in the Jk(a–b–) patient of Pinkerton *et al.*[19]. Some years later two further examples were reported[39, 40]: like the first, they followed transfusion. In all three sera the antibody appeared to be mainly inseparable anti-Jk^{a}Jk^b: in the first[19] some anti-Jk^b component could be demonstrated and in the second[39] some anti-Jk^a.

Arcara et al.[47] describe a family in which a Jk(a−b−) man who had never been transfused had anti-Jk^{a}Jk^b in his serum, apparently of the 'natural' type, while his Jk(a−b−) sister had no Kidd antibody though she had been pregnant seven times.

In letters from Dr Staveley, Mr Albrey and Dr Salmon, we learnt of another nine examples of the antibody; all but one had been found in Polynesians or people with some Chinese ancestry.

That anti-Jk^{a}Jk^b is not merely anti-Jk^a + anti-Jk^b is confirmed by the observations of Marsh et al.[51] that the neutrophil leucocytes of Jk(a+) and Jk(b+) people do not absorb anti-Jk^a or anti-Jk^b, though both types of neutrophil absorb anti-Jk^{a}Jk^b. The conclusion of Marsh et al. that this demonstrates that anti-Jk^{a}Jk^b is detecting a third and distinct antigenic specificity, anti-Jk3, is convincing.

OTHER NOTES ABOUT THE KIDD GROUPS

Dosage

The only quantitative work with anti-Jk^a and anti-Jk^b that we know of is that of Crawford et al.[24] Most anti-Jk^a sera react on the average more strongly with Jk^a homozygotes than with heterozygotes; with some sera the difference may be striking. Anti-Jk^b undoubtedly can make a dosage distinction but with antisera so far available we have found it difficult to elicit with any regularity.

Development of the antigens

Jk^a and Jk^b are well developed in cord blood: we found Jk^a in two '17 weeks' foetuses, and, in 1961, Cleghorn[20] tested 19 foetuses, aged from 17½ to 28 weeks, with both antisera; the results were:

Jk(a+b−)	Jk(a+b+)	Jk(a−b+)	Jk(a−b−)
8	9	2	0

In 1973, Toivanen and Hirvonen[49] reported the results of testing foetuses between 7 and 20 weeks' gestation, 41 of them with anti-Jk^a and 36 with anti-Jk^b: the antigens were present in the proportions expected. The youngest Jk(a+) was 11 weeks and youngest Jk(b+) 7 weeks.

Anthropological differences

The Kidd groups are proving useful in anthropology[50] for there are striking differences in their distribution. Early work showed the phenotype Jk(a+) to occur in about 95% of West Africans[34], about 93% of American Negroes[5, 8], about 77% of Europeans and about 50% of Chinese[5]. Further, there is the remarkable association of the phenotype Jk(a−b−) with Polynesians.

REFERENCES

1   ALLEN F.H., DIAMOND L.K. and NIEDZIELA BEVELY (1951) A new blood-group antigen. *Nature, Lond.*, **167**, 482.
2   RACE R.R., SANGER RUTH, ALLEN F.H., DIAMOND L.K. and NIEDZIELA BEVELY (1951) Inheritance of the human blood group antigen Jk^a. *Nature, Lond.*, **168**, 207.
3   PLAUT GERTRUDE, IKIN ELIZABETH W., MOURANT A.E., SANGER RUTH and RACE R.R. (1953) A new blood-group antibody, anti-Jk^b. *Nature, Lond.*, **171**, 431.
4   SANGER RUTH and RACE R.R. (1953) Unpublished data.
5   ROSENFIELD R.E., VOGEL P., GIBBEL NATALIE, OHNO GRACE and HABER GLADYS (1953) Anti-Jk^a: three new examples of the isoantibody. Frequency of the factor in Caucasians, Negroes, and Chinese of New York City. *Amer. J. clin. Path.*, **23**, 1222–1225
6   LUNDEVALL J. (1956) The Kidd blood group system, *Acta path microbiol scand.*, **38**, 39–42.
7   HALLE G. HÄSSIG A. and ROSIN S. (1955) Über die bildung von Begleitantikörpern gegan das blutgruppenantigen Jk^a im verlaufe einer Rhesusimmunisierung. *Klin. Wschr.*, **33**, 495.
8   SANGER RUTH, RACE R.R., CAHAN A. and JACK J.A. (1955) Unpublished data.
9   RACE R.R., SANGER RUTH and THOMPSON JOAN S. (1953) Quoted in the 2nd edition of this book but not elsewhere published.
10   UNGER L.J. (1951) A method for detecting Rh$_0$ antibodies in extremely low titer. *J. Lab. clin. Med.*, **37**, 825–827.
11   STRATTON F. (1956) The value of fresh serum in the detection and use of anti-Jk^a antibody. *Vox Sang.*, **1**, 160–167.
12   HUNTER LOIS, LEWIS MARION and CHOWN B. (1951) A further example of Kidd (Jk^a) haem-agglutinin. *Nature, Lond.*, **168**, 790.
13   MILNE G.R., WALLACE J., IKIN ELIZABETH W. and MOURANT A.E. (1953) The Kidd (anti-Jk^a) haemagglutinin: a third example. *Lancet*, **i**, 627.
14   HART MIA V.D. and LOGHEM J.J. VAN (1953) A further example of anti-Jk^a. *Vox Sang.*, **3**, 72–73.
15   GREENWALT T.J., SASAKI T. and SNEATH JOAN (1956) Haemolytic disease of the newborn caused by anti-Jk^a. *Vox Sang.*, **1**, 157–160.
16   SANGER RUTH, RACE R.R., ROSENFIELD R.E. and VOGEL P. (1953) A serum containing anti-s and anti-Jk^b. *Vox Sang.* (O.S.), **3**, 71.
17   LOGHEM J.J. VAN, HEIER ANNE-MARGARETHA, HART MIA V.D. and RIBEIRO SANCHES V. (1953) A serum containing anti-Jk^b, anti-C and anti-M. *Vox Sang.* (O.S.), **3**, 115–117.
18   ROSENFIELD R.E., LEY A.B., HABER GLADYS and HARRIS JEAN P. (1954) A further example of anti-Jk^b. *Amer. J. clin. Path.*, **24**, 1282–1284.
19   PINKERTON F.J., MERMOD L.E., LILES BOBBIE ANN, JACK J.A. and NOADES JEAN (1959) The phenotype Jk(a–b–) in the Kidd blood group system. *Vox Sang.*, **4**, 155–160.
20   CLEGHORN T.E. (1961) Unpublished observations.
21   ANDRÉ R., SALMON C. and MALASSENET R. (1956) A propos de trois exemples d'anticorps anti-Jk^a acquis par transfusions observés en association avec des anticorps anti-Fy^a, S, c, E. *Rev. Hémat.*, **11**, 495–502.
22   RACE R.R. and SANGER RUTH (1958) *Blood Groups in Man*, 3rd edition, p. 228 and p. 231, Blackwell Scientific Publications, Oxford.
23   SILVER R.T., HABER JANE M. and KELLNER A. (1960) Evidence for a new allele in the Kidd blood group system in Indians of Northern Mato Grosso, Brazil. *Nature, Lond.*, **186**, 481.
24   CRAWFORD MARY N., GREENWALT T.J., SASAKI T., TIPPETT PATRICIA, SANGER RUTH and RACE R.R. (1961) The phenotype Lu(a–b–) together with unconventional Kidd groups in one family. *Transfusion, Philad.*, **1**, 228–232.

25 POLLEY MARGARET J. and MOLLISON P.L. (1961) The role of complement in the detection of blood group antibodies: special reference to the antiglobulin test. *Transfusion, Philad.*, **1**, 9–22.

26 MOLLISON P.L. (1972) *Blood Transfusion in Clinical Medicine*, 5th edition, p. 329, Blackwell Scientific Publications, Oxford.

27 SIMMONS R.T., GRAYDON J.J., JAKOBOWICZ RACHEL, SANTAMARIA J. and GARSON MARGARET (1957) Immunization by the blood antigen Kidd (Jk^a) in pregnancy and in blood transfusion. *Med. J. Aust.*, **ii**, 933–935.

28 KRONENBERG H., KOOPTZOFF OLGA and WALSH R.J. (1958) Haemolytic transfusion reaction due to anti-Kidd. *Aust. ann. Med.*, **7**, 34–35.

29 BAILEY J.P., HUTCHINSON-SMITH B.H., BARBER MARGARET and DUNSFORD I. (1959) Immunization during pregnancy to the Kidd (Jk^a) red cell antigen. *Brit. med. J.*, **i**, 1329.

30 MATSON G.A., SWANSON JANE and TOBIN J.D. (1959) Severe hemolytic disease of the newborn caused by anti-Jk^a. *Vox Sang.*, **4**, 144–147.

31 PILGÅRD S., LINNET-JEPSEN P. and KISSMEYER-NIELSEN F. (1959) Haemolytisk transfusionreaktion forårsaget of anti-Kidd (anti-Jk^a). *Saertryk af Ugeskr. Laeger*, **121**, 1960–1964.

32 KORNSTAD L. and HALVORSEN K. (1958) Haemolytic disease of the newborn caused by anti-Jk^b. *Vox Sang.*, **3**, 94–99.

33 GECZY A. and LESLIE M. (1961) Second example of hemolytic disease of the newborn caused by anti-Jk^b. *Transfusion, Philad.*, **1**, 125–127.

34 IKIN ELIZABETH W. and MOURANT A.E. (1952) The frequency of the Kidd blood group antigen in Africans. *Man*, **52**, 21.

35 CHOWN B., LEWIS MARION and KAITA HIROKO (1965) The Kidd blood group system in Caucasians. *Transfusion, Philad.*, **5**, 506–507.

36 MOHR J. (1966) Genetics of fourteen marker systems: associations and linkage relations. *Acta genet.*, **16**, 1–58.

37 STEINBERG A., SCHWACHMAN H., ALLEN F.H. and DOOLEY R.R. (1956) Linkage studies with cystic fibrosis of the pancreas. *Amer. J. hum. Genet.*, **8**, 162–176.

38 LEWIS MARION, CHOWN B. and KAITA HIROKO (1963) Inheritance of blood group antigens in a largely Eskimo population sample. *Amer. J. hum. Genet.*, **15**, 203–208.

39 DAY DOROTHY, PERKINS H.A. and SAMS B. (1965) The minus-minus phenotype in the Kidd system. *Transfusion, Philad.*, **5**, 315–319.

40 YOKOYAMA M., MERMOD L.E. and STEGMAIER ANN (1967) Further examples of Jk(a–b–) blood in Hawaii. *Vox Sang.*, **12**, 154–156.

41 SEYFRIEDOWA HALINA, WALEWSKA IRENA and ZUPANSKA BARBARA (1965) Anti-Kidd (Jk^a) antibodies in chronic lymphatic leukaemia with hypogammaglobulinaemia. *Arch. Immunol. et Ther. Exper.*, **13**, 133–141.

42 GECZY A. and MATHESON W.A. (1965) Hemolytic disease of the newborn caused by anti-Jk^a. *Amer. J. Obstet. Gynec.*, **82**, 576 (not seen).

43 DEGNAN T.J. and ROSENFIELD R.E. (1965) Hemolytic transfusion reaction associated with poorly detectable anti-Jk^a. *Transfusion, Philad.*, **5**, 245–247.

44 ZODIN V. and ANDERSON R.E. (1965) Hemolytic disease of the newborn due to anti-Kidd (anti-Jk^b): case report and review of the literature. *Pediatrics*, **36**, 420 (not seen).

45 MORGAN P., WHEELER C.B. and BOSSOM EDITH L. (1967) Delayed transfusion reaction attributed to anti-Jk^b. *Transfusion, Philad.*, **7**, 307–308.

46 CHOWN B., LEWIS MARION and KAITA HIROKO (1973) Unpublished observations.

47 ARCARA P.C., O'CONNOR M.A. and DIMMETTE R.M. (1969) A family with three Jk(a–b–) members. *Transfusion, Philad.*, **9**, 282.

48 HOMBERG J.-C., GERBAL A., BRACQ CHRISTINE, SAINT-PAUL DANIÈLE, BRIZARD C.P. and SALMON C. (1969) Intéret transfusionnel du système Kidd. *Rev. franc. Transf.*, **13**, Suppl. to No. 1, 113–122.

49 TOIVANEN P. and HIRVONEN T. (1973) Antigens Duffy, Kell, Kidd, Lutheran and Xg^a on fetal red cells. *Vox Sang.*, **24**, 372–376.

⁵⁰ MOURANT A.E., KOPEĆ ADA C. and DOMANIEWSKA-SOBCZAK KAZIMIERA (1974) *The Distribution of the Human Blood Groups and other Biochemical Polymorphisms*. 2nd edition, Oxford University Press.
⁵¹ MARSH W.L., ØYEN RAGNHILD and NICHOLS MARGARET E. (1974) Kidd blood-group antigens of leukocytes and platelets. *Transfusion, Philad.*, **14**, 378–381.

Chapter 12
The Diego Blood Groups

The antigen Di^a is practically confined to people of Mongolian extraction.

The antibody, anti-Di^a, was found in Venezuela where it had been the cause of haemolytic disease of the newborn (Layrisse, Arends and Dominguez[1], 1955). In the original family the antigen was found in four generations and was clearly behaving like a dominant character (Levine, Robinson, Layrisse, Arends and Dominguez[2]). It is interesting to read that during the investigation of this white family it was noted, by Layrisse and Arends, that certain members showed physical features suggesting the presence of admixture with native Indians: this observation prompted the investigation of Indian blood which was to prove so fruitful.

A preliminary hint that the antigen was rare in white people was included in the first brief mention of Diego[3], no Di(a+) having been found in 200 samples tested; this number was later[2] increased to 1,000, then, by the addition of two further series[4], to 2,600. However, Simmons *et al.*[28] found the antigen in an Irish-Australian family. On the other hand, Layrisse *et al.*[1] found the antigen to be common in South American Indians—notably in the Carib Indians of Cachama (36%).

It is present in Chinese[5] (about 2·5%) and Japanese[5, 6] (about 8 to 12%) and in Chippewa Indians[6] (11%). These frequencies must all be approximate for most samples were small.

There are now very many papers on the distribution of the antigen in different peoples. The subject has been reviewed in two monographs by Layrisse and Wilbert[7, 25] and a number of references are to be found in Won *et al.*[8]. Since Di^a is considered to be essentially a Mongolian character, its all but absence from Eskimos[9, 20, 21, 22] presents a puzzle.

More than ten years after the finding of anti-Di^a, Thompson, Childers and Hatcher[26] (1967) identified the antithetical anti-Di^b. The symbol for the 'not Di^a' allele used to be Di, but after the finding of anti-Di^b it is promoted to Di^b. As no phenotype Di(a−b−) has yet been reported we may, for the present at any rate, think of a system controlled by only two alleles, Di^a and Di^b.

INHERITANCE OF Di^a

Although so many papers have appeared on the distribution of the antigen Di^a in different populations there are few on the genetics of the character.

372

The four families published by Layrisse, Arends and Dominguez[1] made it appear likely that the antigen was inherited as a dominant character but the final proof had to await the paper of Lewis, Kaita and Chown[10]: in testing 50 Japanese families, nine of which had the antigen, they showed that a Di(a+) × Di(a+) mating could have Di(a–) children and also that all of 111 children from 41 Di(a–) × Di(a–) matings were Di(a–).

We know of only two other series of unselected families. Salazar and Arias[11] tested 30 Tlaxcaltecan Indian families:

Di(a+) × Di(a+) matings 0
Di(a+) × Di(a–) matings 11, children Di(a+) 8, Di(a–) 13
Di(a–) × Di(a–) matings 19, children Di(a+) 0, Di(a–) 41

And Layrisse and Wilbert[7] tested 20 Carib families from an area where the frequency of Di(a+) is 29%:

Di(a+) × Di(a+) matings 0
Di(a+) × Di(a–) matings 9, children Di(a+) 17, Di(a–) 18
Di(a–) × Di(a–) matings 11, children Di(a+) 0, Di(a–) 44

These figures were in good agreement with those calculated on the basis of 29% Di(a+) in the general population.

A series for which no expectations can easily be calculated because the families came from areas of variable frequency of the antigen are also reported by Layrisse and Wilbert[7]:

Di(a+) × Di(a+) matings 2, children Di(a+) 6, Di(a–) 1
Di(a+) × Di(a–) matings 29, children Di(a+) 52, Di(a–) 35
Di(a–) × Di(a–) matings 15, children Di(a+) 0, Di(a–) 45

These results and those of tests on families selected for having Di(a+) members all conspire to establish the antigen Di^a as a straightforward dominant character.

A large Japanese family in which the antigen Di^a is segregating was reported by Mohn and his colleagues[23]. Lewis, Chown and Kaita[22] tested 116 Eskimo families with 364 children without finding a single Di(a+).

The independence of the antigen Di^a

Evidence from the literature and from nine new families was collected by Layrisse, Sanger and Race[12] which showed the antigen to be independent of most of the established systems. In Table 65 the Diego groups are seen to be on the verge of achieving systemic status: Lutheran is the only real hurdle left. To achieve systemic status Diego does not have to be excluded from systems discovered later: subsequent systems such as Yt and Dombrock have, on the other hand, to be shown to be independent of Diego.

13*

The reasoning on which the statement in Table 65 that, for example, Di^a is not part of the ABO system needs some explanation and the following attempt, taken mainly from Layrisse, Sanger and Race[12], will serve for any other dominant character: the treatment of recessive characters will be illustrated by applying it to the rare Ge negative phenotype (page 411). The argument is based on the fact that recombination, which is the outward sign of crossing-over, has never, or hardly ever, been observed between antigens controlled by a gene complex such as that responsible for Rh. If therefore the genes for the Diego system segregate away from the genes for, say, the ABO system we can be sure that the Di^a antigen is not a previously unknown part of that system. The only qualification is that illegitimacy could give a false appearance of separate segregation when the separation is the contribution of the sperm rather than of the ovum.

Table 65. The independence of Diego of other blood group systems: references to families in which separate segregation can be seen

	ABO	MNSs	P	Rh	Luth.	Kell
Di^a	bcdefh	abcefh	bcde	acdef		eg

	Duffy	Kidd	Yt	Domb.	sec.
Di^a	beh	ae		j	d*fi

a. Levine and Robinson[13], 1957; other groups recorded of the large family in which the antigen was first found.
b. Lewis, Kaita and Chown[10, 14], 1957, 1958; one large Japanese pedigree.
c. Allen[15], 1958; 11 Peruvian Indian families.
d. Iseki, Masaki, Furukawa, Mohn, Lambert and Rosamilia[16], 1958; six Japanese families.
e. Layrisse, Sanger and Race[12], 1959; nine Venezuelan families of mixed Indian, Spanish and negro ancestry.
f. Mohn, Lambert, Iseki, Masaki and Furukawa[23], 1963; one large Japanese family.
g. Alter, Gelb and Lee[24], 1964; one Puerto Rican family.
h. Thompson, Childers and Hatcher[26], 1967; one Mexican Indian family, tested with anti-Di^a and anti-Di^b.
i. Iseki, Masaki, Furukawa, Lambert and Mohn[29], 1970; a Japanese family.
j. Lewis, Kaita and Chown, 1974, personal communication.

Many of the families exclude X- or Y-linkage: the existence of Di(a+b+) males also excludes X-linkage.

* Based on Lewis phenotypes of red cells; saliva not tested.

Families of two or more children are needed to show separate segregation of two loci and they have to be of certain mating types. (A one child family can be informative in the somewhat less usual situation where the grandparents have also been tested, see Chapter 27.) The most informative kind of mating is that known as the double back-cross: in this type one parent must be heterozygous at both the loci being investigated and the destination, in the children, of this parent's genes must be clear. The family in Figure 24 serves as an example. The mother, I-2, is of the genotype $Di^a Di^b$ for she has some Di(a−) children (the family was tested before the days of anti-Di^b); she is also heterozygous $A_1 O$ for she has some OO children. Her contribution to the five children has been Di^b, O; Di^a, A_1; Di^a, A_1; Di^b, A_1; Di^a, O. The following is a simple way of seeing whether the children demonstrate that the two systems are not part of each other. The four possible contributions of the doubly heterozygous parent are written down thus:

Di^a	Di^b	Di^b	Di^a
A_1	O	A_1	O
2	1	1	1

The example gives what we call an independence count of 3:2. If, as in this example, there be entries on both sides of the vertical line then the two gene systems being tested are proved not to belong to one and the same system. If all the entries be on one side of the vertical line it is probably a chance finding, but if it were a constant finding in other families then it would show that the two systems were one and the same. If in most families the entries were all on one side but in occasional families entries on both sides were found this would mean that the two

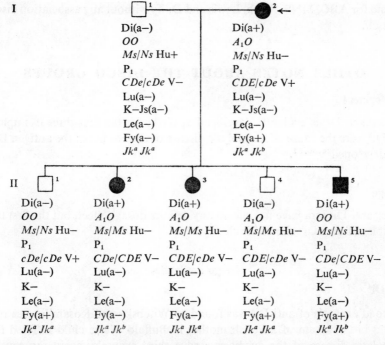

Fig. 24. A family (Lan.) illustrating the independence of the antigen Di^a of the ABO, MNSs, Rh, Duffy and Kidd systems. Black = Di(a+). (From Layrisse, Sanger and Race[12], 1959.)

systems were not part of each other but that their loci were linked in the classical sense; this type of linkage presents quite a separate problem and will be discussed in the chapter on linkage (page 547). So far no linkages between the Diego and other loci have been detected[12].

Incidentally, the family in Figure 24 besides showing that Di^a is not part of the ABO system excludes it from MNSs (3:2), Rh (4:1,) Duffy (4:1) and Kidd (4:1).

Only one family is on record in which the antigen Lu^a and the antigen Di^a are possessed by one person and he handed on his Lu^b allele and his Di^b allele to all three children: an independence count of 3:0, which leaves open the question of a possible association of Diego and Lutheran[17].

For completeness, mention should be made of another way in which a new antigen may be shown to belong to, or at least be influenced by, an old system. If the frequency of the new antigen is not the same in each of the different divisions of a known system then the antigen probably belongs to that system. For example, the observation that the antigen S was more common in samples of blood of group M than of group N gave the first indication that S was part of the MN system. A more extreme example is the antigen Tj^a which was recognized as belonging to the P system when all Tj(a−) persons tested at that time were found to be negative with anti-P_1. The method can only show dependence, it cannot prove independence. Allen[15] applied this method to samples from 308 Peruvian Indians tested for Di^a and for ABO, MNS, P, Rh, Lewis and Duffy without any association disclosing itself.

OTHER NOTES ABOUT THE DIEGO GROUPS

Development

The antigen Di^a is evidently developed at birth, for the first three examples of anti-Di^a were the cause of haemolytic disease of the newborn: the antigen Di^b is well developed[26, 30, 31].

Dosage

So far, anti-Di^a sera have not shown any definite dosage effect, but the first three examples of anti-Di^b showed it clearly.

Diego antibodies

Anti-Di^a

A second example of anti-Di^a was found by Witebsky and Rosamilia (see reference 2) in the serum of a Polish mother in Buffalo whose child suffered from haemolytic disease of the newborn, and a third example, again the cause of haemolytic disease, was reported by Tatarsky, Stroup, Levine and Ernoehazy[18]. A fourth example was found by van Peenen, Scudder, Jack and Awer[19] in the serum of a Puerto Rican mother whose twins were healthy though their direct antiglobulin tests were positive. A fifth example was found in an Australian woman in whom it appeared to be 'naturally occurring'[28]. Many more examples have been found but they no longer get reported.

Anti-Di^b

The first two examples were reported by Thompson, Childers and Hatcher[26]; both were found in Mexican Indian women. One was found during the investigation of jaundice following transfusion, the other at cross-matching. Both women had had many pregnancies but only the first had been previously transfused. A third example (Mermod and Hatcher[27]) was found on cross-matching the serum of a Japanese woman in Hawaii. The first two examples reacted only by the antiglobulin test: the third reacted also by enzyme tests. We know of three more examples[30, 31, 32].

The Venezuelan discovery of Di^a will make a good contribution to human genetics: it has already made an outstanding contribution to the anthropology of the Mongolian world.

REFERENCES

1 LAYRISSE M., ARENDS T. and DOMINGUEZ SISCO R. (1955) Nuevo grupo sanguineo encontrado en descendientes de Indios. *Acta Medica Venezolana*, 3, 132–138.
2 LEVINE P., ROBINSON ELIZABETH A., LAYRISSE M., ARENDS T. and DOMINGUEZ SISCO R. (1956) The Diego blood factor. *Nature, Lond.*, 177, 40–41.
3 LEVINE P., KOCH ELIZABETH A., McGEE R.T. and HILL G.H. (1954) Rare human isoagglutinins and their identification. *Amer. J. clin. Path.*, 24, 292–304.
4 LAYRISSE M. and ARENDS T. (1958) The 'Diego' blood factor distribution: genetic, clinical and anthropological significance. *Proc. 6th Congr. int. Soc. Blood Transf.*, 114–116.
5 LAYRISSE M. and ARENDS T. (1956) The Diego blood factor in Chinese and Japanese. *Nature, Lond.*, 177, 1083–1084.
6 LEWIS MARION, AYUKAWA HIROKO, CHOWN B. and LEVINE P. (1956) The blood group antigen Diego in North American Indians and in Japanese. *Nature, Lond.*, 177, 1084.
7 LAYRISSE M. and WILBERT J. (1960) *El Antigeno del Sistema Sanguineo Diego*, pp. 160, La Fundación Creole y la Fundación Eugenio Mendoza, Caracas.
8 WON C.D., SHIN H.S., KIM S.W., SWANSON JANE and MATSON G.A. (1960) Distribution of hereditary blood factors among Koreans residing in Seoul, Korea. *Amer. J. phys. Anthrop.*, 18, 115–124.
9 LEWIS MARION, CHOWN B. and KAITA HIROKO (1956) Further observations on the blood factor Di^a. *Nature, Lond.*, 178, 1125.
10 LEWIS MARION, KAITA HIROKO and CHOWN B. (1957) The blood groups of a Japanese population. *Amer. J. hum. Genet.*, 9, 274–283.
11 SALAZAR MALLÉN M. and ARIAS TERESA (1959) Inheritance of Diego blood group in Mexican Indians. *Science*, 130, 164–165.
12 LAYRISSE M., SANGER RUTH and RACE R.R. (1959) The inheritance of the antigen Di^a: evidence for its independence of other blood group systems. *Amer. J. hum. Genet.*, 11 17–25.

13 LEVINE P. and ROBINSON ELIZABETH A. (1957) Some observations on the new human blood factor Di^a. *Blood*, **12**, 448–453.

14 CHOWN B., LEWIS MARION and KAITA HIROKO (1958) Diego as an independent blood group system. *Nature, Lond.*, **181**, 1598–1599.

15 ALLEN F.H. (1958) Inheritance of the Diego (Di^a) blood group factor. *Amer. J. hum. Genet.*, **10**, 64–67.

16 ISEKI S., MASAKI S., FURUKAWA K., MOHN J., LAMBERT R.M. and ROSAMILIA H.C. (1958) Diego and Miltenberger blood factor in Japanese. *Gunma J. med. Sci.*, **7**, 120–126.

17 ALLEN F.H. and CORCORAN PATRICIA A. (1960) Blood groups of the Penobscot Indians. *Amer. J. phys. Anthrop.*, **18**, 109–114.

18 TATARSKY J., STROUP MARJORY, LEVINE P. and ERNOEHAZY W.S. (1959) Another example of anti-Diego (Di^a). *Vox Sang.*, **4**, 152–154.

19 PEENEN H.J. VAN, SCUDDER J., JACK J.A. and AWER ERIKA (1961) The Diego factor in a Puerto Rican family: a case of anti-Diego. *Blood*, **17**, 457–461.

20 CHOWN B. and LEWIS MARION (1959) The blood group genes of the Copper Eskimo. *Amer. J. phys. Anthrop.*, **17**, 13–18.

21 CORCORAN PATRICIA A., ALLEN F.H., ALLISON A.C. and BLUMBERG B.S. (1959) Blood groups of Alaskan Eskimos and Indians. *Amer. J. phys. Anthrop.*, **17**, 187–193.

22 LEWIS MARION, CHOWN B. and KAITA HIROKO (1963) Inheritance of blood group antigens in a largely Eskimo population sample. *Amer. J. hum. Genet.*, **15**, 203–208.

23 MOHN J.F., LAMBERT R.M., ISEKI S., MASAKI S. and FURUKAWA K. (1963) The blood group antigen Mi^a in Japanese. *Vox Sang.*, **8**, 430–437.

24 ALTER A.A., GELB A.G. and LEE ST. L. (1964) Hemolytic disease of the newborn caused by a new antibody (anti-Go^a). *Proc. 9th Congr. int. Soc. Blood Transf.*, México 1962, 341–343.

25 LAYRISSE M. and WILBERT J. (1966) *Indian Societies of Venezuela: their Blood Group Types*, pp. 318. Editorial Sucre, Caracas-Venezuela.

26 THOMPSON P.R., CHILDERS D.M. and HATCHER D.E. (1967) Anti-Di^b: first and second examples. *Vox Sang.*, **13**, 314–318.

27 MERMOD L.E. and HATCHER D.E. (1967) Personal communication.

28 SIMMONS R.T., ALBREY J.A., MORGAN J.A.G. and SMITH A.J. (1968) The Diego blood group: anti-Di^a and the Di(a+) blood group antigen found in Caucasians. *Med. J. Aust.*, **1**, 406–407.

29 ISEKI S., MASAKI S., FURUKAWA K., LAMBERT R.M. and MOHN J.F. (1970) The blood group antigen Di^a in Japanese and its independence of the ABH secretor system. *Vox Sang.*, **19**, 483–487.

30 FELLER C.W., SHENKER L., SCOTT E.P. and MARSH W.L. (1970) An anti-Diego^b (Di^b) antibody occurring during pregnancy. *Transfusion, Philad.*, **10**, 279–280.

31 GOTTLIEB A.M. (1971) Hemolytic disease of the newborn due to anti-Di^b. *Vox Sang.*, **21**, 79–80.

32 NAKAJIMA H., HAYAKAWA Z. and ITO H. (1971) A new example of anti-Di^b found in a Japanese woman. *Vox Sang.*, **20**, 271–273.

Chapter 13
The Yt Blood Groups

The antibody defining the very common antigen Yt^a was the cause of a cross-matching difficulty investigated by Eaton, Morton, Pickles and White[1], in 1956. The antibody was not avid: it reacted best with the antiglobulin test or the trypsin antiglobulin test and only certain antiglobulin sera were suitable; it was presumed to be the result of several previous transfusions.

Samples of blood from 1,051 English people were tested and only four negatives were found. The positives showed two grades of strength and the assumption that the weaker reactors were heterozygotes allowed an estimate of the gene frequencies simply by counting. The frequencies were internally consistent and very close to those found later.

Further examples of anti-Yt^a soon followed and in 1964 Giles and Metaxas[2] found the first example of the anticipated anti-Yt^b.

FREQUENCIES

Table 66 shows the combined results of two Oxford series of tests using anti-Yt^a: the original series of Eaton et al.[1] and a later one by Cameron and Pickles[3]. The table also shows the results of tests on Europeans by Giles, Metaxas-Bühler, Romanski and Metaxas[4] using anti-Yt^b. The gene frequencies, calculated in the usual way, agree very well. We propose to take the 'European' figures since the proportion of negatives, on which the calculations are based, is so much higher when anti-Yt^b is used.

Table 66. Tests with anti-Yt^a or anti-Yt^b on unrelated white people

	Phenotypes				Genes	
	Yt(a+)	Yt(a−)	Yt(b+)	Yt(b−)	Yt^a	Yt^b
Eaton et al.[1], 1956 Oxford Cameron and Pickles[3], 1959 Oxford	2,563	5			0·9564	0·0436
Giles et al.[4], 1967 European			113	1,286	0·9587	0·0413

379

The calculated phenotype and genotype frequencies are:

Yt(a+b−)	$Yt^a Yt^a$	0·9192
Yt(a+b+)	$Yt^a Yt^b$	0·0791
Yt(a−b+)	$Yt^b Yt^b$	0·0017

Giles and her colleagues[4] tested 84 Yt(b+) London donors with anti-Yt^a and found two Yt(a−), which fits perfectly with expectation. Only one Yt(b+) was found in testing samples from 69 Negroes, mostly from New York. Wurzel and Haesler[12] tested 714 American Negroes with anti-Yt^b and the gene frequencies were Yt^a 0·9571 and Yt^b 0·0429 which are indistinguishable from those for Europeans.

No example of Yt(a−b−) has yet been found, but experience of other systems suggests that, sooner or later, it will be.

INHERITANCE

Eaton, Morton, Pickles and White[1] tested three families selected for containing Yt(a−) members and showed that the antigen Yt^a was inherited as a dominant character.

Giles and her colleagues[4] tested 56 families with 181 children with anti-Yt^b and often with anti-Yt^a also. The results showed that Yt^b is a dominant character.

Independence of other systems

Using anti-Yt^a Eaton et al.[1] showed, by independent segregation in families, that the Yt system was not part of the ABO, MN or Rh systems: the pedigrees also excluded X or Y linkage. To the systems excluded, Allen, Milkovich and Corcoran[5] added Lutheran; and Giles et al.[4], using anti-Yt^b, added P, Kell, Lewis, secretor, Duffy, Kidd and Dombrock (and, incidentally, the serum groups Hp and Gc). Exclusion from the Scianna system was recorded by Giles et al.[10], in 1970, and from the Colton system by Lewis et al.[11], in 1973. So Yt it all but genetically established as an independent blood group system; its exclusion from the Diego locus may take a long time, depending on whether Mongolian people have an appreciable frequency of Yt^b.

OTHER NOTES ABOUT THE Yt GROUPS

Dosage

A difference in strength of reaction of the original anti-Yt^a was skilfully exploited by Eaton and his colleagues[1] to distinguish between homozygotes and heterozygotes: this allowed them to make a very accurate estimate of the gene frequencies.

Giles and her colleagues[4] record how their two examples of anti-Yt[b] do not give an appreciable dosage effect.

Development

The antigen Yt[a] is present at birth, though weaker than in adults[1]: the antigen Yt[b] appears to be fully developed[4].

Yt antibodies

Anti-Yt[a]

The antibody is evidently immune; it was not found in the serum of six Yt(a−) untransfused people[1].

Towards the end of her life the original patient suffered from severe ascites. Anti-Yt[a] was found in the ascitic fluid and a method of concentrating it was developed. The account of this admirable investigation should be read in the original[1].

Samples of Yt(a−) cells from Oxford were used to identify a second example of anti-Yt[a], in the serum of a Yt(a−) patient in the Memorial Center for Cancer and Allied Diseases, New York[6]. A powerful anti-Yt[a] sent to us by Dr A.A. Alter was found in a non-transfused mother whose newborn child gave a positive direct antiglobulin test but did not show any evidence of haemolytic disease.

Very many examples of anti-Yt[a] were subsequently found, often in the company of other antibodies; some of them were published[7, 9, 12, 16]. The antibody seems usually to do little harm[1, 13, 14] though two cases are reported[9, 16] in which it resulted in the rapid removal of ^{51}Cr labelled Yt(a+) cells.

Anti-Yt[b]

The first example was found by Giles and Metaxas[2] in a much-transfused Swiss woman whose serum also contained separable anti-Fy[b] and anti-Bp[a]. Six months later, a second example[8] was identified in a much-transfused Englishman suffering from nocturnal haemoglobinuria whose serum also contained anti-C. The third example was found three years later, again in a much transfused man and this time accompanied by anti-c. Other examples we know of were found by Mrs Patricia Stiles of Ortho, Ontario and by Dr Salmon and his colleagues in Paris; the former contained anti-Fy[a], the latter contained many other antibodies including Anti-Au[a].

From 1956 to 1964 the antigen Yt[a] was of practical importance only because of the occasional cross-matching problem which it caused. The finding of the antithetical anti-Yt[b] raised the stature of the Yt system to that of a chromosome marker of about the same potential usefulness (see page 507) as the Lutheran system.

REFERENCES

1   EATON B.R., MORTON J.A., PICKLES MARGARET M. and WHITE K.E. (1956) A new antibody anti-Yt^a, characterizing a blood group of high incidence. *Brit. J. Haemat.*, 2, 333–341.
2   GILES CAROLYN M. and METAXAS M.N. (1964) Identification of the predicted blood group antibody anti-Yt^b. *Nature, Lond.*, 202, 1122–1123.
3   CAMERON A. and PICKLES MARGARET M. (1959) Personal communication to Giles *et al.*[4]
4   GILES CAROLYN M., METAXAS-BÜHLER M., ROMANSKI Y. and METAXAS M.N. (1967) Studies on the Yt blood group system. *Vox Sang.*, 13, 171–180.
5   ALLEN F.H., MILKOVICH LUCILLE and CORCORAN PATRICIA A. (1963) A pedigree showing that Yt^a is not in the Lutheran blood-group system. *Vox Sang.*, 8, 376–377.
6   LEY A.B., HARRIS JEAN P., SANGER RUTH and RACE R.R. (1957) Unpublished observation.
7   BERGVALDS HELENA, STOCK ANNE and McCLURE P.D. (1965) A further example of anti-Yt^a. *Vox Sang.*, 10, 627–630.
8   IKIN ELIZABETH W., GILES CAROLYN M. and PLAUT GERTRUD (1965) A second example of anti-Yt^b. *Vox Sang.*, 10, 212–213.
9   BETTIGOLE R., HARRIS JEAN P., TEGOLI J. and ISSITT P.D. (1968) Rapid *in vivo* destruction of Yt(a+) red cells in a patient with anti-Yt^a. *Vox Sang.*, 14, 143–146.
10 GILES CAROLYN M., BEVAN BERYL and HUGHES R.M. (1970) A family showing independent segregation of Bu^a and Yt^b. *Vox Sang.*, 18, 265–266.
11 LEWIS MARION, KAITA HIROKO, GIBLETT ELOISE R. and STEINBERG A.G. (1973). Independence of the Colton and Yt blood group systems. *Vox Sang.*, 25, 540–542.
12 WURZEL H.A. and HAESLER W.E. (1968) The Yt blood groups in American Negroes. *Vox Sang.*, 15, 304–305.
13 DOBBS JOAN V., PRUTTING D.L., ADEBAHR MARGOT E., ALLEN F.H. and ALTER A.A. (1968) Clinical experience with three examples of anti-Yt^a. *Vox Sang.*, 15, 216–221.
14 LAVALLÉE R., LACOMBE M., CHARRON M. and D'ANGELO C. (1970) Un cas d'allo-immunisation foeto-maternelle due à un antigène de haute fréquence Yt^a. *Rev. fr. Transfus.*, 13, 71–76.
15 WURZEL H.A. and HAESLER W. (1968) Another example of anti-Yt^b. *Vox Sang.*, 14, 460–461.
16 GÖBEL U., DRESCHER K.H., PÖTTGEN W. and LEHR H.J. (1974) A second example of anti-Yt^a with rapid *in vivo* destruction of Yt(a+) red cells. *Vox Sang.*, 27, 171–175.

Chapter 14
The Auberger Blood Groups

The antibody which defined the antigen Au^a was found in Paris at the Centre Départmental de Transfusion Sanguine (Salmon, Salmon, Liberge, André, Tippett and Sanger[1], 1961). The investigation was made difficult because in the serum of Madame Au., besides the antibody named after her, were present also anti-A, anti-B, anti-E, anti-K and anti-Fy^b. Madame Au. had been many times transfused, and died in 1961.

It was hoped that donors in Paris and London classified with anti-Au^a would serve as a net to catch further examples of the antibody, but not till 1971 did this succeed when Dr Salmon, Dr Gerbal and Dr Tippett isolated a second example in an extremely complicated serum in which anti-K as well as other antibodies had been found by Dr Vidal of Corbeil. Besides anti-Au^a the serum contained anti-A, anti-Lu^a, anti-K, anti-Fy^b and anti-Yt^b. The patient Mme Tor., had been much transfused and several times pregnant.

In both sera the anti-Au^a worked best by the antiglobulin method, using prepapainized cells.

The antigen is well developed at birth.

FREQUENCIES

Table 67 shows that about 82% of French and English people are Au(a+): the corresponding gene frequencies are

$$Au = \sqrt{0\cdot1801} = 0\cdot4244$$
$$Au^a = 1 - 0\cdot4244 = 0\cdot5756$$

and the genotype frequencies:

Au^aAu^a	0·3313
Au^aAu	0·4886
$AuAu$	0·1801

Of all Au(a+) 0·4041 are expected to be homozygous, Au^aAu^a, and 0·5959 heterozygous, Au^aAu.

It looks as if the frequencies will prove about the same in Negroes: 39 were tested and 34 were Au(a+).

Two by two, two by three, etc., contingency tables disclosed no serological association between the Au groups and ABO, MNSs, P, Rh, Lutheran, Lewis, Duffy and Kidd groups; nor did the distribution differ significantly in the two sexes.

Table 67. Distribution of the Au(a+) phenotype in Paris and London. (After Salmon, Salmon, Liberge, André, Tippett and Sanger[1], 1961)

	Total tested	Au(a+) Absolute	Au(a+) Per cent
Paris	389	315	80·98
London	155	131	84·52
	544	446	81·99

INHERITANCE

The antigen behaves like a dominant character: $+ \times +$ matings produced $+$ and $-$ children, and $- \times -$ matings produced only $-$ children. Owing to the limited amount of serum some of the 33 families tested[1] were selected for the mating type Au(a+) $\times$ Au(a−) in order to get as much information as possible about the genetical independence of Au and the other systems. This plan was rewarded and Au was very nearly established as an independent system. The families showed that the gene responsible for the antigen Au^a segregated away from the genes for ABO, MNSs, P, Rh, Duffy, Kidd and Le^a in saliva; nor was it X- or Y-linked. It remained therefore to be proved independent of Lutheran, Kell and secretor.

In view of the association of Au(a−) with the dominant form of Lu(a−b−), to be described below, the genetical relationship of Auberger and Lutheran became of special interest. Was Auberger part of the Lutheran system? This, mainly due to shortage of anti-Au^a, remained unknown for 11 years. Then, in 1974, Salmon and his colleagues (personal communication) found a family which gave the answer; Au^a is controlled from a locus independent of the Lutheran locus (2 non-recombinants: 2 recombinants).

In(Lu) and the antigen Au^a

That Lu(a−b−) people of the dominant type are too often Au(a−) was observed by Tippett[2,3] in 1963 when testing the Crawford family (Figure 18, page 270). Dr Tippett's present count for families of the dominant Lu(a−b−) type is:

	Au(a+)	Au(aw)	Au(a−)
Lu(a−b−) members	1	2	32
members not Lu(a−b−)	20	0	7

for which the probability is 1 in many millions were there no association between the two phenotypes.

There now seems no doubt that a rare allele at an inhibitor locus, for the present called *In(Lu)*, is responsible for the inhibition of the Au^a antigen as well as for the antigens Lu^a and Lu^b, and that the inhibition also involves the antigens P$_1$ and i (Crawford, Tippett and Sanger[4], 1974). The subject has been dealt with a little more fully in the Lutheran chapter.

The discovery in France of an antibody which reacts with the cells of 82% of Europeans was a useful contribution on its own: of more fundamental importance, however, is the part Auberger has played in showing that the inhibitor first detected by its action on the Lutheran system acts also on other systems.

REFERENCES

[1] SALMON C., SALMON D., LIBERGE G., ANDRÉ R., TIPPETT P. and SANGER R. (1961) Un nouvel antigène de groupe sanguin erythrocytaire présent chez 80% des sujets de race blanche. *Nouv. Rev. franc. Hémat.*, **1**, 649–661.
[2] TIPPETT PATRICIA (1963) *Serological Study of the Inheritance of Unusual Rh and Other Blood Group Phenotypes.* Ph.D. Thesis, University of London.
[3] *Lister Institute, Report of the Governing Body* (1964). Page 35.
[4] CRAWFORD MARY N., TIPPETT PATRICIA and SANGER RUTH (1974) The antigens Au^a, i and P$_1$ of cells of the dominant type of Lu(a–b–). *Vox Sang.*, **26**, 283–287.

Chapter 15
The Dombrock Blood Groups

That this system was not discovered until 20 years after the introduction of the antiglobulin test reflects the heterogeneity of antiglobulin sera. The first example of anti-Do[a], identified in 1965 by Swanson, Polesky, Tippett and Sanger[1], reacts, like two further examples hot on its heels, only with a minority of otherwise good antiglobulin sera. Trial and error has so far been the best guide to choice of appropriate antiglobulin sera.

The expected antithetical antibody, anti-Do[b], was found in 1973 by Molthan, Crawford and Tippett[9].

FREQUENCIES

All the tests on unrelated people recorded in Table 68 were done with the original anti-Do[a] from Mrs Dombrock.

For the calculations we will take the figures for the 755 Northern Europeans because the families to be analysed below are of such stock, and, not a little,

Table 68. Dombrock groups of unrelated people tested with anti-Do[a]

		Total tested	Do(a+)		Do(a−)	
Swanson et al.[1], 1965	Northern Europeans	258	166	64·34%	92	35·66%
Tippett et al.[2], 1967	Northern Europeans	165	105	63·64%	60	36·36%
Tippett[3], 1967	Northern Europeans	332	230	69·28%	102	30·72%
	Total	755	501	66·36%	254	33·64%
Polesky and Swanson[4], 1966	U.S.A. Whites	391	250	63·94%	141	36·06%
Tippett[3], 1967	Israelis	128	83	64·84%	45	35·16%
Polesky and Swanson[4], 1966	U.S.A. Negroes	161	89	55·28%	72	44·72%
Tippett[3], 1967	U.S.A. Negroes	76	34	44·74%	42	55·26%
Polesky and Swanson[4], 1966	American Indians	276	157	56·88%	119	43·12%
Chandanayingyong et al.[8], 1967	Thais	423	57	13·48%	366	86·52%

386

because we may, with no expense of spirit or waste of time, lift them straight from Dr Tippett's paper.[3] The antigen Do^a being a dominant character the calculated gene and genotype frequencies for Northern Europeans are:

Do^a	0·4200	Do^aDo^a	0·1764
Do^b	0·5800	Do^aDo^b	0·4872
		Do^bDo^b	0·3364

The Israelis, who were all non-Ashkenazi and mostly Iraqi, have a distribution of Do^a indistinguishable from the Northern Europeans. American Negroes and American Indians both have a lower incidence of the antigen and the divergencies from the European frequencies are highly significant, and so, of course, are those of the Thais.

After the finding of anti-Do^b by Molthan, Crawford and Tippett[9] (1973) the earlier symbol Do for the allele of Do^a was promoted to Do^b, leaving Do as the symbol for the *Dombrock* locus.

Because of other antibodies present in the anti-Do^b serum relatively few unrelated people have been tested with anti-Do^a and with anti-Do^b. The expectations in the following series of Molthan *et al.*[9] were derived from the gene frequencies based on the 755 tests with anti-Do^a recorded above, and the fit is very close:

	Do^aDo^a	Do^aDo^b	Do^bDo^b	total
Observed	16	46	31	93
Expected	16·4	45·3	31·3	93·0

There is no hint yet of the existence of the phenotype Do(a–b–) though judging by other systems it may be expected to turn up sooner or later.

INHERITANCE

From the genotype frequencies given above the expected incidence of the six genotypically and the three phenotypically different matings can be calculated together with the children expected therefrom. In Table 69 are the expected distributions when anti-Do^a alone is used, and in Table 70 these expectations are compared with the results of testing 201 Northern European families with 573 children (these families include the 52 of the original paper[1]). Tippett[3] gives details of these families and analyses them also by Fisher's method described in the chapter on P: both methods show very good agreement between calculated and observed.

Tippett[3] also gives details of 76 Israeli, mostly Iraqi, families with 224 children:

Do(a+) × Do(a+) matings 28, children Do(a+) 68, children Do(a–) 9
Do(a+) × Do(a–) matings 40, children Do(a+) 76, children Do(a–) 52
Do(a–) × Do(a–) matings 8, children Do(a+) 1, children Do(a–) 18

These families also agreed well with expectation. The one Do(a+) child with both parents Do(a–) is presumed to be extra-marital.

The inheritance of Do[b] is, as expected, straightforward: the many families tested in our Unit were often selected and therefore not suitable for analysis.

Table 69. The expected distribution of the Dombrock groups, defined by anti-Do[a], in Northern European parents and offspring. (From Tippett[3], 1967)

Phenotypes			
Matings		Proportion of children from each mating	
Type	Frequency	Do(a+)	Do(a−)
Do(a+) × Do(a+)	0·4403	0·8652	0·1348
Do(a+) × Do(a−)	0·4465	0·6329	0·3671
Do(a−) × Do(a−)	0·1132	—	1·0000
	1·0000		

Table 70. The Dombrock groups of 201 Northern European families with 573 children. (From Tippett[3], 1967)

Matings				Children						
	Number				Do(a+)		Do(a−)			
Type	obs.	exp.	χ^2	Total	obs.	exp.	obs.	exp.	χ^2	d.f.
Do(a+) × Do(a+)	77	88·5	1·49	216	192	186·9	24	29·1	1·03	1
Do(a+) × Do(a−)	98	89·7	0·77	270	177	170·9	93	99·1	0·60	1
Do(a−) × Do(a−)	26	22·8	0·45	87	1*	0	86	87		
	201		2·71 for 2 d.f.	573					1·63	2

* Presumed extra-marital.

Genetical independence of the antigen Do[a]

That Dombrock is an independent blood group system was very thoroughly established by Tippett, from whose paper[3] the following is extracted.

'Genetic recombination in the families showed that the gene *Do[a]* is not sited at the loci for any of the established red cell systems: ABO, MNSs, P, Rh, Lutheran, Kell, Lewis, Duffy, Kidd, Yt, or for the secretor system, and that it is not X- or Y-linked. Recombination also dissociates the locus for Do[a] from the loci for the following genetic characters of the blood: haptoglobins acid phosphatase, phosphoglucomutase, 6-phosphogluconate dehydrogenase, lactate dehydrogenase, serum cholinesterase E_1 and C_5, adenylate kinase.

'*Do[a]* has not yet been shown to segregate away from the Auberger genes. Unhappily, the few available families known to segregate for Auberger did not segregate for Dombrock. However, the incidence of Do(a+) and Do)a−) within Au(a+) and Au(a−) groups does not differ significantly from that in the general population.'

Do^a was subsequently excluded from the *Colton* locus[10] and from the *Diego* locus (Chown, Lewis and Kaita, personal communication) and, from our own records, from *Sid*.

Linkage relations

Tippett's families[3] not only showed that the *Dombrock* locus is not part of the loci for any of the systems mentioned above, they further showed that the *Dombrock* locus is not close to any of them.

Three counts gave very faint hints that linkage might be measurable between *Dombrock* and *MNSs* or *Rh* or *Duffy*. After about five years Tippett *et al.*[10] had tested enough families to justify a second analysis and this ruled out *Rh* and *Duffy* but made linkage between *Dombrock* and *MNSs* look somewhat more likely than before. If there is linkage θ', the male recombination rate, is around 0·35 which represents such a long distance that it will take years of testing families to get a definite answer either way. Linkage between *Do* and other blood group loci either was ruled out or made unlikely.

OTHER NOTES ABOUT THE DOMBROCK GROUPS

Dosage

In reporting the second example of anti-Do^a, Webb, Lockyer and Tovey[5] record how it gave strong, medium and weak, and negative reactions in good agreement with the calculated frequencies of the three genotypes. However, they quote Tippett (personal communication) who had found that while most medium and weak reactors were heterozygotes, as judged by family tests, some similarly proved heterozygotes gave strong positive reactions.

The single example of anti-Do^b also shows a good dosage effect[9].

Development

The original paper[1] records how the antigen Do^a was found in normal strength in two samples of cord blood, and later samples confirmed this. The antigen Do^b also is well developed at birth[9].

Anti-Do^a

In less than a year, second (Webb, Lockyer and Tovey[5]) and third (Williams and Crawford[6]) examples of anti-Do^a were found, and we had heard of a fourth[7]. All were in transfused patients and were accompanied by other immune antibodies. The fifth example of anti-Do^a was stimulated by pregnancy[11]; again it was accompanied by several other immune antibodies, as was the sixth example which was found in Paris by Dr Salmon and his colleagues.

Polesky and Swanson[4] showed by survival tests that anti-Do^a is active *in vivo*: labelled injected Do(a+) cells had a very short survival time and were condemned to the spleen rather than to the liver.

Anti-Do^b

The single example of anti-Do^b was made by a white woman who had had monozygotic twins in 1949 and had subsequently been much transfused[9]. Crossmatching difficulty in 1972 led to the identification of anti-Do^b, anti-E, anti-C^w and anti-K in her serum. Her cells could not be tested with anti-Do^a for they had developed a strong direct antiglobulin reaction.

The recognition of the Dombrock system gave particular pleasure for it was the first autosomal system to make useful distinctions between white people to be found since the discovery of the Kidd system 14 years before. If anti-Do^a alone is available, Dombrock comes sixth amongst the autosomal systems in 'usefulness' in discriminating between white people. If anti-Do^b is used as well, Dombrock is practically level in fourth place, with Duffy and Kidd, in the order of usefulness, being beaten only by A_1A_2BO, MNSs and Rh.

REFERENCES

1   SWANSON JANE, POLESKY H.F., TIPPETT PATRICIA and SANGER RUTH (1965) A 'new' blood group antigen, Do^a. *Nature, Lond.*, 206, 313.
2   TIPPETT PATRICIA, SANGER RUTH, SWANSON JANE and POLESKY H.F. (1967) The Dombrock blood group system. *Proc. 10th Congr. europ. Soc. Haemat.*, Strasbourg 1965. Part II, 1443–1446. Karger, Basel/New York.
3   TIPPETT PATRICIA (1967) Genetics of the Dombrock blood group system. *J. med. Genet.*, 4, 7–11.
4   POLESKY H.F. and SWANSON JANE L. (1966) Studies on the distribution of the blood group antigen Do^a (Dombrock) and the characteristics of anti-Do^a. *Transfusion, Philad.*, 6, 268–270.
5   WEBB A.J., LOCKYER J.W. and TOVEY G.H. (1966) The second example of anti-Do^a. *Vox Sang.*, 11, 637–639.
6   WILLIAMS CATHERINE H. and CRAWFORD MARY N. (1966) The third example of anti-Do^a. *Transfusion, Philad.*, 6, 310.
7   SPEISER P. and GILES CAROLYN M. (1966) Personal communication.
8   CHANDANAYINGYONG D., SASAKI T.T. and GREENWALT T.J. (1967) Blood groups of the Thais. *Transfusion, Philad.*, 7, 269–276.
9   MOLTHAN LYNDALL, CRAWFORD MARY N. and TIPPETT PATRICIA (1973) Enlargement of the Dombrock blood group system: the finding of anti-Do^b. *Vox Sang.*, 24, 382–384.
10 TIPPETT PATRICIA, GAVIN JUNE and SANGER RUTH (1972) The Dombrock system: linkage relations with other blood group loci. *J. med. Genet.*, 9, 392–395.
11 POLESKY H.F., SWANSON JANE and SMITH ROSALYN (1968) Anti-Do^a stimulated by pregnancy. *Vox Sang.*, 14, 465–466.

Chapter 16
The Colton Blood Groups

The finding of a 'public' antibody in Oslo, in 1965, started an investigation which tied together two other antibodies studied in Minneapolis, Oxford and London a few months before (Heistö, van der Hart, Madsen, Moes, Noades, Pickles, Race, Sanger and Swanson[1], 1967). The antigen, Co[a], was first shown to be an inherited character by tests on the family of the Oslo patient.

The antithetical antibody anti-Co[b] was found in 1970 by Giles, Darnborough, Aspinall and Fletton[2], and this finding made the Colton system a useful one in human genetics.

FREQUENCIES

The results of a great many tests are set out in Table 71. Since there is a hint[3] that U.S.A. Negroes may have a lower incidence of Co(a−) we have confined the

Table 71. Tests with anti-Co[a] or anti-Co[b] on various unrelated people

Antibody	Investigators	Population	Total tested	Negatives
Anti-Co[a]	Heistö et al.[1], 1967	N. Europeans	3,030	8
	Crawford[3], 1967	Philadelphia Whites	1,083	1
	Wray et al.[4], 1968	Canadian donors	1,843	3
	Brocteur[8], 1972	Belgians	5,683	8
			11,639	20
				0·0017
	Heistö et al.[1], 1967	Minneapolis donors	1,727	4
	Crawford[3], 1967	Philadelphia Negroes	1,706	0
Anti-Co[b]	Giles et al.[2], 1970	London	203	185
		Cambridge	669	623
	Ikin et al.[5], 1970	Zurich	62	56
	Case[6], 1971	Sydney and Dunedin	2,471	2,247
			3,405	3,111
				0·9137

analysis to unrelated people of European extraction: 11,639 tested with anti-Co^a and 3,405 tested with anti-Co^b. The results dovetail most happily; the gene and genotype frequencies are practically the same whether based on the tests with anti-Co^a or with anti-Co^b:

		using anti-Co^a	using anti-Co^b
genes	Co^a	0·9588	0·9559
	Co^b	0·0412	0·0441
genotypes	Co^aCo^a	0·9193	0·9137
	Co^aCo^b	0·0790	0·0843
	Co^bCo^b	0·0017	0·0020

This, together of course with the fact that all Co(a−) people tested were Co(b+), leaves no doubt about the allelism of Co^a and Co^b. The figures calculated from the anti-Co^b results should be taken as the better estimate, for the smaller class, Co(b+), numbered 294 whereas with anti-Co^a the smaller class, Co(a−), numbered only 20.

INHERITANCE

The number of families tested is so far small, but it does not matter very much for the gene frequencies have so solidly established the manner of inheritance: Co^a and Co^b are alleles and the antigens Co^a and Co^b are dominant characters. Tests on families will confirm the main truth but, sooner or later, will show that it is not the whole truth: as in other systems no doubt 'silent' alleles will be shown to exist and modifying or regulator loci found. (We wrote this sentence before Rogers, Stiles and Wright[15] found a Co(a−b−) person, honestly we did; this late arrival will be tucked in a section on anti-Co^{a}Co^b below.)

Heistö et al.[1] and his colleagues tested the relatives of five Co(a−) propositi and this, besides illustrating the dominant inheritance of the antigen Co^a, showed by segregation that the Co locus is not sited at the loci for ABO, MNSs, P, Rh, Duffy, Kidd and Dombrock, and ruled out X- and Y-linkage. Three families tested with anti-Co^a by Wray and Simpson[4] confirmed some of these and added secretor. Lewis et al.[7] reported two families, tested with both anti-Co^a and anti-Co^b, and the loci for Lutheran and Kell were added to the list of exclusions. Another fine family from Winnipeg (Lewis et al.[9], 1973) tested with both antisera excluded Yt.

So Colton is a system on its own, provided that it comes to be similarly separated from the remaining established system, Diego.

OTHER NOTES ABOUT COLTON

Development

The antigen Co^a appears to be fully developed at birth[1, 10], but we have not found any information about Co^b.

Dosage

Anti-Co[a] may show a good dosage effect[1] but we can find no information about anti-Co[b].

Anti-Co[a]

Three[1] of the six known examples were stimulated by transfusion: the background of the first[1] and fifth[10] was hazy and pregnancy probably caused the sixth[14]. All six antisera react well by the antiglobulin test and better still if the cells are papainized beforehand. Unlike anti-Co[b] these examples of anti-Co[a] have been relatively free of other antibodies.

Anti-Co[b]

Eight examples have been found that we know of[2, 5, 6, 7, 11, 12, 13]. Since Co(b−) people are common (about 91 % in Whites) the antibody must be difficult to make and this is supported by the host of antibodies the eight people have made in addition to their anti-Co[b]. It is probably due to the practical serological difficulties presented by these additional antibodies that so few families have been tested with anti-Co[b].

Like anti-Co[a], anti-Co[b] reacts well by the antiglobulin test and better still if the cells are papainized beforehand.

Before anti-Co[b] presented itself active attempts to find it had been made: in testing 461 random sera Dr Cleghorn found no example of an agglutinin active in saline with a sample of Co(a−) cells. Further, at Ullevål Hospital[1] the sera of seven patients known to have been transfused with blood from Co(a−) donors, and the sera of 1,430 transfused and non-transfused patients picked out at random, were tested against Co(a−) cells using the antiglobulin and the papain-antiglobulin methods, without a glimmer of anti-Co[b].

Anti-Co[a]Co[b]

Anti-Co[a]Co[b] was recently identified by Rogers, Stiles and Wright[15] in the serum of a French Canadian woman whose red cells were Co(a−b−): it reacted with all cells tested save her own and those of two of her four sibs, who are also Co(a−b−). Both parents, her other two sibs and her twin children are Co(a+b−). Absorption and elution tests confirmed that the propositus' cells really are Co(a−b−) and that her anti-Co[a]Co[b] is not separable into anti-Co[a] and anti-Co[b] components. No antibody was found in the serum of the Co(a−b−) sibs.

The cells of Co(a−b−) members of this family showed that an 'unpublished' antibody, listed in our last edition as Swarts, was presumably anti-Co[a]Co[b]. Swarts died in 1964, before the Colton groups were recognized, but her serum, sent to us by Dr van den Berghe of Antwerp, continued to be tried against problem red cell samples for 10 years and the only negative reactions were given by the cells of these Canadian Co(a–b–) people.

With the finding of anti-Co^b the Colton system became potentially the ninth most useful of the autosomal blood groups, exceeding Lutheran, Kell and Yt in its powers of discriminating between European people.

REFERENCES

[1] HEISTÖ H., VAN DER HART MIA, MADSEN GRETHE, MOES MIEKE, NOADES JEAN, PICKLES MARGARET M., RACE R.R., SANGER RUTH and SWANSON JANE (1967) Three examples of a new red cell antibody, anti-Co^a. *Vox Sang.*, **12**, 18–24.

[2] GILES CAROLYN M., DARNBOROUGH J., ASPINALL P. and FLETTON M.W. (1970) Identification of the first example of anti-Co^b. *Brit. J. Haemat.*, **19**, 267–269.

[3] CRAWFORD MARY N. (1967) Personal communication.

[4] WRAY ELIZABETH and SIMPSON SHIRLEY (1968) A further example of anti-Co^a and two informative families with Co(a–) members. *Vox Sang.*, **14**, 130–132.

[5] IKIN E.W., METAXAS-BÜHLER M., METAXAS M.N., BOWLEY C.C. and STAPLETON R. (1970) Two further examples of anti-Co^b. *Vox Sang.*, **19**, 537–539.

[6] CASE J. (1971) A pure example of anti-Co^b and frequency of the Co^b antigen in New Zealand and Australian blood donors. *Vox Sang.*, **21**, 447–450.

[7] LEWIS M., KAITA H., ANDERSON C. and CHOWN B. (1971) Independence of Colton blood group. *Transfusion, Philad.*, **11**, 223–224.

[8] BROCTEUR J. (1972) Personal communication.

[9] LEWIS MARION, KAITA HIROKO, GIBLETT ELOISE R. and STEINBERG A.G. (1973) Independence of the Colton and Yt blood group systems. *Vox Sang.*, **25**, 540–542.

[10] SMITH D.S., STRATTON F., HOWELL P. and RICHES R. (1970) An example of anti-Co^a found in pregnancy. *Vox Sang.*, **18**, 62–66.

[11] CLAUSEN J. (1972) Another example of anti-Co^b in the presence of multiple antibodies. Abstracts AABB and ISH Meeting, Washington, p. 45.

[12] MILLER W.V. (1973) Personal communication.

[13] MANN JULIA (1971) Personal communication.

[14] THOMAS MARTHA J., DEVENEY LINDA and WURZEL H.A. (1971) A new example of anti-Co^a Abstracts AABB Meeting, Chicago, p. 100.

[15] ROGERS MARGARET J., STILES PATRICIA A. and WRIGHT J. (1974) A new minus–minus phenotype: three Co(a–b–) individuals in one family. AABB Abstracts Transfusion, Philad., **14**, 508.

Chapter 17
The Sid Groups

A rather vague antigen antibody system had been investigated for years at Dundee, Oxford and London. The antibody, later called anti-Sd^a, reacted well with a few cell samples, weakly with most and negatively with some: the antibody distinguished itself, right from the start, by agglutinating only a proportion of cells even of strong positive reactors (making a picture like that first seen with anti-Lu^a).

However, in 1967 improved techniques enabled Macvie, Morton and Pickles[1] in Oxford, and Renton, Howell, Ikin, Giles and Goldsmith[2] in Manchester and London to bring more order to the system. The system was named Sid, after Mr Sidney Smith of the Lister Institute, whose cells had, over many years, given the clearest positive reaction with the emerging class of antibodies.

Morton, Pickles and Terry[3] (1970) then went on to find that the antigen Sd^a is widely distributed in the tissues and fluids of mammals but is not present in birds.

Another step was the recognition in our own and no doubt other laboratories of the existence of rare families in which an extremely strong Sd^a antigen was inherited: so strong were these examples of Sd^a antigens that they were sent to us as 'private' antigen problems. At about the same time Cazal, Monis, Caubel and Brives[4] (1968), in a paper of outstanding interest, reported their investigation in Montpellier of the remarkable Mauritian family 'Cad'. The cells of certain members of this family, though not group A, were strongly agglutinated by preparations of *Dolichos biflorus*, previously thought to be only anti-A$_1$ in specificity. Then Sanger, Gavin, Tippett, Teesdale and Eldon[5]. (1971) showed that such non-A$_1$ *Dolichos* positive samples were the extremely strong reactors with anti-Sd^a, and concluded that the Cad antigen is Sd^a *in excelsis*.

In this account the red cell phenotype notation Sd(a++) is used for the rare outstandingly strong reactors ('super Sid' in rather convenient laboratory jargon), and Sd(a+) for positives of the ordinary sort. There are grades of strength in the Sd(a+) range as there are in the Sd(a++) range and we suspect that given enough measurements strength would be seen to be distributed in one continuous curve.

FREQUENCIES

Sd(a+) and Sd(a−)

In 1967 the two groups of workers found an almost identical incidence of the antigen. Macvie *et al.*[1] used a tube test followed by incubation on a slide and Renton *et al.*[2] an antiglobulin test using 'antiglobulin reagents which contained either a powerful anti-γM or an anti-complement antibody'. The two groups of workers found an almost identical incidence of the antigen:

	Macvie *et al.*[1]	Renton *et al.*[2]	Total
Sd(a+)	265 (91·38%)	131 (90·97%)	396 (91·24%)
Sd(a−)	25 (8·62%)	13 (9·03%)	38 (8·76%)
	290	144	434

However, red cell tests must be missing some weaker Sd(a+) people because, in 1970, when Morton *et al.*[3] found Sd^a in body tissues and fluids, the presence or absence of Sd^a in urine was seen to give a truer idea of the antigenic constitution; and in tests on the urine of 361 people they found

Sd^a present	347	0·9612
Sd^a absent	14	0·0388
	361	

The corresponding gene frequencies are: *Sd^a* 0·8030 and *Sd* 0·1970, and the genotype frequencies are: *Sd^{a}Sd^a* 0·6448, *Sd^{a}Sd* 0·3164 and *SdSd* 0·0388.

To their series of tests on red cells Renton *et al.*[2] applied 2 × 2 contingency tables which showed no disturbance in the proportion of Sd(a+) and Sd(a−) samples within the ABO, MNSs, P, Rh, Lutheran, Kell, Lewis (red cells), Duffy, Kidd, Yt, Dombrock and Xg groups; nor was there any difference between the sexes.

Sd(a++)

An estimate of the frequency of Sd(a++) can be gathered from the reactions of group O and group B cells with *Dolichos biflorus*. As far as we know *Dolichos* positive O and B cells are Sd(a++) provided Tn polyagglutinability has been ruled out, which is easy to do (page 488). But it must be remembered that the label Sd(a++) is arbitrary and represents an attempt to cut off the right hand end of a distribution curve of increasing Sd^a strength. Just where the cut between no reaction and reaction with *Dolichos* is made will depend somewhat on the strength of the *Dolichos* preparation, so it is not easy to compare the frequencies of Sd(a++) found in different laboratories. As will be seen below, the agglutinin in *Dolichos* for Sd(a++) cells is the same as that for A$_1$ cells: therefore some comparison could be made between Sd(a++) frequencies found in different places if the Sd(a++) strength were recorded in terms of so much above or so much below that of A$_1$ cells, just as Cazal *et al.*[6] recorded their measurements of the Cad and other families.

The phenotype Sd(a++) is certainly rare: in France, Professor Cazal estimates that in his laboratory about 250,000 group O and group B donors and patients had been tested with *Dolichos* without a positive being found[4]. Several European

Sd(a++) have been found but they had selected themselves out of unknown thousands by the trouble their strong antigen had caused at cross-matching against sera containing the quite frequent antibody anti-Sd^a.

At Winnipeg the Rh Laboratory found 2 examples in testing 1,425 group O and B random Canadians, an incidence of 0·0014. One of the two *Dolichos* positives was the propositus in the family with Wr(a+) as well as Sd(a++) members, to be mentioned below (Lewis *et al.*[7], 1973): the other was a sample which we would only just have classed as Sd(a++); in our hands it reacted with *Dolichos* and with anti-Sd^a only a little more strongly than did a control sample from Mr Sid., the original strong Sd(a+). In Toronto, Dr Moore (personal communication) found one *Dolichos* positive in testing 2,191 group O and B donors.

In Japan, Yamaguchi, Okubo, Ogawa and Tanaka[8, 9, 28] found 15 in 51,420 group O and B samples, a frequency of 0·0003. It is of interest that as long ago as 1962 Ikuta *et al.*[10] found a sample of O cells which was agglutinated by *Dolichos*, and in 1967 Murakami found another[11].

The highest incidence so far is in Thailand: Sringarm and her colleagues[12, 13] found 37 in 14,261 group O and B samples, a frequency of 0·0026.

INHERITANCE

Using human anti-Sd^a serum Macvie *et al.*[1], in 1967, tested the red cells of 55 Oxford families with 168 children and found the antigen Sd^a to be inherited as a dominant character. The families showed that the *Sd* locus cannot be part of, or closely linked to, the loci for ABO, MNSs, P, Rh, Kell and Duffy, nor is *Sd* X- or Y-borne: to these exclusions were later added Dombrock, Gm and PGM$_1$ (Lewis *et al.*[7]), Auberger (Salmon, unpublished), Kidd and secretor (from our records). So at least it can be that Sid is not closely linked to any of these other markers.

From tests on families in France[4, 6], in Japan[8, 9, 28], in Thailand[13], in Canada[7] and in our Unit there is general agreement that Sd(a++) as measured by *Dolichos* (with or without anti-Sd^a tests) is a dominant character. These Sd(a++) families show the dominance very clearly without any problem of deciding whether members are Sd^a weak or Sd^a negative. We have tested 4 Sd(a++) families, in which the propositus was noted, and the following counts were made: sibs of propositi Sd(a++) 4: not Sd(a++) 4; children of Sd(a++), excluding the propositus were he amongst them, Sd(a++) 11: not Sd(a++) 11; which merely confirms the obvious pedigree appearance of the dominance of Sd(a++).

Sometimes all the Sd(a++) members of a particular family give very similar scores with *Dolichos* but sometimes their scores vary within the family[9, 7] (discounting, of course, any A$_1$ and A$_1$B members). We do not find the variation surprising: if sensitive measurement of antigen strength in the Sd(a++) families were made, like that of P$_1$ antigen strength made by Henningsen (page 148), the variability of the Sd(a++) reaction might be seen to be due to different Sd^a rating

14

of the alleles partnering the super strong one. Our limited family tests, using both *Dolichos* and anti-Sd^a support this possibility.

Incidentally an example of what we consider to be Sd(a++) travelling through three generations of a family has been reported as a weak A, first[26] called A$_{xx}$ then[27] A$_{lae}$.

A hint of linkage

In a Canadian Sd(a++) family[7] a very rare antigen, Wr^a, is segregating. The segregation of the two characters is informative: the family shows six non-recombinants and no recombinant. The lod score (page 555) at $\theta = 0{\cdot}00$ is $1{\cdot}806$ which is tantalizingly suggestive of linkage but does not reach the significant lod score of 3. However, as Lewis and her collaborators[7] note, the lod score might be pointing not towards linkage in the usual sense but towards Wright and Sid being controlled from the same complex locus. In this family there was also a hint of some association between Sid and the glutamic phosphate transaminase, GPT, polymorphism.

VARIATIONS IN STRENGTH OF Sd^a

Variation of Sd^a antigen strength between people was a notable feature from the earliest days of its investigation. The Oxford workers[1] retested second samples from 100 people who, with a few exceptions, were placed in their original grade: the exceptions involved only 'the weak and doubtful class'.

The strength of reaction of the cells of Sd(a++) people, as noted in previous sections, also varies, whether measured by *Dolichos* or by anti-Sd^a. An example from our records is given in Table 72 which shows only three of the many grades of Sd(a++) antigen strength. In all our tests the strength of reaction with *Dolichos* has mirrored that with anti-Sd^a though the spread of scores with *Dolichos* has been greater than that with anti-Sd^a.

The classification of some samples into Sd(a+) or Sd(a++) is bound to be

Table 72. An example of the parallel reactions of *Dolichos biflorus* and human anti-Sd^a with Sd(a++) cells: titration scores for tests made on one day

Cells		*Dolichos biflorus*	Anti-Sd^a human
Cad propositus, B	Sd(a++)	110	79
Århus propositus, A$_2$	Sd(a++)	88	59
sister, A$_2$	Sd(a++)	89	59
daughter, O	Sd(a++)	91	59
Manchester propositus, O	Sd(a++)	26	39
Control, O	Sd(a+)	0	7
Control, A$_1$	Sd(a−?)	73	0

arbitrary depending on the *Dolichos* preparation in use. We once tested in parallel our home-made extract and three others given to us, two of them commercial preparations, and they scored:

A_1 cells	80	41	59	62
O Sd(a++), of modest strength	46	15	26	16

We guess that the last three extracts would not have detected the Manchester Sd(a++) listed in Table 72.

POLYAGGLUTINABILITY IN THE CAD FAMILY

So far in this account no mention has been made of the extraordinarily interesting observation, recorded in the original paper of Cazal, Monis, Caubel and Brives[4] (1968), that in the Cad family the cells of the *Dolichos* positive (non-A_1) members were polyagglutinable, and polyagglutinability of cells had never before been found as an inherited character. None of five subsequent *Dolichos* positive, non-A_1, propositi tested by Cazal *et al.*[6] (1971) had polyagglutinable cells nor have others tested since shown it, at any rate to the extent of the Cad family. The serum of the three *Dolichos* positive members of the Cad family did not contain the poly-agglutinating factor and the polyagglutinability of the cells was shown to be sero-logically distinct from that due to T or Tn (Cazal *et al.*[4], Bird *et al.*[14, 15], Gunson *et al.*[16], Myllylä *et al.*[17] and Tables 81 and 82, page 488).

After the recognition that the Cad antigen was Sd(a++) we formed the opinion, first expressed at a meeting[18] in 1971, that the polyagglutinability in the Cad family is not polyagglutinability in the usual sense of the word but is due to the presence of anti-Sd^a in the serum of the great majority of people–anti-Sd^a which can be demonstrated only by the strongest Sd(a++) cells, as found in the Cad family.

The opinion was based on the observation in our Unit that sera from Sd(a++) people do not agglutinate Cad cells, while sera from other people do agglutinate them in varying degree. It appears that the Cad agglutinating power of a serum is roughly in inverse proportion to the strength of the donor's Sd^a antigen. This was confirmed by absorption of a serum having strong 'polyagglutinating' power for Cad cells. This serum was absorbed by cells representing eight steps of Sd^a strength, ranging from Sd(a++) of the Cad family, through lesser Sd(a++), through Sd(a+) strong, medium and weak to Sd(a–): the strength of the 'poly-agglutinating' factor left in the serum was in inverse proportoin to the Sd^a strength of the absorbing cells.

Our opinion gained further support from the work of Sringarm, Chiewsilp, Tubrod and Sriboonruang[13]. In Thailand they found Sd(a++) samples that were weakly polyagglutinable by a proportion of normal sera, and the examples giving the highest score with *Dolichos* were those agglutinated by the greater proportion of the sera: in other words there was a direct relation between the Sd(a++) strength and the polyagglutinability of these cells.

To picture anti-Sd^a in the serum of Sd(a+) people, as required by the theory, is a little difficult, but precedents may be found in the anti-A$_1$ in A$_2$ or A$_2$B people and the anti-H detectable in most people when suitably sensitive tests are used[19].

Other notes about the Cad family

The electrophoretic mobility of the cells of the propositus was only slightly reduced[17], in marked contrast to T and Tn polyagglutinable cells. Professor Cazal generously sent us samples from all available members of the remarkable family and a few points from our records may be mentioned.

The T antigen of the Sd(a++) members was notably weaker than that of the rest of the family and of controls, as measured by *Arachis hypogaea*, and somewhat weaker as measured by human anti-T.

The M and N antigens of the Sd(a++) members were depressed, whether measured by human, rabbit or plant reagents. Furthermore, after RDE treatment the Sd(a++) cells gave abnormally weak reactions with *Vicia* and *Bauhinia* extracts compared with the cells of the rest of the family and of controls.

It may be that this extreme limit of Sd^a antigen strength is accompanied by some surface change, but there was no sign of a change in the cells of somewhat lesser Sd(a++) people such as the members of the Århus family included in Table 72 whose M and N and T antigens gave normal reactions.

OTHER NOTES ABOUT Sd^a

Distribution of Sd^a

That a variable amount of Sd^a was to be found in saliva was recognized in the early days, but a fine investigation by Morton, Pickles and Terry[3] showed how short that was of the whole story. Sd^a is present in the saliva of adults but there is much more of it in the saliva of newborn infants. Sd^a is to be found in urine, and at present urine tests make the best distinction between weak Sd(a+) and Sd(a−) people, as mentioned in the earlier section on frequencies. It is present also in meconium and in milk. Of tissues the kidney has the greatest amount but none could be detected in liver or spleen.

Turning to other creatures that abound in Oxford, Morton and his colleagues[3] found rich sources of Sd^a in the kidneys of moles and hedgehogs, though lamb kidneys lacked it; but the best source of all was guinea pig kidney and guinea pig urine; and guinea pig urine became a prized reagent in blood grouping laboratories.

On the other hand the birds of Oxford, the chicken, the turkey, the pheasant, the wood pigeon and the tawny owl (*Strix aluco*) lack the antigen; and here again was an important observation, for it led to the successful making in several laboratories of immune anti-Sd^a in chicken, as noted below.

Returning to man, Morton and his colleagues found only slight amounts of Sd^a in the serum of Sd(a+) people but they would have found much more if they had had the serum of the rare Sd(a++) people to work with.

Other sources of 'anti-Sd^a'

Dolichos, although it detects Sd(a++), can hardly be called anti-Sd^a. From inhibition tests[5] it seems that *Dolichos* is reacting with terminal N-acetyl-D-galactosamine present in Sd(a++) and A$_1$ cells alike.

That one and the same agglutinin in *Dolichos* reacts with O or B Sd(a++) and with A$_1$ cells has been shown in other ways. Though we agree with the original observation of Cazal *et al.*[4] that absorption of *Dolichos* with A$_1$ cells can leave 'anti-Cad', we found that continued absorption with the same A$_1$ cells did remove all antibody for these strongest of Sd(a++) cells. In our opinion the apparent splittability of the antibody was due to the Cad cells being stronger reactors than A$_1$ cells, and a stage had been reached when A$_1$ no longer reacted but Cad cells did; and the same effect is achieved by simple dilution of the extract. We found that repeated absorption of *Dolichos* by A$_1$ Sd(a+) and A$_1$ Sd(a−) removes the agglutinin for O Sd(a++) and A$_1$ Sd(a−) cells in parallel. Another pointer towards the unity of the agglutinin is that papain, ficin or RDE treatment of O Sd(a++) and A$_1$ cells results in mutual enhancement of their reaction with *Dolichos*, whereas trypsin treatment leaves the reactions of both unaltered.

Other anti-A$_1$ lectins, notably *Phaseolus lunatus* and *Phaseolus limensis*, fail to react even with Cad cells, the strongest Sd(a++)[17, 20, 21]; this surprised some workers[20, 21], for *Phaseolus lunatus* was thought, like *Dolichos*, to be specific for α-linked N-acetyl-D-galactosamine. *Salvia horminum* and *Salvia farinacea* seed extracts contain an agglutinin, separable from their anti-Tn, which reacts with Sd(a++) cells[29, 30].

On the other hand, most snail anti-A reagents do agglutinate Sd(a++) cells[17, 20, 21, 6, 22]. Everyone agrees that *Helix pomatia* and *Helix aspersa* extracts react splendidly. We[17] and others[6, 22] find, however, that *Cepaea nemoralis* does not react (thus making a useful quick distinction between Cad and Tn polyagglutinability) but a German snail of this make behaved differently[21].

In 1968 Dr M. Kitahama sent, from Tokyo, serum from a chicken which had been immunized with human red cells, and the antibody proved to be anti-Sd^a. This was surprising at the time but was later made understandable by the Oxford report[3] that birds lacked the antigen Sd^a. Incidentally this chicken antibody reacted by the antiglobulin test with anti-human globulin, and it was only after some time that we woke up to the alien specificity of the antiglobulin. We then bought some anti-chicken globulin but it did not work as well as the anti-human variety, perhaps it was not a very good one.

Bizot and Cayla[23] immunized chicken with red cells of the Cad family propositus: in saline tests the resulting antibody agglutinated only Sd(a++) cells but in antiglobulin tests it agglutinated Sd(a+) cells as well. The interesting observation

was made that before immunization the chicken had 'natural' anti-Sd(a++) but
no detectable anti-Sd^a.

Inhibitions

The presence of Sd^a in saliva and urine of people of the phenotype Sd(a+) has been
referred to earlier in the chapter. Some other inhibition results from our records
show:

1 N-acetyl-D-galactosamine inhibits the reaction of Dolichos, of Helix pomatia
and of Helix aspersa with Sd(a++) and with A$_1$ cells: it does not inhibit the reaction
of human anti-Sd^a with Sd(a+) or with Sd(a++) cells, nor of human anti-A with
A cells.

2 N-acetyl-D-glucosamine inhibits the reaction of Helix pomatia and Helix
aspersa with Sd(a++) cells and with A cells: it does not inhibit the reaction of
Dolichos with these cells, nor does it inhibit the reaction of human anti-Sd^a or
anti-A.

3 Guinea pig urine inhibits the reaction of human anti-Sd^a with Sd(a+) and
Sd(a++) cells and of Dolichos with Sd(a++) cells and with A$_1$ cells.

4 Serum from Sd(a++) people inhibits human anti-Sd^a but not the reaction of
Dolichos with Sd(a++) cells. This failure to inhibit Dolichos was surprising but it
was also the finding of Bizot[22] in a paper giving further details of inhibitions of the
reactions of snail extracts with Sd(a++) and with A cells.

Chemistry of Sd^a

The observation that the reaction of Dolichos with Sd(a++) cells was inhibited by
N-acetyl-D-galactosamine alone of many sugars tried led to the suggestion that
Sd^a, like A, depends on terminal N-acetyl-D-galactosamine[5]: others, with more
chemical knowledge[20, 21], agreed and added 'in the α-linked position'.

For a deeper look at the biochemical properties of Sd^a the reader is referred to
the paper by Morton and Terry[24] who worked on material with high Sd^a activity
concentrated from pooled human urine of group A secretor people. A partial
separation of the A and Sd^a substances was achieved.

Development of Sd^a

All the 75 cord red cell samples so far reported[1, 2] gave the reaction Sd(a−). However, the Oxford workers[3] found plenty of Sd^a in the saliva, the urine and the
meconium of newborn infants. As far as we know, no cord sample from an
Sd(a++) family has yet been tested.

When those cells of an Sd(a+) person which were left unagglutinated by the
first exposure to anti-Sd^a were separated and exposed to more anti-Sd^a they gave,
once again, the mixed cell picture[2]. From this it was assumed that the majority of
cells of an Sd(a+) person do carry the antigen, though perhaps unequally shared

out. No difference in reaction with anti-Sd^a was found between the older and the more recently launched Sd(a+) cells after their separation by centrifugation[2], and we find this to be true also of Sd(a++) cells, whether measured by *Dolichos* or by human anti-Sd^a.

Sd^a in pregnancy

There is a change to the red cell Sd^a in pregnancy: the incidence of Sd(a−) amongst the pregnant is far too high[1]; however, there is still plenty of Sd^a in the urine, and the antigen reappears on the red cells soon after delivery[3].

Here may be noted that the Oxford workers[1] found that Sd(a−) cells incubated with the plasma of Sd(a+) people acquired no Sd^a antigen, and this we found to be so even after incubation with the plasma of Sd(a++) people, rich in Sd^a substance.

Anti-Sd^a in man

Anti-Sd^a, an IgM antibody, is estimated to occur 'naturally' in about 1% of donors[1, 2] when Sd(a+) cells are used for its detection. People with useful anti-Sd^a are true Sd(a−), that is people who have no Sd^a in their urine[3]. When Sd(a++) cells are used in the search it seems that almost all people have a trace of the antibody (page 399).

Anti-Sd^a, again IgM, caused a haemolytic transfusion reaction (Peetermans and Cole-Dergent[25], 1970). Dr Peetermans later traced the group O donor whose cells had caused the reaction and we found them to be Sd(a++) though not in the highest range, for their reaction with *Dolichos* was less strong than that of A$_1$ cells.

Usually, however, anti-Sd^a causes no trouble in transfusion[1] though it presumably would cause cross-matching trouble when confronted with the rare Sd(a++) donor: indeed, it is through cross-matching that most of the European Sd(a++) have been identified.

This chapter is more diffuse than some because Sid is a fairly new and probably important system and we are still uncertain what detail to put in and what to leave out of the account. But Sd^a must be an important antigen, otherwise why those Mauritians with it so abundantly and those owls so completely without it?

REFERENCES

[1] MACVIE S.I., MORTON J.A. and PICKLES M.M. (1967) The reactions and inheritance of a new blood group antigen, Sd^a. *Vox Sang.*, **13**, 485–492.

[2] RENTON P.H., HOWELL P., IKIN ELIZABETH W., GILES CAROLYN M. and GOLDSMITH K.L.G (1967) Anti-Sd^a, a new blood group antibody. *Vox Sang.*, **13**, 493–501.

[3] MORTON J.A., PICKLES M.M. and TERRY A.M. (1970) The Sd^a blood group antigen in tissues and body fluids. *Vox Sang.*, **19**, 472–482.

4   CAZAL P., MONIS M., CAUBEL J. and BRIVES J. (1968) Polyagglutinabilité héréditaire domi-
    nante: antigène privé (Cad) correspondant à un anticorps public et à une lectine de
    Dolichos biflorus. *Rev. franc. Transf.*, **11**, 209–221.
5   SANGER RUTH, GAVIN JUNE, TIPPETT PATRICIA, TEESDALE PHYLLIS and ELDON K. (1971)
    Plant agglutinin for another human blood-group. *Lancet* **i**, 1130.
6   CAZAL P., MONIS M. and BIZOT M. (1971) Les antigènes Cad et leurs rapports avec les anti-
    gènes A. *Rev. franc. Transf.*, **14**, 321–334.
7   LEWIS MARION, KAITA HIROKO, CHOWN B., TIPPETT PATRICIA, GAVIN JUNE, SANGER RUTH,
    GIBLETT ELOISE and STEINBERG A.G. (1973) A family with the rare red cell antigens Wr^a
    and 'super' Sd^a. *Vox Sang.*, **25**, 336–340.
8   YAMAGUCHI H., OKUBO Y. and TANAKA M. (1971) (1) Dolichos positive O- and B-group
    families. *Jnl. Jap. Soc. Bld. Transf.*, **18** (3, 4), 85–86 (in Japanese).
9   YAMAGUCHI H., OKUBO Y. and TANAKA M. (1972) Families with group O and B red cells
    agglutinable by *Dolichos biflorus* extract. Abstracts AABB and ISH Meeting,
    Washington, p. 41.
10 IKUTA S. *et al.* (1962) *Jnl. Jap. Soc. Bld. Transf.*, **9**, 37–38 (in Japanese).
11 MURAKAMI S. (1967) The rare blood types and variants in Japanese. *Act. Crim. Japon.*, **33**,
    138–145.
12 SRINGARM SOMMAI, CHUPUNGART C. and GILES CAROLYN M. (1972) The use of *Ulex euro-
    paeus* and *Dolichos biflorus* extracts in routine ABO groupings of blood donors in
    Thailand. *Vox Sang.*, **23**, 537–545.
13 SRINGARM SOMMAI, CHIEWSILP P., TUBROD J. and SRIBOONRUANG N. (1972) Cad receptors in
    Thai blood donors. Abstracts AABB and ISH Meeting Washington, p. 45, and *Vox.
    Sang.* (1974) **26**, 462–466.
14 BIRD G.W.G. (1970) Comparative serological studies of the T, Tn and Cad receptors. *Blut*,
    21, 366–370.
15 BIRD G.W.G. SHINTON N.K. and WINGHAM JUNE (1971) Persistent mixed-field polyaggluti-
    nation. *Brit. J. Haemat.*, **21**, 443–453.
16 GUNSON H.H., STRATTON F. and MULLARD G.W. (1970) An example of polyagglutinability
    due to the Tn antigen. *Brit. J Haemat.* **18**, 309–316.
17 MYLLYLÄ G., FURUHJELM U., NORDLING S., PIRKOLA ANNA, TIPPETT PATRICIA, GAVIN JUNE
    and SANGER RUTH (1971) Persistent mixed field polyagglutinability: electrokinetic and
    serological aspects. *Vox Sang.*, **20**, 7–23.
18 SANGER RUTH and RACE R.R. (1971) Discussion at 'Journée d'études sur la membrane du
    globule rouge', Paris. *Nouv. Rev. franc. Hémat.*, **11**, 878–884.
19 CRAWFORD HAL, CUTBUSH MARIE and MOLLISON P.L. (1953) Specificity of incomplete 'cold'
    antibody in human serum. *Lancet*, **i**, 566.
20 BIRD G.W.G. and WINGHAM JUNE (1971) Some serological properties of the Cad receptor.
    Vox Sang., **20**, 55–61.
21 UHLENBRUCK G., SPRENGER I., HEGGEN M. and LESENEY A.M. (1971) Diagnosis of the 'Cad'
    blood group with agglutinins from snails and plants. *Z. Immun.-Forsch.*, **141**, 290–
    291.
22 BIZOT M. (1972) Comportement de quelques extraits de gastéropodes terrestres vis-à-vis
    des substances de spécificité Sd^a. *Rev. franc. Transf.*, **15**, 371–375.
23 BIZOT M. and CAYLA J.-P. (1972) Hétéro-anticorps anti-Cad du poulet. *Rev. franc. Transf.*,
    15, 195–202.
24 MORTON J.A. and TERRY A.M. (1970) The Sd^a blood group antigen. Biochemical properties
    of urinary Sd^a. *Vox Sang.*, **19**, 151–161.
25 PEETERMANS M.E. and COLE-DERGENT J. (1970) Haemolytic transfusion reaction due to
    anti-Sd^a. *Vox Sang.*, **18**, 67–70.
26 SCHUH V., VYAS G.N. and FUDENBERG H.H. (1971) A$_{xx}$, a new variant of blood group A.
    Proc. 12th Congr. int. Soc. Blood Transf., Moscow 1969, in *Bibl. haemat.*, No. 38, part I,
    81–83.

THE SID GROUPS 405

27 SCHUH V., VYAS G.N. and FUDENBERG H.H. (1972) Study of a French family with a new variant of blood group A: A_{1ae}. *Amer. J. Hum. Genet.*, **24**, 11–17.
28 YAMAGUCHI H., OKUBO Y., OGAWA Y. and TANAKA M. (1973) Japanese families with group O and B red cells agglutinable by *Dolichos biflorus* extract. *Vox Sang.*, **25**, 361–369.
29 BIRD G.W.G. and WINGHAM JUNE (1974) Haemagglutinins from *Salvia. Vox Sang.*, **26**, 163–166.
30 POOLE JOYCE (1973) Personal communication.

Chapter 18
The Scianna Blood Groups

Last time this chapter told a story about a very common antigen called Sm and a very rare one called Bu[a] and how they were seen to be related. Now that their allelic relationship is clear and the notation rationalized[8] the story is a little spoilt, for the new names make rather obvious what once was very difficult to see: Sm is called Sc1 and Bu[a] Sc2 and the two antigens are 'allelic'.

In 1962 Schmidt, Griffitts and Northman[1] described an antibody, anti-Sm, which they had studied intermittently for some years. All cells tested contained the new antigen except those of the person in whose serum the antibody was found and those of three of her five sibs.

On the other hand, in 1963, Anderson, Hunter, Zipursky, Lewis and Chown[2] described an antibody, anti-Bu[a], which reacted with the cells of only a very small proportion of people.

The observation[3] that an Sm negative person, a member of the original family, was Bu(a+) started some beautiful work in Winnipeg and Miami which showed that the antigens Sm and Bu[a] were, in all probability, controlled by allelic genes: the alternative being that they were controlled by two separate but closely linked loci.

FREQUENCIES

In our last edition we quoted the 600 tests by Schmidt et al.[1], using anti-Sc1 (then anti-Sm) without the finding of a single negative reactor; and nearly 4,000 tests by Anderson et al.[2], Lewis et al.[4] and Seyfried et al.[5] using anti-Sc2 (then anti-Bu[a]) with the finding of about 30 positive reactors.

Now it is more convenient to quote the figures of Lewis et al.[8] who used both antisera on 1,000 unrelated 'caucasian' adults with these results:

anti-			phenotype	genotype
Sc1	Sc2		notation	notation
+	+	17	Sc: 1,2	Sc^1Sc^2
+	−	983	Sc: 1,−2	Sc^1Sc^1

It was not surprising that no example of the phenotype Sc:−1,2 was found in a sample of this size, for the calculated gene and genotype frequencies are:

Sc^1	0·9915	Sc^1Sc^1	0·9831
Sc^2	0·0085	Sc^1Sc^2	0·0168
		Sc^2Sc^2	0·0001

The Canadian workers[2,4] found the antigen Sc2 to be more frequent in Mennonites than in other Canadians; tests in London and Warsaw[5] suggested that the antigen is present in 1 in about 130 Northern Europeans. Though no Sc2 was found in the 212 Negroes tested in Canada, it can be present in these people[7].

INHERITANCE AND INDEPENDENCE OF OTHER SYSTEMS

Schmidt and her colleagues[1], testing the family of the maker of anti-Sc1, showed the Sc:−1 phenotype to be a recessive condition and the antigen Sc1 to segregate independently of the ABO, MNSs and Kidd groups, and of secretor and of sex. The authors added 'nor is it the reciprocal of known low incidence antigens', a perfectly correct statement—at the time.

Anderson and her colleagues[2] showed Sc2 to be inherited as a dominant character, and this was put beyond all doubt by Lewis and her colleagues[4] who tested 145 families, some of them selected for having Sc:2 members: there were 134 Sc:−2 × Sc:−2 matings from which all 361 children were Sc:−2.

The Canadian workers[2,4,6], with great energy, found enough families to make clear that Sc2 segregates independently of ABO, MNSs, P, Rh, Lutheran, Kell Duffy, Kidd, Dombrock, Wr^a and sex, to which Yt was added later[9].

The acute observation, by Lewis, Chown, Schmidt and Griffitts[3] that the thawed stored frozen cells of the original Sc:−1 propositus reacted strongly with anti-Sc2, led to the retesting of the living members of the family of the propositus, with the following results:

	Sc1	Sc2
the propositus and three of her sibs	−	+
another sib of the propositus	+	+
another sib of the propositus	+	−
the child of the propositus	+	+

Sc:−1,2 members reacted more strongly with anti-Sc2 than did the two Sc:1,2 members.

The catching in one family of two very rare phenotypes, Sc:−1 and Sc:2, immediately suggested an allelic control and this was greatly supported by the stronger and weaker reactions with anti-Sc2 just cited. Further support came when Lewis and her colleagues[6] found, in part of a large inbred kindred of Mennonites, three Sc:1,2 × Sc:1,2 matings (all consanguineous) which had

produced 3 Sc:−1,2 and 11 Sc:1,2 and 7 Sc:1,−2 offspring: near enough to the
1:2:1 ratio of children expected of a mating of two heterozygotes.

Assuming that there is only one locus (or even if there were two loci close
together) Sc^1 and Sc^2 do not share loci with those for any of the established red
cell antigen systems, save Diego and Colton for which there is yet no information.

The minus-minus phenotype, Sc:−1,−2

The phenotype Sc:−1,−2 was found by McCreary and his crew[10] in two members
of a kindred living in Likiep Atoll, of the Marshall Islands (10·00 N., 169·08 E.).
The patient had been transfused without cross-matching difficulty, but 7 months
later one of her cousins was the only compatible donor to be found: she also was
Sc:−1,−2.

Search for linkage between Sc and other autosomal markers

Lewis, Kaita and Chown[8] submitted their extensive family results to the
computer system devised by Professor J.H. Edwards. The lod scores ruled out any
close linkage between Sc and ABO, MN, P, Fy, Jk or Do and made unlikely
linkage with Rh, Lu and K.

OTHER NOTES ABOUT Sc1 AND Sc2

Development

The antigen Sc1 was presumed to be developed in uterine life because the first
example of anti-Sc1 appeared to have been made in response to pregnancy; the
antigen is well developed in cord cells.

Anderson and her colleagues[2] tested the cord cells of a baby born into one of
the Sc2 families which they were investigating: the cells gave an Sc2 reaction every
bit as good as that of its Sc2 elders.

Anti-Sc1

Schmidt and her colleagues[1] noted that the Sc:−1 sibs of their propositus had no
antibody, and concluded that the anti-Sc1 in the serum of the propositus was
probably stimulated by her pregnancies, for she had not been transfused or
injected with blood. The antibody reacted by the antiglobulin method.

In the original paper a second example of anti-Sc1, found in an Sc:−1 person,
is briefly mentioned. And, more recently, a third example, again stimulated by
pregnancy, was found by Dr H. Simard, of Chicoutimi, Quebec.

Anti-Sc2

The first example[2] was undoubtedly immune in origin: a patient, Mr Char., was transfused with blood compatible by the antiglobulin test, but 14 days later the donor's blood was found to be incompatible by the same test.

Four further examples of anti-Sc2 were induced by extraordinary chance (Seyfried et al.[5], 1966). Fourteen Rh negative volunteers in Warsaw were injected with Rh positive blood to provide anti-D for routine purposes, but it so happened that the donor was Sc2 and four examples of anti-Sc2 resulted, one of them powerful. A no less powerful example of anti-Sc2 was sent to us from the States[7]. Mollison et al.[11] found Sc2 to be less antigenic than D: of seven subjects given at least two injections of Rh positive Sc2 red cells four formed anti-D and only one anti-Sc2.

Though the high frequency of the one antigen and the low frequency of the other make the Scianna system of little practical use in genetical work, the bringing of order out of disorder, by the researches in Winnipeg and Miami, gives a lot of pleasure.

REFERENCES

[1] SCHMIDT R. PAULINE, GRIFFITTS J.J. and NORTHMAN F.F. (1962) A new antibody, anti-Sm, reacting with a high incidence antigen. Transfusion, Philad., 2, 338–340.

[2] ANDERSON CATHERINE, HUNTER JOY, ZIPURSKY A., LEWIS MARION and CHOWN B. (1963) An antibody defining a new blood group antigen, Bu^a. Transfusion, Philad., 3, 30–33.

[3] LEWIS MARION, CHOWN B., SCHMIDT R. PAULINE and GRIFFITTS J.J. (1964) A possible relationship between the blood group antigens Sm and Bu^a. Amer. J. hum. Genet., 16, 254–255.

[4] LEWIS MARION, CHOWN B., KAITA HIROKO and PHILIPPS SYLVIA (1964) Further observations on the blood group antigen Bu^a. Amer. J. hum. Genet., 16, 256–260.

[5] SEYFRIED HALINA, FRANKOWSKA KRYSTYNA and GILES CAROLYN M. (1966) Further examples of anti-Bu^a found in immunized donors. Vox Sang., 11, 512–516.

[6] LEWIS MARION, CHOWN B. and KAITA HIROKO (1967) On the blood group antigens Bu^a and Sm. Transfusion, Philad., 7, 92–94.

[7] WILLIAMS CATHERINE, HAIST ANNA and GAVIN JUNE (1967) Unpublished observations.

[8] LEWIS MARION, KAITA HIROKO and CHOWN B. (1974) Scianna blood group system. Vox Sang., 27, 261–264.

[9] GILES CAROLYN M., BEVAN BERYL and HUGHES R.M. (1970) A family showing independent segregation of Bu^a and Yt^b. Vox Sang., 18, 265–266.

[10] McCREARY J., VOGLER A.L., SABO B., ECKSTEIN E.G. and SMITH T.R. (1973) Another minus-minus phenotype: Bu(a−) Sm- two examples in one family. Transfusion, Philad., 13, 350 (Abstract).

[11] MOLLISON P.L., FRAME MARION and ROSS MARGARET E. (1970) Differences between Rh(D) negative subjects in response to Rh(D) antigen. Brit. J. Haemat., 19, 257–266.

Chapter 19
Some Very Frequent Antigens

Very common antigens, or 'public' antigens as they have been called, may, like the 'private' antigens, herald new systems or they may be part of established systems. For example, Tj^a was not at first recognized to be part of the P system nor U part of the MNSs system: Kp^b, on the other hand, was brilliantly shown right from the start to belong to the Kell system.

Some of these 'public' antigens have almost reached systemic state but the reason why they are not given separate chapters is that, though important in transfusion they are not useful polymorphic characters (this is true for all populations studied with the extraordinary exception of the antigen Ge in some Melanesians).

We have made our own rules for entry into the list of 'public' antigens given in Tables 73 and 74. The antigens must of course be possessed by the vast majority of people, and they must be proved inherited characters (shown by two sibs lacking the antigen). The antigens must be serologically distinct from each other and distinct from the antigens defined by the following antibodies: anti-H, -U, -P, -PP$_1$P^k, -Luke, -LW, -Lu^b, -Lu^{a}Lu^b (-Lu3), -k, -Kp^b, -Js^b, -Ku, -KL, -Le^{a}Le^b, -Fy3, -Jk^{a}Jk^b, -Di^b, -Yt^a, -Sc1, -Wr^b, -Co^a, -Co^{a}Co^b, -I, -Cs^a, -Chido; antibodies in the serum of Rh$_{null}$ (or immunized people homozygous for $-D-$, C^wD- or $cD-$), and the para-Lutheran and para-Kell antibodies should be remembered.

The antigens listed in Table 73 are not known to be the hypothetical antigens antithetical to any of the 'private' antigens of Chapter 20.

FREQUENCIES AND INHERITANCE

How distinguished it is to lack the antigens of this chapter is shown in Table 73 or, in the case of Vel, in the text. Persons lacking any of these antigens are presumed to be either (i) homozygous for a rare allele of the gene responsible for the antigen, or (ii) homozygous for the absence of a very common allele of a modifying gene necessary for the production of the antigen. Whatever the explanation, the absence of these antigens behaves as a recessive character; this may ultimately need slight qualification for we are beginning to suspect that the Vel negative state may in a minority of families be controlled by a dominant inhibitor, in the way the Lutheran antigens can be.

410

Table 73. 'Public' or 'high incidence' antigens (for Vel see text)

Name of antigen	Investigators	Unrelated people tested		
		Population	Total	Negative
Ge (Gerbich)	Rosenfield et al.[10], 1960	New Yorkers*	11,000	0
		Danish	500	0
	Cleghorn[5], 1961	English	22,331	0
	Hindmarsh et al.[18], 1962	Californians	500	0
	Booth et al.[44], 1970	Australians	700	0
	McLoughlin et al.[45], 1970	New Zealanders	>5,000	0
	Muller et al.[46], 1973	French	5,912	1
			>45,943	1
	Booth et al.[47], 1972	Middle Sepik (Melanesian extreme)	70	45
Lan	van der Hart et al.[11], 1961	Dutch	4,000	1
	Grindon et al.[55], 1968	U.S.A.	400	0
	Smith et al.[56], 1969	English	2,268	0
	Frank et al.[57], 1970	U.S.A.	>500	0
	Clancey et al.[58], 1972	Canadian	407	1
Gy^a (Gregory)	Swanson et al.[30], 1966	Minneapolis Whites	9,459	0
		Minneapolis Indians	611	0
		Minneapolis Negroes	75	0
At^a (August.)	Applewhaite et al.[24], 1967	New Yorkers†	>6,600	0
Jr^a	Gellerman et al.[68], 1974	Pittsburgh donors	9,145	0
		Asiatics	1,041	0
		Eskimos	75	0
	Staveley[69], 1974	New Zealanders	937	0
Kn^a (Knops)	Helgeson et al.[64], 1970	Minneapolis donors	2,091	4
El	Frank et al.[57], 1970	Miami donors	3,000	0
Dp	Frank et al.[57], 1970	Miami donors	600	0
Gn^a (Gonsowski)	Fox et al.[65], 1969	Minnesota donors	2,600	0

* Of whom it is estimated that at least 1,500 must have been Negroes and at least 100 Asiatics, mostly Chinese.

† Of whom at least 2,200 were Negroes.

Genetical independence of other systems

Table 74 shows how far the antigens have been excluded from belonging to the established systems. There are two arguments behind these exclusions involving a very common antigen. The first applies to all families and the second only to families in which the parents of the propositus are consanguineous.

1 If two sibs be, say, Ge— and differ in their groups on another system, then Ge cannot be part of that system. For example, if the gene responsible for the antigen Ge belonged to the ABO locus (it does not) then the two sibs, II-2 and II-4, in Figure 25 (page 418) would have to have the same ABO groups because both would

Table 74. Separate segregation of the genes responsible for certain very common antigens and those for established systems

		ABO	MNSs	P	Rh	Lu	K	Fy	Jk	Do	Sec.	X-borne
Vel	v. Loghem et al.[12], 1958		×		×							
	Strickel et al.[14], 1959	×	×		×						×*	×
	Tate and Schmidt[15], 1959	×	×		×						×*	×
	Clegorn[5], 1961		×		×	×		×	×			
	Wiener et al.[20], 1961		×		×		×		×			×
	Albrey et al.[8], 1965	×	×		×			×	×			×
	Cedergren et al.[39], 1974	×	×	×	×			×	×		×*	×
Ge	Rosenfield et al.[10], 1960	×	×	×	×				×			×
	Cleghorn[5], 1961		×	×	×		×		×			×
	Hindmarsh et al.[18], 1962		×	×	×							
	Nunn et al.[25], 1967		×		×				×			
	Muller et al.[46], 1973		×		×			×				×
	Brocteur[49], 1973							×		×	×*	×
	Colpitts et al.[67], 1974	×	×					×		×		×
Lan	van der Hart et al.[11], 1961	×	×		×	×			×			
	Grindon et al.[55], 1968		×		×			×	×			×
	Smith et al.[56], 1969							×	×			×
	Frank et al.[57], 1970		×	×	×			×	×			
	Clancey et al.[58], 1972	×	×	×	×			×	×			
Gyᵃ	Swanson et al.[23,30], 1966	×	×	×				×	×			
	Swanson[35], 1967			×	×				×			×
Atᵃ	Applewhaite et al.[24], 1967	×	×	×	×				×			
	Gellerman et al.[61], 1970		×	×					×			×
Jrᵃ	Gellerman et al.[68], 1974	×	×				×				×	×
Knᵃ	Helgeson et al.[64], 1970	×	×		×	×					×	×
El	Frank et al.[57], 1970										×*	×
Dp	Frank et al.[57], 1970		×		×			×			×*	×

Crosses represent separate segregation in families (information from the original papers or from our records).

* Based on Lewis phenotypes of red cells; saliva not tested.

There is no information yet about the genetical relationship of any of these antigens to the Diego, Yt, Auberger, Colton, Sid or Scianna systems.

have received their father's 'not-Ge' *ABO* gene and their mother's 'not-Ge' *ABO* gene. The groups given in Figure 25 are sufficient to show that Ge does not belong to the ABO, MNSs, P or Kell systems.

2 If a person who is, say, Vel–, came from a consanguineous mating, then Vel cannot be part of any system for which that person is heterozygous. The argument is that cousins heterozygous for a very rare gene may be assumed to have identical copies of that gene, since it has come to each from one grandparent: if Vel were part of Rh (it is not) then the homozygous Vel– offspring of a cousin mating would have to be homozygous for Rh too. Cleghorn[5] records a family (Cooper) to which this argument applies: one member only is Vel– and her parents are cousins; she is *Ms/Ns*, *CDe/cde*, *Lu^aLu^b* and *Jk^aJk^b*, thus demonstrating that Vel cannot be part of any of these four systems.

Exclusion of sex-linkage

We are assuming, for the present purpose, that crossing-over does not happen between the X and the Y chromosomes. 'Public' antigens cannot be Y-linked characters because females have these antigens.

X-linkage of a 'public' antigen is excluded if a female lacking the antigen has a father or son with it. Conversely, if a 'public' antigen were X-linked the fathers and sons of females lacking the antigen would lack it too and, furthermore, males would greatly outnumber females amongst people lacking the antigen.

THE ANTIGEN VEL

In 1952 Sussman and Miller[1] investigated the serum of a patient called Vel who had suffered a transfusion reaction. The serum agglutinated all but four of ten thousand samples of group O but otherwise unselected blood: it did not agglutinate the patient's own red cells. No other negatives were found amongst eight available sibs of the five Vel–people. However, it was assumed that Vel was inherited and the negativeness was a recessive character.

No light on the inheritance came with the second example of anti-Vel (Levine, Robinson, Herrington and Sussman[2]) but the antibody had haemolytic as well as agglutinating properties. This haemolytic faculty, though not found in all anti-Vel sera, can be a useful guide to the identification of the antibody. The third example[3] again gave no clue to the inheritance.

Six years after the finding of the first Vel–, van Loghem and van der Hart[12] investigated a family (Woud.) in which two sibs were Vel–, thus demonstrating that the character was inherited and launching the work on the exclusion of Vel from established systems. Thereafter the tempo increased and a great many examples of anti-Vel have now been found.

Several of the earlier papers recorded variation of strength of the antigen in Vel positive people. Weak reactors to anti-Vel sera certainly exist, and without the help of powerful antisera it is easy to get false negative reactions. Cleghorn, in his thesis,[5] remarks of anti-Vel sera:

'These are the most difficult and unreliable of all the reagents with which the author has worked. Cells which appear Vel-negative must be tested with as many reagents as can be assembled, and should never be accepted as such until a fresh sample has been obtained from the donor. The author has wasted many weeks in following families of persons who were not in fact Vel-negative, before this simple truth became apparent.'

Albrey et al.[8] also note the variability in strength of reaction of the cells of different Vel positive people, a difference that cannot possibly, on frequency grounds, be attributed simply to that between heterozygotes and homozygotes.

We would guess from our limited experience that titrations would show the strength of the Vel antigen to make a normal distribution curve. However, in 1968 Issitt and his colleagues[21] in New York postulated that anti-Vel sera are of two kinds (anti-Vel1 plus anti-Vel2 and anti-Vel2) which corresponded to three Vel phenotypes, Vel:1,2; Vel:1,−2 and Vel:−1,−2. The case is beautifully made yet we are not convinced that the answer is as crisp as this: for using many anti-Vel sera we were unable to achieve such a neat pattern.

Frequencies

Well over 50,000 people have been tested with anti-Vel sera[1-8, 32, 33] and the incidence of negative reactors seems to be of the order of 1 in 2 to 4 thousand. It is not known how the anti-Vel sera used by the majority of workers would now be classified according to Issitt et al.[21]. The original anti-Vel of Sussman and Miller[1] was later classified[21] as perhaps anti-Vel1 plus anti-Vel2, at any rate not anti-Vel2, and it had reacted negatively with 4 in 10,000 New Yorkers, an incidence of 1 in 2,500, and Battaglini et al.[32] also found 4 in testing 10,000 French; Cleghorn[5] found 4 in 16,548 English, an incidence of 1 in 4,137 but Nevanlinna[33] found no negatives in testing 18,920 Finns. Cedergren[22] in the other hand, found 52 negatives in 91,605 people around Umeå in the north of Sweden, an incidence of 1 in 1762, while Kornstad[34] found 4 in testing 5,009 Norwegians.

Issitt and his collaborators[21] using their anti-Vel2 serum found 24 negatives in 31,139, an incidence of 1 in 1297: the people were New York blood donors of whom the Caucasian fraction was estimated to be 'no higher than 75%'.

To give some idea of the gene frequencies we may compare Cleghorn's figures for England[5] with those of Issitt et al.[21] for New York; the calculations are based on the assumption that Vel negativeness is a recessive character though, as will be seen below, we think it unlikely that all Vel negatives are recessive, but supposing they are:

England		New York	
Ve^a	0·9859	$Vel^{1,2}$	0·97 'probably about'
Ve	0·0141	$Vel^{-1,-2}$	0.016
		$Vel^{1,-2}$	0·012

Inheritance and independence

The absence of the Vel antigen must usually be a recessive condition but a few families are known with Vel— members in two[8, 38, 39] or even three[6] generations. Chance seems so improbable an explanation that we are beginning to wonder whether there may be, as in the Lutheran system, two causes of the negativeness: one due to a recessive allele at the *Vel* locus and the other due to an inhibitor gene dominant in effect and perhaps genetically independent of the *Vel* locus.

In the families showing Vel negatives in only one generation it is surprising how many lack information about one[3, 5, 8, 14] or both[1, 2, 5, 12, 13, 20] parents of the propositus. The information given by sibs usually fits best a recessive mode of inheritance but in two families[13, 20] a dominant mode is perhaps more likely.

Counts of the sibs and the children of Vel negative propositi are peculiar, but we think it better not to make an issue of this because of the increased likelihood of a family being published if it includes one or more Vel negative sib of the propositus.

The Vel antigen (or antigens) has been shown, by segregation in families, not to be controlled from the loci for other blood group systems as recorded in Table 74. It should be said that these exclusions are based on the assumption of recessive inheritance.

At the time of our last edition the independence of the P system had not been established and we thought, mainly because of the lytic powers of some anti-Vel sera, that there might be an association: but Cedergren and Giles[39] have now been able to rule this out.

Vel can therefore be considered practically an established system: it remains only to rule out membership of the Diego, Yt, Auberger, Dombrock, Colton and Sid systems.

Development of the antigen Vel

Sussman[9] records difficulty in grouping cord cells, because of the weakness of the antigen. We, on the other hand, found it quite well developed though rather weaker than in the adult (mean score for five cord samples = 33, mean score for five adult samples = 52). Cleghorn[5] found the antigen in foetuses aged between $17\frac{1}{2}$ and 28 weeks. But the last word seems to be with Toivanen and Hirvonen[40] (1969) who found the antigen well developed in 12 out of 12 foetuses, the youngest of whom was 12 weeks.

Anti-Vel

Though the Vel— phenotype is so rare many examples of anti-Vel have been identified (some published[1–3, 5, 6, 8, 9, 13, 14, 20, 41, 42], and more not). This reflects the acute transfusion emergency that the antibody can cause: identification is essential, for the chance of finding a donor, if sibs have failed to provide one, is slight by random cross-matching, and the aid of a rare donor panel will be needed.

Our own tests and those of Dr Cleghorn using 14 anti-Vel sera gave no evidence that these examples were heterogeneous, though the more recent work of Issitt and his collaborators[21] makes it probable that there are at least two kinds of anti-Vel. In our last edition we wondered whether anti-Vel may be a complicated antibody like anti-Luke (page 164) and many anti-I (page 452) whose reactions are influenced by the presence of antigens belonging to systems genetically independent of each other, but we still have no evidence to support this possibility.

The antibody is usually of the IgM type; it is not 'regularly occurring' for it has not been found in the Vel− sibs of propositi. The known examples can all be attributed to immunization by transfusion, with one exception: Szalóky and van der Hart[42] found one which appeared to be 'auto'.

Anti-Vel has been responsible for haemolytic reaction to transfusion[6]. The antibody has not yet been blamed for haemolytic disease of the newborn[43] though it can be stimulated by pregnancy[41]. Drachmann and Lundsgaard[41], in reporting an IgG anti-Vel which did not affect the Vel positive foetus, consider that 'it is not unlikely that a high titred maternal IgG anti-Ve will occur in a pregnancy, in which the foetus has a strong Ve antigen, and will cause erythroblastosis foetalis'.

Some anti-Vel sera react in saline tests but usually react better by albumin, enzyme or anti-globulin tests, but a 'two-stage' antiglobulin test seems to be the method of choice: negative results, especially of saline tests, are only to be trusted with fresh cells. Cleghorn[5] found that all of his and of our collection of anti-Vel sera reacted by the antiglobulin test if anti-IgM sera were used: he was unable to restore, by the addition of human or animal complement, the lytic activity of once lytic anti-Vel sera. This also was the experience of Sussman but, as he pointed out, not of all workers[9]. Evidently sera vary in this respect. Cleghorn[5] found, and we agreed, that the absorption test is not very helpful in deciding the Vel negative status of a doubtful sample: anti-Vel can be very difficult to absorb—so much so that Cleghorn successfully removed anti-A and anti-B, leaving anti-Vel, by absorption with cells which he later found to be weak Vel+. Issitt and his collaborators[21], on the other hand, did not experience this difficulty with the sera they were using.

We guess that something of basic interest will emerge from the study of the inheritance of the Vel system of Sussman and Miller.

THE ANTIGEN Ge (GERBICH)

Three examples of the antibody defining this antigen were found at about the same time in the serum of three mothers, an American of Italian extraction (Mrs Ge.), a Mexican (Snra Es.) and a Dane (Fru St.); their babies all gave positive direct anti-globulin reactions though none required treatment (Rosenfield, Haber, Kissmeyer-Nielsen, Jack, Sanger and Race[10], 1960).

Two of the propositi had available families and in both of them one sib was, like the propositus, Ge–, thus demonstrating that the antigen is an inherited character. The pedigree of one of the families is given in Figure 25. None of the three propositi was the product of a consanguineous marriage.

A fourth example was found by Barnes and Lewis[19]: it came from a Turkish Cypriot, Mrs Yus., whose serum had powerfully agglutinated all cells tested save her own. Cleghorn[5] found that the serum did not agglutinate Ge– cells; all three examples of Rosenfield et al.[10] were tried. The cells of Mrs Yus. were negative with the serum of Snra Es. and of Fru St. but, unexpectedly, they were strongly positive with the serum of Mrs Ge.: thus, very soon after their first description, the Ge groups were shown to be subdivisible.

Absorption by the cells of Mrs Yus., unlike other Ge– cells, removed all antibody from the serum of Mrs Ge. The serum of Mrs Ge. evidently has some factor in addition to that present in the serum of the other three: the cells of Mrs Yus., alone of the four, possess the corresponding antigen. Cleghorn[5] pointed out that a parallel with Rh is useful in giving a picture of what is happening, though he considered it almost certainly an over-simplification: if the cells of Ge., Es. and St. be thought of as cc and the antibodies in Es., St. and Yus. be likened to anti-C then the Ge antibody can be thought of as anti-CC^w and the cells of Yus. as $C^w c$ or $C^w C^w$.

We propose to call cells of the Yus. type Ge– though they are in fact positive with perhaps a quarter of anti-Ge sera which includes that from the mother who happened to give her name to the groups.

We are going to tell the story first in terms of the tests on people of the continents of Europe and America; and then to describe the astonishing findings of Booth[44] and his colleagues in Melanesians.

Frequencies

These are given in Table 73. The New Yorkers, the Australians and the French were tested with anti-Ge sera which react with cells of the Yus type: the Danish, English, Californians and New Zealanders with anti-Ge sera which do not react with the Yus type of cells.

Ge– is indeed a rare state, not till after 17 years and more than forty thousand tests was the first random example found[46], outside Melanesia that is. Many Ge– people were, of course, known, but they were propositi (or their sibs) who had selected themselves out of the million by having anti-Ge in their serum. We know of 20 such propositi drawn from 10 non-Melanesian countries; they were of European, Mexican, South American Indian and negro extraction. Some details of 12 examples were given in our last edition and the references have been retained (they are 5, 10, 18, 25–29, 31 and 37): of the remaining 8 propositi 3 have been published[45, 46, 48].

Of 17 propositi tested in our Unit 5 were of the Yus type.

Inheritance and independence

The original paper[10] included two pedigrees (Figure 25 is one of them) which showed that the antigen Ge is an inherited character, and Rosenfield and his collaborators wrote 'The simplest solution is that the antigen Ge is a dominant character and its absence recessive. Less simple would be the proposition that the absence of Ge is due to the presence of a modifying gene in the homozygous state'. The absence of consanguinity between the parents of the three original propositi was commented on.

Since that time there has been little change of outlook. Other (non-Melanesian) families have been tested and 9 propositi have 12 Ge+ sibs and 8 Ge− sibs. This is not a significant deviation, and the theory that the absence of Ge is a recessive condition is not contradicted. (The probability of observing deviations

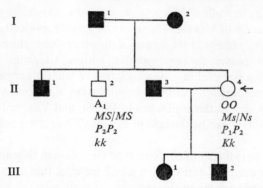

Fig. 25. A family with two Ge− sibs. White = Ge−, black = Ge+. The other recorded groups show that the antigen Ge is independent of the systems they represent. (From Rosenfield, Haber, Kissmeyer-Nielsen, Jack, Sanger and Race[10], 1960.)

from expected Mendelian ratios 1:1, 1:3, etc., can conveniently be found for totals up to 50 in *Probability Tables for Mendelian Ratios with Small Numbers*, Texas Agricultural Experiment Station Bulletin No. 463, 1932.)

For 10 propositi there is parental information: 9 were not consanguineous and 1 pair were second cousins. Considering the great rarity of Ge− it is rather surprising that the incidence of consanguinity was not higher.

The genetical independence of Ge and established systems is dealt with in Table 74.

Although Ge− seems clearly a recessive condition there are a few hints that its background may be rather more complicated. The count of sibs of the propositi does not differ significantly from that expected of a recessive character but nor does it from that expected of a dominant. There is not a great deal of family information: we know of five families[10, 18, 46, 49, 5] in which both parents of a Ge− propositus are Ge+, as expected of a recessive.

In testing the family of a Ge− woman from Moncton, New Brunswick, with anti-Ge in her serum, Colpitts and her colleagues[67] were surprised to find that the mother of the propositus was also Ge–. This, and the fact that two of the four sibs of the propositus were also Ge–, made the Ge negative condition, had it been judged by this pedigree alone, appear to be a dominant character. The explanation was that the parents of the propositus are cousins and the father of the propositus must be a heterozygote. The maternal grandparents were not known to be related. The sibs of the propositus were, of course, excluded from the sib count above.

An association with the Kell system

In at any rate three families, one French, one Italian-Belgian and one Canadian, an association between Ge– and depression of the Kell antigens is established (Muller, André-Liardet, Garretta, Brocteur and Moullec[46], 1973; Brocteur[49], 1973; Colpitts, Cornwall and Moore[67], 1974). Samples were distributed to a number of laboratories and there is no doubt about the depression: it has been shown to involve the antigens K, k, Kp^b, Js^b, Ku and KL of all 8 Ge– members of the three families. For the curious, the para-Kell antigens (see page 299) appeared normal.

That the *Gerbich* locus is not part of the *Kell* locus was shown by one of the original families, which is reproduced in Figure 25. In the original testing of this family we had not noticed any depression of Kell antigens in either II-2 or II-4 and were relieved when, on retesting the samples recently, Dr Carolyn Giles agreed that their Kell phenotypes were both correct and normal.

Is this a further hint of heterogeneity of the Ge– condition? It makes one wonder whether Ge– may on occasion reflect activity at an inhibitor locus rather than at the *Gerbich* locus.

Development of the antigen Ge

The antigen is well developed at birth[10] and Cleghorn has found it well developed in 19 foetuses, aged $17\frac{1}{2}$ to 28 weeks (personal communication).

Anti-Ge

The first three examples of the antibody may have been stimulated by pregnancy for serologically they behaved like immune antibodies, reacting best by the antiglobulin method and producing one strong and two weak positive direct antiglobulin reactions in the cells of the three healthy infants. The fourth example, that of Mrs Yus., was probably 'naturally occurring': it strongly agglutinated cells in saline at room temperature, but at 37° it reacted only feebly by all methods; the direct antiglobulin test on the baby's cells was negative. None of the examples was haemolytic. No anti-Ge could be detected in the serum of the Ge– sibs of Mrs Ge., Fru St. or Mrs Yus.

The anti-Ge in the serum of Mr Mon.[18] was certainly 'naturally occurring': he had never been transfused and, furthermore, anti-Ge was present in the serum

of his two Ge– sibs. The antisera of these brothers reacted in saline at room
temperature: they did not react by straightforward anti-globulin tests but Dr
Tippett found good reactions using the two-stage antiglobulin test (involving
EDTA and complement). The antibody of Mr Arm., on the other hand, though
believed to be 'naturally occurring', reacted best by the straightforward antiglobulin method[29]. A slight transfusion reaction[25] was attributed to anti-Ge.
From Newfoundland came a dramatic story of the management of placenta
praevia and erythroblastosis in a pregnancy of a woman with anti-Ge in her
serum.[48]

All examples of anti-Ge we have tested were of the IgG type.

The difference of specificity of anti-Ge, the minority reacting with the Yus type
of cells, is discussed above and will be returned to below.

The Gerbich groups in New Guinea

The serum of a transfused native woman, Mrs Imp., living about 100 miles from
Lae up the Markham Valley was found to contain a strong anti-Ge of the IgG
type (Booth, Albrey, Whittaker and Sanger[44], 1970). The use of Mrs Imp.'s
serum brought to light the astonishing frequency in those parts of the phenotype
Ge–, and launched a huge anthropological survey by Booth and his colleagues[47, 52–54]. The story is fascinating: it is summarized by Booth and
McLoughlin[47] from which the following paragraph is taken.

'The Gerbich gene frequencies . . . show a mixture of what may be clinal variations (e.g. *Ge*
decreasing from the head of the Markham Valley to the Morobe Coast) and sharp lines of de-
marcation (e.g. between the head of the Markham Valley and the upper Ramu, or above the
Kassam Pass). Any clinal variation might be related to *Ge* spread by intermarriage, though in
general both among the Wapei (Lumi) and Atzera (Markham Valley) peoples, marriages are
still limited for any one village to a group of perhaps 4 surrounding villages. This would involve
groups of not more than a thousand people, and often much less. Such spread of *Ge* as seems to
exist occurs in the direction where natural barriers are least effective—along large rivers and the
coast. In New Guinea, geographical barriers usually also divide peoples of differing cultures or
languages, as might be expected, and this is true at the head of the Markham Valley, and also
where the Torricelli Mountains meet the coastal plain. Thus the abrupt transfer from peoples
possessing a high *Ge* frequency to those with apparently no *Ge* is explicable.'

This gold mine of Ge– people made contribution to the serology and genetics of
the system as well as to population genetics.

In testing[47] the sera of 664 Ge– people 89, or 13 %, were found to contain anti-
Ge. The incidence of the antibody 'appears to be much the same in males and
females'. The majority were 'naturally occurring' but some were immune and
both types reacted with IgG but not with IgA or IgM antiglobulin. The reaction
was unaffected by the addition of saliva, hydatid cyst fluid or by a variety of sugars.

Seven out of 71 anti-Ge sera were, like Mrs Gerbich herself, of the kind which
reacts with Yus cells, and Booth and McLoughlin called this type anti-Ge1,2,3.
Most of the sera were of the common type which do not react with Yus cells, and

these were called anti-Ge1,2. One of the 71 sera (and another found later[50]) was of a new specificity which was called anti-Ge1. Accordingly the proposed pattern of antibody antigen interaction was:

anti-Ge,1,2,3	anti-Ge1,2	anti-Ge1	
+	+	+	most people
+	+	−	some Melanesians
+	−	−	no Melanesians, rare elsewhere
−	−	−	some Melanesians, rare elsewhere

and further divisions were expected[50].

Just as Yus type cells (+−−) removed all activity from anti-Ge1,2,3 so also did ++− Melanesian cells remove all activity from anti-Ge1,2,3 and anti-Ge1,2.

Booth and Hornabrook[51] report the testing of 30 New Guinea families with both parents available and 64 families with only one parent available. Having ingeniously made an allowance for the gene frequencies in the area from which each family came, expectations for the proportion of Ge+ or Ge− children were calculated for the whole. The observed distribution of the children in the families in which both parents were tested fitted very well that expected, and confirmed that in these people also the antigen Ge is a dominant character. Furthermore, tests on 26 families showed that the phenotypes Ge1,2,3 (+++) and Ge2,3 (++−) and Ge (−−−) were inherited straightforwardly and were compatible with a three allele Gerbich system, of the A_1A_2O pattern, in New Guinea.

THE ANTIGEN Lan

The antibody defining the antigen Lan was found by van der Hart, Moes, van der Veer and van Loghem[11] (1961) in the serum of a man who suffered a reaction to his third transfusion. The antibody was avid and worked only by the antiglobulin method. The Lan antigen was evidently very common for only 1 Lan negative was found in testing 4,000 random Dutch people (Table 73). The antigen was an inherited character, for one of the two sibs of the propositus also lacked it. The Lan negative phenotype was assumed to be a recessive character and this was supported by the late parents of the two negatives being consanguineous. The other groups of the family showed the *Lan* locus not to belong to the loci for ABO, MNSs, Rh or Kidd (Table 74). Both the propositus and his Lan negative sib suffered from retinitis pigmentosa: it is unlikely that there is any direct association for no subsequent Lan negative has had it. Concerning the possibility of linkage between the two conditions nothing can be said: to find other families with autosomal recessive retinitis pigmentosa and Lan negatives must be a forlorn hope.

Seven years passed before a second example of anti-Lan was found (Grindon et al.[55], 1968) in a woman two weeks after her first transfusion. Her serum reacted with all of 400 random samples of red cells: the cells of one of her three sibs were negative. Her parents were dead. The family confirmed certain exclusions and added X-linkage (Table 74).

In 1969 a third example of anti-Lan was found (Smith *et al.*[56]). One of the patient's two sibs was also Lan negative and some exclusions were confirmed (Table 74): it was stated that Kell was excluded but this was a mistake. The patient had been transfused at the birth of her first child and her second had mild haemolytic disease of the newborn: he had a direct positive antiglobulin reaction and anti-Lan was detected in his serum. The mother's serum was used to screen 2,268 donors but without finding a negative.

The fourth example (Frank *et al.*[57], 1970) was found in a patient who had not been transfused but has four children: four of her sibs were tested with her serum and one was negative. Certain exclusions were confirmed (Table 74). No compatible donor was found in more than 500 tests.

In 1972, Clancey *et al.*[58] found another example of the antibody in a boy three months after his first transfusion. His family, and the family of one Lan negative found in testing 407 random donors, both filled a gap: it was the first time that both parents of a Lan negative person had been tested, and both, as expected, were Lan positive. The two families between them confirmed certain exclusions and added P (Table 74). Of the sibs of the two propositi 2 were Lan negative and 3 positive.

We were kindly given details of a family investigated by Miss Delores McGuire and Mr W.L. Marsh in which the Lan negative propositus had 3 Lan positive sibs, and this, added to the published families, makes the count of the sibs of propositi:

Lan negative 6, Lan positive 13

which is very close to the 1 in 4 expected of the sibs if the character were a recessive.

The Ig type of anti-Lan in all examples in which its determination was recorded is IgG: this aspect was particularly studied in the patient of Smith *et al.*[56]. Anti-Lan has not been found 'naturally occurring' but the antigen is efficiently antigenic when transfused.

We have found the antigen Lan to be well developed in cord cells and this was to be expected because of the mild haemolytic disease of the newborn described by Smith *et al.*[56]

A dosage effect was looked for by Smith *et al.*[56], but Lan heterozygotes appeared to react as well as homozygotes.

Unlike Vel and Gerbich the Lan antigen is, so far, pleasantly free from subdivision.

THE ANTIGEN Gy^a (GREGORY)

Anti-Gy^a, yet another Minneapolis find, presented itself at ante-natal testing (Swanson, Zweber and Polesky[23, 30], 1966, 1967). The anti-Gy^a in the serum of

Mrs Gregory reacted with all random samples tested (Table 73). It also reacted with the cells of her parents, her husband, her five children, and three of her six sibs. Of the three compatible sibs two are male and their serum does not contain anti-Gy^a but the third is a female with two Gy(a+) children, and anti-Gy^a is present in her serum too. Although the antibody is avid and works well by the antiglobulin test none of the seven children of the two Gy(a−) mothers showed any evidence of haemolytic disease of the newborn.

The parents of Mrs Gregory are of Czechoslovakian descent and are second cousins.

This one family is extraordinarily informative and shows not only that Gy(a−) is a recessive condition but also that the locus responsible is distinct from the loci for ABO, MNSs, P, Rh, Duffy and Kidd and that it is not X-linked (Table 74).

Swanson and her colleagues[30] were able to detect a difference in strength of reaction with anti-Gy^a between the cells of the presumed homozygous and heterozygous Gy(a+) members of the family. The antibody is of the IgG type. The antigen Gy^a is developed at birth.

A second family of Czechoslovakian descent with Gy(a−) was investigated by Swanson[35]. The propositus and her Gy(a−) sister both have been pregnant and both have anti-Gy^a in their serum. A Gy(a−) brother has no anti-Gy^a. The family adds Lutheran to the list of systems excluded (Table 74).

A further example of anti-Gy^a was reported at a congress in Bal Harbour in 1973 by Massaquoi and Cornwall[59] who mentioned a previous example found on the South Coast of Newfoundland in 1967, but we know no details of this: their own propositus was found in the same area in 1972, and extensive investigation of her kindred showed that she was probably related to the previous propositus; it also unearthed three more Gy(a−) people.

Moulds, Ellisor, Reid and Harrison[60] reported, at the same congress, that the antigen Hy (Holley)[35, 36] was related to Gy in that the cells of Hy negative people gave weak reactions with anti-Gy^a and anti-Hy did not react with Gy(a−) cells. This suggested sub-division within the Gy system, which therefore seems to be going the way of Gerbich. The phenotype Gy(aw) appears to be a negro character.

THE ANTIGEN At^a (AUGUST)

Attention was drawn to the antibody in the serum of Mrs August., a Negress, when the cells of her third baby gave a weak positive direct antiglobulin reaction (Applewhaite, Ginsberg, Gerena, Cunningham and Gavin[24], 1967). The antibody was powerful and worked best by the antiglobulin test; the reaction was not inhibited if the cells were first treated with papain.

Table 73 shows that no random person has yet been found to be At(a−), consequently no estimate of the frequency of At^a is possible.

The antigen At^a is inherited, for Mrs August.'s brother is, like her, At(a−). The parents were not consanguineous. Mrs August.'s mother, sister and baby girl were all At(a+) as, presumably, was her father who is dead. The other groups of Mrs August. and her brother show that the antigen At[a] is not a hitherto unrecognized member of the MNSs, Rh, Kidd or Xg systems. (That the *At* locus is independent of the *Xg* locus does not, of course, give any evidence for or against X-linkage.)

The antigen At[a] is well developed in cord cells. The antibody in the serum of Mrs August. was presumably caused by pregnancy for she had never been transfused and there was no anti-At[a] in the serum of her At(a−) brother.

Nothing more was heard of At[a] until 1973 when Gellerman, McCreary, Yedinak and Stroup[61] of the Philip Levine Laboratories, Raritan, reported the finding of six more examples of anti-At[a]. All six propositi were Negroes and all had been pregnant or transfused. All the antibodies were of the IgG type.

Some relatives of five of the propositi could be tested and confirmed that the *At* locus is not part of the *MNSs* locus and added exclusion from the *P* locus and from X-linkage (Table 74). A count of the sibs of the At(a−) propositi[24, 61] showed that 7 were At(a+) and 2 At(a−), almost exactly what was to be expected if At(a−) were a recessive character. None of the parents of the propositi was known to be consanguineous. Though the antigen At[a] was shown to be well developed at birth[24,61] it had not caused haemolytic disease in childen of the 5 of the propositi who were mothers[61]. That anti-At[a] is not 'naturally occurring' was confirmed by the two At(a−) sibs of the propositi in whose serum no antibody could be found.

THE ANTIGEN Jr[a]

Unfortunately, little has been published so far about this important antigen which Stroup and MacIlroy[62] spoke of at San Francisco in 1970. At that stage, five examples of the antibody had been found and families of the Jr(a−) propositi had shown the phenotype to be inherited. Stroup and Gellerman (née MacIlroy) write that they have now tested 18 propositi (seven of whom are Japanese) and some of their relatives. No random white or Asiatic Jr(a−) person has yet been found (Table 73).

Jr(a−) appears to be a straightforward recessive condition for, at the latest count we know of[68, 69], among 51 sibs of propositi 10 were Jr(a−) and 41 Jr(a+). *Jr[a]* was shown to be independent of almost all the established blood group loci[68] (Table 74).

Anti-Jr[a] is not 'regularly occurring' in Jr(a−) people: it evidently can be stimulated by pregnancy but has not so far been the cause of haemolytic disease of the newborn[62]; anti-Jr[a] has caused a cross-matching problem before heart surgery on a male who had previously been transfused[63].

THE ANTIGEN Kn[a] (KNOPS-HELGESON)

Lack of this antigen is not quite such a rarity as lack of the other antigens in this chapter. Mrs Kn. who had made the 'new' antibody, presumably as the result of her previous transfusions, was in urgent need of blood. By extraordinarily happy fortune Miss M. Helgeson, working in the Minneapolis War Memorial Blood Bank, found her own blood to be compatible: so the donor problem was solved (Helgeson, Swanson and Polesky[64], 1970).

Investigation of the Helgeson family showed the antigen Kn^a to be inherited and to be independent of the loci for ABO, MNSs, Rh, Lutheran, Kidd and secretor and not to be X-linked, a splendid beginning.

Several other examples of anti-Kn^a were later found, as mentioned in the original paper.

In testing 2,091 unrelated donors 4 Kn(a−) were found, from which an estimate of the gene frequencies in Minneapolis is

$$Kn^a \ 0 \cdot 956 \text{ and } Kn \ 0 \cdot 044$$

Miss Helgeson's blood has generously been distributed to a number of laboratories and as a result complexities are beginning to appear: for example, Dr Tippett and Dr Contreras in our Unit find that several 'public' antisera fail to react with Helgesen's cells but also fail to react with some cell samples which are Kn(a+). In their hands these latter 'anti-Kn^a-like' sera, unlike true anti-Kn^a, are inactive against prepapainized Kn(a+) cells.

This behaviour made us wonder whether Kn^a should perhaps have been placed in Chapter 23, and the doubt was increased on reading in Mrs Swanson's unpublished thesis that she considers Helgeson type of antigens to be primarily of the leucocytes. No HL-A activity was found in our anti-Kn^a and 'anti-Kn^a-like' sera; nevertheless absorption with buffy coat cells removed both types of antibody.

OTHER VERY FREQUENT ANTIGENS

The antigen El

Anti-El, described by Frank, Schmidt and Baugh[57] in 1970 was found in a non-transfused Negress, Mrs El., during her seventh pregnancy: it reacted by the antiglobulin and by enzyme tests. No compatible donor was found amongst 3,000 unrelated people (Table 73). Like Mrs El., one of her three sisters was also El negative, showing that the antigen is inherited: it is a dominant character, for all of Mrs El.'s seven children were positive. The only other information to be gained from the family was that El is independent of the $secretor$ locus and is not X-borne (Table 74). The antibody has been referred to as anti-Eldridge: a second example has yet to be found.

The antigen Dp

The maker of anti-Dp, which again reacts by antiglobulin and by enzyme methods, is white and her parents are first cousins (Frank $et\ al.$[57]). Anti-D was also present but was removed by absorption with the cells of an Rh positive Dp negative brother of the propositus, leaving anti-Dp. No Dp negative was found among 600 unrelated donors. The groups of the family showed *Dp* to segregate independently of the loci for MNSs, Rh, Duffy and secretor and not to be X-borne. Two of Mrs Dp.'s sibs were Dp negative and four positive. This antibody is sometimes referred to as anti-Dupuy; a second example has yet to be found.

The antigen Gn^a (Gonsowski)

Fox and Taswell[65], 1969, found anti-Gn^a in the serum of a white blood donor, a non-transfused mother of six children: the antibody reacted best by the antiglobulin method and was separable from weak anti-D also present in the serum. No Gn(a−) samples were found among 2,600 random Rh negative donors (Table 73). The parents of the propositus are dead: their parents came from the same region in the Krackow province of Poland. Both living sibs of the propositus are Gn(a−), as is one of the 5 children of a dead brother. If, with this unusual distribution of Gn(a−) in the family, we allow Gn^a to be thought of as a dominant character, then *Gn^a* segregates independently of the loci for ABO, MNSs, P, Kell, Duffy and Kidd and it is not X-borne.

Strictly, the antigen Gn^a does not qualify for this chapter since it has not been excluded from identity with Kn^a. From its mode of reaction and its unusual inheritance we wonder whether we should perhaps have placed Gn^a in Chapter 23.

The antigen Jo^a (Joseph)

Anti-Jo^a, found in the serum of two Negroes, both previously transfused and one of them twice pregnant, is described by Jensen *et al.*[66] (1972). No compatible donor was found among 3,000 unselected donors, mostly white, or among 768 Negroes. Only one sib of the two propositi was available for testing and he is Jo(a+) so, as the authors point out, Jo^a is not yet proved to be inherited. Anti-Jo^a has been beautifully worked out and the only things that prevent Jo^a from being a fully paid up member of this chapter are the lack of proof of inheritance and the lack of exclusion of identity with El, another apparently negroid character. No doubt these hurdles will soon be surmounted.

SOME NOTES ABOUT 'PUBLIC' ANTIGENS

Unpublished antibodies

Most blood grouping laboratories have a long list of antibodies to 'public' antigens to which no label can be given other than the names of the owners. It seems that these lists are not much use until the independence of these antigens from those of this chapter, and those belonging to established systems, are worked out.

This is very hard work, as may be the demonstration that they are inherited characters. The ruling out of the T antigen[17, 16, 10] and the Tn antigen is now relatively simple (Chapter 24).

Serological independence of 'private' antigens

It should be remembered that a 'public' antigen may be antithetical to one of the 'private' antigens, so the cells of people lacking a 'public' antigen should be tested with all available antibodies to 'private' antigens. Such testing was brilliantly successful in the tying together of Sm and Bu[a] (Chapter 18) and in preventing what turned out to be, in all probability, anti-Wr[b] (Chapter 20) from appearing in this one.

The 'public' antigens of the present chapter were tested as well as they could be to exclude any relationship of this sort, but, of course, the extent of the cross-testing depends on cells and antisera being available.

The 'public' antigens may not be examples of a balanced polymorphism: they may represent Ford's frankly advantageous alleles which have swept through the populations so far studied. If they are advantageous there is no clue yet to the nature of the advantage: haemolytic disease of the newborn does not seem to be selecting against the negative alleles, at least not noticeably.

REFERENCES

1   SUSSMAN L.N. and MILLER E.B. (1952) Un nouvaeu facteur sanguin 'Vel'. *Rev. Hémat.*, 7, 368–371.
2   LEVINE P., ROBINSON ELIZABETH A., HERRINGTON L.B. and SUSSMAN L.N. (1955) Second example of the antibody for the high-incidence blood factor Vel. *Amer. J. clin. Path.*, 25, 751–754.
3   BRADISH ELIZABETH B. and SHIELDS WILMA F. (1959) Another example of anti-Vel. *Amer. J. clin. Path.*, 31, 104–106.
4   CORCORAN PATRICIA, ALLEN F.H., ALLISON A.C. and BLUMBERG B.S. (1959) Blood groups of Alaskan Eskimos and Indians. *Amer. J. phys. Anthrop.*, 17, 187–193.
5   CLEGHORN T.E. (1961) *The Occurrence of Certain Rare Blood Group Factors in Britain*, M.D. Thesis, University of Sheffield.
6   LEVINE P., WHITE JANE A. and STROUP MARJORY (1961) Seven Ve[a] (Vel) negative members in three generations of a family. *Transfusion, Philad.*, 1, 111–115.
7   WALKER MARY E. and sixteen others (1961) Tests with some rare blood-group antibodies. *Vox Sang.*, 6, 357.
8   ALBREY J.A., McCULLOCH W.J. and SIMMONS R.T. (1965) Inheritance of the Vel blood group in three families. *Med. J. Aust.*, 2, 662–665.
9   SUSSMAN L.N. (1962) Current status of the Vel blood group system. *Transfusion, Philad.*, 2, 163–171.
10 ROSENFIELD R.E., HABER GLADYS V., KISSMEYER-NIELSEN F., JACK J.A., SANGER RUTH and RACE R.R. (1960) Ge, a very common red-cell antigen. *Brit. J. Haemat.*, 6, 344–349.
11 HART MIA V.D., MOSE MEIKE, VEER M. V.D. and LOGHEM J.J. VAN (1961) Ho and Lan—two new blood group antigens. Paper read at VIIIth Europ. Cong. Haemat.
12 LOGHEM J.J. van and HART MIA V.D. (1958) Personal communication.

13   WHITE JANE A. and REINERT IRENE (1962) A family with five *VeVe* individuals. *Transfusion, Philad.*, **2**, 269–270.

14   STRICKEL PATTI, BROWN W.G. and JACK J.A. (1959) Two sisters lacking the blood group antigen Vel. *Program. Amer. Ass. Blood Banks*, *12th Ann. Meeting*, Chicago.

15   TATE HERMINE and SCHMIDT R. PAULINE (1959) Personal communication.

16   SANGER RUTH and RACE R.R. (1958) Evidence that the antigen T is independent of certain blood group antigens of very frequent occurrence. *Vox Sang.*, **3**, 379–380.

17   FRIEDENREICH V. (1930) *The Thomsen hemagglutination phenomenon*, Levin and Munksgaard, Copenhagen.

18   HINDMARSH CORINNE, JENNINGS E.R., TIPPETT PATRICIA and SANGER RUTH (1962) Anti-Ge: a report of two additional examples. *Program. Amer. Ass. Blood Banks*, *15th Ann. Meeting*, Memphis.

19   BARNES R. and LEWIS T.L.T. (1961) A rare antibody (anti-Ge) causing haemolytic disease of the newborn. *Lancet*, **ii**, 1285–1286.

20   WIENER A.S., GORDON EVE B. and UNGER L.J. (1961) Sensitization to the very high frequency blood factor Vel, with observations on the occurrence of the very rare vel-negative type among siblings. *Bull. Jew. Hosp.*, Brooklyn, **3**, 46–51.

21   ISSITT P.D., ØYEN RAGNHILD, REIHART JUDITH K., ADEBAHR MARGOT E., ALLEN F.H. and KUHNS W.J. (1968) Anti-Vel 2, a new antibody showing heterogeneity of Vel system antibodies. *Vox Sang.*, **15**, 125–132.

22   CEDERGREN B. (1972) Rare blood in Northern Sweden. Abstracts AABB and ISBT Congress, Washington, p. 11.

23   SWANSON JANE, ZWEBER MARY and POLESKY H.F. (1966) An antibody defining a new public antigenic determinant Gy^a (Gregory). *Transfusion, Philad.*, **6**, 525–526. (Abstract.)

24   APPELWHAITE F., GINSBERG V., GERENA J., CUNNINGHAM C.A. and GAVIN JUNE (1967) A very frequent red cell antigen, At^a. *Vox Sang.*, **13**, 444–445.

25   NUNN HILARY D., GILES CAROLYN M. and SEIDL S. (1967) Anti-Ge, as a transfusion problem. *Vox Sang.*, **13**, 23–26.

26   COOK A.L., ROSENFIELD R.E. and STROUP MARJORY (1961) Unpublished observations.

27   FISHER NATHALIE (1963) Unpublished observations.

28   KONUGRES ANGELYN and CLEGHORN T.E. (1963) Unpublished observations.

29   MARNETTE BETTY LOU (1964) Unpublished observations.

30   SWANSON JANE, ZWEBER MARY and POLESKY H.F. (1967) A new public antigenic determinant Gy^a (Gregory). *Transfusion, Philad.*, **7**, 304–306.

31   FERMEPIN G.H., PEREZ-PRADO A., DE PIPPIG TERESA F., BRITO J. and DE AVENA CLARA S. (1968) Anti-Ge in a transfused male. *Vox Sang.*, **14**, 228–229.

32   BATTAGLINI P.F., RANQUE J., BRIDONNEAU C., SALMON C. and NICOLI R.M. (1965) Etude du facteur Vel dans la population marseillaise à propos d'un cas d'immunisation anti-Vel. *Proc. 10th Congr. int. Soc. Blood Transf.*, Stockholm 1964, 309–311.

33   NEVANLINNA H. (1966) Personal communication.

34   KORNSTAD L. (1970) Unpublished observations.

35   SWANSON JANE (1967) Unpublished observations.

36   SCHMIDT R. PAULINE, FRANK SALLY and BAUGH MARIE (1967) New antibodies to high incidence antigenic determinants (anti-So, anti-El, anti-Hy and anti-Dp). *Transfusion, Philad.*, **7**, 386. (Abstract.)

37   FENTON ELIZABETH and MOORE B.P.L. (1967) Personal communication.

38   LEISEN GRETCHEN (1970) Personal communication.

39   CEDERGREN B. and GILES CAROLYN (1974) Personal communication.

40   TOIVANEN P. and HIRVONEN T. (1969) Fetal development of red cell antigens K, k, Lu^a, Lu^b, Fy^a, Fy^b, Vel and Xg^a. *Scand. J. Haemat.*, **6**, 49–55.

41   DRACHMANN O. and LUNDSGAARD ANNE (1970) Prenatal assessment of blood group antibodies against 'public' antigens. An example of anti-Ve (Vel) in pregnancy. *Scand. J. Haemat.*, **7**, 37–42.

42 SZALOKY AGNES and VAN DER HART MIA (1971) An auto-antibody anti-Vel. *Vox Sang.*, **20**, 376–377.
43 SUSSMAN L.N. and PRETSHOLD HANNAH (1972) The Vel blood group system. *Haematologia*, **6**, 129–133.
44 BOOTH P.B., ALBREY J.A., WHITTAKER JOAN and SANGER RUTH (1970) Gerbich blood group system: a useful genetic marker in certain Melanesians of Papua and New Guinea. *Nature*, **228**, 462.
45 MCLOUGHLIN K. and ROGERS JAN (1970) Anti-Ge[a] in an untransfused New Zealand male. *Vox Sang.*, **19**, 94–96.
46 MULLER A., ANDRÉ-LIARDET J., GARRETTA M., BROCTEUR J. and MOULLEC J. (1973) Observations sur un anticorps rare: l'anti-Gerbich. *Rev. fr. Transf.*, **16**, 251–257.
47 BOOTH P.B. and MCLOUGHLIN K. (1972) The Gerbich blood group system, especially in Melanesians. *Vox Sang.*, **22**, 73–84.
48 PEDDLE L.J., JOSEPHSON J.E. and LAWTON A. (1970) Auto-donation in the management of placenta previa and erythroblastosis in a pregnancy complicated by Gerbich isoimmunization. *Vox Sang.*, **18**, 547–550.
49 BROCTEUR J. (1973) Unpublished observations.
50 MACGREGOR A. and BOOTH P.B. (1973) A second example of anti-Ge1 and some observations on Gerbich subgroups. *Vox Sang.*, **25**, 474–478.
51 BOOTH P.B. and HORNABROOK R.W. (1973) The inheritance of the Gerbich blood groups: an analysis of New Guinean families. *Hum. Biol. Oceania*, **2**, 72–78.
52 BOOTH P.B., WARK LYNETTE, MCLOUGHLIN K. and SPARK R. (1972) The Gerbich blood group system in New Guinea. I. The Sepik district. *Hum. Biol. Oceania*, **1**, 215–222.
53 BOOTH P.B., MCLOUGHLIN K., HORNABROOK R.W., MACGREGOR A. and MALCOLM L.A. (1972) The Gerbich blood group system in New Guinea. II. The Morobe district and north Papuan coast. *Hum. Biol. Oceania*, **1**, 259–266.
54 BOOTH P.B., MCLOUGHLIN K., HORNABROOK R.W. and MACGREGOR A. (1972) The Gerbich blood group system in New Guinea. III. The Madang district, the highlands, the New Guinea islands and the south Papuan coast. *Hum. Biol. Oceania*, **1**, 267–272.
55 GRINDON A.J., MCGINNISS MARY H., ISSITT P.D., REIHART JUDITH K. and ALLEN F.H. (1968) A second example of anti-Lan. *Vox Sang.*, **15**, 293–296.
56 SMITH D.S., STRATTON F., JOHNSON T., BROWN R., HOWELL P. and RICHES R. (1969) Haemolytic disease of the newborn caused by anti-Lan antibody. *Brit. Med. J.*, **3**, 90–92.
57 FRANK S., SCHMIDT R.P. and BAUGH M. (1970) Three new antibodies to high-incidence antigenic determinants (anti-El, anti-Dp and anti-So). *Transfusion, Philad.*, **10**, 254–257.
58 CLANCEY M., BONDS S. and VAN EYS J. (1972) A new example of anti-Lan and two families with Lan-negative members. *Transfusion, Philad.*, **12**, 106–108.
59 MASSAQUOI J.M. and CORNWALL SHEILA (1973) The Gregory blood group. AABB Abstracts, *Transfusion, Philad.*, **13**, 362–363.
60 MOULDS J.J., ELLISOR SANDRA S., REID MARION E. and HARRISON MARLENE (1973) Association of Holley-Gregory blood group systems. AABB Abstracts, *Transfusion, Philad.*, **13**, 363.
61 GELLERMAN M.M., MCCREARY J., YEDINAK E. and STROUP M. (1973) Six additional examples of anti-At[a]. *Transfusion, Philad.*, **13**, 225–230.
62 STROUP MARJORY and MACILROY MIJA (1970) Jr, five examples of an antibody defining an antigen of high frequency in the Caucasian population. Program 23rd Ann. Meet. AABB, San Francisco, p. 86.
63 VERSKA J.J. and LARSON N.L. (1973) Autologous transfusion in cardiac surgery: a case report of a patient with a rare antibody. *Transfusion, Philad.*, **13**, 219–220.
64 HELGESON M., SWANSON J. and POLESKY H.F. (1970) Knops-Helgeson (Kn[a]), a high-frequency erythrocyte antigen. *Transfusion, Philad.*, **10**, 137–138.
65 FOX J.A. and TASWELL H.F. (1969) Anti-Gn[a], a new antibody reacting with a high-incidence erythrocytic antigen, *Transfusion, Philad.*, **9**, 265–269.

15

[66] JENSEN L., SCOTT E.P., MARSH W.L., MACILROY M., ROSENFIELD R.E., BRANCATO P. and FAY A.F. (1972) Anti-Jo^a: an antibody defining a high-frequency erythrocyte antigen. *Transfusion, Philad.*, **12**, 322–324.

[67] COLPITTS PEARL, CORNWALL SHEILA and MOORE B.P.L. (1974) Unpublished observations.

[68] GELLERMAN MIJA and STROUP MARJORY (1974) Personal communication.

[69] STAVELEY J.M. (1974) Personal communication.

Chapter 20
Some Very Infrequent Antigens

Being so rare, the antigens of this chapter can seldom be useful as genetic markers; but their very existence raises grand if unanswered evolutionary questions.

Since there is no difficulty in finding donors for patients with antibodies to 'private' antigens there is no need to identify the antibody, as there so urgently is to identify antibodies to 'public' antigens. It is all the more praiseworthy that the antibodies to 'private' antigens have been, with much labour, polished to their present state, reflecting the high spirit of scientific curiosity present in transfusion laboratories.

Occasionally an antigen in this private category is found to be a member of one of the established systems and it may then enlarge the understanding of that system as a whole; such an antigen on its elevation to the establishment may still be thought of as 'private' but does not qualify for this chapter. (We prefer the term 'private' to the perhaps more correct circumlocutions 'very infrequent' or 'of low incidence'.) Several antigens of our last edition have been thus elevated: Be^a, Go^a and Evans to Rh and Stobo to Bg.

With the help of Dr Cleghorn we made rules for admission to the list of 'private' antigens given in Tables 75 and 76. Such antigens:
i   Must be shown to be dominant characters.
ii   Must not be known to be controlled by 'established' blood group loci: infrequent antigens known to be part of other systems are dealt with in the appropriate chapters.
iii   Must have an incidence of less than 1 in 400 in populations so far sampled.
iv   Must be defined by a specific antibody.
v   Must be shown, by serological means, not to duplicate others already on the list. (It is almost impossible to show genetical independence.)
vi   Must still be extant: this is satisfied if a donor with the antigen is available or if some of the antiserum still exists, at least *in vitro*.

The investigation of an antibody which reacts only with rare samples of red cells is laborious. Two approaches are involved: the testing of the cells which disclosed the presence of antibody, usually those of a donor or a husband, with a battery of antisera to antigens known to be rare, and the testing of the serum containing the antibody with a range of cells known to carry rare antigens. By one or the other way the following have to be excluded:

Table 75. 'Private' or 'very infrequent' antigens

The antigens of this table have been shown to be inherited as dominant characters and to be serologically distinct from each other and from known antigens of the established systems: all have an incidence of less than 1 in 400, at any rate in white people. The information is from the original papers or from our records or, more often, from those of Dr Cleghorn

Name of antigen	Investigators	Unrelated people tested			Notes about the antibody
		Population	Total	Positive	
An^a (Ahonen)	Furuhjelm, Nevanlinna, Gavin and Sanger[63], 1972	Finnish	10,000	6	Caused cross-matching difficulty: IgG. Further examples found in about 1 in 1,000 normal people: no evidence of stimulation by transfusion or pregnancy.[63]
		Swedish	3,266	2	
Bi (Biles)	Wadlington, Moore and Hartmann[37], 1961	Americans	1,110	0	Stimulated by pregnancy[37].
		American Whites	179	0	
		American Negroes	140	0	
		Cherokee Indians	181	0	
Bp^a (Bishop)	Cleghorn[31], 1964; Ørjasaeter et al.[51], 1966; Kornstad[84], 1974	English	75,000	1	Found in random tests[31] with serum Gu. (see anti-Sw^a below) and in 2 other a.h.a. sera. 2 examples found in 2,796 normal sera[31].
		Tibetans	42	0	
		Norwegians	7,000	0	
Bx^a (Box)	Jenkins and Marsh[43], 1961; Cleghorn[31], 1967	English	3,000	1	Found during tests on a 'stored cell' antibody in an a.h.a. patient, separable. No further example in more than 8,000 normal sera[31].
		English	4,445	0	
By (Batty)	Simmons and Were[19], 1955	Australian Whites	500	0	Caused mild h.d.n.[19]. 8 examples found since: 5 in patients with acquired haemolytic anaemia (a.h.a.) and 1 in patient with carcinoma of colon (all 6 also had anti-Wr^a and most had anti-Sw^a as well as other antibodies[31]), 1 in pregnant woman[26] 1 in papain tests on 7,987 normal sera[31]. None in saline tests on 2,000 normal sera[31].
		Aborigines	24	0	
	Chown et al.[10], 1959	Eskimo, Copper	299	0	
	Cleghorn[14], 1960	English	31,522	2	
	Cleghorn[15], 1961	Negroes	157	0	
	Walker et al[35], 1961	Bostonians	78	0	
Chr^a	Kissmeyer-Nielsen[20], 1955, et al.[70], 1973	Danish	500	1	Found in routine screening, 'naturally occurring': second example found 20 years later[70].

Table 75—*continued*

Name of antigen	Investigators	Unrelated people tested			Notes about the antibody
		Population	Total	Positive	
Good	Frumin, Porter and Eichman[22], 1960	Pennsylvanians	308	0	Found in pregnant negro woman[22], caused severe h.d.n., studied up till 12th pregnancy[30,32];
	Cahan, cited in[22]	New Yorkers	1,395	0	8 examples found in 2,718 normal sera[30].
	Molthan and Eichman[30], 1967	Pennsylvanians	2,382	0	
	Cleghorn[31], 1962	English	397	0	
Gf (Griffiths)	Cleghorn, Grant and Pickles[31], 1966	English	6,886	0	Found in a.h.a. serum. 2 further examples in 2,000 normal sera[31].
Heibel	Ballowitz et al.[50], 1968	Germans	>500	0	Caused h.d.n.
Hey	Yvart, Gerbal and Salmon[64], 1974	French	8,127	2	Found during routine screening. 3 other examples found in patients, but none in 3,061 donors[64].
Hov	Szaloky, Sijpesteijn and v.d. Hart[65], 1973	Dutch	1,155	2	Found with anti-Fy^a in a mother[65].
Ht^a (Hunt)	Jahn and Cleghorn[31], 1962	English	453	0	Caused h.d.n.
Je^a (Jensen)	Skov[66], 1972	Danish	>1,000	0	Found in ABO serum check. IgM. One more found in >100,000 sera.
Jn^a	Kornstad et al.[48], 1967	Norwegian	4,767	0	Found in an anti-Wr^a serum; 2 further examples found. All 3 sera contained other 'private' antibodies[48].
	Ørjasaeter et al.[51], 1966	Norwegian	1,906	0	
		Tibetans	42	0	
	Kornstad[84], 1974	Norwegian	7,000	0	
Levay	Callender and Race[1], 1946	English	350	0	Stimulated by transfusion[1]; now mainly incomplete, still reacted well after 23 years; stock insufficient for large scale tests (because for many years this serum was the only source of anti-C^w and anti-Lu^a); no example found in 5,774 normal sera[31].
	Sanger and Race[39], 1958	English	124	0	
		Venezuelan Negro-Indians	10	0	
	Cleghorn[31], 1963	English	676	0	

Table 75—*continued*

Name of antigen	Investigators	Unrelated people tested			Notes about the antibody
		Population	Total	Positive	
Ls^a (Lewis II)	Cleghorn and Dunsford[31], 1963	English	5,887	0	Found in an anti-B serum; no other example in 2,557 normal sera[31].
		Finnish	60	1	
		Other Europeans	226	0	
		Negroes, U.S.A.	110	1	
		Negroes, West Indies	878	9	
		Negroes, West Africa	81	2	
Mo^a (Moen)	Kornstad and Brocteur[67], 1972	Norwegians	9,000	0	Found in an anti-Jn^a serum. Another example found in 5,010 Oslo donors and five in 'multiple antibody sera'.
		Belgians	9,793	2	
Or (Orriss)	Cleghorn, Jenkins and Koster[31], 1964	English	887	0	Found in a.h.a. serum. No example in 1,405 normal sera[31].
		Negroes, U.S.A.	163	1	
Pt^a (Peters)	Pinder, Staveley, Douglas and Kornstad[68], 1969	New Zealanders	14,500	0	Found in an anti-Vw+anti-Wr^a serum. 6 further examples found in 460 random antenatal sera, all with other naturally occurring antibodies. 10 found in sera known to contain anti-Wr^a or anti-Vw.
		Norwegians	14,674	0	
		Tibetans	43	0	
		Chinese	83	0	
	Kornstad[84], 1974	Norwegians	7,000	0	
Rd (Radin)	Rausen et al.[42], 1967	N.Y. Jewish	562	3	5 examples[42], all caused h.d.n., 4 found in Whites, 1 in a Negro; all 5 react best by antiglobulin method. No example found in 2,443 random sera[42].
		Assorted people	6,773	0	
Re^a (Reid)	Lundsgaard and Jensen[78], 1968 Lewis[82], 1973	Danes	4,933	24	2 Danish examples, one caused by transfusion the other 'naturally occurring'; no anti-Rd in 30,000 donors[78].
		Canadians	634	3	
		Ukranians	170	1	
	Guévin, Taliano, Fiset, Bérubé and Kaita[69], 1971	Canadians	>10,000	0	Caused slight h.d.n. IgG

Table 75—*continued*

Name of antigen	Investigators	Unrelated people tested			Notes about the antibody
		Population	Total	Positive	
Rlᵃ (Rosenlund)	Kornstad[84], 1974	Norwegians	4,400	7	Found in two sera with antibodies to other private antigens.
Swᵃ (Swann)	Cleghorn[21, 14, 15]1959, 1960, 1961	English	31,522	5*	Found in cross-matching test[21, 25]; serum from the a.h.a. patient, Gu, contained other, separable, 'private' antibodies[14, 24]. Not uncommon in pathological sera[15, 21], usually accompanied by anti-Wrᵃ, -Byᵃ, -Cˣ, -Miᵃ, -Mᵍ.
	Cleghorn[31], 1963	Negroes	157	0	
		English	23,888	4	
Toᵃ (Torkildsen)	Kornstad *et al.*[49], 1968	Norwegian	6,461	1	Found in an anti-Stᵃ serum, then detected in 66 of 5,704 normal sera[49] (1·2%) IgM anti-Toᵃ found in 16% of 300 random donors[77].
Trᵃ (Traversu)	Cleghorn[24], 1962	English	38,069	2	Found in random tests[24] with the serum Gu. (see anti-Swᵃ above); present[24], and separable, in 12 of 18 anti-Wrᵃ sera and in 1 of 700 random sera, again with anti-Wrᵃ.
	Kornstad[84], 1974	Norwegians	9,500	0	
Wb (Webb)	Simmons and Albrey[38], 1963	Australian Whites	3,550	2	Found in an ABO grouping serum[38]; no further example in 2,000 Australian[38], but 3 in 2,400 English[31], normal sera.
		Australian Aborigines	92	0	
		New Guinea Natives	105	0	
	Cleghorn[31], 1963	English (adults)	15,815	3	
		English (cords)	395	0	
	Ikemoto *et al.*[40], 1964	Japanese	513	0	
	Nakajima *et al.*[41], 1965	Japanese	2,957	0	
	Ørjasaeter *et al.*[51], 1966	Tibetans	42	0	

Table 75—*continued*

Name of antigen	Investigators	Unrelated people tested			Notes about the antibody
		Population	Total	Positive	
Wr[a] (Wright)	Holman[5], 1953	English	1,004	0	First[5] and second[6] examples caused h.d.n.; has caused severe transfusion reaction[9,27]; commonly found in sera containing immune antibodies (for refs. see Kornstad[13]). Cleghorn[15] found 11 examples in serum of 2,316 normal donors (saline tests); 12 in the serum of 173 women with Rh antibodies; 6 in the serum of 16 a.h.a. patients; 11 in 117 other pathological sera. McGuire and Funkhouser[57], using anti-globulin, albumin and enzyme tests, found 77 examples of anti-Wr[a] in 1,000 random donors.
	Wiener and Brancato[6], 1953	U.S.A. Whites	48	0	
	Dunsford[7], 1954	English	273	1	
	Wallace and Milne[8], 1958	Scots	1,000	1	
	Chown and Lewis[10], 1959	Eskimo, Copper	299	1	
	Corcoran et al.[11], 1959	Eskimo, Alaskan	241	0	
		Alaskan Indians	255	0	
	Juel[12], 1959	Norwegian	5,138	0	
	Kornstad[13], 1961	Norwegian	3,140	2	
		Lapps	433	0	
	Cleghorn[14], 1960	English	31,522	24	
	Cleghorn[15], 1961	English	14,109	12	
		Negroes	157	0	
	Walker et al.[35], 1961	Bostonians	2,784	3	
	Metaxas et al.[27], 1963	Swiss	3,753	2	
	Kout[28], 1962	Czechoslovakians	1,500	1	
	Ørjasaeter et al.[51], 1966	Tibetans	42	0	
	McGuire and Funkhouser[57], 1967	Ohio donors	7,000	0	
	Glasgow et al.[74], 1968	Bhutanese	30	0	
	Harvey et al.[75], 1969	Caribs, Dominica	c. 100	0	
	Liotta et al.[76], 1970	Italians	6,350	7	
Wu (Wulfsberg)	Heistö[44], 1966	Norwegian	652	0	Found in routine screening for antibodies when Wu's cells happened to be used. 3 further examples found in serum of 8,406 patients[44] and 1 in 1,228 Oslo donors[58], but 10 of 700 Swedish donors[85]. Occasional cause of cross-matching problem[86,87], once when cells were from a Negro[85].
	Kornstad and Wolthuis,[58] 1967	Norwegian	1,511	0	
	Kornstad[84], 1974	Norwegian	7,000	1	

Most of the antibodies in this table have been found not to react with cells lacking common antigens (Fy(a−b−), Jk(a−b−), K_o, Ge− etc. etc.) thus showing they are not detecting theoretically possible antigens resulting from the alleles replacing the familiar ones.

* Two of these were found to be related to each other.

Table 76. Separate segregation of the genes responsible for certain rare antigens and those for established polymorphic systems

Antigen	Reference	ABO	MNSs	P	Rh	Lu	K	Fy	Jk	Yt	Do	Sec	Le	X	Y
An^a (Ahonen) 15*	Furuhjelm et al.[63], 1972	×	×	×	×	×	×	×	×	×	×	×*		×	×
By (Batty)	Simmons and Were[19], 1955	×				×	×	×				×*		×	×
Bi (Biles)	Cleghorn[15], 1961				×									×	×
	Wadlington et al.[37], 1961				×										×
Bp^a (Bishop)	Cleghorn[31], 1964	×	×	×	×			×	×					×	×
Bx^a (Box)	Jenkins et al.[43], 1961														×
Chr^a	Jørgensen et al.[70], 1973		×											×	×
Good	Molthan et al.[30], 1966				×									×	×
Gf (Griffiths)	Cleghorn et al.[31], 1966		×		×						×			×	×
Heibel	Ballowitz et al.[50], 1968		×											×	×
Hey	Yvart et al.[64], 1974		×												×
Hov	Szaloky et al.[65], 1973		×	×	×			×	×			×*		×	×
Ht^a (Hunt)	Jahn and Cleghorn[31], 1962		×		×									×	×
Je^a (Jensen)	Skov[66], 1972	×	×	×	×	×		×	×			×*			×
Jn^a	Kornstad et al.[48], 1967		×	×	×		×	×	×					×	×
Levay	Callender and Race[1], 1946		×	×	×									×	×
Ls^a (Lewis II)	Cleghorn and Dunsford[31], 1963	×	×		×	×			×					×	×
Mo^a (Moen)	Kornstad and Brocteur[67], 1972	×	×		×			×	×			×		×	×
Or (Orriss)	Cleghorn et al[31], 1964	×			×							×		×	×
Pt^a (Peters)	Pinder et al.[68], 1969		×												×

Table 76—continued

	ABO	MNSs	P	Rh	Lu	K	Fy	Jk	Yt	Do	Sec	Le	X	Y
Rd (Radin) Rausen et al.[42], 1967	×	×	×	×	×†	×	×	×					×	×
Lundsgaard et al.[78], 1968; Lewis et al.[81], 1973		×	×	×		×	×	×			×*		×	×
Re^a (Reid) Guévin et al.[69], 1971		×	×	×	×	×	×	×	×				×	×
Rl^a (Rosenlund) Kornstad[84], 1974	×	×	×	×		×	×						×	×
Sw^a (Swann) Cleghorn[25,31], 1960, 1967	×	×	×	×	×	×	×	×			×		×	×
To^a (Torkildsen) Kornstad et al.[49], 1968	×	×	×	×			×				×*		×	×
Crossland et al.[88], 1974	×	×		×			×				×*		×	×
Tr^a (Traversu) Cleghorn[24], 1962	×	×	×	×			×	×			×			×
Wb (Webb) Simmons and Albrey[38], 1963	×	×	×	×	×		×						×	×
Cleghorn[31], 1963	×	×	×	×		×	×	×					×	×
Wr^a (Wright) Holman[5], 1953	×	×	×	×			×	×					×	×
Kornstad[13], 1961	×	×	×	×	×	×	×	×					×	×
Cleghorn[15,24], 1961	×	×	×	×	×	×	×	×			×	×	×	×
Allen[33], 1961		×			×		×							×
Stout et al.[34], 1961	×	×	×	×	×		×							×
Metaxas et al.[27], 1963		×		×			×				×*		×	×
Lewis et al.[72], 1973		×		×						×			×	×
Wu (Wulfsberg) Heistö[44], 1966														
Kornstad[84], 1974		×												
Howell and Giles[87], 1974				×	×									
Jørgensen[86], 1974	×							×					×	×

Crosses represent separate segregation in one or more families. Most of the independence counts have been made by us from the original data.

* Based on Lewis phenotypes of red cells: saliva not tested.

† With a 4% possibility of error introduced by a missing parent.

There is no information yet about the genetical relationship of any of these antigens to the Diego, Auberger, Colton, Sid (Wr^a excepted) or Scianna systems.

a   Rare antigens belonging to established systems, for example A_x, the many MNSs 'satellite' antigens, P^k, the rare Rh antigens such as E^w, C^x, Be^a, Go^a and Evans, and antigens which are rare in Whites such as Js^a and Di^a. Cells with a very strong P_1 antigen may, by reacting with a weak and otherwise undetectable anti-P_1, simulate a private antigen-antibody system.

b   The private antigens of Table 75 and, if possible, also those listed below which do not qualify for Table 75. A private antigen may in the long run be seen to represent the allele of a public antigen, a brilliant example was the recognition that Bu^a and Sm were thus related: they became the Scianna groups (page 406).

We hope that Tables 75 and 76 will explain themselves. A very great many of the distinctions there recorded are from the work of Dr Cleghorn and Miss June Gavin.

Concerning some of the antigens of Tables 75 and 76

Wr^a (Wright)

It will be seen from Tables 75 and 76 that Holman's Wr^a antigen[5] is virtually established as an independent system and the only reason why we have not given it a chapter of its own is that its 'usefulness' (page 507) is so low. Progress towards independence was much forwarded by Cleghorn[14, 15, 24] who tested over 45 thousand London donors, and the families of 30 of the Wr(a+) propositi thereby found. All families supported the original view that Wr^a is a dominant character, notable amongst them is the extremely rare one[15, 24] in which both father and mother are Wr(a+) and a child is Wr(a−); the parents are not consanguineous.

In 1971, Adams, Broviac, Brooks, Johnson and Issitt[71] described an antibody found in the serum of a white woman who had been once pregnant but never transfused: it reacted with the cells of all of 2,114 random donors. The propositus was Wr(a+) as were her child and 3 of her 5 sibs: her parents who were dead were not known to have been consanguineous. The red cells of the propositus reacted more strongly with anti-Wr^a sera than did those of her Wr(a+) relatives or those of unrelated Wr(a+) people. The case for the antibody being anti-Wr^b thus seems very strong, but Adams and her colleagues showed modest caution in claiming it to be so.

A Canadian family in which Wr^a and the very strong Sd^a antigens are segregating is described by Lewis et al.[72], 1973 (see page 398). The lod scores are suggestive, but not significantly so, of either close linkage of the two loci or of the two antigens being controlled from one complex locus, but chance has yet to be ruled out as the cause of the apparent association.

From the genetical point of view, if not from the medical, it is a pity that Wr^a is not a more frequent antigen: anti-Wr^a is a fairly common antibody and a very good case has been made for the existence of anti-Wr^b.

Swᵃ (Swann)

This antigen also has been so well investigated (Cleghorn, 1959 onwards[21, 14, 15, 31]) that it looks like an independent system. However, in 1960 Cleghorn[25] found a strong hint that the loci for Swᵃ and for secretor might be linked. In view of the known linkage between *secretor* and *Lutheran* he pointed out that the linkage relation of *Swᵃ* to *Lutheran* needed particular attention.

Twelve years later Metaxas-Bühler, Metaxas and Giles[73] found a family in which *Swᵃ* and *Luᵃ* and *Se* were segregating with no recombination in four generations. The lod scores provided by this family were suggestive, but not significant of linkage between *Sw* and *Lu* and thus in support of Cleghorn's hint that *Sw* might belong to the *Lutheran* locus.

But all was called in question again when Metaxas and his collaborators (personal communication, 1973) found another family in which *Swᵃ* and *Luᵃ* were segregating, but this time with evidence strongly against linkage, 4 non-recombinants and 3 recombinants, or *vice-versa*: so we think we must leave Swann in this chapter, and change the subject.

Other antigens heading for systemic status

Table 76 shows the following to be hopefuls: Anᵃ (Ahonen), Rd (Radin), Trᵃ (Traversu) and Wb (Webb), but only Rd and Wb have been shown to be free of the grasping Kell system.

Notes on 'private' antigens which do not qualify for Tables 75 and 76

Beᵃ (Berrens) (Davidsohn, Stern, Strauser and Spurrier[16, 17], 1953)

Antibody stimulated by transfusion of husband's blood and caused h.d.n. Antibody successfully stimulated in volunteers[17]. Since 1953 many thousand people tested with anti-Beᵃ but no further Be(a+) propositus found[10, 11, 35, 36, 29] until 1973 when two more brought to light by h.d.n. (McCreary *et al.*[79], and Ducos *et al.*[80]): the family of the last propositus[80] showed Beᵃ to be part of Rh (see page 204).

Stobo (Wallace and Milne[46], 1959)

Antigen not present in parents of propositus, nor shown to be inherited in two other families[46]; inherited as a dominant in three generations in family tested by Dunsford[47]. Antigen present in two out of 3,000 Scottish people[46]; distinguished from most of the antigens in Table 75. Antibody first found in an anti-E serum, later in 20 out of 1,078 'non-immune' and 15 out of 469 'immune' sera. Antigen now known to be part of the Bg complex (see page 475).

Goᵃ (*Gonzalez*) (Alter, Gelb and Lee[54], 1962)

Antigen a negro character with frequency approaching 2%, but no Go(a+) found in testing many thousand Whites[55]. In 1967 Goᵃ shown to belong to the Rh system (Lewis *et al.*[56], Lovett and Crawford[60]). Dr Tippett finds Goᵃ one aspect of Category IV type of unusual D (page 194).

Evans (W. Weiner[52], 1966)

A dominant character; caused h.d.n. Outside the family of the propositus one positive found in 480 random British. The antigen was assumed to belong to Rh when Wrobel and Gavin (unpublished observations, 1968, see page 210) found that all 4 Evans positive members of the original family have an Rh complex like, but not identical to, $-D-$, whereas all 3 Evans negative blood relatives do not (P = 1 in about 35).

Jobbins (Gilbey[2], 1947)

A dominant character; 120 random people tested, all negative; antibody no longer active[31]; cells of propositus negative[31] for all those antigens of Table 75 known before 1968.

Becker (Elbel and Prokop[3], 1951)

A dominant character; caused h.d.n.; no positive found in 122 random people; distinguished only from By of Table 75.

Ven (van Loghem and v. d. Hart[4], 1952)

A dominant character; caused h.d.n.; no positive found in tests on 170 random people; distinguished only from Wrᵃ.

Rm (v.d. Hart, Bosman and van Loghem[18], 1954)

A dominant character; caused h.d.n.; no positive found in 200 random people; distinguished from Levay, Wrᵃ, Beᵃ and By. We understand that the family is now out of touch.

Kamhuber (Speiser *et al.*[59, 45], 1965–66)

Inherited, but not shown to be a dominant character. The antibody was the result of a patient receiving blood for the second time from the same donor, Herr Kamhuber, after an interval of 11 years. No positive found in 1,100 random Viennese; distinguished[45, 31] from all the antigens in Table 75 before 1968.

Skjelbred (Kornstad, Øyen and Cleghorn[49], 1968)

Many examples of antibody found in normal sera. Antigen not present in 4 sibs or 2 children of propositus. No further Skjelbred positive found among 12,753 Norwegians, 42 Tibetans or 58 Chinese.

Ts (*Tsunoi*) (Nakajima, Kuniyuki and Takahara[61], 1967)

Antibody found in serum of a.h.a. patient. Antigen not strictly private being present in 2 of 150 Japanese tested. Dominant character segregating independently of Kidd; not X- or Y-borne. Anti-Ts not found in early 2,000 sera from normal people.

Zd (Švanda, Procházka, Kout and Giles[62], 1970)

Antibody caused h.d.n. Zd not found in 270 random Czechoslovakians. A dominant character, probably independent of Lewis and not X- or Y-borne. The 3 generation family strongly suggests *Zd* is part of the Rh complex, in this family travelling with *cde*.

Unpublished antigens

Most specialist laboratories have a list of private antigens known by, so far, parochial names. Sometimes the lack of evidence of inheritance has been the reason for their not being published. The length of these lists at least adds to the wonder at the infinite hospitality of the red cell surface.

Anthropological differences

Nothing so dramatic as the immense difference in distribution of the public antigen Gerbich between New Guinea and the rest of the tested world has turned up in the distribution of the private antigens. However, we hope that remote populations will continue to be tested for the private antigens. The search should surely be rewarded: Js^a for example would masquerade as a private antigen in Whites but is nevertheless a useful marker in Negroes.

It may be possible to interpret the existence of these very infrequent antigens in terms of natural selection. Perhaps they are not examples of a balanced polymorphism but of Ford's frankly harmful alleles which are being reduced towards that level at which they can be maintained only by recurrent mutation. Haemolytic disease of the newborn must, at any rate in the past, have operated strongly against some of them.

Some parallels are perhaps to be found in the isozymes where Harris, Hopkinson and Robson[83] (1974) find evidence that rare alleles are as frequent in the polymorphic as in the 'monomorphic' systems. If this applied also to blood groups we could expect antigens of private frequencies to occur as often in polymorphic systems like ABO and MNSs as in 'monomorphic' systems like Swann or Radin. But this may not apply because the electrophoretic variants are thought by some to be selectively neutral whereas rare antigens are known to be the occasional cause of haemolytic disease of the newborn.

The relatively very high frequency of the antibodies to these very rare antigens is a mystery. Cleghorn[15] commenting on his finding of anti-Sw^a, anti-By, anti-Wr^a, anti-C^x, anti-Mi^a and anti-M^g all together in a number of sera from patients suffering from acquired haemolytic anaemia says:

'The finding of this particular combination of antibodies in these sera is strange. Anti-Wr^a, -Vw and -M^g are all to be found quite frequently in the serum of normal persons; anti-Sw^a and anti-Mi^a usually only when some other antibody stimulant is at work, in the author's experience. It is possible that all are present in most human sera in undetectable strength, and that the hyperactivity of the reticulo-endothelial system associated with acquired haemolytic anaemia supplies some "non-specific" boost.'

It is probably right to suppose that each of this seemingly endless procession of 'private' antigens stakes its site on the red cell, a site which is usually occupied by an antithetical antigen yet to be recognized. Already exhausted in believing that the established systems are each represented by an average of perhaps 10,000 antigen sites on every red cell, we now have to picture no fewer sites devoted to each of these 'private' antigens. When one is not equipped to think in molecular terms such over-crowding crushes the imagination.

REFERENCES

1 CALLENDER SHEILA T. and RACE R.R. (1946) A serological and genetical study of multiple antibodies formed in response to blood transfusion by a patient with lupus erythematosus diffusus. *Ann. Eugen., Lond.*, **13**, 102–117, and see ref. 23.
2 GILBEY B.E. (1947) A new blood group antigen, 'Jobbins'. *Nature, Lond.*, **160**, 362.
3 ELBEL H. and PROKOP O. (1951) Ein neues erbliches Antigens als Ursache gehaufter Fehlgeburten. *Zeitschr. f. Hygiene*, **132**, 120–130.
4 LOGHEM J.J. VAN and HART MIA V.D. (1952) Een zeldzaam voorkomende bloedgroep (Ven.). *Bull. cen. Lab. Bloedtransf Dienst ned. Rode Kruis*, **2**, 225–229.
5 HOLMAN C.A. (1953) A new rare human blood-group antigen (Wr^a). *Lancet*, **ii**, 119.
6 WIENER A.S. and BRANCATO G.J. (1953) Severe erythroblastosis fetalis caused by sensitization to a rare human agglutinogen. *Amer. J. hum. Genet.*, **5**, 350–355.
7 DUNSFORD I. (1954) The WRIGHT blood group system. *Vox Sang.* (O.S.), **4**, 160–163.
8 WALLACE J. and MILNE G.R. (1956) Personal communication.
9 LOGHEM J.J. VAN, HART MIA V.D., BOK J. and BRINKERINK P.C. (1955) Two further examples of the antibody anti-Wr^a. *Vox Sang.* (O.S.), **5**, 130–134.
10 CHOWN B. and LEWIS MARION (1959) The blood group genes of the Copper Eskimos. *Amer. J. phys. Anthrop.*, **17**, 13–18.
11 CORCORAN PATRICIA A., ALLEN F.H., ALLISON A.C. and BLUMBERG B.S. (1959) Blood groups of Alaskan Eskimos and Indians. *Amer. J. phys. Anthrop.*, **17**, 187–193.
12 JUEL E. (1959) Personal communication to Kornstad.[13]
13 KORNSTAD L. (1961) Some observations on the Wright blood group system. *Vox Sang.*, **6**, 129–135.

[14] CLEGHORN T.E. (1960) The frequency of the Wr^a, By and M^g blood group antigens in blood donors in the South of England. *Vox Sang.*, **5**, 556–560.

[15] CLEGHORN T.E. (1961) *The Occurrence of Certain Rare Blood Group Factors in Britain.* M.D. thesis, University of Sheffield.

[16] DAVIDSOHN I., STERN K., STRAUSER E.R. and SPURRIER WILMA (1953) Be, a new 'private' blood factor. *Blood*, **8**, 747–754.

[17] STERN K., DAVIDSOHN I., JENSEN F.G. and MURATORE R. (1958) Immunologic studies on the Be^a factor. *Vox Sang.*, **3**, 425–434.

[18] HART MIA V.D., BOSMAN HELENE and LOGHEM J.J. VAN (1954) Two rare human blood group antigens. *Vox Sang.* (O.S.), **4**, 108–116.

[19] SIMMONS R.T. and WERE S.O.M. (1955) A 'new' family blood group antigen and antibody (By) of rare occurrence. *Med. J. Aust.*, **ii**, 55–58.

[20] KISSMEYER-NIELSEN F. (1955) A new rare blood group antigen: Chr^a. *Vox Sang.* (O.S.), **5**, 102–103.

[21] CLEGHORN T.E. (1959) A 'new' human blood group antigen, Sw^a. *Nature, Lond.*, **184**, 1324.

[22] FRUMIN A.M., PORTER MARY M. and EICHMAN MARY F. (1960) The Good Factor as a possible cause of hemolytic disease of the newborn. *Blood*, **15**, 681–682.

[23] CALLENDER SHEILA RACE R.R. and PAYKOÇ Z.V. (1945) Hypersensitivity to transfused blood. *Brit. med. J.*, **ii**, 83.

[24] CLEGHORN T.E. (1962) Personal communication.

[25] CLEGHORN T.E. (1960) The inheritance of the antigen Sw^a, and evidence for its independence of other blood group systems. *Brit. J. Haemat.*, **6**, 433–438.

[26] JAKOBOWICZ RACHEL, ALBREY J.A., McCULLOCH W.J. and SIMMONS R.T. (1960) A further example of anti-By (Batty) in the serum of a woman whose red cells are of the A$_x$ (A$_0$) subgroup of group A. *Med. J. Aust.*, **ii**, 294–296.

[27] METAXAS M.N. and METAXAS-BÜHLER M. (1963) Studies on the Wright blood group system. *Vox Sang.*, **8**, 707–716.

[28] KOUT M. (1962) The incidence of the C^w, M^g and Wr^a agglutinogens in the population of Prague. *Vox Sang.*, **7**, 242–244.

[29] CHOWN B., LEWIS MARION, KAITA HIROKO and PHILLIPS SYLVIA (1963) Some blood group frequencies in a Caucasian population. *Vox Sang.*, **8**, 378–381.

[30] MOLTHAN LYNDALL and EICHMAN MARY F. (1967) The blood group antibody 'Good'. 1966. Part I: clinical aspects, routine serologic studies, further search for antigen and antibodies. *Transfusion Philad.*, **7**, 327–329.

[31] CLEGHORN T.E. (1962 to 1967) Unpublished observations.

[32] ABELSON NEVA M. and RAWSON A.J. (1967) The blood group antibody 'Good'. 1966 Part II: physico-chemical studies. *Transfusion, Philad.*, **7**, 330–335.

[33] ALLEN F.H. (1961) Notes on the inheritance of Wr^a. *Transfusion, Philad.*, **1**, 124.

[34] STOUT T.D., MOORE B.P.L. and KAITA HIROKO (1961) Independent segregation of the antigen Wr^a. *Transfusion, Philad.*, **1**, 393.

[35] WALKER MARY E., TIPPETT PATRICIA A., ROPER JUDITH M., OSTHOLD MARGARETHE D., MUNN MARILYN J., MATHIESON ANNE, LEWIS SHEILA J., KRABBE SISSEL M.R., GILLIS MARY, FARRENKOPF CLARE F., DOWNS JUNE M., CRAWCOUR PAMELA, CORCORAN PATRICIA A., CASPERSEN KARI, VON BERCKEN TRAUTE, BALL RITA and ALLEN F.H. (1961) Tests with some rare blood-group antibodies. *Vox Sang.*, **6**, 357.

[36] CLEGHORN T.E. (1961) Unpublished observations.

[37] WADLINGTON W.B., MOORE W.H. and HARTMANN R.C. (1961) Maternal sensitization due to Bi: a presumed 'new, private' red cell antigen. *Amer. J. Dis. Ch.*, **101**, 623–630.

[38] SIMMONS R.T. and ALBREY J.A. (1963) A 'new' blood group antigen Webb (Wb) of low frequency found in two Australian families. *Med. J. Aust.*, **i**, 8–10.

[39] SANGER RUTH and RACE R.R. (1958) Not elsewhere published.

[40] IKEMOTO S., NAKAJIMA H. and FURUHATA T. (1964) The Webb (Wb) blood antigen among the Japanese. *Proc. Japan Acad.*, **40**, 432–433.

41 NAKAJIMA H., IKEMOTO S., TOKUNAGA E. and FURUHATA T. (1965) Further investigation of the Webb (Wb) blood antigen among the Japanese. *Proc. Japan Acad.*, **41**, 86–87.

42 RAUSEN A.R., ROSENFIELD R.E., ALTER A.A., HAKIM S., GRAVEN S.N., APOLLON CORA J., DALLMAN P.R., DALZIEL JOAN C., KONUGRES ANGELYN A., FRANCIS BETTY, GAVIN JUNE and CLEGHORN T.E. (1967) A 'new' infrequent red cell antigen, Rd (Radin). *Transfusion, Philad.*, **7**, 336–342.

43 JENKINS W.J. and MARSH W.L. (1961) Autoimmune haemolytic anaemia: three cases with antibodies specifically active against stored red cells. *Lancet*, **ii**, 16–18.

44 HEISTÖ H. (1967) Personal communication.

45 SPEISER P., KÜHBÖCK J., MICKERTS D., PAUSCH V, REICHEL G., LAUER D., POREMBA I., DOERING I. and HAMACHER H. (1966) 'Kamhuber' a new human blood group antigen of familial occurrence, revealed by a severe transfusion reaction. *Vox Sang.*, **11**, 113–115.

46 WALLACE J. and MILNE G.R. (1959) A 'new' human blood group antigen of rare frequency. *Proc. 7th Congr. int. Soc. Blood Transf.*, 587–589.

47 DUNSFORD I. (1962) Unpublished observations.

48 KORNSTAD L., KOUT M., LARSEN A.M.H. and ØRJASAETER H. (1967) A rare blood group antigen, Jn^a. *Vox Sang.*, **13**, 165–170.

49 KORNSTAD L., ØYEN R. and CLEGHORN T.E. (1968) A new rare blood group antigen To^a (Torkildsen) and an unsolved factor Skjelbred. *Vox Sang.*, **14**, 363–368.

50 BALLOWITZ L., FIELDER H., HOFFMAN C. and PETTENKOFER H. (1968) 'Heibel' a new rare human blood group antibody, revealed by a haemolytic disease of the newborn. *Vox Sang.*, **14**, 307–309.

51 ØRJASAETER H., KORNSTAD L. and LARSEN A.M.H. (1966) A contribution to the blood group frequencies of Tibetans. *Vox Sang.*, **11**, 726–729.

52 WEINER W. (1966) Unpublished observations.

53 LOCKYER J.W. and TOVEY G.H. (1967) Personal communication.

54 ALTER A.A., GELB A.G. and LEE ST L. (1964) Hemolytic disease of the newborn caused by a new antibody (anti-Go^a). *Proc. 9th Congr. int. Soc. Blood Transf.*, Mexico 1962, 341–343.

55 ALTER A.A., GELB A.G., CHOWN B., ROSENFIELD R.E. and CLEGHORN T.E. (1967) Gonzales (Go), a new blood group system. *Transfusion, Philad.*, **7**, 88–91.

56 LEWIS M., CHOWN B., KAITA H., HAHN D., KANGELOS M., SHEPEARD W.L. and SHACKELTON K. (1967) Blood group antigen Go^a and the Rh system. *Transfusion, Philad.*, **7**, 440–441.

57 MCGUIRE DELORES and FUNKHOUSER J.W. (1967) A study of the Wright blood group system as found in a normal donor population. *Transfusion, Philad.*, **7**, 385. (Abstract.)

58 KORNSTAD L. and WOLTHUIS KARI (1967) Unpublished observations.

59 SPEISER P., KÜHBÖCK J., MICKERTS D., PAUSCH V., REICHEL G., LAUER D., POREMBA I., DOERING I. and HAMACHER H. (1965) Über ein neues Erbmerkmal, das Familienantigen Kamhuber. *Wien. klin. Wschr.*, **40**, 710–712.

60 LOVETT D.A. and CRAWFORD M.N. (1967) Js^b and Go^a screening of negro donors. *Transfusion, Philad.*, **7**, 442.

61 NAKAJIMA H., KUNIYUKI M. and TAKAHARA N. (1967) An infrequent blood antigen 'Tsunoi (Ts)' defined by the serum from a patient with acquired haemolytic anaemia. *Jap. J. Hum. Genet.*, **12**, 187–189.

62 ŠVANDA M., PROCHAZKA R., KOUT M. and GILES CAROLYN M. (1970) A case of haemolytic disease of the newborn due to a new red cell antigen, Zd. *Vox Sang.*, **18**, 366–369.

63 FURUHJELM U., NEVANLINNA H.R., GAVIN JUNE and SANGER RUTH (1972) A rare blood group antigen An^a (Ahonen). *J. Med. Genet.*, **9**, 385–391.

64 YVART J., GERBAL A. and SALMON C. (1974) A new 'private' antigen: Hey. *Vox Sang.*, **26**, 41–44.

65 SZALOKY AGNES, SIJPESTEIJN N.K. and VAN DER HART, MIA (1973) A new blood group antigen, Hov. *Vox Sang.*, **24**, 535–541.

66 SKOV F. (1972) A new rare blood group antigen, Je^a. *Vox Sang.*, **23**, 461–463.

67 KORNSTAD L. and BROCTEUR J. (1972) A new, rare blood group antigen, Mo^a (Moen). Abstracts AABB and ISH Meeting, Washington, p. 58.
68 PINDER L.B., STAVELEY J.M., DOUGLAS R. and KORNSTAD L. (1969) Pt^a—a new private antigen. *Vox Sang.*, **17**, 303–305.
69 GUÉVIN R.-M., TALIANO V., FISET D., BÉRUBÉ P. and KAITA H. (1971) L'antigène Reid, un nouvel antigène privé. *Rev. fr. Transf.*, **14**, 455–459.
70 JORGENSEN J. and KISSMEYER-NIELSEN F. (1973) Unpublished observations.
71 ADAMS J., BROVIAC M., BROOKS W., JOHNSON N.R. and ISSITT P.D. (1971) An antibody, in the serum of a Wr(a+) individual, reacting with an antigen of very high frequency *Transfusion, Philad.*, **11**, 290–291.
72 LEWIS MARION, KAITA HIROKO, CHOWN B., TIPPETT PATRICIA, GAVIN JUNE, SANGER RUTH, GIBLETT ELOISE and STEINBERG A.G. (1973) A family with the rare red cell antigens Wr^a and 'super' Sd^a. *Vox Sang.*, **25**, 336–340.
73 METAXAS-BÜHLER M., METAXAS M.N. and GILES C.M. (1972) A Swiss family showing inheritance of the Swann antigen with Lu^a. *Vox Sang.*, **23**, 429–432.
74 GLASGOW BRIDGET G., GOODWIN MARILYN J., JACKSON F., KOPEĆ ADA C., LEHMANN H., MOURANT A.E., TILLS D., TURNER R.W.D. and WARD M.P. (1968) The blood groups, serum groups and haemoglobins of the inhabitants of Lunana and Thimbu, Bhutan. *Vox Sang.*, **14**, 31–42.
75 HARVEY R.G., GODBER MARILYN J., KOPEĆ A.C., MOURANT A.E. and TILLS D. (1969) Frequency of genetic traits in the Caribs of Dominica. *Hum. Biol.*, **41**, 342–364.
76 LIOTTA I., PURPURA M., DAWES B.J. and GILES C.M. (1970) Some data on the low frequency antigens Wr^a and Bp^a. *Vox Sang.*, **19**, 540–543.
77 GRALNICK MARY ANN, SHERWOOD G.K., DE PERALTA FLORENTINA and SCHMIDT P.J. (1971) Torkildsen: experience with the low-incidence antigen in the United States. Program, AABB Meeting, Chicago, 105–106.
78 LUNDSGAARD ANNE and JENSEN K.G. (1968) Two new examples of anti-Rd. A preliminary report on the frequency of the Rd (Radin) antigen in the Danish population. *Vox Sang.*, **14**, 452–457.
79 MCCREARY J., MACILROY M., COURTENAY D.G. and OHMART D.L. (1973) The second example of anti-Be^a causing hemolytic disease of the newborn. *Transfusion, Philad.*, **13**, 428–431.
80 DUCOS J. and others (1974) In preparation.
81 LEWIS MARION, JENSEN K.G. and HOPPE ANN (1973) Personal communication.
82 LEWIS MARION (1973) Personal communication.
83 HARRIS H., HOPKINSON D.A. and ROBSON ELIZABETH R. (1974) The incidence of rare alleles determining electrophoretic variants: data on 43 enzyme loci in man. *Ann. Hum. Genet.*, **37**, 237–253.
84 KORNSTAD L. (1974) Personal communication.
85 BROMAN B. (1973) Personal communication.
86 JØRGENSEN J. (1974) Personal communication.
87 HOWELL P. and GILES CAROLYN M. (1974) Personal communication.
88 CROSSLAND J.D., KORNSTAD L. and GILES C.M. (1974) Third example of the blood group antigen To^a. *Vox Sang.*, **26**, 280–282.

Chapter 21
The I and i Antigens

The agglutinin in the serum of patients suffering from acquired haemolytic anaemia of the 'cold antibody' type has been studied for years. The corresponding antigen was looked on as a species antigen common to all human beings, and this view still seems to have a part of the truth in it. Work in the last 20 years has gradually exposed a complicated blood group-like system which is serologically related in some way to the ABH system, a relationship which the biochemists are beginning to clarify.

Even when the serological difficulties are settled the Ii system will not, because of the great rarity of I negatives, qualify as a polymorphism. It will not be a useful autosomal marker, its contribution seems to lie more in the direction of immunology than genetics.

THE ANTIGEN I

The name I was given to the antigen by Wiener, Unger, Cohen and Feldman[1], in 1956, who recognized for the first time that very rare people existed who had very little I and this phenotype was denoted i.

This paper gives a fascinating account of the difficulties met in transfusing a patient with acquired haemolytic anaemia with powerful anti-I in her serum. The I antigen of normal people was found to be of varying strength.

The antigen I in adults

Our first introduction to anti-I was when Professor Prokop sent us serum from a patient called Steg. suffering from acquired haemolytic anaemia. Titration tests[7], using this powerful serum and cells from 79 of our colleagues at the Institute, showed that there was a great range of I antigen strength and that it fitted a normal distribution curve (the lowest score was 74 and the highest 129). Repeated tests showed that I strength was a constant property of the cells—at least over the period of about six months during which the investigation lasted. Representative samples were tested also with titrations of the anti-I of Wiener et al.[1] and of the antibodies described by Crookston, Dacie and Rossi[6] (1956) and were placed in the order given by the serum Steg.

447

Two samples of blood with anti-I in the serum and very little I on the red cells—one found in a donor to the National Blood Transfusion Service, Brentwood, and the other in a donor to the Knickerbocker Foundation, New York—precipitated an investigation which led to at least the partial unravelling of the system (Jenkins, Marsh, Noades, Tippett, Sanger and Race[2], 1960; Tippett, Noades, Sanger, Race, Sausais, Holman and Buttimer[3], 1960). Much interest was contributed by the finding by Marsh and Jenkins[4, 5] (1960, 1961) of the antibody anti-i.

The antigen I in cord cells

We and our colleagues (Jenkins et al.[2], Tippett et al.[3]) found that cord cells gave relatively very weak reactions with powerful anti-I and failed to react at all with the less powerful anti-I. The development of the antigen strength was studied by Marsh[5] who found that it reached the adult strength by 18 months. Qualitative and quantitative differences in the I antigen of cord and adult cells are reported by Marsh, Nichols and Reid[46].

Weak I antigen in i adults

There are two distinct grades of weak I divided by a wide gulf from the weaker end of the normal distribution curve. Both grades are extremely rare: the weaker has so far been found only in Whites and the not quite so weak mainly in Negroes. In the earlier papers[2, 3] we called both of these phenotypes and that of cord cells i, but Marsh and Jenkins[4, 5] suggested the following notation. In the order of increasing strength of I the symbols are:

i_1 as found so far as a rarity in Whites
i_2 as found so far as a rarity in Negroes, rarer still in Whites
$i_{(cord)}$ as found so far in all cord samples
$I_{(int)}$ as found in people thought to be heterozygous for I
I as found in adults

Apart from the fairly definite agglutination difference, i_1 and i_2 can be distinguished by absorption tests: if an anti-I from an i_1 donor (see antibody section below) be absorbed with i_1 cells no antibody is removed; if it be absorbed with i_2 cells some anti-I is removed; while I cells remove all the anti-I in a single absorption.

However, Marsh et al.[46] subsequently found the I antigen to have two main components I^F (foetal) and I^D (developed), I^F being present in foetal cells and in the cells of i adults.

Not long after the finding of the Brentwood i_1 blood, further examples were found by Dr T.J. Greenwalt in Milwaukee and by Dr J. Wallace in Glasgow. Since that time, although there has been a flood of papers about Ii antibodies we know of disappointingly few reports of the finding of the i phenotype in adults[11–13, 47–51].

THE ANTIGEN i

For a short time i remained merely the absence of I until Marsh and Jenkins[4, 5] reported two examples of anti-i. The stronger of the two examples had an average agglutination titre for ordinary adult cells of about 16, but for adult i cells and for cord cells the titre was 32,000 and more. The finer i differences detected by anti-I were confirmed, in a converse way, by anti-i: the order of increasing strength of i was found to be I adults, $I_{(int)}$, $i_{(cord)}$, i_2 and i_1. Later, Jenkins and Marsh[9] tested foetal cells with anti-I and anti-i and found them to react like cord cells.

Marsh[5] gives a very interesting graph which shows how during the earlier months of life the amount of I antigen on the red cells increases as the amount of i antigen falls, until the adult levels are reached at about 18 months. The influence of marrow stress on the strength of the i antigen[14] is mentioned on page 457.

FREQUENCIES OF THE I PHENOTYPES
IN ADULTS

Though the rule in cord samples, the phenotype i must be extremely rare in adults. Wiener et al.[1] found five examples in testing 22,000 New York donors. Since four of the five were Negroes we may guess that they were what we are now calling i_2. Jenkins et al.[2] tested 17,000 London donors without finding a single example of i. Wallace[10], on the other hand, in a search for donors for his i_1 patient, found two i_2 in 6,000 random donors tested in Glasgow: one was a white American airman and the other was a Scot, and both had anti-I in their serum. Yamaguchi et al.[47] tested 1,017 Japanese adults without finding an example of i. All the adult i propositi that we have tested have disclosed themselves by problems caused by the 'natural' anti-I in their serum.

INHERITANCE OF THE I GROUPS

The family in Figure 26 gave the first evidence that the I groups were, as expected, inherited characters. The fact that the cells of the mother gave less than an ordinary adult reaction with anti-I suggested that she was a heterozygote and her i_2 children were homozygotes. The family in Figure 27 shows that, as expected, i_1 is also a recessive condition. In a family tested by Marsh[5] with anti-i as well as anti-I, the one available parent and the daughter of an i_2 propositus were intermediate in their reactions with both antisera.

The three i_2 sibs in Figure 26 differ between each other in the groups shown in the pedigree: this means that the genes responsible for the I groups are not alleles of, nor very closely linked to, the genes for ABO, MNSs, P or secretion (translating the Lewis phenotypes of the red cells into secretion). The family in Figure 27 confirms ABO, MNSs and secretion and adds Rh and sex. (The argument behind such deductions is given on page 411.)

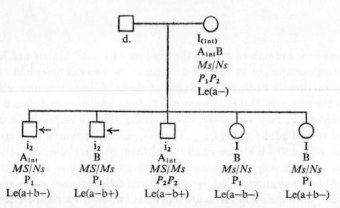

Fig. 26. A negro family showing that i_2 is an inherited character. (After Tippett, Noades, Sanger, Race, Sausais, Holman and Buttimer[3], 1960.) Note the unusual entry of two propositi: the two brothers presented themselves at the same donor session for the Baltimore City Hospitals.

Since 1960, though there has been such a flood of papers about the antibodies, there has been disappointingly little information about the inheritance of the antigens. Claflin[11], Jakobowicz and Simmons[12], Marsh et al.[50], Dzierzkowa-Borodej et al.[49] and Burnie[51] have all recorded the groups of white families with i propositi and Yamaguchi et al.[47, 48] those of four Japanese families. These families, together with an unpublished one tested by the late Dr Ivor Dunsford, confirm the exclusions of ABO, MNSs, P, Rh, secretor and sex and they add Duffy and Kidd.

It is of note that the I groups are not controlled from the *AB, H* or *P* loci but it will be seen below that anti-I, at any rate in the auto form, can be much entangled with these systems.

If the i phenotype really is a recessive character one in four of the sibs of an i propositus would be expected to be i. The present count, excluding the propositus,

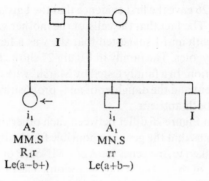

Fig. 27. The family M-D: evidence that i_1 is a homozygous condition. (Dr J. Wallace, personal communication 1960.)

is: sibs I 23, i 16. The excess of i sibs is beginning to be disturbing (P = 0·02). However, there is always the question whether a family is more likely to be published if the propositus has at least one sib with the rare condition.

In 10 families about which we have information, the parents of the propositi were known to be consanguineous in one.

Jørgensen[74] (1968) investigated a family in which the propositus had a 'new' Ii phenotype: she was I weak and i negative while her parents and three sibs were all normal I+. She was found in a survey which included patients with primary amenorrhoea: she has Turner's syndrome though having two apparently normal X chromosomes (perhaps 1 in 5 patients with Turner's syndrome are of this sort). She had no haematological disorder. Just as there was doubt whether straight linkage was the explanation of the 8 i members of 4 Japanese families who had a cataract[48] (discussed on page 567), so in the present family there is doubt whether Turner's syndrome and the Ii peculiarity are associated by chance alone. Jørgensen tested several other patients with Turner's syndrome but found no I or i upset.

In most blood group systems we can picture the genes putting the stamp of specificity on preformed substrate, but with I it is not so simple: the genes which have been identified have to be thought of as not themselves concerned with Ii specificity but with the assistance or non-assistance in the development of i into I. Jenkins and Marsh[9] suggest that a very common gene, say Z, is necessary for the development of foetal i antigen into I; the very rare i adult is not, as was first supposed, homozygous ii but homozygous for z which does nothing to assist the moulding of i into I. The Z gene evidently acts very early in foetal life, for Jenkins and Marsh[9] found that the cells from four '14 weeks' foetuses had, like cord cells, more I than have the cells of i_1 or i_2 adults.

ANTIBODIES OF THE I SYSTEM

Anti-I

Now that it can be identified (by means of cord cells or i adult cells) anti-I is found to be quite a common auto-antibody: the 'natural' or iso form is of necessity rare owing to the rarity of i people.

Auto anti-I

In the serum of people suffering from acquired haemolytic anaemia of the cold antibody type the antibody is usually anti-I[1-3, 6-9, 15]. Such antisera, for example Steg., may vary in strength of reaction with cells of the same ABO group—a faculty to be distinguished from their fairly frequent ability to discriminate between different ABO groups, to be referred to below. The red cells of these patients may, on occasion, appear to be i, but this is due to blocking by the auto-antibody, presumably in an incomplete form[8]: this may explain the apparent I negativeness of the original patient[1].

The commonest source must be the sera which in the past were said to contain a 'non-specific complete cold auto-agglutinin': Jenkins et al.[2] found the antibody in more than 50 consecutive examples to be anti-I.

'Natural' or iso anti-I

In our experience this occurs regularly in the serum of i_1 or i_2 adults, though enzyme tests may be needed to show it. The antibody varies a little according to its source: anti-I from i_2 people does not react with i_1 or i_2 cells; anti-I from i_1 people does react weakly with i_2 cells and, as already mentioned, i_2 cells can absorb some anti-I from these sera. 'Natural' anti-I tend not to reveal the gradation of antigen strength in I people so clearly shown by some auto anti-I sera.

'Natural' anti-I apparently does not cross the placenta: it could not be found in the serum or on the cells of the normal baby of an i_1 mother (Wallace[10]) or that of an i_2 mother (Marsh[5]). Marsh et al.[50] report that the strongest iso anti-I they had met was active at $37°C$, had haemolytic properties but was exclusively IgM and was not present in the newborn child of the propositus.

Heterogeneity of anti-I

Jenkins and Marsh[9] consider the I antigen a mosaic and distinguish two main types of anti-I directed at different parts of the mosaic: some anti-I react relatively strongly with i_1 cells and such sera react more strongly with $i_{(cord)}$ cells; other anti-I sera, though reacting strongly with adult I, scarcely react at all with cord cells. The heterogeneity of anti-I sera, as shown by the niceties of their agglutinating reactions and by the variety of their response to inhibitory substances, is noted in many subsequent papers (see particularly McGinniss, Grindon and Schmidt[81], 1974).

Anti-I and the ABO groups

There is no obvious disturbance of the distribution of the ABO groups in people with anti-I in their serum, but from the time that I was emerging it was realized that the reactions of some anti-I sera could be influenced by the ABO groups of the test cells[2, 3]; that some sera previously called 'anti-O' were in fact anti-I was reported for the first time in our fourth edition[16]. The first clear example[3] of the influence of the ABO groups was the iso anti-I in the serum of the Knickerbocker propositus mentioned on the first page of this chapter. It was surprising in that it reacted more strongly with A_1 than with A_2 or O cells. Absorption with OI cells, or mere dilution, resulted in a pseudo anti-A_1. This pseudo anti-A_1 differed from a proper anti-A_1 in the following ways. (1) It did not agglutinate A_1i cells. (2) It was not inhibited by A_1 secretor saliva. (3) It was inhibited by hydatid cyst fluid. (4) It came from a person whose red cells had an apparently normal A_1 antigen.

Reports on anti-I sera (all but one auto) sensitive to the ABO groups of the red cells illustrate one aspect of the heterogeneity of these sera. They may be listed thus:

i   Stronger with OI than with A_1I cells: references 2, 15, 17–22, 52, 53.
ii Stronger with A_1I than with OI cells: references 3, 17, 20, 54, 57.
iii Stronger with BI than with cells lacking B: references 20, 41, 42.
iv Positive reaction with O_hI cells: references 2, 3, 12, 17, 18, 20–23, 53, 56.
v   Negative with O_hI cells: references 17–20, 22, 23, 52, 53.

A very perplexing crop of names has sprung up in attempts to describe the varying reactions of anti-I sera with cells of different ABO and H groups.

One antiserum is reported by Tegoli et al.[55]: it agglutinates only group O or A_2, I, Le(a−b+) cells.

Anti-I and the P groups

Tippett et al.[3] observed that certain anti-I sera were inhibited or partly inhibited by hydatid cyst fluid, and this has been confirmed[41, 51]. Another link with the P system, and one of practical importance, was recorded by Issitt et al.[41, 45]. In testing four anti-P_1 sera they found two which reacted with P_1 cells only if the cells also contained I. They point out that in testing the cells of newborns it is necessary not to use this anti-IP_1 type of antiserum.

The Luke antigen (page 163) relates, in some way not understood, the P to the ABO system, and I relates to both ABO and to P; furthermore i is related to Lutheran, to Auberger and to P, but in this case a common inhibitor is thought to be the link (page 267).

Anti-i

By including the cells of Mr M., their original i_1 donor, as a routine in tests on serum, Marsh and Jenkins[4, 5] found, within a year, two examples of a new antibody, anti-i; a third example they found later: all three were from patients suffering from some kind of reticulosis; one of the patients died with haemolytic anaemia. A fourth example was found by van Loghem and his colleagues[15] in the serum of a patient suffering from myeloid leukaemia.

Later, transient auto anti-i was found in the serum of some sufferers from infectious mononucleosis: Jenkins, Koster, Marsh and Carter[25] found it in about 8% of 85 cases, and Rosenfield, Schmidt, Calvo and McGinniss[26] in about 66% of 33 cases. For other reports see Capra et al.[58] (1969) and Wilkinson et al.[59] (1973).

Anti-i is usually of the IgM type but can[58] be IgG and has even been blamed for haemolytic disease of the newborn (Gerbal et al.[60], 1971).

An antibody which reacted more strongly with cord cells than with the cells of adults, and therefore presumed to be anti-i, was found by Rubin and Solomon[27] to be not uncommon in the serum of sufferers from alcoholic cirrhosis.

Some of the reactions of anti-i have been briefly rehearsed in the section above on the antigen i.

The strength of reaction of anti-i has not, as far as we know, been found to be influenced by the presence or absence of A and B antigens on the cells. The first two examples of anti-i were found by Marsh[5] to give normal adult reactions with O_h cells. However, Crookston and Giles[38] subsequently showed that the *Hh* genes influence the reactions of some anti-i sera and this was confirmed by Bhatia[39]: some anti-i react as strongly with O_h cells as with cord cells. So the same O_h cells can be of any of four phenotypes, I+i−, I+i+, I−i+, I−i−, depending on the anti-I and anti-i sera used. Though anti-i has been found in the serum of O, A, B and AB people, we do not know whether the heterogeneity of anti-i sera is connected with these groups of the donors.

In testing a series of cold agglutinins which appeared not to be specific for any one of the various I or i antigens Jackson *et al.*[77] (1968) showed by absorption and elution methods that all of 22 such sera contained separable anti-I and anti-i.

Anti-I^T

Cold autoagglutinins are found in the serum of a high proportion of Melanesians and the Ii system was incriminated (Curtain, Baumgarten, Gorman, Kidson, Champness, Rodrigue and Gajdusek[28], 1965; Booth and MacGregor[29], 1966). Booth, Jenkins and Marsh[30] (1966) found cold agglutinin in about 76% of 'the coastal populations of Papua and New Guinea'. Six examples were studied intensively: one was an ordinary anti-I and the other five had a specificity related to the Ii system. The general pattern of reaction of the five was: strong with cord cells, weaker with adult normal I cells and weaker still with adult i cells. Booth *et al.*[30] conclude that their results suggest 'that the antibody is aimed at a developing I antigen present in maximal amount during the transition from i to I, though still present in minimal amount in cells of the mature adult; accordingly, we have named it anti-I^T'.

Booth[83] found a weak form of I^T antigen in some Melanesian samples and it was associated with a significant depression of the antigens LW, D, C, e, S, s and U but not with other antigens measured. He writes 'a likely explanation of the phenomenon would be that the series of depressed determinants all depend, for their full expression, upon the membrane component(s), the proper synthesis of which is being genetically affected'.

Layrisse and Layrisse[61] (1968) found anti-I^T in the serum of 84% of 90 Yanomama Indians in the upper Orinoco River of Venezuela.

Garratty *et al.*[62, 63] (1972) found anti-I^T for the first time in Whites: three of 24 sufferers from Hodgkin's disease had an IgG form of the antibody.

FURTHER NOTES ABOUT THE I SYSTEM

Other sites of I and i antigens

Facts about the distribution of these antigens in the human body have been slow to emerge presumably due to the heterogeneity of anti-I and anti-i sera.

Lymphocytes

Shumak, Rachkewich, Crookston and Crookston[64], 1971, demonstrated very clearly that both I and i are present on adult and on cord lymphocytes. That the i present on adult lymphocytes was the same antigen as detected on cord red cells was neatly shown by absorption tests using adult and cord red cells.

Saliva

Early workers[2, 3] agreed that anti-I sera, whether auto or iso, were not inhibited by saliva. However, in 1971, Dzierzkowa-Borodej and her colleagues[65] described a powerful cold auto anti-I which was inhibited by all salivas whether from I or i people or from newborn babies. However anti-I sera that are appreciably inhibited by saliva are a rarity[66, 51]. The amount of I substance in the saliva was not associated with the presence of ABH, Lewis or Sd[a] substances[65].

Marsh[5] in the original work on anti-i found the antibody not to be inhibited by saliva, and this was thought to be the general case. However de Boissezon et al.[67] and Abbal[68] did find i in saliva, and Burnie[51] found that one of two salivas inhibited only one of seven anti-i sera.

Milk, amniotic fluid and urine

Marsh, Nichols and Allen[66] (1970) showed that human milk contains more I substance than does saliva and this could be demonstrated by inhibition tests using iso or auto anti-I sera. Dzierzkowa-Borodej and Osińska[69] found I substance together with anti-I in the milk of four women. Marsh et al.[50] capped this by finding I in the milk of a i woman in amounts comparable to I milk: the i woman's iso anti-I was inhibited by her own milk.

Convincing inhibition of anti-i with I and i milk could not be demonstrated by Marsh et al.[50] or by Burnie[51] but was by Abbal[68].

Cooper[70] showed amniotic fluid to contain I inhibiting substance with the same properties as that in milk. Urine from adults, pregnant women and newborn babies also had some I substance, though not so much. Abbal[68] confirmed this and found i inhibiting substance in both fluids.

Burnie[51] tested one example of ovarian cyst fluid and it inhibited an anti-I and an anti-i serum.

Under the heading anti-I and the P groups it was recorded that hydatid cyst fluid inhibits some anti-I sera[3, 41, 51]: here we could add that three anti-i sera[5, 51] were not inhibited.

Chiewsilp et al.[71] showed water soluble I substance to be present in the milk and saliva of rhesus monkeys though I is not on their red cells.

Serum

No convincing case has been made for the presence of I in serum[65, 51] but there are technical difficulties in the search[51].

On the other hand, i substance was clearly shown by de Boissezon, Marty, Ducos and Abbal[67] (1970) to be present in the serum of all but one of several hundred samples from normal adults or newborns: the exception was one of 100 cord samples. However, i is not present in the serum of patients with strong anti-i, and it is suggested[67] that 'toute la substance i a été déjà consommée *in vivo* ou bien que seuls les sujets dépourvus de substance i sont susceptibles de développer un anti-i de titre élevé'. De Boissezon and his colleagues showed i to be in the same chromatographic fraction as that in which Cooper[70] had found amniotic I: further, anti-i, eluted from red cells, gave sharp precipitin lines with human serum in Ouchterlony tests[67, 68]. (Incidentally, in the same year, Feizi and Marsh[72] found such precipitin tests useful for certain I:anti-I reactions.)

This French work on i in serum had obviously not been seen by Cooper and Brown[73] (1973) who in a most erudite paper showed normal serum to contain a glycoprotein which strongly and specifically inhibits anti-i. Nor had the French work been seen by Burnie[51] (1973) who independently found normal serum to contain i as measured by 6 out of 7 anti-i sera.

The antigen i was found[67, 68] also in the serum of baboons, sheep, rabbits, a horse and a goose (only the first being known to have i on their red cells[33]) but not in the serum of pigs, cattle, dogs or goats.

Ii antigens on the red cells of animals

Wiener, Moor-Jankowski, Gordon and Davis[33] (1965) tested a very wide range of animals for these antigens and point out that the distribution they found suggests a heterophile behaviour, for it cuts across taxonomic lines. This definitive work must be consulted in the original: over 160 animals were involved.

Jenkins and his colleagues[25] found the red cells of the Cynamolgus monkey to be particularly rich in i and, therefore, useful in the detection of weak examples of anti-i.

Marsh, Nichols and Reid[46] using selected anti-I sera showed that rhesus monkey cells behaved very like human cord cells in that they lacked the I^D (I developed) antigen. Chiewsilp, Colledge and Marsh[71] state that in a limited series of tests on the cells of cats, dogs, guinea pigs and java monkeys they found no evidence of a developmental change in the Ii antigens similar to that which occurs in man. As for kangaroos, wallabies and wombats, their I antigen and antibody status is dealt with by Curtain[40].

The Ii antibodies and antigens in haematological disorders

What a vast amount of work has been done on high titre cold autoantibodies can be seen from Dacie's classical book[31] *The Haemolytic Anaemias, Congenital and Acquired*, 2nd edition, 1962, Part 2. Many subsequent references will be found in the 5th edition of Mollison's *Blood Transfusion in Clinical Medicine* (1972).

Most of these acquired haemolytic disease cold antibodies must be of the anti-I type. We have already mentioned that the serum of sufferers from infectious mononucleosis often contains auto anti-i.

The strength of the I antigen of red cells has been found to be decreased in certain cases of leukaemia (Jenkins and Marsh[9]; McGinniss, Schmidt and Carbone[13]); and in one case the I antigen was found to be decreased and the i increased (Jenkins, Marsh and Gold[44]).

In certain haematological disorders the i antigen strength of the patient's red cells was found to be increased beyond the normal, without any complementary decrease in the strength of the I antigen (Giblett and Crookston[32], 1964; Giblett, Hillman and Brooks[21] (1965). In a most important paper Hillman and Giblett[14] report that the i condition 'can be induced in normal adults by submitting their marrow to the stress of repeated phlebotomy so that the intramarrow maturation time is progressively decreased. After bleeding is discontinued, newly developed cells are no longer i positive.' And they conclude 'We suggest that the bone marrow environment may be a decisive factor in normal red cell maturation, and that the persistent i activity of prematurely released cells may represent retention of a property that normally disappears at an early developmental stage within the marrow.'

It is of interest that as the marrow transit time shortens, and the i appears and increases, there is no change in the strength of the I or the H antigens.

Cooper, Hoffbrand and Worlledge[24] found increased i and increased I antigens in the cells of most of their patients suffering from sideroblastic or megaloblastic anaemia. The raised i strength of Hempas cells is noted on page 485.

Rochant et al.[76] (1973) report the results of a quantitative investigation of I and i antigen strength in over 250 patients mostly suffering from malignant blood diseases.

The association of Ii with the ABO system

The two pedigrees in Figures 26 and 27 provide evidence that the locus for the control of development of i into I is not part of, or closely linked to, the *ABO* locus. However, at the time of the early genetical work[3] it was realized that there was some interrelation with the ABO system and the pointers in this direction were listed[3, 35].

The subsequent work on many examples of anti-I (page 452) has confirmed the association but has not thrown light on its background.

Nor has the testing of adult i cells with anti-H reagents shown any clear picture: most, if not all, A_1i_1 and A_1i_2 samples reacted outstandingly more weakly with *Ulex* anti-H than did cells of ordinary A_1 people[2, 3, 10, 19]; one Bi_2 reacted normally with *Ulex*[3] while another was a weak reactor[5]; Oi cells so far have reacted like OI cells with *Ulex* and with anti-H from O_h donors[36, 19] but are much weaker than OI cells when other anti-H reagents are used, a difference which is less marked if papainized cells are used[36].

Dzierzkowa-Borodej[80], from extensive tests with Oi and Bi_2 cells against well classified anti-H, -HI, -I sera and anti-H lectins, concluded there must be a close structural relationship between the Ii and ABH systems.

A competition, between the genes converting i to I and the *Hh* and *ABO* genes, for some common precursor substance seems unlikely. Were there such a straight-forward competition, O_h cells would be expected to be notably rich in I, and i cells notably rich in H; but neither is the case.

Chemistry

Marcus, Kabat and Rosenfield[37] started the ball rolling, in a paper which showed that treatment with an enzyme from *Clostridium tertium* destroyed the I of A_1 cells more rapidly and completely than that of O or B cells. The I antigen was considered to contain carbohydrate.

Feizi, Kabat, Vicari, Anderson and Marsh[78, 79] worked on a partially purified I substance from human milk together with various ovarian cyst substances and they conclude[78] 'I specificity appears at intermediate stages in the biosynthesis of the A, B, H, Le^a and Le^b substances', and again[79], 'The various I specificities are concealed in interior structures of the blood group A, B, H, Le^a and Le^b sub-stances and may be exposed by stepwise periodate oxidation and Smith degrada-tion of A, B and H substances or by mild acid hydrolysis of B substance'.

An extract from red cell stroma prepared by Gardas and Kościelak[82] (1974) was found to contain a single antigenic material in which all A, B, H and I blood group activities were located on the same molecule. The authors write 'This conclusion offers the explanation for the occurrence of anti-I serums which are influenced by the ABH group of the test erythrocytes in that the adjacent A-, B-, H- and I-active structures may give rise to antibodies of mixed ABH and I specificity'.

Cooper and Brown[73], as mentioned above, isolated a glycoprotein with i specificity from normal human serum.

These four papers[73, 78, 79, 82] must be read by those trying to get to the roots of the biochemical make-up of the system. The biochemical investigations, like the serological, are made difficult by the heterogeneity of the indicator tools, the anti-I and anti-i sera.

The very many papers about I and i, only perhaps half of which are cited in this chapter, rather echo the flood of writing about O, H, Le^a and Le^b which pre-ceded the dispersal of the serological clouds by the biochemists: it looks as if they are going to rescue us again.

REFERENCES

[1] WIENER A.S., UNGER L.J., COHEN L. and FELDMAN J. (1956) Type-specific cold auto-anti-bodies as a cause of acquired hemolytic anemia and hemolytic transfusion reactions: biologic test with bovine red cells. *Ann. intern. Med.*, **44**, 221–240.

2 JENKINS W.J., MARSH W.L., NOADES JEAN, TIPPETT PATRICIA, SANGER RUTH and RACE R.R. (1960) The I antigen and antibody. *Vox Sang.*, **5**, 97–106.
3 TIPPETT PATRICIA, NOADES JEAN, SANGER RUTH, RACE R.R., SAUSAIS LAIMA, HOLMAN C.A. and BUTTIMER R.J. (1960) Further studies of the I antigen and antibody. *Vox Sang.*, **5**, 107–121.
4 MARSH W.L. and JENKINS W.J. (1960) Anti-i: a new cold antibody. *Nature, Lond.*, **188**, 753.
5 MARSH W.L. (1961) Anti-i: a cold antibody defining the Ii relationship in human red cells. *Brit. J. Haemat.*, **7**, 200–209.
6 CROOKSTON J.H., DACIE J.V. and ROSSI V. (1956) Differences in the agglutinability of human red cells by the high-titre cold antibodies of acquired haemolytic anaemia. *Brit. J. Haemat.*, **2**, 321–331.
7 RACE R.R. and SANGER RUTH (1958) *Blood Groups in Man*, 3rd edition, p. 328, Blackwell Scientific Publications, Oxford.
8 WEINER W., SHINTON N.K. and GRAY I.R. (1960) Antibody of blood-group specificity in simple ('cold') haemolytic anaemias. *J. clin. Path.*, **13**, 232–236.
9 JENKINS W.J. and MARSH W.L. (1961) Unpublished observations.
10 WALLACE J. (1960) Personal communication.
11 CLAFLIN ALICE J. (1963) Three members of one family with the phenotype i; one with an anti-I antibody. *Transfusion, Philad.*, **3**, 216–219.
12 JAKOBOWICZ RACHEL and SIMMONS R.T. (1964) The identification of anti-I agglutinins in human serum: an atypical antibody which simulates a non-specific cold agglutinin. *Med. J. Aust.*, **i**, 194–195.
13 McGINNISS M.H., SCHMIDT P.J. and CARBONE P.P. (1964) Close association of I blood group and disease. *Nature, Lond.*, **202**, 606.
14 HILLMAN R.S. and GIBLETT ELOISE R. (1965) Red cell membrane alteration associated with 'marrow stress'. *J. clin. Invest.*, **44**, 1730–1736.
15 LOGHEM J.J. VAN, HART MIA V.D., VEENHOVEN-VAN RIESZ E., MARGA V.D., ENGELFRIET C.P. and PEETOOM F. (1962) Cold auto-agglutinins and haemolysins of anti-I and anti-i specificity. *Vox Sang.*, **7**, 214–221.
16 RACE R.R. and SANGER RUTH (1962) *Blood Groups in Man*, 4th edition, p. 54, Blackwell Scientific Publications, Oxford.
17 GOLD E.R. (1964) Observations on the specificity of anti-O and anti-A₁ sera. *Vox Sang.*, **9**, 153–159.
18 VOAK D. (1964) Anti-HI, a new cold antibody of the H.O.I. complex. A preliminary report. *Scand. J. Haemat.*, **1**, 238–239.
19 ROSENFIELD R.E. and SCHROEDER RUTH, BALLARD RACHEL, HART MIA V.D., MOES MIEKE and LOGHEM J.J. VAN (1964) Erythrocytic antigenic determinants characteristic of H, I in the presence of H (IH), or H in the absence of i (H(−i)). *Vox Sang.*, **9**, 415–419.
20 SALMON C., HOMBERG J.C., LIBERGE G. and DELARUE F. (1965) Autoanticorps a spécificités multiples, anti-HI, anti-AI, anti-BI, dans certain éluats d'anémie hémolytique. *Revue fr. Étud. clin. biol.*, **10**, 522–525.
21 GIBLETT ELOISE R., HILLMAN R.S. and BROOKS LUCY E. (1965) Transfusion reaction during marrow suppression in a thalassemic patient with a blood group anomaly and an unusual cold agglutinin. *Vox Sang.*, **10**, 448–459.
22 SCHMIDT P.J. and McGINNISS MARY H. (1965) Differences between anti-H and anti-OI red cell antibodies. *Vox Sang.*, **10**, 109–112.
23 BHATIA H.M. and GOLD E.R. (1964) Observations on the O antigen. *Vox Sang.*, **9**, 622–624.
24 COOPER A.G,, HOFFBRAND A.V. and WORLLEDGE S.M. (1968) Increased agglutinability by anti-i of red cells in sideroblastic and megaloblastic anaemia. *Brit. J. Haemat.*, **15**, 381–387.
25 JENKINS W.J., KOSTER H.G., MARSH W.L. and CARTER R.L. (1965) Infectious mononucleosis: an unsuspected source of anti-i. *Brit. J. Haemat.*, **11**, 480–483.

26 ROSENFIELD R.E., SCHMIDT P.J., CALVO R.C. and McGINNISS MARY H. (1965) Anti-i, a frequent cold agglutinin in infectious mononucleosis. *Vox Sang.*, **10**, 631–634.

27 RUBIN H. and SOLOMON A. (1967) Cold agglutinins of anti-i specificity in alcoholic cirrhosis. *Vox Sang.*, **12**, 227–230.

28 CURTAIN C.C., BAUMGARTEN A., GORMAN J., KIDSON C., CHAMPNESS L., RODRIGUE R. and GAJDUSEK D.C. (1965) Cold haemagglutinins: unusual incidence in Melanesian populations. *Brit. J. Haemat.*, **11**, 471–479.

29 BOOTH P.B. and MACGREGOR A. (1966) The incidence of cold autohaemagglutinins in Melanesian children and adults. *Vox Sang.*, **11**, 720–723.

30 BOOTH P.B., JENKINS W.J. and MARSH W.L. (1966) Anti-I^T: a new antibody of the I blood-group system occurring in certain Melanesian sera. *Brit. J. Haemat.*, **12**, 341–344.

31 DACIE J.V. (1962) *The Haemolytic Anaemias, Congenital and Acquired.* 2nd edition, Part 2, J. and A. Churchill, London.

32 GIBLETT ELOISE R. and CROOKSTON MARIE C. (1964) Agglutinability of red cells by anti-i in patients with thalassaemia major and other haematological disorders. *Nature, Lond.*, **201**, 1138–1139.

33 WIENER A.S., MOOR-JANKOWSKI J., GORDON EVE B. and DAVIS J. (1965) The blood factors I and i in primates including man, and in lower species. *Amer. J. phys. Anthrop.*, **23**, 389–396.

34 BROCTEUR J., ANDRÉ A., OTTO-SERVAIS M., BOUILLENNE J.C. and NICOLAS E. (1965) Utilisation d'un serum anti-I dans la serologie de routine de l'isoimmunisation foeto-maternelle. Paper read at 10th Congr. Europ. Soc. Haemat., Strasbourg.

35 RACE R.R. and SANGER RUTH (1962) *Blood Groups in Man*, 4th edition, p. 334, Blackwell Scientific Publications, Oxford.

36 GOLD E.R. and BHATIA H.M. (1964) Observations on the H antigen. *Vox Sang.*, **9**, 625–628.

37 MARCUS D.M., KABAT E.A. and ROSENFIELD R.E. (1963) The action of enzymes from *Clostridium tertium* on the I antigenic determinant of human erythrocytes. *J. exp. Med.* **118**, 175–194.

38 CROOKSTON MARIE and GILES CAROLYN M. (1966) Personal communication.

39 BHATIA H.M. (1966) Personal communication.

40 CURTAIN C.C. (1969) Anti-I agglutinins in non-human sera. *Vox Sang.*, **16**, 161–171.

41 TEGOLI J., HARRIS JEAN P., ISSITT P.D. and SANDERS C.W. (1967) Anti-IB, an expected 'new' antibody detecting a joint product of the *I* and *B* genes. *Vox Sang.*, **13**, 144–157.

42 DRACHMANN O. (1968) An autoaggressive anti-BI(O) antibody. *Vox Sang.*, **14**, 185–193.

43 ISSITT P.D. (1967) I blood group system and its relation to other blood group systems. *J. med. Lab. Tech.*, **24**, 90–97.

44 JENKINS W.J., MARSH W.L. and GOLD E.R. (1965) Reciprocal relationship of antigens 'I' and 'i' in health and disease. *Nature, Lond.*, **205**, 813.

45 ISSITT P.D., TEGOLI J., JACKSON VALERIE, SANDERS C.W. and ALLEN F.H. (1968) Anti-IP$_1$: antibodies that show an association between the I and P blood group systems. *Vox Sang.*, **14**, 1–8.

46 MARSH W.L., NICHOLS MARGARET E. and REID MARION E. (1971) The definition of two I antigen components. *Vox Sang.*, **20**, 209–217.

47 YAMAGUCHI H., OKUBO Y., TOMITA T., YAMANO H. and TANAKA M. (1970) A rare i (I-negative) phenotype blood found in Japanese families. *Proc. Jap. Acad.*, **46**, 889–892.

48 YAMAGUCHI H., OKUBO Y. and TANAKA M. (1972) A note on possible close linkage between the Ii blood locus and a congenital cataract locus. *Proc. Jap. Acad.*, **48**, 625–628.

49 DZIERZKOWA-BORODEJ WANDA, KAZMIERCZAK ZDZISLAWA and ZIEMNIAK J. (1972) The antigens of Ii blood group system in a further case of i$_2$ (Bi$_2$) adult person. *Arch. Immunol. et Ther. Exp.*, **20**, 851–859.

50 MARSH W.L., JENSEN L., DECARY F. and COLLEDGE K. (1972) Water-soluble I blood group substance in the secretions of i adults. *Transfusion, Philad.*, **12**, 222–226.

51 BURNIE KATHERINE (1973) Ii antigens and antibodies. *Can. J. med. Technol.*, **35**, 5–26.

52 LODGE T.W. and VOAK D. (1968) An example of inhibitable anti-HI in a group B donor. *Vox. Sang.*, **14**, 60–62.
53 VOAK D., LODGE T.W., HOPKINS JEAN and BOWLEY C.C. (1968) A study of the antibodies of the H′O′I-B complex with special reference to their occurrence and notation. *Vox Sang.*, **15**, 353–366.
54 BAUMGARTEN A., CURTAIN C.C., GOLAB T., GORMAN J.G., KIDSON C. and RUTGERS CAROL F. (1968) Endemic autoimmunity: cold auto-agglutinins in Melanesia. *Brit. J. Haemat.*, **15**, 567.
55 TEGOLI J., CORTEZ MYRNA, JENSEN LEILA and MARSH W.L. (1971) A new antibody, anti-ILe^{bH}, specific for a determinant formed by the combined action of the I, Le, Se and H gene products. *Vox Sang.*, **21**, 397–404.
56 LOPEZ M., GERBAL A. and SALMON C. (1972) Excès d'antigène I dans les érythrocytes de phénotypes O$_h$, A$_h$ et B$_h$. *Rev. fr. Transf.*, **15**, 187–193.
57 BAUMGARTEN A. and CURTAIN C.C. (1970) A high frequency of cold agglutinins of anti-IA specificity in a New Guinea highland population. *Vox Sang.*, **18**, 21–26.
58 CAPRA J.D., DOWLING P., COOK S. and KUNKEL H.G. (1969) An incomplete cold-reactive γG antibody with i specificity in infectious mononucleosis. *Vox Sang.*, **16**, 10–17.
59 WILKINSON L.S., PETZ L.D. and GARRATTY G. (1973) Reappraisal of the role of anti-i in haemolytic anaemia in infectious mononucleosis. *Brit. J. Haemat.*, **25**, 715–722.
60 GERBAL A., LAVALLÉE R., ROPARS C., DOINEL C., LACOMBE M. and SALMON C. (1971) Sensibilisation des hématies d'un nouveau-né par un auto-anticorps anti-i d'origine maternelle de nature IgG. *Nouv. Rev. fr. Hemat.*, **11**, 689–700.
61 LAYRISSE Z. and LAYRISSE M. (1968) High incidence cold autoagglutinins of anti-I^T specificity in Yanomama Indians of Venezuela. *Vox Sang.*, **14**, 369–382.
62 GARRATTY G., PETZ L.D., WALLERSTEIN R. and FUDENBERG H.H. (1972) I^T, a new specificity associated with autoimmune hemolytic anemia and Hodgkin's disease. Abstracts AABB and ISBT Meeting, Washington. And (1974) *Transfusion, Philad.*, **14**, 226–231.
63 GARRATTY G., HAFFLEIGH B., DALZIEL J. and PETZ L.D. (1972) An IgG anti-I^T detected in a Caucasian American. *Transfusion, Philad.*, **12**, 325–329.
64 SHUMAK K.H., RACHKEWICH ROSE A., CROOKSTON MARIE C. and CROOKSTON J.H. (1971) Antigens of the Ii system on lymphocytes. *Nature New Biol.*, **231**, 148–149.
65 DZIERZKOWA-BORODEJ WANDA, SEYFRIED HALINA, NICHOLS MARGARET, REID MARION and MARSH W.L. (1970) The recognition of water-soluble I blood group substance. *Vox Sang.*, **18**, 222–234.
66 MARSH W.L., NICHOLS MARGARET E. and ALLEN F.H. (1970) Inhibition of anti-I sera by human milk. *Vox Sang.*, **18**, 149–154.
67 DE BOISSEZON J.-F., MARTY YVONNE, DUCOS J. and ABBAL M. (1970) Presence constante d'une substance inhibitrice de l'anticorps anti-i dans le serum humain normal. *C.R. Acad. Sci., Paris*, **271**, 1448–1451.
68 ABBAL M. (1971) Les substances inhibitrices des anti-I et anti-i des liquides biologiques humains et animaux. Thesis Université Paul Sabatier, Toulouse.
69 DZIERZKOWA-BORODEJ WANDA and OSIŃSKA MARIA (1971) Anti-I antibodies in human milk. *Arch. Immunol. et. Ther. Exp.*, **19**, 609–612.
70 COOPER A.G. (1970) Soluble blood group I substance in human amniotic fluid. *Nature, Lond.*, **227**, 508–509.
71 CHIEWSILP P., COLLEDGE KATHERINE I. and MARSH W.L. (1971) Water soluble I blood group substance in the secretions of rhesus monkeys. *Vox Sang.*, **21**, 30–36.
72 FEIZI T. and MARSH W.L. (1970) Demonstration of I-anti-I interaction in a precipitin system. *Vox Sang.*, **18**, 379–382.
73 COOPER A.G. and BROWN M.C. (1973) Serum i antigen: a new human blood-group glycoprotein. *Biochem. biophys. Res. Commun.*, **55**, 297–304.
74 JØRGENSEN J.R. (1968) A new phenotype in the Ii blood group system. *Vox Sang.*, **15**, 171–176.

16

[75] MOLLISON P.L. (1972) *Blood Transfusion in Clinical Medicine*, 5th ed. Blackwell Scientific Publications, Oxford.

[76] ROCHANT H., TONTHAT H., MAN NGO M., LEFAOU J., HENRI A. and DREYFUS B. (1973) Étude quantitative des antigènes érythrocytaires I et i en pathologie. *Nouv. Rev. fr. Hemat.*, **13**, 307–318.

[77] JACKSON VALERIE A., ISSITT P.D., FRANCIS BETTY J., GARRIS MARY LOU and SANDERS C.W. (1968) The simultaneous presence of anti-I and anti-i in sera. *Vox Sang.*, **15**, 133–141.

[78] FEIZI TEN, KABAT E.A., VICARI G., ANDERSON B. and MARSH W.L. (1971) Immunochemical studies on blood groups. XLVII. The I antigen complex-precursors in the A, B, H, Le^a and Le^b blood group system-hemagglutination-inhibition studies. *J. Exp. Med.*, **133**, 39–52.

[79] FEIZI TEN, KABAT E.A., VICARI G., ANDERSON B. and MARSH W.L. (1971) Immunochemical studies on blood groups. XLIX. The I antigen complex: specificity differences among anti-I sera revealed by quantitative precipitin studies; partial structure of the I determinant specific for one anti-I serum. *J. Immunol.*, **106**, 1578–1592.

[80] DZIERZKOWA-BORODEJ WANDA (1971) *HI* and I^s fractions in the expression of *H* activity in human erythrocytes. *Ann. Immunol.*, **III**, 3–4, 85–107.

[81] MCGINNISS M.H., GRINDON A.J. and SCHMIDT P.J. (1974) Evidence for two anomalous I blood group determinants. *Transfusion, Philad.*, **14**, 257–260.

[82] GARDAS A. and KOŚCIELAK J. (1974) I-active antigen of human erythrocyte membrane. *Vox Sang.*, **26**, 227–237.

[83] BOOTH P.B. (1974) Depressed blood group antigens among Melanesians. In preparation.

Chapter 22
The En Blood Groups and Some Other Phenotypes Affecting the Cell Surface

In this chapter are collected certain conditions that have in common some physico-chemical change to the cell surface and some abnormality of expression of the MN antigens. The common factor is evidently a loss of sialic acid and a consequent reduction of the negative charge of the red cell surface. There are examples of polyagglutinability which might have been included but we decided to leave them to Chapter 24.

THE En BLOOD GROUPS

Darnborough, Dunsford and Wallace[1] at a meeting of the British Society for Haematology in 1965 described the first family: an antibody, named anti-En^a, was present in the serum of the propositus (M.P.) which reacted strongly with all cells tested, 7,000 at the time, but which did not react with her own cells or those of two of her eight sibs. The propositus was pregnant and had been transfused two years before. In the admirable abstract of the paper[1, 2] is recorded: 'The reactions of various unrelated blood group antigens are modified, in some cases enhanced and in others depressed, the total picture being strongly reminiscent of the effects of proteolytic enzyme treatment. It is suggested that these effects can only be due to some factor affecting the red cell structure possibly by modifying the cell envelope'. The En of the notation stood for envelope.

This account enabled a further antibody to be recognized as anti-En^a in 1968: the finding of a second example, Mr V.B., this time in Finland, greatly stimulated interest in the system and a long investigation followed in Helsinki and in London (Furuhjelm, Myllylä, Nevanlinna, Nordling, Pirkola, Gavin, Gooch, Sanger and Tippett[3], 1969). In 1970 a third example was found, Mr G.W., again in Finland (Furuhjelm, Nevanlinna and Pirkola[4], 1973). Like the first, both Finnish antibodies were attributed to previous transfusion.

Frequency

The phenotype En(a−) is extremely rare. No random example was found in testing 12,500 English[2], 8,800 Finnish[3] and 200 Estonians[3] with anti-En^a. En(a−) cells

463

might be recognized in another way: one of their attributes, as will be explained below, is to react, though suspended in saline, with appropriate incomplete Rh antisera; but no example of En(a–) has been caught this way in tests on many thousand people in our own and other[2, 5] laboratories.

The only En(a–) people so far found are the three propositi and four of their sibs: the En(a–) condition is undoubtedly a recessive character, genotype *EnEn*.

Serological reactions of En(a–) and heterozygous En(a+) cells

En(a–) cells apart from not reacting with anti-En[a] are peculiar in other ways, of which the following are the most striking:

1   Their M and N antigens are notably depressed, as judged by human, animal and some seed anti-M and anti-N reagents, yet their S or s antigens give normal[3] or even enhanced reactions[2].

We were kindly sent samples from the English M En(a–) sibs and they reacted positively with all our human and animal anti-M sera, though less strongly than did control cells, but with none of our human and animal anti-N sera: the cells of the Finnish MN En(a–) cells reacted with only about half the anti-M but with almost all the anti-N sera. The relative weakness of the M antigen may be shown by, for example, titration scores with a human anti-M: 2 English M En(a–), 29, 28, Finnish MN En(a–) 5, control M 75, control MN 50, control N 0. (Another human anti-M, not showing such a marked dosage effect, scored thus with the same cells: 30, 30, 19, 45, 40, 0.) The MN reactions of the 4 En(a+) heterozygotes, all M, that we have tested[3] gave normal reactions with anti-M. Lectins are not reliable as MN reagents for En(a–) cells as will be seen below.

2   Their Rh reactions are surprising, En(a–) cells though suspended in saline have the property of being strongly agglutinated by *incomplete* Rh antisera of appropriate specificity[2, 3].

All En(a–) cells so far found happen to have the antigen D and they reacted when suspended in saline more strongly with incomplete anti-D than did –*D*–/–*D*– cells. Only selected incomplete anti-Rh sera are efficient at detecting in this way heterozygous En(a+), *En[a]En*, cells. In the second Finnish family[4] this test, as well as the seed extract test to be described, failed to pick out two of nine people who must be heterozygotes on pedigree evidence (Figure 28). That these two were the only N S– *En[a]En* samples yet to be tested may or may not be significant.

3   En(a–) cells are agglutinated more strongly than are normal cells by non-immune animal sera[3].

We have tried sera from rabbit, horse, cow, sheep, dog, cat, orang, baboon, toad and water buffalo. One exception should be mentioned: En(a–) cells, one example, unlike all other human cells tested, were not agglutinated by the plasma of one of two coelacanths[6], so here it seems we had stumbled on a way to distinguish at least some coelacanths from, say, water buffaloes.

4   En(a–) cells are agglutinated more strongly than are normal cells by certain seed extracts[3, 18].

An extract from the seeds of *Sophora japonica*, absorbed with A_1B cells to remove its known anti-A+B component, was particularly useful in that it reacted thereafter strongly with En(a−) cells and quite strongly with En^aEn heterozygous cells but scarcely at all with cells of the En^aEn^a multitude[3].

Many seed extracts, whether they have blood group specificity or not, can recognize En(a−) cells[3, 18]. All anti-H extracts tried react more strongly with En(a−) than with En(a+) cells but this was due to their anti-H, and not to any specific 'anti-En' component. Three seed extracts stand out in not reacting with En(a−) cells[3]: *Dolichos biflorus* (anti-A_1), *Phaseolus lunatus* (anti-A), *Arachis hypogea* (anti-T).

An extract of the seeds of *Bauhinia purpurea*, like *Sophora*, reacted strongly with En(a−) cells and less strongly with heterozygous En(a+) cells; the agglutinin for En(a−) cells reacted also with rabbit cells and could be separated from the anti-N present in the extract, hinting that *Bauhinia* has at least two components[3], but other workers concluded that *Bauhinia* has but one agglutinin[18]. Perhaps all *Bauhinia* extracts do not behave alike: in our experience *Vicia graminea* extracts vary in their ability to agglutinate M En(a−) cells.

We do not feel competent to assess the importance of the evidence from the seed reactions of En(a−) concerning red cell membrane topography (Bird and Wingham[18]).

En(a+) heterozygotes cannot be distinguished from the common En(a+) homozygotes by dosage tests with human or rabbit (see below) anti-En^a sera, for these sera react equally strongly with both types of cells. However, with two exceptions mentioned earlier, clear distinctions were made between heterozygotes and homozygotes by appropriate incomplete Rh antisera and by the *Sophora japonica* preparation.

The En(a−) condition was, of course, shown not to be the same as any of the phenotypes previously described lacking 'public' antigens[2, 3]. It was readily dissociated serologically[7, 3] from T and Tn and Pr (syn. Sp_1, HD).

The En(a−) state affected the reactions with antisera of other blood group systems but the four listed above were the most striking. All the reactions were those expected of normal, En(a+), cells after treatment with proteolytic enzymes, which suggested that they would prove to have a single common background and prompted the work in Helsinki now to be described.

Physicochemical reactions of En(a−) and heterozygous En(a+) cells

The increased agglutinability of enzyme treated cells was known to be due, at least in part, to the removal of sialic acid and consequent reduction of negative surface charge (shown by reduced electrophoretic mobility). This aspect of En(a−) cells clearly required investigation, and very extensive tests in Helsinki are briefly summarized in Table 77; but those interested should read the section in the original paper[3].

Compared with normal cells En(a−) cells showed a markedly decreased electrophoretic mobility and a more than 50% reduction in sialic acid content. Heterozygous En(a+) cells differed less in these respects but even they showed a significant reduction in mobility and sialic acid content. It was further shown that the electrophoretic mobility of En(a−) cells was just about that of normal cells treated with pronase or trypsin.

Table 77. The En system: summary of physicochemical measurements
(after Furuhjelm *et al.*[3], 1969)

Cells	Genotype	Approximate percentage of normal	
		Electrophoretic mobility	Sialic acid
En(a−)	*EnEn*	58%	33%
heterozygous En(a+)	*En^aEn*	88%	78%
homozygous En(a+)	*En^aEn^a*	100%	100%

The decreased surface charge of En(a−) cells adequately explains their increased agglutinability with incomplete Rh antisera, with seed extracts and with animal sera; the shortage of sialic acid reasonably accounts for their depressed MN activity, for sialic acid is known to be closely involved in the M and N antigens (page 121). This is a simple interpretation of the discussion in the original paper[3].

Though untreated En(a−) cells in many respects behave like ordinary cells treated with proteolytic enzymes there is a chemical difference: in 1972 Herz *et al.*[8] found the acetylcholinesterase of En(a−) cells to be normal, whereas acetylcholinesterase is inactive in normal cells treated with proteolytic enzymes.

Inheritance

Pedigrees of the three En(a−) propositi are given in Figure 28. En(a−) is undoubtedly a recessive condition, the sib count strongly suggests it and the consanguinity rate of parents supports it. The sibs of the three propositi fit a recessive expectation:

	En(a−)	En(a+)
observed	4	12
expected	*4*	*12*

Furthermore, heterozygotes can usually be distinguished, as explained below, and their incidence fits too.

The parents of the English propositus were not known to be consanguineous but came from Grimsby in Yorkshire, a fishing port noted for a high rate of intermarriage[2]. The parents of the first Finnish propositus were not known to be related, but church records showed them to have been second cousins[3]. Church records then showed that the parents of the second Finnish propositus were third cousins. These amazing church records, in the Vaasa area, excelled themselves in further showing that the two Finnish propositi had both descended from a couple born in the early 18th century[4]. The pedigree (Figure 29) gives rein to many genealogical excursions, for example, if we are not mistaken:

V.B. and G.W. are related in six different ways: they are 2nd cousins once removed, 3rd cousins once removed, 4th cousins and, via three different paths, 4th cousins once removed. The parents of V.B., besides being 2nd cousins, are 3rd cousins once removed: the parents of G.W., besides being 3rd cousins, are also 4th cousins. Furthermore, G.W.'s paternal grandparents were 3rd cousins and his paternal maternal great grandparents 2nd cousins.

ENGLISH FAMILY

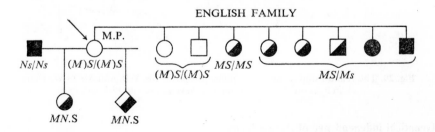

FIRST FINNISH FAMILY

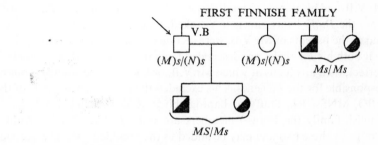

SECOND FINNISH FAMILY

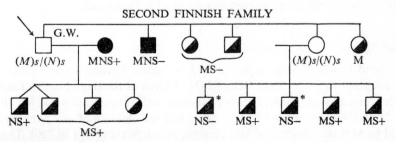

Fig. 28. The families of the three propositi lacking the antigen En[a], and their MNSs genotypes or, when anti-s was not used, phenotypes. English family, after Darnborough et al.[2]; first Finnish family, after Furuhjelm et al.[3]; second Finnish family, after Furuhjelm et al.[4].

Hollow   = En(a−), genotype *EnEn*
Half black = En(a+) heterozygote, genotype *En^aEn*
Black   = En(a+) homozygote, genotype *En^aEn^a*
Asterisk = heterozygotes by pedigree but not, unlike the other heterozygotes, detected serologically (see text)
Brackets = depressed antigens
The birth order of sibs is not necessarily correct.

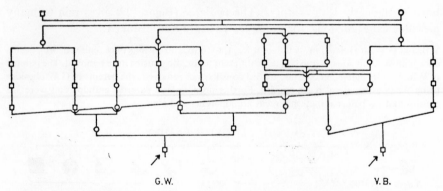

G.W.   V. B.

Fig. 29. The relationship of the two Finnish propositi Mr V.B. and Mr G.W. from church records; from Furuhjelm, Nevanlinna and Pirkola[4].

Genetical independence of the *En* locus

Mr V.B. and his En(a–) sister differed in their Duffy groups, so *En* is not controlled from the *Duffy* locus, nor is it Y-linked. Since the allele *En* is so extremely rare and as the parents of Mr V.B. were second cousins the chances must be very high that both his *En* alleles are descended from one and the same *En* allele. If this be correct, then any locus at which Mr V.B. or his sister are heterozygous cannot be responsible for the *En* genes. This excluded the *En* locus being part of the loci for ABO, MNSs, Rh, Duffy or haptoglobins; it also excluded X-linkage. In the English family the En(a–) members are not all alike in their Kidd and Gm groups so these two loci may be added to the excluded list. The second Finnish family confirms several of the exclusions and adds Dombrock.

En and MN

The second Finnish family, reported by Furuhjelm, Nevanlinna and Pirkola[4], drew attention to a significant lack of MN children of the three Finnish En(a–) people who had issue: all three are MN, though both antigens are weak, but all of their 11 children are either M or N. Since half the children of any MN parent should be MN this absence of MN children is significant ($P = 1$ in 250). This is disturbing and makes one wonder whether En(a–) people have no *M* or *N* alleles, a possibility suggested by Dr and Mrs Metaxas, and whether their weak M and N reactions are false and due to some serological artefact. If this were so, *En* could be thought of as a silent allele at the *MN* locus and the children of an *EnEn* parent as hemizygous *M* or *N*. However, much against this is the fact that all three En(a–) sibs in the English family have quite respectable M antigens as may be seen from certain titration scores given above (page 464). Furthermore, it recently became known that both children of the English En(a–) propositus (M.P.) are MN.S (Mr R.R. Stapleton, personal communication, 1973) thus proving that in this family a silent allele is not operating.

Though the *En* and *MN* loci appear to be genetically independent there is clearly an association between the lack of the antigen En^a and the MN antigens, and presumably sialic acid is the link, but insight into the nature of the MN defect of En(a−) cells will probably have to await chemical analysis. Perhaps En(a−) cells are imperfect in some MN precursor substance, resembling O$_h$ cells in the ABO system which are practically devoid of H.

Anti-En^a

The three human examples found so far were undoubtedly immune in origin: the result of transfusion in the two Finnish male propositi[3,4] and of transfusion perhaps aided by pregnancy in the English female propositus[2]. The 1964 baby of M.P. showed no symptoms of haemolytic disease though the cord cells gave a positive direct antiglobulin reaction. The 1971 baby, however, did have haemolytic disease and was transfused with blood from her En(a−) uncle (Mr R.R. Stapleton, personal communication, 1973). No anti-En^a was detected in the serum of the four En(a−) sibs of the propositi, none of whom had been transfused.

As noted above anti-En^a has reacted with all of many thousand samples tested but not with the cells of the three propositi and four of their sibs; and it does not show a dosage effect. All three examples of the antibody showed some agglutinating ability for cells suspended in saline but reacted more strongly by enzyme on antiglobulin methods.

Tests with the anti-En^a of Mr V.B. were particularly extensive[3]: the reactions with En(a+) cells suspended in saline were notably increased by previous treatment of the cells with ficin, papain, bromelin and pronase, whereas trypsin and neuraminidase had little effect. The reaction was enhanced by the use of IgG antiglobulin but not by IgA or IgM sera. Elaborate absorption and inhibition tests appeared to demonstrate the presence in the serum of Mr V.B. of two separable forms of anti-En^a.

Of a great range of cells representing rare genotypes, Rh$_{null}$ samples alone stood out in reacting with anti-En^a sera slightly but definitely more strongly than the rest[9]. This might be something to do with the known slight surface change of these cells but, on the other hand, M^gM^g and M^k cells, with their more severe physico-chemical changes, reacted normally with anti-En^a.

Immunization of rabbits

A rabbit was injected with MN, En(a+) cells[3] and the resulting antiserum, after absorption with En(a−) cells, reacted with En(a+) but not En(a−) cells. The antibody was presumed to be anti-En^a and appropriate absorptions did not indicate that it contained any anti-M or anti-N component. Rabbit, like human, anti-En^a showed no dosage effect.

Injection of En(a−) cells into a rabbit[3] greatly increased the agglutinin previously active for En(a−) cells only, but now En(a+) cells reacted also. That the
16*

agglutinin was not specific, in the serological sense, for En(a−) cells was shown by successive absorptions with En(a+) cells which removed in parallel the reaction for En(a−) and En(a+) cells.

Other notes about En[a]

The antigen En[a] is well developed at birth[2, 3]: anti-En[a] reacts as strongly with cord cells as with adult cells.

The antigen En[a] appeared not to be present on platelets; tests on white cells were doubtful but brain cells seemed to have it[3].

The antigen En[a] is not present on the red cells of rabbit, horse, sheep, kitten or gibbon[3], as judged by the failure of one sample of each to absorb human anti-En[a].

As one of us wrote[10] 'It would be satisfying if a simple genetical model could be thought of which would cope with the lack of the antigen En[a] and the shortage of sialic acid. A regulator locus could be postulated which cuts down sialic acid, and sialic acid shortage might result in inability to make En[a]. But it is difficult to see how this simplest explanation fits the observation that neuraminidase, and the proteolytic enzymes, have no [depressing] effect on the En[a] antigen of normal cells.' Furuhjelm and his colleagues, no less perplexed, ended their account[3]: 'The basis of the changes to the red cell surface caused by the En allele is unknown, though it may be guessed that some enzyme needed for the building of the normal surface is defective. If this were so the En(a−) condition could be thought of as an "inborn error of metabolism".'

OTHER PHENOTYPES AFFECTING THE CELL SURFACE

M[k] and M[g]

Introduction, by En[a], to the curious effects of sialic acid shortage prompted the workers[3, 11] in Helsinki and London to look more closely at some of the rarer MN variants because of the known particular relationship of MN to sialic acid. M[k] and M[g] suggested themselves, for they possess little or no M or N antigen (pages 105 and 104).

Dr Phillip Sturgeon provided samples from a fine Chinese family in Los Angeles in which M[k] was segregating. The cells of the M[k] members, though suspended in saline, were agglutinated by appropriate incomplete Rh antisera and reacted preferentially to selected seed extracts[11]. Indeed, the M[k] members, all heterozygotes, were thus recognized as M[k] in our laboratory before any MN tests were done. The family was later described in detail by Sturgeon et al.[12], a harrowing immigration story but with a happy ending. Further M[k] samples, all heterozygous, from Zurich, gave the same serological reactions and in Helsinki were shown to have reduced electrophoretic mobility and sialic acid content. The extent of the reduction equalled that shown by En(a+), En^aEn, heterozygotes, as may be seen from our simplified summary (Table 78) of the original results[11].

In view of the M^k reactions it was decided to look at M^g cells: M^g heterozygous cells, also from Zurich, when suspended in saline, reacted positively with the incomplete Rh antisera and the extract of *Sophora japonica*, though the reactions were not as strong as those of M^k heterozygotes. The electrophoretic mobility and sialic acid content of the M^g heterozygotes were both significantly reduced[11] but not to the extent shown by M^k heterozygotes (Table 78).

Table 78. M^k and M^g heterozygotes: summary of physicochemical measurements (after Nordling *et al.*[11], 1969)

	Approximate percentage of normal	
Cells	electrophoretic mobility	sialic acid
M^k heterozygotes	88%	79%
M^g heterozygotes	94%	88%
En heterozygotes	88%	78%
controls	100%	100%

No M^kM^k homozygote has yet been found, but a Swiss M^gM^g child is known (Metaxas-Bühler *et al.*[13], and page 105): in 1963 Dr and Mrs Metaxas had sent us a sample of cord blood from this child the cells of whom though suspended in saline had reacted strongly with incomplete anti-D, a reaction to which, though repeated, we had turned a blind eye in our excitement over the MN reactions of these precious cells.

In 1971 Dr Metaxas was able to trace the M^gM^g homozygote, then aged eight, and samples from her and her mother and a control were sent to Helsinki: the mother's heterozygous M^gM cells had a mobility 93% of normal while the child's M^gM^g cells were about 90% of normal (personal communication, Drs Nordling and Metaxas, 1971).

It perhaps should be repeated that these M^gM^g cells, like M^k cells, give normal positive reactions with anti-En^a.

Metaxas and Metaxas-Bühler[5] (1972) then used the incomplete Rh antisera saline test as a trap for MN variants. In testing 6,202 donors 6 M^k were amongst the strongest reactors, but 4 M^g heterozygotes known to be amongst these donors were missed, which is not surprising considering their weaker reaction with incomplete anti-Rh. From this investigation emerged two other MN variants with surface effects, Mi-V and St^a.

Mi-V and St(a+)

Three examples of Mi-V cells of the Miltenberger series were caught in the 6,202 survey[5], two of them Ms/Ns^{Mi-V} and one Ns/Ns^{Mi-V} (page 113); this was the first record that such cells had any surface alteration. One sample was measured and found to have a reduced electrophoretic mobility very like that of M^k heterozygotes.

Six St(a+) samples (page 116) were also caught in the 6,202 survey but their reactions were not as strong as those of M^k or Mi-V.

So M^k, Mi-V and, to a lesser degree, M^g heterozygotes share some of the serological and physicochemical peculiarities of En^aEn heterozygotes, and shortage of sialic acid is presumably the common factor. Notable difference within the four phenotypes in relation to the MNSs system are summarized in Table 79. St(a+) heterozygotes are not included in the table for their electrophoretic mobility or sialic acid content has yet to be measured and, further, St(a+) is a heterogeneous group.

Table 79. Distinctions between some phenotypes showing sialic acid shortage

	Haplotypes			
	M^k	Mi-V	M^g	En
MN antigens	−	w	−	w
Ss antigens	−	+	+	+
M^g antigen	−	−	+	−
Hil antigen	−	+	−	−
Genetic relationship to MNSs	+	+	+	−

Inherited direct positive antiglobulin reaction

As noted in the MNSs chapter (page 106) four families, Australian, Danish, Swiss and East German, have been found in which a direct positive antiglobulin reaction is inherited as a dominant character. In two of the families[14,15] the reaction is segregating with a weak N, in one[16] with a weak M and in one[17] the segregation is not disclosed, for a mother and her son, both showing the reaction, appeared to be normal M.

Jensen and Freiesleben[14] found that anti-IgG was not involved in the reaction: Jeannet, Metaxas-Bühler and Tobler[15], during the investigation of a large family, excluded anti-IgG, anti-IgA and anti-β_{1c} and showed that the presence of anti-IgM is needed to bring about the reaction. None of the 14 positive members of the two families showed any sign of anaemia. The Swiss authors concluded that the primary abnormality was probably an alteration in red cell sialic acid metabolism.

We were given the opportunity to test samples from two of the four families at about the same time, two members of the Swiss family of Jeannet et al.[15], through the kindness of Professor Alfred Hässig, and the two members of the East German family of Fünfhausen and Velhagen[17]. All four samples reacted strongly with five British rabbit antiglobulin sera in routine use. In agreement with the Swiss findings the samples failed to react with specific anti-IgG sera, from rabbit, sheep and horse, and with specific anti-IgA sera, from sheep and rabbit. Surprisingly, all four samples failed to react with all of three excellent routine rabbit antiglobulin reagents made commercially in the United States. We cannot help wondering whether this is connected with the fact that no inherited anti-globulin reaction has yet, as far as we know, been found in America.

The direct positive antiglobulin reaction was no longer positive after treatment of the four samples with papain but, surprisingly, it was still strongly positive after the cells had been treated with neuraminidase: Jensen and Freiesleben[14] had reported abolition of the reaction, and Jeannet et al.[15] diminution, by treatment with neuraminidase.

Though the Swiss and the East German cells had required so precisely the same antiglobulin sera to show their direct positive reaction there were slight serological differences between them. The Swiss cells, R_1r and rr, when suspended in saline reacted with selected incomplete anti-Rh sera but the East German, R_1R_2, cells did not. The Swiss and East German cells were alike in giving the normal En(a+) reaction, and all four samples were negative with extracts of Sophora japonica.

It is difficult to say what is the primary cause of this inherited positive direct antiglobulin reaction: the Swiss authors[15] suggested that an alteration of red cell sialic acid metabolism has led to the antiglobulin reaction and to the weak M or N. If this were so the gene controlling the alteration of sialic acid must be part of, or very closely linked to, the MN locus, otherwise we would expect to find weak M and weak N members of the same family. This has not been observed: in each informative family the same weak M or weak N has travelled with the anti-globulin reaction though had linkage not been close the families could have shown recombination on eight occasions. So perhaps it is easier to think that the rare MN alleles are themselves responsible for the reaction, by changing the cell surface, perhaps by failing to contribute some substance related to sialic acid which normal MN alleles provide.

REFERENCES

1 DARNBOROUGH J., DUNSFORD I. and WALLACE JOSEPHINE A. (1965) The En factor. A genetical modification of human red cells affecting their blood grouping reactions. Programme, Brit. Soc. Haemat. Meeting, p. 28.
2 DARNBOROUGH J., DUNSFORD I. and WALLACE JOSEPHINE A. (1969) The En^a antigen and antibody. A genetical modification of human red cells affecting their blood grouping reactions. Vox Sang., 17, 241–255.
3 FURUHJELM U., MYLLYLÄ G., NEVANLINNA H.R., NORDLING S., PIRKOLA ANNA, GAVIN JUNE, GOOCH ANN, SANGER RUTH and TIPPETT PATRICIA (1969) The red cell phenotype En(a–) and anti-En^a: serological and physicochemical aspects. Vox Sang., 17, 256–278.
4 FURUHJELM U., NEVANLINNA H.R. and PIRKOLA ANNA (1973) A second Finnish En(a–) propositus with anti-En^a. Vox Sang., 24, 545–549.
5 METAXAS M.N. and METAXAS-BÜHLER M. (1972) The detection of MNSs 'variants' in serial tests with incomplete Rh antisera in saline. Vox Sang., 22, 474–477.
6 TIPPETT PATRICIA and TEESDALE PHYLLIS (1973) Limited blood group tests on samples from two coelacanths (Latimeria chalumnae). Vox Sang., 24, 175–178.

[7] MYLLYLÄ G., FURUHJELM U., NORDLING S., PIRKOLA ANNA, TIPPETT PATRICIA, GAVIN JUNE and SANGER RUTH (1971) Persistent mixed field polyagglutinability. Electrokinetic and serological aspects. *Vox Sang.*, **20**, 7–23.

[8] HERZ F., KAPLAN E. and FURUHJELM U. (1972) Acetylcholinesterase activity in En(a−) red cells. *Vox Sang.*, **23**, 228–231.

[9] SANGER RUTH and RACE R.R. (1971) Immunogenetics of certain antigens of the red cell membrane. *Nouv. Rev. franc. Hémat.*, **11**, 878–884.

[10] SANGER RUTH (1970) Genetics of blood groups. In: *Blood and Tissue Antigens*, ed. D. Aminoff, N.Y. Acad. Press Inc., pp. 17–31.

[11] NORDLING S., SANGER RUTH, GAVIN JUNE, FURUHJELM U., MYLLYLÄ G. and METAXAS M.N. (1969) M^k and M^g: some serological and physicochemical observations. *Vox Sang.*, **17**, 300–302.

[12] STURGEON P., METAXAS-BÜHLER M., METAXAS M.N., TIPPETT PATRICIA and IKIN E.W. (1970) An erroneous exclusion of paternity in a Chinese family exhibiting the rare MNSs gene complexes M^k and Ms^{III}. *Vox Sang.*, **18**, 395–406.

[13] METAXAS-BÜHLER M., CLEGHORN T.E., ROMANSKI J. and METAXAS M.N. (1966) Studies on the blood group antigen M^g. II. Serology of M^g. *Vox Sang.*, **11**, 170–183.

[14] JENSEN K.G. and FREIESLEBEN E. (1962) Inherited positive Coombs' reaction connected with a weak N-receptor (N_2). *Vox Sang.*, **7**, 696–703.

[15] JEANNET M., METAXAS-BÜHLER M. and TOBLER R. (1963) Anomalie héréditaire de la membrane érythrocytaire avec test de Coombs positif et modification de l'antigène de groupe N. *Schweiz. med. Wschr.*, **93**, 1508–1509, and (1964) *Vox Sang.*, **9**, 52–55.

[16] JAKOBOWICZ RACHEL, BRYCE LUCY M. and SIMMONS R.T. (1949) The occurrence of unusual positive Coombs reactions and M variants in the blood of a mother and her first child. *Med. J. Aust.*, **2**, 945–948.

[17] FÜNFHAUSEN G. and VELHAGEN H. (1970) Personal communication.

[18] BIRD G.W.G. and WINGHAM JUNE (1973) The action of seed and other reagents on En(a−) erythrocytes. *Vox Sang.*, **24**, 48–57.

Chapter 23
Some Other Antigens

In this chapter we have collected certain antigens which have presented special difficulties and have been the cause of a great deal of rather frustrating work. Troublesome characteristics common to most of them are: (i) The antigens may 'skip' a generation though they appear to be dominant characters: the gene or genes responsible may be said to be incomplete in their penetrance. (ii) There may be intermediate reactions which are difficult to classify and these weaker reactions may be observed amongst the relatives of strong reactors: the gene or genes responsible may be said to be variable in their expressivity. (iii) The weaker reactions are not always reproducible.

However, the air has been cleared by the use of newer techniques and by the growing realization that the antigens properly belong to the white cells and have merely spilled over onto the red.

THE Bg ANTIGENS

In our fourth edition we ventured the opinion that three difficult antigens known for years and called Ot[1], Ho[2] and 'Bennett-Goodspeed-Sturgeon or Donna'[3, 4] belonged to the same complex. Beautiful work at Oxford[5] on this rather intractable material established and clarified the relationship. The key to this success was the use by Seaman, Benson, Jones, Morton and Pickles[5] (1967) of the Auto-Analyser (optical density system) and in this original paper three antibodies are distinguished, and a fourth, anti-Bg^{b+c} was added later[9]; and a fifth, previously called anti-Stobo[6], was shown very probably to belong to the Bg system. The following scheme could be drawn:

	anti-Bg^a	anti-Bg^{a+b}	anti-Bg^{a+b+c}	anti-Bg^{b+c}
Bg(a+)	+	+	+	−
Bg(b+)	−	+	+	+
Bg(c+)	−	−	+	+
Bg neg	−	−	−	−

The antigen Bg^a was found to be much commoner than Bg^b or Bg^c and if the system

475

is reduced to two phenotypes Bg(a+) and Bg(a−) it becomes a manageable poly-morphism. In tests on 72 Oxonians 21 were Bg(a+), and an estimate of the gene frequencies is Bg^a 0·159 and Bg 0·841. Thirty families showed the antigen Bg^a to be inherited as a dominant character and showed the Bg locus not to be part of the loci for ABO, MNSs, P, Rh, Lutheran, Kell, Duffy and Kidd and not to be X-borne. The Bg^a antigen was found to be only partially developed at birth.

The next advance came again from Oxford, when it was shown that the Bg antigens were rather pale reflections on the red cells of HL-A antigens on the leucocytes. Morton, Pickles and Sutton[10] (1969) found that the Bg^a group 'shows almost complete concordance with the histocompatibility group HL-A7'. This and the earlier discovery of Rosenfield et al.[17] (1967) that anti-leucocyte sera could have haemagglutinating properties was a great step towards understanding this difficult Bg system. In 1971 Morton, Pickles, Sutton and Skov[11] found that while Bg^a corresponded to HL-A7, so Bg^b corresponded to W17 (Te57) and Bg^c to W28 (Ba* Da15). A further haemagglutinin in some multispecific antisera reacted with the red cells of HL-A10 positive donors.

Swanson[12] (1973) in confirming this work detected further HL-A antigens on red cells. No attempt was made to correlate the additional HL-A types with the Bg subgroups. That HL-A substances are present in normal serum has evidently been known for some time and Swanson makes the interesting observation that Bg(a−) red cells can be changed into Bg(a+) by incubation in Bg(a+) plasma. An interesting account of the Bg system is to be found in Joan Marshall's thesis[22].

The incidence of Bg antibodies in routine blood grouping sera[23] and in the sera of donors and patients[24] has recently been estimated.

The Bg antibodies have emerged as potentially useful and certainly interesting, after years of being merely troublesome contaminants of routine grouping sera. Their importance may be judged from the concluding paragraph of Morton et al.[11]

'The Bg^b and Bg^c antigens as well as Bg^a are important in transplantation immunology in that the presence of haemagglutinins may draw attention to the presence of antibodies which give feeble reaction in the cytotoxic test. Prospective recipients with preformed cytotoxic anti-bodies should be tested on the AutoAnalyzer using strongly reacting cells and matched with their donors for the antigens W28 and W17 and HL-A7 and HL-A10 since it is possible that they may have antibodies only reacting by haemagglutination. It would also be interesting to look for haemagglutinating antibodies in recipients who have rejected apparently compatible kidneys.'

THE ANTIGEN CHIDO (Ch^a)

Several examples of an antibody which had caused a lot of worry at cross-matching were brought together by Harris, Tegoli, Swanson, Fisher, Gavin and Noades[8] (1967). It was described as 'nebulous' and called anti-Chido because its haziness seemed scarcely to justify a more concrete symbol. The authors wrote 'More than 2,000 prospective donors were tested in New York and only two, or perhaps three, fairly convincing negatives were found. However, we may assume that the makers of the Chido type of antibody are themselves truly negative.'

The next steps were taken in Canada: Middleton[13] showed that Chido positive people had Chido substance in their plasma, independent in amount of the strength of the Chido reactivity of their red cells. Using plasma inhibition of anti-Chido as an index Middleton and Crookston[14] found 11 of 639 (1·7%) Toronto donors to be Chido negative which agreed well with later series[15, 16]. The red cells of newborn children too often lacked the antigen but their plasma had it as frequently and as strongly as in adults.

Molthan[15] converted Chido negative red cells by incubating them with Chido positive plasma, and this was confirmed by Swanson[12]. However, Crookston and her colleagues (personal communication, 1974) found that transfused O, Chido negative cells did not take up Chido substance *in vivo*, though they did take up A_1Le^b, after 12 days in the circulation of a Chido positive, A_1, Le(b+) recipient.

Swanson[12] further showed that anti-Chido could be absorbed by leucocytes from Chido positive, but not from Chido negative people.

Humphreys et al.[16] reported that families classified for the presence or absence of Chido antigen in their plasma showed *Chido* to be genetically independent of the loci for ABO, MNSs, Rh, Duffy, Kidd and secretor.

A family tested at the Toronto General Hospital by Miss Janice Middleton and Mrs Marie Crookston in 1972 gave a strong hint of linkage between *Chido* and *HL-A*, and this led to a large combined investigation in several countries (Middleton et al.[21], 1974). The triumphant outcome was the clear demonstration that *Chido*, now awarded the symbol *Ch*, is indeed linked to *HL-A*, the odds in favour of linkage being calculated to be 1,450,000 to 1. The estimate of the recombination fraction between *Ch* and *LA* was $4\frac{1}{2}\%$, and that between *Ch* and *Four* was $1\frac{1}{2}\%$. On the assumption that the recombination fraction between *LA* and *Four* is 1%, the most likely order of the loci was thought to be *LA, Four, Ch*.

The HL-A groups of unrelated Ch(a−) people gave a hint of an association, in that there seemed to be too many with the Four antigens W5 and 12. If this were not due to chance the authors[21] suggested it could be explained by linkage disequilibrium.

The finding by Middleton and Crookston of Chido substance in serum or plasma of Chido positive people and the development of a routine method for detecting it made a sharp genetical tool of the nebulous red cell antigen first recognized by Miss Jean Harris and her colleagues five years before.

THE ANTIGENS Cs^a AND Yk^a

These two antigens have much in common and very skilled work is going on to tease out their relationships.

Cs^a

In a very thorough investigation Giles, Huth, Wilson, Lewis and Grove[7] (1965) showed the Cs^a : anti-Cs^a system to be serologically distinct from practically every blood group antigen and antibody known at the time.

Anti-Cs^a reacted with the red cells of 354, or 97·5%, of 363 unrelated Europeans and from these figures the estimate of the gene frequencies was Cs^a 0·84 and Cs 0·16.

Tests on the families of three Cs(a−) propositi showed that the antigen Cs^a is, in all probability, a dominant character. Assuming this to be correct, the other groups of the families showed that the antigen Cs^a is not controlled by genes at the loci for Rh, MNSs, Duffy or Kidd: the pedigrees also excluded it being X- or Y-borne.

Marked variation in strength of the antigen was noted[7], a variation which did not correspond to the homozygous and heterozygous state. The antigen is developed at birth[7].

The antigen Yk^a (York)

This antigen from the start (Molthan, Crawford, Giles, Chudnoff and Eichman[18], 1969) was spoken of in the same breath as Cs^a. Anti-Yk^a, many examples of which were found, is evidently stimulated by transfusion but does not cause transfusion reactions. The antibody was found to react with the red cells of 95% of random donors in the United States: there was much variation in the strength of the reaction and this was not related to zygosity.

An association between Yk^a and Cs^a was assumed[18] because, although makers of anti-Yk^a were all Cs(a+) Yk(a−), the three examples of anti-Cs^a known at the time were from Cs(a−) Yk(a−) people.

Little has been published about Cs^a and Yk^a since the original papers and we gather there is some disagreement about what has been published[12]: this is not surprising, for difficulties are to be expected if the present opinion that Cs^a and Yk^a are primarily white cell antigens is correct. We hope clarification will come in time for the Addenda to this book.

Other antigens which should perhaps have found their way to this chapter are Kn^a and Gn^a (in Chapter 19).

We did not know where to place the antigen Sf^a (Stoltzfus) described by Bias et al.[19] (1969): it was used as a marker character in a linkage investigation of the nail-patella syndrome and the enzyme adenylate kinase (Schleutermann et al.[20], 1969) but there were many exceptions to straightforward dominant inheritance in the families. Perhaps Sf^a is primarily an antigen of the white cells.

REFERENCES

[1]   DORFMEIER HANNY, HART MIA V.D., NIJENHUIS L.E. and LOGHEM J.J. VAN (1959) A 'new' blood group antigen of rare occurrence (Ot). *Proc. 7th Congr. int. soc. Blood Transf.*, 608–610.

2   HART MIA V.D., MOES MEIKE, VEER MARGA V.D. and LOGHEM J.J. VAN (1961) Ho and Lan-
    two new blood group antigens. Paper read at the VIIIth Europ. Cong. Haemat.

3   BUCHANAN D.I. and AFAGANIS A. (1963) The Bennett-Goodspeed-Sturgeon or 'Donna' red
    cell antigen and antibody. Vox Sang., 8, 213–218.

4   CHOWN B., LEWIS MARION and KAITA HIROKO (1963) The Bennett-Goodspeed antigen or
    antigens. Vox Sang., 8, 281–288.

5   SEAMAN M.J., BENSON R., JONES M.N., MORTON J.A. and PICKLES M.M. (1967) The reac-
    tions of the Bennett-Goodspeed group of antibodies with the Auto Analyser. Brit. J.
    Haemat., 13, 464–473.

6   WALLACE J. and MILNE G.R. (1959) A 'new' human blood group antigen of rare frequency.
    Proc. 7th Congr. int. Soc. Blood Transf., 587–589.

7   GILES CAROLYN M., HUTH M.C., WILSON T.E., LEWIS H.B.M. and GROVE G.E.B. (1965)
    Three examples of a new antibody anti-Cs^a, which reacts with 98 % of red cell samples.
    Vox Sang., 10, 405–415.

8   HARRIS JEAN P., TEGOLI J., SWANSON JANE, FISHER NATHALIE, GAVIN JUNE and NOADES JEAN
    (1967) A nebulous antibody responsible for cross-matching difficulties (Chido). Vox Sang.,
    12, 140–142.

9   KISSMEYER-NIELSEN F. and GAVIN JUNE (1967) Unpublished observations.

10 MORTON J.A., PICKLES M.M. and SUTTON L. (1969) The correlation of the Bg^a blood group
    with the HL-A7 leucocyte group: demonstration of antigenic sites on red cells and leuco-
    cytes. Vox Sang., 17, 536–547.

11 MORTON J.A., PICKLES M.M., SUTTON L. and SKOV F. (1971) Identification of further anti-
    gens on red cells and lymphocytes. Vox Sang., 21, 144–153.

12 SWANSON JANE L. (1973) Laboratory problems associated with leukocyte antibodies. In
    A Seminar on Recent Advances in Immunohematology. AABB, Bal Harbour, Florida,
    121–155.

13 MIDDLETON J. (1972) Anti-Chido: a cross-matching problem. Can. J. med. Technol., 34, 41–62.

14 MIDDLETON JANICE and CROOKSTON MARIE C. (1972) Chido-substance in plasma. Vox
    Sang., 23, 256–261.

15 MOLTHAN L. (1972) The Chido antigen—some developments. Abstracts AABB and ISH
    Meeting, Washington, p. 57.

16 HUMPHREYS JUNE, STOUT T.D., MIDDLETON JANICE and CROOKSTON MARIE C. (1972) The
    identification of Chido-negative donors by a plasma-inhibition test. Abstracts AABB,
    and ISH Meeting, Washington, p. 57.

17 ROSENFIELD R.E., RUBINSTEIN P., LALEZARI P., DAUSSET J. and VAN ROOD J.J. (1967)
    Hemagglutination by human anti-leukocyte serums. Vox Sang., 13, 461–466.

18 MOLTHAN L., CRAWFORD M.N., GILES C.M., CHUDNOFF A. and EICHMAN M.F. (1969) A
    new antibody, anti-Yk^a (York) and its relationship to anti-Cs^a (Cost-Sterling). Trans-
    fusion, Philad., 9, 281.

19 BIAS WILMA B., LIGHT-ORR JEANNETTE K., KREVANS J.R., HUMPHREY R.L., HAMILL P.V.V.,
    COHEN BERNICE H. and MCKUSICK V.A. (1969) The Stoltzfus blood group, a new poly-
    morphism in man. Amer. J. hum. Genet., 21, 552–558.

20 SCHLEUTERMANN DONNA A., BIAS WILMA B., LAMONT-MURDOCH J. and MCKUSICK V.A.
    (1969) Linkage of the loci for the nail-patella syndrome and adenylate kinase. Amer. J.
    hum. Genet., 21, 606–630.

21 MIDDLETON JANICE, CROOKSTON MARIE C., FALK JUDITH A., ROBSON ELIZABETH B., COOK
    P.J.L., BATCHELOR J.R., BODMER JULIA, FERRARA G.B., FESTENSTEIN H., HARRIS R.
    KISSMEYER-NIELSEN F., LAWLER SYLVIA D., SACHS J.A. and WOLF EVA (1974) Linkage
    of Chido and HL-A. Tissue Antigens, 4, 366–373.

22 MARSHALL JOAN V. (1973) The Bg antigens and antibodies. Can. J. med. Technol., 35, 26–35.

23 PAVONE BEVERLEY G. and ISSITT P.D. (1974) Anti-Bg antibodies in sera used for red cell
    typing. Brit. J. Haemat., 27, 607–611.

24 ESKA PATRICIA L. and GRINDON A.J. (1974) The high frequency of anti-Bg^a. Brit. J. Haemat.,
    27, 613–615.

Chapter 24
Miscellany

Under this heading are collected some subjects which do not easily fit into other chapters.

FISHER'S 'EXACT' METHOD FOR 2 × 2 TABLES

The two simple probability tests, the 'exact' method for 2 × 2 tables and the χ^2 test[1], are of enormous help in interpreting the results of blood group tests: they tell us what the chance is that an apparent association which we have found is merely a coincidence.

Let us take as an example the use of the 'exact' method in deciding whether a certain antibody is present in a serum when the number of tests has been rather small. Say a serum has given the following reactions:

	Known cells		
	E	*ee*	
unknown serum+	3	0	3
unknown serum−	0	2	2
	3	2	5

then we want to know whether this is convincing proof of the presence of anti-E. The answer is that the results probably do mean that anti-E is present; but they are not adequate proof, for the probability of getting such a distribution by chance alone, if the antibody had nothing to do with anti-E, is as high as 1 in 10. This is how the probability, P, is found:

$$P = \frac{3!2!2!3!}{5!} \times \frac{1}{3!2!0!0!} = \frac{1}{10}$$

For the calculation to be as straightforward as this, one of the figures for the four observations must be 0. If there is not a 0 then the calculation has to be repeated, reducing each of the two diagonal figures which are smaller than expected by one and adjusting the other two to keep the marginal totals as before. This reduction by one is repeated until 0 is reached. The probabilities are then added up. Take as an example another serum:

                        Known cells
                        E   *ee*
unknown +   4   3 | 7
serum   −   2   5 | 7
                        ───────────── $P = \dfrac{7!\,7!\,8!\,6!}{14!} \times \dfrac{1}{4!\,3!\,5!\,2!}$
                        6   8 | 14

to which must be added the probability of the more extreme cases:

                        5   2 | 7
                        1   6 | 7
                        ───────────── $P = \dfrac{7!\,7!\,8!\,6!}{14!} \times \dfrac{1}{5!\,2!\,1!\,6!}$
                        6   8 | 14

and:

                        6   1 | 7
                        0   7 | 7
                        ───────────── $P = \dfrac{7!\,7!\,8!\,6!}{14!} \times \dfrac{1}{6!\,1!\,7!\,0!}$
                        6   8 | 14

We make the answer $P = 0 \cdot 2961$; that is to say, the slight hint of association of the unknown antibody with the antigen E would be found merely by chance in about one in three such investigations.

For those with as little mathematical knowledge as the writers we may add, without, we hope, giving offence, that factorial 4 or 4! equals $4 \times 3 \times 2 \times 1$, and factorial 3 equals $3 \times 2 \times 1$, etc., though factorial 0, 0!, seems, surprisingly enough, to be 1, or nothing at all, anyhow not 0.

We have put in the 0's to show exactly where the figures in the 2×2 tables are placed in the fractions.

When larger figures are being dealt with, too large for the convenient application of this exact method, the χ^2 test is used. These two statistical methods have been of immense use to us in sorting the certain from the doubtful, in prompting the judgement.

THE χ^2 TEST

An example has already been given on page 93, and the often puzzling problem of the number of degrees of freedom has been touched upon on page 95.

The χ^2 test can also conveniently be used to decide whether two sets of data differ significantly. As an example we will take the comparison of Canadians of English descent with those of Hebrew descent (Table 80) made by Chown *et al.*[23] This method is not suitable when the figures are small, the expectation in each group should be greater than five, therefore smaller groups should be pooled. Chown and his co-workers pooled six small phenotype groups called 'the rest' in Table 80.

Table 80. Comparison of two sets of Rh data

	Observed			Expected		χ^2 $\dfrac{(o-e)^2}{e}$	
	Hebrew	English	Total	Hebrew	English	Hebrew	English
R_1r	49	265	314	$314 \times \dfrac{140}{932}$	$314 \times \dfrac{792}{932}$	0·0710	0·0125
R_1R_1	41	140	181	$181 \times \dfrac{140}{932}$	$181 \times \dfrac{792}{932}$	7·0142	1·2399
rr	11	134	145		etc.	5·3356	0·9431
R_2	7	117	124			7·2602	1·2836
R_1R_2	24	107	131			0·9483	0·1676
The rest	8	29	37			1·0708	0·1894
Total	140	792	932			25·5362 for 5 d.f.	

The dotted line can be ignored; it is an elementary aid, which we have found useful, to finding the number of degrees of freedom. It was suggested to us by Professor Penrose. The number is given by the entries to the left of the line—in this case five.

On the assumption that there is no difference between the two populations an expectation is found for each of the twelve entries. The fraction $\dfrac{(\text{obs.}-\text{exp.})^2}{\text{exp.}}$ is worked out for each of the twelve entries, and the twelve answers when added up give the total χ^2 value, for five degrees of freedom. The figure is then looked up in the table of χ^2 (page 636) from which the probability is obtained. If the probability be greater than 1 in 20 then the observed results are considered to be consistent with the assumption that there is no real difference between the samples. When the probability is very small, as it is in the present example, it is considered that a real difference exists between the samples. In the present example $\chi^2 = 25\cdot54$ for five degrees of freedom. This is off the table of χ^2. The probability of the difference being due to chance is therefore less than 1 in 1,000. The curious may want to know how much less: Professor W.C. Boyd[24] worked out a very useful nomogram for χ^2 probabilities, the probability is 1 in about 6,700.

LEVELS OF PROBABILITY

In general biological work it is customary to take 1 in 20 as the level of 'significance', that is to say, the level at which interest begins to focus on the problem and more work to be planned; this level is suited to the result of an experiment which has set out to compare two things. In blood group work we usually do not set out to compare anything, but make the comparisons *after* the work is done; the results may then be compared in many ways (fifty-five different ways in one example). The number of ways in which the work has been compared makes a big difference to the level of probability at which an observed association is considered to be 'significant'. Our general rule is not to get too excited until the probability is less than 1 in 100, but, at about that level, to begin the investigation again, on fresh material, with the one comparison in mind. Since the second investigation sets out to compare only two things, the 1 in 20 level of probability can now be considered 'significant'. However, a much lower probability should be obtained— usually with but little more work.

These reservations apply when some totally unexpected association is stumbled on. In the identification of familiar antibodies we are usually satisfied with a probability of 1 in 40 or so.

COUSIN MARRIAGES

When a person is homozygous for a rare allele, whether it be a blood group allele or not, it will often be found that his parents are cousins. This is because a rare allele is bound to be more common in the family of a person possessing it than in the general population. Conversely, on several occasions the fact that the parents of a person with a novel blood group were cousins has given a useful clue that we were dealing with a homozygote.

In England the cousin marriage rate, for hospital patients, in 1930 was about 0.6%, and there is some evidence[58] that the rate is falling, which is what we would expect to happen as people move about more and more.

Fraser Roberts[59] gives the following Lenz-Dahlberg formula for the expected percentage of cousin marriages in the parents of people homozygous for a rare gene, which we have on occasion found useful:

$$\frac{a}{a + 16p}$$

where a equals the frequency of first cousin marriages in the population as a whole and where p equals the frequency of the recessive gene in that population.

SOME SEROLOGICAL ODDITIES

This section is very incomplete, it includes only a few curiosities which have interested us over the years.

An agglutinating factor for all cells suspended in albumin

Two examples of a very rare and apparently innocuous agglutinating property in human serum were described by W. Weiner, Tovey, Gillespie, Lewis and

Holliday[2]. These sera agglutinated all cells, including the donor's own, provided they were suspended in albumin. The agglutinating factor was at first thought not to be an antibody. W. Weiner and Hallum[3] reported two more examples, and so did Marsh and Jenkins[4] who showed that the agglutinating property had neither anti-I nor anti-i specificity.

A great many publications followed. Lovett and Moore[15] (1968) considered the agglutinating factor to be an antibody of the IgG type directed against albumin adsorbed on red cells. In 1969 Golde, McGinniss and Holland[16] went further and found that the IgG antibody was directed at an antigen-antibody complex adsorbed on red cells, the antigen being albumin altered by the addition of caprylate as a stabilizer.

Agglutinating factors for all trypsinized cells

Hurley and Dacie[5] described a serum which was capable of agglutinating and lysing all samples of trypsinized cells including the donor's own (on which, incidentally, the direct antiglobulin test was negative).

An observation which was hoped to have important applications in human genetics was reported by Heistö, Harboe and Godal[28] at Stockholm in 1964. Certain normal freshly taken sera haemolysed trypsinized red cells: the ability to do so was commoner in the serum of females than of males. The frequencies fitted perfectly with those expected if the haemolytic property were an X-linked dominant character and this was supported by the few families tested: however, after much pursuit[18, 20] the X-linked discrimination could not be recaptured; the original batch of trypsin must have had a rare eclectic property (see page 594).

Agglutinating factors for all 'stored' cells

Brendemoen[6] found, in the serum of an anaemic patient, an antibody which did not agglutinate any cells freshly shed but which did agglutinate the same cells after they had been kept at 37°C. for 48 hours. The antibody could be absorbed only by the old cells.

Similar sera were described by Hougie et al.[27] and by Stratton et al.[7] who demonstrated that the reaction occurred whether the cells had aged in vivo or in vitro. Three more examples were reported by Jenkins and Marsh[29], and one more by Ozer and Chaplin[30].

Agglutinating factors for washed cells

Freiesleben and Jensen[21] reported three sera with the curious faculty of agglutinating all red cells, including the donor's own, if they had recently been washed in saline. The responsible factor behaved like an antibody.

Another serum which agglutinated red cells after they had been washed in saline was intensively studied by Harboe, Reinskou, Heistö and Björnstad[22] who concluded that the responsible factor was a γ-globulin of high molecular weight having some of the properties of the rheumatoid factor.

Antibody to cells exposed to penicillin

An antibody has been described which may agglutinate, or sensitize, red cells which have been exposed to penicillin (Ley, Harris, Brinkley, Liles, Jack and Cahan[8-10]). The antibody was found in the serum of eight out of 55 hospital patients: it was found in the serum of four out of 1,893 normal blood donors. All eight patients and two of the four donors were known to have had penicillin injections, the other two donors were not available for questioning.

The antibody was subsequently studied by others[11, 17, 19, 31-33].

The Matuhasi-Ogata phenomenon

The Matuhasi-Ogata phenomenon of non-specific antibody adherence to an antibody-antigen complex as an explanation of apparent cross-reactivity of blood group antibodies[25, 26, 34, 35] was referred to in the ABO chapter, page 50. It has been invoked to explain some unexpected eluates involving anti-I (Svardal et al.[36]), anti-Bg^a (Furuhjelm et al.[61]), anti-Bg^b (Wilkinson et al.[100]) and various multispecific antisera (Allen et al[85]). Bove, Holburn and Mollison[86], 1973, using Iodine-labelled reagents, provided a fresh outlook on the phenomenon and they conclude:

'In confirmation of much previous work, it was found that red cells took up appreciable amounts of IgG non-specifically; however, this uptake was not increased by previous coating of the red cells with specific antibody. When the IgG taken up non-specifically included a blood-group antibody in relatively high concentration, an eluate subsequently prepared from the red cells contained sufficient of the antibody to be detectable. Thus, the finding of unexpected antibodies in eluates may be due to non-specific uptake of IgG rather than to adherence of antibodies to antigen–antibody complexes.'

Hybrid antigen in the rabbit

In the rabbit there is a series of alleles Hg^A, Hg^D and Hg^F which produce distinct red cell antigens: however, the heterozygote $Hg^A Hg^D$ produces antigen A and D and a third antigen called I (Cohen[12-14]). This kind of trans interaction has not yet been recognized in man but it should be looked out for.

The HEMPAS abnormality

This is an abbreviation for hereditary erythroblastic multinuclearity with positive acidified serum test, and it is an uncommon recessive type of anaemia investigated by the Crookstons and their colleagues[87, 88]: it is of interest from the blood grouping point of view because the cells of affected people are agglutinated, and lysed, by an antibody present in the serum of most adults. Although HEMPAS cells have elevated i antigen, anti-i is not the culprit because the antibody in normal sera is removed by absorption with HEMPAS cells but not by absorption by adult or or cord i cells. It is hard to know where to place this well investigated phenomenon. HEMPAS cells do not fit any of the classes of polyagglutinability described below; T was excluded at an early stage[87] and our Unit, amongst no doubt other laboratories, who have been given the chance to test such cells, find no relation to Tn, Sd^a, En^a or Pr (Sp$_1$, HD).

Cold agglutinins recognizing Pr (Sp$_1$ or HD)

In 1968 and 1969 Marsh and Jenkins[89] and Roelcke[90] independently described the reactions of cold auto-agglutinins which were different from anti-I or anti-i (Chapter 21): the former workers called the culprit antigen Sp$_1$, the latter HD, but the name now seems to be settling down to Pr.

Anti-Pr, so far as we know not yet found in healthy people, may easily be distinguished from other cold agglutinins because its reaction is completely inhibited if the test cells are pretreated with ficin (or several other enzymes). Anti-Pr is sensitive to variations of the pH and ionic strength of the red cell suspending medium, maximum activity being around pH 6·2.

The placing of Pr in this book was difficult, for strictly and genetically speaking it is not a blood group in that no person lacking the antigen has been found. However, Pr must be remembered whenever antisera to 'public'antigens are being investigated. For example, we found that En(a−) cells can appear to be Pr negative with some anti-Pr sera, but En(a−) cells have the attribute of behaving like enzyme treated normal cells: however, if the pH of the suspending fluid is adjusted to 6·2, then En(a−) cells are clearly Pr positive[94].

Since Pr is not a polymorphic blood group, we shall confine ourselves to giving some further informative references to the subject[91−99, 101].

POLYAGGLUTINABILITY

Red cells which have been altered in some way and have become agglutinable by normal ABO compatible sera are said to be polyagglutinable. The condition, a rare cause of blood grouping difficulty, has been investigated for more than forty years but has come in for much attention during the last five or so years.

T and anti-T

It seems that this type of polyagglutinability is usually associated with infection by micro-organisms: it can happen *in vitro* or *in vivo*.

In vitro infection of a sample of blood may change the cells in such a way that they can thereafter be agglutinated by all sera. This has come to be known as the

Hübener-Thomsen-Friedenreich phenomenon (see Friedenreich[37], 1930). Filtrates of certain bacteria contain an enzyme which acts on human red cells and transforms a latent antigen into an active one; this antigen Friedenreich called T. Friedenreich[37] found anti-T to be present in all adult sera but 'absent in serum of newborns and infants'. Anti-T can be removed from the serum by absorption with cells whose T antigen has been activated. The enzyme used nowadays to activate the T antigen of red cells, one produced by many viruses and bacteria, is neuraminidase (the 'receptor destroying enzyme' RDE): neuraminidase splits neuraminic acid from sialo-mucoproteins exposing the T antigen on the cell surface (for many references see Klenk and Uhlenbruck[62], Uhlenbruck[55], Springer[63]).

An observation of great practical importance was that extracts of peanuts (*Arachis hypogea*) contained powerful anti-T agglutinin for RDE treated cells (Bird[57]). Apart from being a research tool *Arachis* can sometimes be very useful in detecting infection as a cause of unusual blood group reactions given by old or much travelled samples. Work with this extract and with human and animal anti-T led Uhlenbruck *et al.*[64] to conclude that 'Terminal non-reducing β-D-galactoside structures are involved in the specificity of the so called T antigen.'

In vivo polyagglutinability of red cells was first described by Levine and Katzin[38] in 1938. In this and most of the subsequent cases there is a story of infection by some organism. The proportion of normal sera which can agglutinate such cells may vary during the course of the illness. If the patient recovers the polyagglutinability wears off. The agglutination does not usually occur at temperatures as high as 37°C. Polyagglutinable cells can absorb their corresponding agglutinin from the sera that agglutinate them. An example from our records is included in Table 81.

Many cases of polyagglutinable cells of the *in vivo* type have been described[38-54]. Henningsen[43] concluded that the antibody active for the cells of his case was the anti-T agglutinin of Friedenreich; so did Holländer[46], van Loghem and his colleagues[44, 51], and Chorpenning and Hayes[54]. Jørgensen[60] investigated a newborn infant of whose red cells about 10% were polyagglutinable: at two weeks of age very few polyagglutinable cells were to be found.

Examples of T activation are seldom nowadays reported except when they are included as controls in Tn investigations[75, 71]. Dr Halvorsen of Bergen sent us a sample from a patient with two populations of red cells, but other facts did not fit a chimera. It turned out that this group O patient's cells were polyagglutinable and the polyagglutinability, of the T type, was wearing off: newly launched cells, separated by centrifugation, unlike the older cells, were not polyagglutinable. The polyagglutination was, on the average, more clearly shown by sera containing anti-A than by sera lacking anti-A, hence giving the appearance of an A:O mixture. We first noticed this affinity of polyagglutinable cells (O or B) for anti-A in work[65] on Tn.

In 1972, Bird and Wingham[66] reported a case of transient polyagglutinability, associated with gross infection, which did not fit the T:anti-T situation in all respects. The patient's cells were agglutinated by sera from which anti-T had been removed. The antigen and antibody involved were named Tk and anti-Tk.

Table 81. Effects of absorbing an AB serum by various cells: normal, RDE treated normal, T, Tn and Cad (from MRC Blood Group Unit records)

Cells	AB serum from adult					
	unab-sorbed	abs. × normal	abs. × RDE	abs. × T poly.	abs. × Tn poly.	abs. × Cad
normal	−	−	−	−	−	−
normal RDE treated	+	+	−	−	+	+
T polyagg.	+	+	−	−	+	
Tn polyagg.	+	+	+	+	−	+
Cad	+	+	+	+	+	−

Tn and anti-Tn

This kind of polyagglutinability differs from that due to the antigen T not only serologically but in being persistent and not transient: it is not associated with gross infection, but rather with haematological upsets such as acquired haemolytic anaemia, leucopenia and thrombocytopenia and may be found in people described as always healthy. Some of the ways of distinguishing Tn from T are shown in Tables 81 and 82.

Table 82. Some simple distinctions between T, Tn and Cad cells (from MRC Blood Group Unit records)

Reagent	Normal cells		Polyagglutinable cells		
	un-treated	RDE treated	T	Tn	Cad
AB serum	−	+	+	+	+
AB serum v. papainized cells	−	+	+	−	+
Arachis extract	−	+	+	−	−
Dolichos extract*	−	−	−	+	+
Bauhinia extract**	−			+	−

* For non-A_1 cells.
** Used at dilution at which the anti-N component is no longer active.

Moreau, Dausset, Bernard and Moullec[56, 67] in 1957 and 1959 reported a fine investigation of a patient with acquired haemolytic anaemia who for 9 years had polyagglutinable cells. The agglutination was due not to T but to a previously unknown antigen which they named Tn. All adult sera (490 were tested) contained anti-Tn. The antigen Tn was not found in 23 relatives of the patient.

Two further examples of polyagglutinability due to Tn were reported by van der Hart et al.[68], again in patients with acquired haemolytic anaemia. The next example was of particular interest: in 1962 Freiesleben, Jensen and Knudsen[69] described a healthy blood donor, investigated for over two years, who persisted in showing a 'mixed field' polyagglutinability, only one fifth of his cells being affected. The agglutination was shown not to be due to anti-T. Neither parent had the condition, nor had a sister.

The finding of another example of persistent mixed field polyagglutinability, in Finland, precipitated an investigation which lasted over four years in Helsinki and, towards the end, in London and which resulted in several new contributions to the subject: for example, the polyagglutinable cells, about 50 % of the total, were found to have reduced electrophoretic mobility and sialic acid content[70]. The histogram in Figure 30 shows the result of mobility tests on the native cell sample and on samples following attempts to separate the two components. It was further

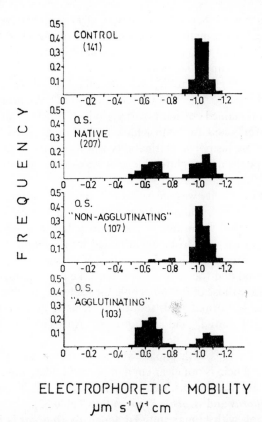

Fig. 30. Electrophoretic mobility of the cells of a donor (Mr OS) with mixed field polyagglutinability due to Tn. Measurements before and after attempts to separate the two components by serological means. The figures in brackets show the number of cells timed. (From Myllylä et al.[71], 1971.)

observed that group O and group B cells with the T or Tn type of polyagglutinability were on the average more strongly agglutinated by sera containing anti-A
than by sera lacking it. This is an important practical point for the predilection for
anti-A led to what was thought to be an A:O chimera[72] being recognized as a case
of group O mixed cell polyagglutinability[65, 71, 73]. We suspect that it also led to the
report of a case of polyagglutinability with acquired A, though the investigators
did not agree with this, and for a good reason[77], but still we are in doubt.

At about the same time, 1969 onwards, there was a burst of activity in this
previously rather neglected field and it is almost impossible to sort out who found
what first: Tn was being investigated in Finland[70, 71], England[75, 76, 78] and the
States[72–74, 77]. Although it was pointed out that Tn might be an umbrella name
covering more than one antigen antibody system[71] the examples about to be referred to have reacted, almost without exception, alike in the many tests to which
they have been exposed. From these and the earlier papers the main points to
emerge are:

1 The condition is not inherited: 88 relatives of 11 propositi were all normal.
2 Haematological abnormalities were found in 8 of the 11, 4 had haemolytic
anaemia[56, 67, 68, 77], 4 had thrombocytopenia and or leucopenia[74–76, 78] but were
mostly in good health, and 3 were healthy[69–73].
3 In 6 cases the polyagglutinability was general[56, 67, 68, 74, 75, 77] and in 5 it was
of the mixed-field type[69–73, 76, 78]. With one exception[76], the proportion of polyagglutinable cells remained constant over periods of observation never less than
one year. (However, one case[74] must have been normal when he was a blood
donor 10 years before his polyagglutinability was recognized.) In one example of
the mixed field type the non-agglutinable cells were intensively studied and found
not to be normal[71].
4 Electrophoretic mobility was measured in 6 cases and found to be reduced in
all of them[70, 71, 73, 74, 76, 78]. Sialic acid was estimated in 4 cases and in all of them
it was reduced[70, 71, 74, 77, 78]; in one of these cases sialic acid shortage was confirmed by failure of the cells to be agglutinated by polybrene[78].
5 The T antigen of the red cells and the anti-T of the serum of practically all the
propositi were tested and found to be normal. Like anti-T, anti-Tn was present
in all adult sera, save those of the Tn people themselves: it is absent from or very
weak in cord sera. In normal adult sera there seems to be no relationship[79] between the titre of anti-T and of anti-Tn. Anti-Tn can be induced in
rabbits[56, 67, 71, 75].
6 Treatment of Tn cells with papain abolishes their polyagglutinability, the
effect of trypsin and ficin is not clear cut and neuraminidase has no effect[71, 75].
7 Seed extracts are useful in distinguishing Tn from T[71, 78, 80], particularly those
from *Dolichos biflorus* and *Arachis hypogea* (see Table 82).
8 The Tn reaction with human anti-Tn and with *Dolichos* is inhibited by *N*-
acetyl-D-galactosamine alone of many sugars tried[71, 78].
9 The survival of a Tn person's cells in his own circulation was found to be normal, which was not surprising for he lacked anti-Tn. The survival of the same cells

in a normal volunteer was notably shortened, presumably because of his anti-Tn[71]. Normal cells were found to survive normally in a Tn polyagglutinable person, indicating that the defect originates in the marrow[74]; and this fitted the observation, in another case[71], that newly launched cells showed the same mixed field picture as did older cells.

Since this rather condensed summary was written more papers on Tn have appeared[102-109], some of them emphasize the effect of the Tn condition on the M and N antigens[103, 104, 109], a subject which we have not included in our summary: others[106-108] report the usefulness of various *Salvia* seed extracts as a diagnostic tool in helping to distinguish the various kinds of polyagglutinability.

Cad 'polyagglutinability'

So far, outside Tables 81 and 82, there has been no mention in this account of polyagglutinable red cells of the Cad type described by Cazal, Monis, Caubel and Brives[81] (1968) in a paper which helped to stimulate much of the recent enthusiasm for polyagglutination in general.

The Cad type of polyagglutination, which is unlike the other types in being an inherited character, appears in Tables 81 and 82 because it is usually brought into discussions of the diagnosis of different types of polyagglutinability[71,75,78,80,82,83]. However, following the recognition of the relationship of Cad to the Sid blood group system by Sanger, Gavin, Tippett, Teesdale and Eldon[84] (1971) it became clear that Cad polyagglutination is fundamentally different from that of T and Tn, and our account has been given in Chapter 17 on the Sid groups.

REFERENCES

[1] FISHER R.A. *Statistical Methods for Research Workers*, many editions, Oliver & Boyd Edinburgh.

[2] WEINER W., TOVEY G.H., GILLESPIE E.M., LEWIS H.B.M. and HOLLIDAY T.D.S. (1956) 'Albumin' auto-agglutinating property in three sera. 'A pitfall for the unwary'. *Vox Sang.*, **1**, 279–288.

[3] WEINER W. and HALLUM JEAN L. (1957) A further 'albumin' auto-agglutinating serum, *Vox Sang.*, **2**, 38–42.

[4] MARSH W.L. and JENKINS W.J. (1961) A possible specificity of albumin auto-antibodies. *Nature Lond.*, **190**, 180.

[5] HURLEY T.H. and DACIE J.V. (1953) Haemolysis and reversible agglutination of trypsinized normal red cells by a normal human serum. *J. clin. Path.*, **6**, 211–214.

[6] BRENDEMOEN O.J. (1952) A cold agglutinin specifically active against stored red cells. *Acta path. microbiol. scand.*, **31**, 574–578.

[7] STRATTON F., RENTON P.H. and RAWLINSON VIOLET I. (1960) Serological difference between old and young cells. *Lancet*, **i**, 1388–1390.

[8] LEY A.B., HARRIS JEAN P., BRINKLEY MARY, LILES BOBBIE, JACK J.A. and CAHAN A. (1957) An agglutinin active against penicillin-treated normal human erythrocytes. *Prog. 10th Ann. Meeting Amer. Ass. Blood Banks*, Chicago.

[9] LEY A.B., HARRIS JEAN P., BRINKLEY MARY, LILES BOBBIE, JACK J.A. and CAHAN A. (1958) Circulating antibody directed against penicillin. *Science*, **127**, 1118–1119.

[10] LEY A.B., CAHAN A. and MAYER K. (1959) A circulating antibody directed against penicillin. *Proc. 7th Congr. int. Soc. Blood Transf.*, 539–541.

[11] BIRD G.W.G. (1960) Penicillin antibody. *J. clin. Path.*, **13**, 51–53.

[12] COHEN C. (1956) Occurrence of three red blood cell antigens in rabbit as the result of interaction of two genes. *Science*, **123**, 935–936.

[13] COHEN C. (1958) Influences upon the agglutinability of rabbit erythrocytes in the presence of iso-antibody: genetic factors. *J. Immunol.*, **80**, 73–76.

[14] COHEN C. (1960) A second example of a rabbit red blood cell antigen resulting from the interaction of two genes. *J. Immunol.*, **84**, 501–506.

[15] LOVETT CECILE A. and MOORE B.P.L. (1968) Pan- and auto-agglutination in albumin: a serological and immunochemical study of five cases. *Immunology*, **14**, 357–365.

[16] GOLDE D.W., McGINNISS M.H. and HOLLAND P.V. (1969) Mechanism of the albumin agglutination phenomenon. *Vox Sang.*, **16**, 465–469.

[17] ASCARI W.Q. and GORMAN J.G. (1969) Hemagglutinating antipenicillin antibodies (HAPA). Incidence and significance in four groups of patients. *Transfusion, Philad.*, **9**, 35–42.

[18] HEISTØ H., JENSEN LEILA and KNUDS F. (1971) Studies on trypsin treatment of red cells with special reference to differences between trypsin preparations. *Vox Sang.*, **21**, 115–125.

[19] WATSON K.C., JOUBERT S.M. and BENNETT M.A.E. (1960) The occurrence of haemagglutinating antibody to penicillin. *Immunology*, **3**, 1–10.

[20] HEISTØ H., JENSEN LEILA and KNUDS F. (1972) Warm haemolysins active against trypsinized red cells. Stability in the frozen state, reproduceability of results and fluctuations *in vivo*. *Vox Sang.*, **22**, 131–136.

[21] FREIESLEBEN E. and JENSEN K.G. (1960) An antibody specific for washed red cells. *Proc. 7th Congr. europ. Soc. Haemat.*, part II, 1156–1158.

[22] HARBOE M., REINSKOU T., HEISTÖ H. and BJÖRNSTAD P. (1961) Studies on a serum with peculiar haemagglutinating properties. *Vox Sang.*, **6**, 409–428.

[23] CHOWN B., PETERSON R.F., LEWIS MARION and HALL ANN (1949) On the ABO gene and Rh chromosome distribution in the White population of Manitoba. *Canad. J. Res., E.*, **27**, 214–225.

[24] BOYD W.C. (1965) A nomogram for chi-square. *J. Amer. statist. Ass.*, **60**, 344–346.

[25] MATUHASI T. (1959) Plasma protein and antibody fractions observed from the serological point of view. *Proc. 15th Gen. Assembly Jap. med. Congr.*, Tokyo, **4**, 80–87. Not seen.

[26] OGATA T. and MATUHASI T. (1962) Problems of specific and cross reactivity of blood group antibodies. *Proc. 8th Congr. int. Soc. Blood Transf.*, Tokyo 1960, 208–211.

[27] HOUGIE C., DANDRIDGE JANET and BOBBITT O.B. (1959) A new autoagglutinin against stored erythrocytes. *Proc. 7th Congr. int. Soc. Blood Transf.*, Rome 1958, 252–254.

[28] HEISTÖ H., HARBOE M. and GODAL H.C. (1965) Warm haemolysins active against trypsinized red cells; occurrence, inheritance, and clinical significance. *Proc. 10th Congr. int. Soc. Blood Transf.*, Stockholm 1964, 787–789.

[29] JENKINS W.J. and MARSH W.L. (1961) Autoimmune haemolytic anaemia. Three cases with antibodies specifically active against stored red cells. *Lancet*, **ii**, 16–18.

[30] OZER F.L. and CHAPLIN H. (1963) Agglutination of stored erythrocytes by a human serum. Characterization of the serum factor and erythrocyte changes. *J. clin. Invest.*, **42**, 1735–1752.

[31] FUDENBERG H.H. and GERMAN J.L. (1960) Certain physical and biologic characteristics of penicillin antibody. *Blood*, **15**, 683–689.

[32] WATSON K.C. (1964) The nature of antiglobulin reactivity of antibody to penicillin. *Immunology*, **7**, 97–109.

[33] CLAYTON E.M., ALTSHULER J. and BOVE J.R. (1965) Penicillin antibody as a cause of positive direct antiglobulin tests. *Amer. J. clin. Path.*, **44**, 648–653.

[34] MATUHASI T. and USUI M. (1963) Further studies on nonspecific antibody adhesion onto the antigen-antibody complex. *Proc. 1st Asian Congr. Blood Transf.*, Hakone, Japan 1963, 209–213.

[35] OGATA T. and MATUHASI T. (1964) Further observations on the problems of specific and cross reactivity of blood group antibodies. *Proc. 9th Congr. int. Soc. Blood Transf.*, Mexico 1962, 528–531.

[36] SVARDAL JANET M., YARBRO J. and YUNIS E.J. (1967) Ogata phenomenon explaining the unusual specificity in eluates from Coombs positive cells sensitized by autogenous anti-I. *Vox Sang.*, **13**, 472–484.

[37] FRIEDENREICH V. (1930) *The Thomsen Hemagglutination Phenomenon*, pp. 128, Levin and Munksgaard, Copenhagen.

[38] LEVINE P. and KATZIN E.M. (1938) Temporary agglutinability of red blood cells. *Proc. Soc exp. Biol. N.Y.*, **39**, 167–169.

[39] GAFFNEY J.C. and SACHS H. (1943) Polyagglutinability of human red blood cells. *J. Path. Bact.*, **55**, 489–492.

[40] BASIL-JONES B., SANGER RUTH and WALSH R.J. (1946) An agglutinable factor in red blood cells. *Nature, Lond.*, **157**, 802.

[41] BOORMAN KATHLEEN E., LOUTIT J.F. and STEABBEN D.B. (1946) Poly-agglutinable red cells. *Nature, Lond.*, **158**, 446–447.

[42] ENGELSON G. and GRUBB R. (1949) Abnormal agglutinability of red cells in pyogenic infections. *Amer. J. clin. Path.*, **19**, 782–787.

[43] HENNINGSEN K. (1949) A case of polyagglutinable human red cells. *Acta path. microbiol. scand.*, **26**, 339–344.

[44] LOGHEM J.J. VAN, HART MIA V.D. and HEIER ANNA MARGRETHE (1951) Een geval van poly-agglutinabele rode bloedlichaampjes. *Bull, cent. Lab. Bloedtransf-Dienst. ned. Rode Kruis*, **1**, 43–50.

[45] LOGHEM J.J. VAN (1951) Polyagglutinabilité de globules rouges. *Rev. Belg. Path.*, **21**, 213–217.

[46] HOLLÄNDER L. (1951) Polyagglutinabilität der Erythrocyten bei einer Pneumokokken-meningitis. *Helv. paediat. acta*, **2**, 149–155. (Perhaps vol. 6, not clear from reprint.)

[47] GASSER C. and HOLLÄNDER L. (1951) Anémie hémolytique acquise aigue provoquée par des auto-anticorps, accompagnée de purpura thrombocytopénique chez un nourrisson de 7 semaines. *Rev. Hémat.*, **6**, 316–333.

[48] REEPMAKER J. (1952) The relation between polyagglutinability of erythrocytes *in vivo*, and the Hübener-Thomsen-Friedenreich phenomenon. *J. clin. Path.*, **5**, 266–270.

[49] MURALT G. DE, HÄSSIG ROSINA and REYNIER H. DE (1952) Un cas de polyagglutinabilité transitoire des érythrocytes chez une patiente du group A. *Rev. Hémat.*, **7**, 372–380.

[50] MITRA S. and CHOUDHURI P. (1955) Polyagglutinability of human red blood cells. *Brit. med. J.*, **i**, 887–888.

[51] LOGHEM J.J. VAN, HART MIA V.D. and LAND MADELEINE E. (1955) Polyagglutinability of red cells as a cause of severe haemolytic transfusion reaction. *Vox Sang.* (O.S.), **5**, 125–128.

[52] HENDRY P.I.A. and SIMMONS R.T. (1955) An example of polyagglutinable erythrocytes, and reference to panagglutination, polyagglutination and autoagglutination as possible sources of error in blood grouping. *Med. J. Aust.*, **i**, 720–723.

[53] STRATTON F. and RENTON P.H. (1958) *Practical Blood Grouping*, Blackwell Scientific Publications, Oxford, pp. 331.

[54] CHORPENNING F.W. and HAYES J.C. (1959) Occurrence of the Thomsen-Friedenreich phenomenon *in vivo*. *Vox Sang.*, **4**, 210–224.

[55] UHLENBRUCK G. (1961) Zur Definition der Panhaemagglutination unter besonderer Berücksichtigung des Thomsen-Friedenreich'schen Phänomens. *Zbl. Bakt.*, **179**, 229 or 155–250 or 176.

[56] MOREAU R., DAUSSET J., BERNARD J. and MOULLEC J. (1957) Anémie hémolytique acquise avec polyagglutinabilité des hématies par un nouveau facteur présent dans le sérum humain normal (anti-Tn). *Bull. Soc. med. Hôp.* Paris. Séance, May 17th, 569–587.

[57] BIRD G.W.G. (1964) Anti-T in peanuts. *Vox Sang.*, **9**, 748–749.

17

[58] ROBERTS J.A.F. (1955) Cousin marriage. *The Medical Journal of the South-West*, **70**, 142–149.

[59] ROBERTS J.A.F. (1967) *An Introduction to Medical Genetics*, 4th edition, Oxford University Press.

[60] JØRGENSEN J.R. (1967) Prenatal T-transformation? A case of polyagglutinable cord blood erythrocytes. *Vox Sang.*, **13**, 225–232.

[61] FURUHJELM U., NEVANLINNA H.R., NURKKA RIITTA, GAVIN JUNE, TIPPETT PATRICIA, GOOCH ANN and SANGER RUTH (1968) The blood group antigen Ul^a (Karhula). *Vox Sang.*, **15**, 118–124.

[62] KLENK E. and UHLENBRUCK G. (1960) Über neuraminsäurehaltige Mucoide aus Menschenerythrocytenstroma, ein Beitrag zur Chemie der Agglutinogene. *Hoppe-Seyl. Z.*, **319**, 151–160.

[63] SPRINGER G.F. (1963) Enzymatic and nonenzymatic alterations of erythrocyte surface antigens. *Bact. Rev.*, **27**, 191–227.

[64] UHLENBRUCK G., PARDOE GRACE I. and BIRD G.W.G. (1969) On the specificity of lectins with a broad agglutination spectrum. II. Studies on the nature of the T-antigen and the specific receptors for the lectin of *Arachis hypogoea* (ground-nut). *Z. ImmunForsch. All. klin. Imm.*, **138**, 423–433.

[65] SANGER RUTH, RACE R.R., NEVANLINNA H. and FURUHJELM U. (1970) Letter to the Editor, *Blood*, **35**, 883.

[66] BIRD G.W.G. and WINGHAM JUNE (1972) Tk: a new form of red cell polyagglutination. *Brit. J. Haemat.*, **23**, 759–763.

[67] DAUSSET J., MOULLEC J. and BERNARD J. (1959) Acquired hemolytic anemia with polyagglutinability of red blood cells due to a new factor present in normal human serum (anti-Tn). *Blood*, **14**, 1079–1093.

[68] HART MIA VAN DER, MOES MIEKE, LOGHEM J.J. VAN, ENNEKING J.H.J. and LEEKSMA C.H.W. (1961) A second example of red cell polyagglutinability caused by the Tn antigen. *Vox Sang.*, **6**, 358–361.

[69] FREIESLEBEN E., JENSEN K.G. and KNUDSEN E.E. (1962) Permanent mixed field polyagglutinability. *Proc. 8th Congr. europ. Soc. Haemat.*, Vienna 1961, 506, vol. II (Karger, Basel).

[70] MYLLYLÄ G., NORDLING S., FURUHJELM U. and PIRKOLA ANNA (1969) Mixed field polyagglutinability of red cells due to Tn antigen. *Proc. 12th Int. Congr. Blood Transf.*, 194–195, 'MIR' Publishers, Moscow.

[71] MYLLYLÄ G., FURUHJELM U., NORDLING S., PIRKOLA ANNA, TIPPETT PATRICIA, GAVIN JUNE and SANGER RUTH (1971) Persistent mixed field polyagglutinability. Electrokinetic and serological aspects. *Vox Sang.*, **20**, 7–23.

[72] STURGEON P., McQUISTON DOROTHY T., SPARKES R., SOLOMON J. and BARNETT E.V. (1969) Atypical immunologic tolerance in a human blood group chimera. *Blood*, **33**, 507–526.

[73] STURGEON P. and McQUISTON D. (1972) Persistent mixed field polyagglutinability. Abstracts: *XIV Int. Congr. Haemat.*, São Paulo.

[74] HAYNES C.R., DORNER I., LEONARD G.L., ARROWSMITH W.R., and CHAPLIN H. (1970) Persistent polyagglutinability *in vivo* unrelated to T-antigen activation. *Transfusion, Philad.*, **10**, 43–51.

[75] GUNSON H.H., STRATTON F. and MULLARD G.W. (1970) An example of polyagglutinability due to the Tn antigen. *Brit. J. Haemat.*, **18**, 309–316.

[76] GUNSON H.H., BETTS J.J. and NICHOLSON J.T. (1971) The electrophoretic mobility of Tn polyagglutinable erythrocytes. *Vox Sang.*, **21**, 455–461.

[77] BERMAN H.J., SMARTO J., ISSITT C.H., ISSITT P.D., MARSH W.L. and JENSEN L. (1972) Tn-activation with acquired A-like antigen. *Transfusion, Philad.*, **12**, 35–45.

[78] BIRD G.W.G., SHINTON N.K. and WINGHAM JUNE (1971) Persistent mixed-field polyagglutination. *Brit. J. Haemat.*, **21**, 443–453.

[79] ISSITT P.D., ISSITT C.H., MOULDS J. and BERMAN H.J. (1972) Some observations on the T, Tn and Sd^a antigens and the antibodies that define them. *Transfusion, Philad.*, **12**, 217–221.

80   BIRD G.W.G. (1970) Comparative serological studies on the T, Tn and Cad receptors. *Blut*, **21**, 366–370.

81   CAZAL P., MONIS M., CAUBEL J. and BRIVES J. (1968) Polyagglutinabilité héréditaire dominante: antigène privé (Cad) correspondant à un anticorps public et à une lectine de *Dolichos biflorus*. *Rev. franc. Transf.*, **11**, 209–221.

82   BIRD G.W.G. (1971) Erythrocyte polyagglutination. *Nouv. Rev. franc. Hémat.*, **11**, 885–896.

83   BIRD G.W.G. (1972) Membrane abnormalities in polyagglutinable erythrocytes. *Acta Haemat.*, **47**, 193–199.

84   SANGER RUTH, GAVIN JUNE, TIPPETT PATRICIA, TEESDALE PHYLLIS and ELDON K. (1971) Plant agglutinin for another human blood-group. *Lancet*, **i**, 1130.

85   ALLEN F.H., ISSITT P.D., DEGNAN T.J., JACKSON VALERIE A., REIHART JUDITH K., KNOWLIN R.J. and ADEBAHR MARGOT E. (1969) Further observations on the Matuhasi-Ogata phenomenon. *Vox Sang.*, **16**, 47–56.

86   BOVE J.R., HOLBURN A.M. and MOLLISON P.L. (1973) Non-specific binding of IgG to antibody-coated red cells. (The 'Matuhasi-Ogata phenomenon') *Immunology*, **25**, 793–801.

87   CROOKSTON J.H., CROOKSTON MARIE C., BURNIE KATHERINE L., FRANCOMBE W.H., DACIE J.V., DAVIS J.A. and LEWIS S.M. (1969) Hereditary erythroblastic multinuclearity associated with a positive acidified-serum test: a type of congenital dyserythropoietic anaemia. *Brit. J. Haemat.*, **17**, 11–26.

88   CROOKSTON J.H., CROOKSTON MARIE C. and ROSSE W.F. (1972) Red-cell abnormalities in HEMPAS (Hereditary erythroblastic multinuclearity with a positive acidified-serum test). *Brit. J. Haemat.*, **23**, 83–91.

89   MARSH W.L. and JENKINS W.J. (1968) Anti-Sp$_1$: the recognition of a new cold auto-antibody. *Vox Sang.*, **15**, 177–186.

90   ROELCKE D. (1969) A new serological specificity in cold antibodies of high titre: anti-HD. *Vox Sang.*, **16**, 76–79.

91   ROELCKE D., UHLENBRUCK G. and BAUER K. (1969) A heterogeneity of the HD-receptor, demonstrable by HD-cold antibodies: HD$_1$/HD$_2$. Immunochemical aspects. *Scand. J. Haemat.*, **6**, 280–287.

92   MARSH W.L. and NICHOLS MARGARET E. (1969) The effect of bacterial T-activating enzymes on the red cell Sp$_1$ antigen. *Vox Sang.*, **17**, 217–220.

93   BECK M.L. and MARSH W.L. (1970) Red cell Sp$_1$ antigen change associated with *in vivo* poly-agglutinability. *Vox Sang.*, **19**, 91–93.

94   HOMBERG J.C., KRULIK M., HABIBI B. and DEBRAY J. (1971) Une agglutinine froide anti-Sp$_1$, au cours d'une leucémie lymphoide chronique compliquée de cirrhose hépatique. *Nouv. Revue fr. Hemat.*, **11**, 489–495.

95   ROELCKE D., ANSTEE D.J., JUNGFER H., NUTZENADEL W. and WEBB A.J. (1971) IgG-type cold agglutinins in children and corresponding antigens. Detection of a new Pr antigen: Pr$_a$. *Vox Sang.*, **20**, 218–229.

96   ROELCKE D., EBERT W., METZ J. and WEICKER H. (1971) I-, MN- and PR$_1$/Pr$_2$-activity of human erythrocyte glycoprotein fractions obtained by ficin treatment. *Vox Sang.*, **21**, 352–361.

97   ROELCKE D. (1973) Serological studies on the Pr$_1$/Pr$_2$ antigens using dog erythrocytes. *Vox Sang.*, **24**, 354–361.

98   GARRATTY G., PETZ L.D., BRODSKY I. and FUDENBERG H.H. (1973) An IgA high-titer cold agglutinin with an unusual blood group specificity within the Pr complex. *Vox Sang.*, **25**, 32–38.

99   BELL C.A., ZWICKER HELEN, SPIRA SUSAN and FISCHER MARY LOU (1973) Transfusion in the presence of anti-Sp$_1$. *Vox Sang.*, **25**, 271–280.

100 WILKINSON S.L., VAITHIANATHAN T. and ISSITT P.D. (1974) The high incidence of anti-HL-A antibodies in anti-D typing reagents. Illustrated by a case of Matuhasi-Ogata phenomenon mimicking a 'D with anti-D' situation. *Transfusion, Philad.*, **14**, 27–33.

101 ROELCKE D. and UHLENBRUCK G. (1970) Letter to the Editor. *Vox Sang.*, **18**, 478–479.

[102] POSCHMANN A., FISCHER K., REUTHER K. and MYLLYLÄ G. (1973) Persistent mixed field polyagglutinability: an immunofluorescence study in genetically abnormal red cells. *Vox Sang.*, **24**, 489–501.

[103] STURGEON P., MCQUISTON DOROTHY T., TASWELL H.F. and ALLAN C.J. (1973) Permanent mixed-field polyagglutinability (PMFP): I. Serological observations. *Vox Sang.*, **25**, 481–497.

[104] STURGEON P., LUNER S.J. and MCQUISTON DOROTHY T. (1973) Permanent mixed-field polyagglutinability (PMFP): II. Hematological, biophysical and biochemical observations. *Vox Sang.*, **25**, 498–512.

[105] LALEZARI P. and AL-MONDHIRY H. (1973) Sialic acid deficiency of human red blood cells associated with persistent red cell, leucocyte, and platelet polyagglutinability. *Brit. J. Haemat.*, **25**, 399–408.

[106] BIRD G.W.G. and WINGHAM JUNE (1973) Seed agglutinin for rapid identification of Tn polyagglutination. *Lancet*, **i**, 677.

[107] POOLE JOYCE (1973) Personal communication.

[108] BIRD G.W.G. and WINGHAM JUNE (1974) Haemagglutinins from *Salvia*. *Vox Sang.*, **26**, 163–166.

[109] BIRD G.W.G. and WINGHAM JUNE (1974) The M, N and N_{vg} receptors of Tn-erythrocytes. *Vox Sang.*, **26**, 171–175.

Chapter 25
Blood Groups and Problems of Parentage and Identity

Any well-established polymorphic character such as the serum groups or the iso-zymes may solve several types of problem, but we shall confine ourselves to red cell antigens.

1. *Problems of parentage*

The question whether two babies have been accidentally interchanged in a mater-nity ward arises as a rarity and there is a good chance that blood groups will sort them out.

Disputed paternity is the commonest type of parentage problem and blood groups have, of course, been used for many years in an enormous number of affiliation cases.

There must be many facets to the problem: Schatkin, Sussman and Yarbrough[1] describe how a sudden increase of visa applications from Chinese claiming American citizens as their parents led to checks by blood groups. A very high rate of exclusion led to the exposure of an 'immigration ring'.

Exclusion of parentage may be useful scientifically as well as legally. For example, in the working out of the inheritance of a 'new' antigen it is important to avoid being misled by information from extra-marital children. Platt and Stratton[2] used blood groups to exclude parthenogenesis as a theoretically possible background for certain cases of ovarian agenesis with male skin sex; this, of course, was before the days of accurate human cytogenetics.

2. *Problems of identity*

Blood groups help to distinguish between monozygotic and dizygotic twins and a good deal of the next chapter is devoted to the subject.

The groups are, of course, very effective in distinguishing individuals within a race, though not yet so good as fingerprints, and they are very effective in distin-guishing between races.

We do not propose to do more than mention the grouping of blood stains. This has become a fine art of which we have no experience and cannot usefully comment on, but we can refer the reader to the works of Dodd and Lincoln[3-5] where references will be found to papers by other experts such as Ducos, Ruffié Pereira and Henningsen and Kind.

PARENTAGE

A character that is to give unequivocal evidence concerning parentage must be simply inherited, and its mode of inheritance must be known with certainty; it must be adequately developed at birth or soon thereafter; it must retain its character throughout life, unobscured by climate, disease, age or by any other environmental or genetical agency. If the character is to be used to settle a dispute it must be objective.

The blood groups, assuming proper tests and interpretation, fit these criteria. Certain extremely rare apparent exceptions, none of which should cause error, will be mentioned under the appropriate systems: one practical importance is that they may be used in legal argument.

One theoretical cause of error that cannot be circumvented is mutation. If a child, for example, has an antigen not possessed by either parent it can be argued that a mutation has occurred. The argument is worth very little: extremely rough estimates of the mutation rates of several human disease genes have been made[6, 7], which suggest that their frequency is of the order of 1 in 50,000. However, more recently, Stevenson and Kerr[8] (1967) give reasons for thinking that the general mutation rate may be nearer one in a million. In other species it is known that different genes have different rates. The evidence for mutation is so slight in blood groups, and on the two or three occasions when it has been suspected there has always been a somewhat more probable explanation. This makes us think that the blood group genes have a much lower mutation rate than that estimated for the few disease genes studied in this respect. If the child has two antigens lacked by both parents then the argument of mutation is absurd, for the huge improbability of one mutation having happened has now to be squared.

The few examples that could represent mutation can be better explained by recombination (see pages 97–99 in the MNSs chapter and page 188 in the Rh chapter). Mutation could cause a mistaken judgment in the first class of exclusion distinguished below but no convincing example has ever been caught. Recombination can only cause a mistake of judgment in the second class of exclusion; mutation could also cause a mistake in this class and so could the existence of rare or unknown alleles. However, these possible sources of error have to be taken into account before an opinion is given.

The use of any of the blood groups in problems of parentage, whether legal cases or not, is dependent on the antisera being available, and should depend on the tests being done by an expert constantly engaged in such work. Such an expert would always test the three samples of blood with the same antisera and, having found an exclusion, would check it with at least a second example of the excluding antibody.

The main reason for using two or more examples of the antiserum is to rule out the possibility of false positive reactions due to the presence of other, unsuspected, antibodies in a test serum. (For example, anti-Bg, page 476, is not an uncommon contaminant of immune sera and, by ordinary methods of testing, Bg+ children often have apparently Bg– parents. At the time of writing our most avid anti-Lu^a serum and a powerful anti-Fy^a serum each contain anti-Bg which we cannot remove by absorption.)

The two classes of exclusion

There are two classes of exclusion: the first applies to all systems; the second applies only to those systems in which antibodies are available which can detect 'allelic' antigens. In distinguishing the two classes we will assume that the mother is the mother and that only paternity is in question.

1   A man is excluded if he and the mother both lack an antigen which the child has. This follows from the fact that a child cannot have an antigen lacked by both parents. A well-known exception is the Le^a antigen of red cells—but the Lewis system is not used in paternity testing. A few other very rare exceptions to the rule will be mentioned in the sections below: all disclose themselves by recognizable peculiarities which should prevent their being the cause of false exclusion.

2   A man is excluded if antigens which he must hand on are not present in the child. For example, an AB man cannot have an O child. (As will be seen, there is an exception to this also, but again associated peculiarities should prevent mistakes.) This second class of exclusion needs to be employed with caution in most of the other blood group systems.

The ABO groups

Most workers are cautious in using the subgroups of A in legal medicine.

Apparent exceptions

The O$_h$ or 'Bombay' phenotype

This extremely rare kind of blood is discussed on page 20; it cannot fail to disclose itself provided that the sera of all people involved in a case are tested against O cells as well as A cells and B cells—this should never be omitted. In several O$_h$ families there are men who would have been excluded from the parentage of their children had only their *cells* been tested.

The phenotype A$_m$

All examples so far described have disclosed themselves by a 'missing' agglutinin (pages 15, 17, 27) and no exclusion would be based on such an abnormal result. It has been estimated that the frequency of this type of blood in healthy English people is one in about a quarter or half a million. The form of A_m occasionally associated with leukaemia is hardly likely to be involved in paternity proceedings, but it too discloses itself by a 'missing' agglutinin.

The phenotype A_x

This very rare kind of blood is recognized by tests with group O serum in combination with anti-A and anti-B (see page 16). As the inheritance of A_x is still in doubt (page 28) no exclusion would be based on it. The frequency of A_x has been estimated as one in about 40,000 French blood donors.

Acquired B

It is hardly likely, though theoretically possible, that a person with an acquired B antigen (see page 31) would be involved in paternity proceedings, but in any case the condition is easily recognizable on account of the anti-B present in the serum.

A and B inherited together from one parent

The very rare but theoretically very important families in which an AB child has one O parent are discussed on page 34; they do not invalidate the use of ABO groups in paternity tests: the weakness of the B antigen and the simultaneous presence of some kind of anti-B in the serum of these AB people make the condition easily recognizable.

The MNSs groups

Anti-s is now often available for use in paternity problems though it contributes but little to the first class of exclusion and the results have to be interpreted very cautiously in the second class of exclusion in white people and not at all in Negroes (because of the fairly common S^u).

Apparent exceptions

These all involve the second class of exclusion and this class needs to be interpreted with particular caution in complex systems such as MNSs or Rh.

The antigen M^g

M^g, described on page 104, is bound to be invoked, sooner or later, by the prosecution in affiliation cases when the accused man has been exonerated by the MN groups alone. The argument could be applied only to the following exclusions:

accused man M, mother MN, child N,
accused man M, mother N,   child N,
accused man N, mother M,   child M,
accused man N, mother MN, child M.

The argument will be that the accused man is really of the genotype MM^g or NM^g, as the case may be. Such a theoretical possibility is of course ruled out when the tests have included the use of anti-M^g with negative result. If anti-M^g has not been available then the argument of improbability has to be resorted to: no example of the antigen was found in testing 105,128 random English and Bostonian people, but in Switzerland ten examples were found in testing 6,530 unrelated people. M^g is an example of an antigen that could practically prove paternity.

The allele M^k

This allele, which produces no M, N, S or s antigen, is described on page 105; it presents the same sort of problem as M^g except that specific anti-M^k has not been found. In 60,000 Danish mother-child combinations Henningsen[9] found that M^k explained the appearance of false maternity in only one. In Zurich, M^k is not quite so extremely rare (see page 106).

Other MNSs antigens

Complications occasionally arise due to the presence of rare MNSs 'satellite' antigens some of which can cause depression or, more rarely, exaltation of certain MNSs antigens. The antigens involved are described on pages 109–116: they include St^a, M^V, Mi.III, Mi.IV and Mi.V.

The antigen Mi.III in particular needs to be remembered in cases involving Asiatics, for it occurs in 5 to 10 % of these people. A very interesting case, with a happy ending, is reported by Sturgeon et al.[28] involving $Ms^{Mi.III}$ and M^k in a Chinese family (page 470).

Recombination

This must indeed be a rare event (page 97): it would affect only the second class of exclusion.

The P groups

These groups need to be used with great caution in paternity cases. If a child had a strongly developed P_1 antigen and the mother and presumptive father lacked all trace of the antigen, then paternity could be excluded with some confidence: if the child's antigen was only a weak one, no great weight should be given to the evidence it provided. There is only one type of exclusion: a mating $P_2 \times P_2$ with a P_1 child, and this type of mating has a frequency of only 4 to 5 % in Europeans.

17*

We are a little hesitant to point out the academic argument that the presence in a parent of the dominant form of Lu(a−b−) may complicate the picture[10] (page 147): Lu(a−b−) is extremely rare, but in a case where P showed an exclusion a positive test with anti-Lu^b would rule out this theoretical complication.

The Rh groups

The usefulness of the Rh groups depends on the antisera available. Anti-D used alone hardly contributes at all to the problem, for the only exclusion is that of a D child from a supposed mating $dd \times dd$ and the frequency of this mating is only about 2·5 % in white people, and much less in coloured people. Generally the four sera, anti-D, anti-C, anti-c and anti-E are used and, when appropriate, anti-e, and anti-C^w. In cases involving Negroes, anti-V and anti-VS are often informative. Anti-Ce and anti-CE may prove useful[11], and so may anti-ce.

Apparent exceptions

The gene complex −D−

In an Rh exclusion of the second class this rare complex must be remembered and tested for. Fortunately it can usually be detected in the heterozygous state because the cells suspended in saline are agglutinated by suitable incomplete anti-D (page 214).

In 1954 we were involved in investigating a family in which the father had been 'excluded' from paternity by the Rh groups: tests with incomplete anti-D against cells suspended in saline showed that both father and child had, in fact, −D− and paternity, far from being excluded, was, on the contrary, virtually proved. Superficially, the genotypes had appeared to be: mother *CDe/cde*, child *CDe/cde* and father *CDE/cDE*. We found the groups to be: mother *CDe/cde*, child −D−/cde and father −D−/cDE. The appearance of C in father and child was due to incomplete anti-D in the anti-C sera used in the earlier tests.

Henningsen[12] reported a family in which maternity would have been falsely excluded in a paternity case had −D− not been remembered; a number of interesting cases in which this pitfall was avoided have been published[13−15].

Rh$_{null}$ and gene complexes producing no antigen

As an extreme rarity these conditions can cause error: they are described on pages 220 to 228.

Depressed antigenic complexes

The very rare depressed antigens described on pages 217–219 can give a false appearance of exclusion of the second class, particularly if the test antibodies are not strong.

The antigen e in Negroes

Variations on e are not a rarity in Negroes (see page 209), and some anti-e sera can give a false exclusion of paternity (Shapiro[16], Rosenfield, Haber, Schroeder and Ballard[17]). These appear as exclusions of the second class.

Position effects

The *Cde* gene complex can cause an ordinary *D* of its partner chromosome to express itself as a 'high grade' D^u (see page 233). This, of course, must be remembered before an exclusion based on D^u is considered.

Rare forms of D, C and E

Difficulties can be avoided by testing all three blood samples with the same anti-D, anti-C and anti-E sera.

The Lutheran groups

In populations of European extraction these groups should detect 3 to 4 % of false accusations by an exclusion of the first class. The extremely rare dominant inhibitor of Lu^a and Lu^b (page 267) should be kept in mind[18], but if anti-Lu^b is used as well the involvement of the inhibitor would become apparent and misinterpretation prevented.

Exclusions of the second class could be falsified by the presence of the rare 'silent' allele *Lu*.

The Kell groups

Tests with anti-K (anti-K1) can suitably be applied to paternity problems, provided an antiglobulin technique is used. Anti-k is of but little use because of the high incidence of its positive reactions and because a negative reaction does not inevitably indicate the genotype *KK* (page 292). Anti-Js^a (anti-K6) is more useful in Negroes than is anti-K in Whites. Anti-Kp^a (anti-K3) would be useful were the antigen more frequent.

In Britain, at any rate, anti-K (anti-K1) should detect about 4 to 5 % of false accusations.

Again the second class of exclusion, which might follow the additional use of anti-k, anti-Kp^b and anti-Js^b, needs to be interpreted with caution (page 292).

The Lewis groups

The Lewis phenotypes of the red cells can play no part in paternity tests and it does not seem likely that the saliva phenotypes will be of any practical use because of the rarity of the only mating capable of showing an exclusion—nL × nL.

Secretors and non-secretors

Now that group O saliva can easily be classified by means of *Ulex* extract the secretor-non-secretor distinction is ripe for application to problems of parentage. Only the mating non-sec. × non-sec. could show an exclusion.

The Duffy groups

Both anti-Fy^a and anti-Fy^b are of great power in exclusions of the first class: the matings that could show an exclusion are $Fy(a-) \times Fy(a-)$ and $Fy(b-) \times Fy(b-)$ for which the frequencies in white people are about 11 per cent and 4 per cent respectively. Information from the results of both antisera combined cannot be used for exclusions of the second class because of the existence in white people of the gene *Fy* which makes neither Fy^a nor Fy^b (page 351). Similarly, and much more so, in Negroes only exclusions of the first class can be made.

The Kidd groups

Good anti-Jk^a and -Jk^b sera are rare but when they are available both are useful for exclusions of the first class. The matings $Jk(a-) \times Jk(a-)$ and $Jk(b-) \times Jk(b-)$, which can show exclusions, have frequencies in Whites of about 6 per cent and 7 per cent respectively. Information from the use of both antisera combined, for exclusion of the second class, should be treated with caution (page 366), because of the existence of the allele *Jk*, present as a rarity in white people but commoner in Pacific areas.

Other systems

Anti-Di^a is of use only in Mongolian people. Anti-Do^a and anti-Do^b will be useful when the sera become more generally available, and the same applies to anti-Yt^b and anti-Co^b.

Anti-Xg^a can only exclude men from the paternity of female children. An $Xg(a+)$ man cannot have an $Xg(a-)$ daughter (normal XX); and an $Xg(a-)$ man cannot have an $Xg(a+)$ (normal XX) daughter if the mother is $Xg(a-)$.

The chances of exclusion in false accusations of paternity

Table 83 shows that an expert laboratory equipped with the antisera listed could exonerate about 62% of gentlemen in England wrongfully accused of paternity.

As an example of the method of calculating the exclusions the simple case of the Kell groups will serve. The only alleged mating that could show an exclusion is K− × K− and the frequency of such pairs in the population is 0·8294. Only a K+ child could exclude, and the chance of the successful spermatozoon of the real father carrying the gene *K* is the gene frequency of *K*, or 0·0457. The chance of exclusion by this system is 0·8294 × 0·0457 or 0·0379. Only the calculation for Rh is really complicated: the exclusion figure 0·2520 was calculated by Fisher in 1944. In the first and second editions of this book Fisher's table was given: it showed among other things the chances of non-exclusion run by each of the 12 kinds of men defined by the use of anti-D, -C, -c and anti-E when falsely accused by the 12 kinds of women. Boyd[19-21] has published formulae for the calculations involving Rh and MNS.

Table 83. The chance of an Englishman being exonerated, by the blood groups, of a false charge of paternity brought by an Englishwoman

	Exclusion by each system	Combined exclusion
1. ABO	0·1760	0·1760
2. MNSs	0·2390	0·3729
3. Rh	0·2520	0·5309
4. Kell	0·0379	0·5487
5. Lutheran	0·0333	0·5637
6. Duffy	0·0700	0·5942
7. Kidd	0·0611	0·6190

SOURCES

1. Schiff and Boyd[22]; based on German gene frequencies which are sufficiently close to the English for the present purpose.
2. Frequencies given on page 94; based on the use of anti-M, -N, -S.
3. Fisher (see text); based on the use of anti-C, -c, -D, -E.
4. Frequencies given on page 284; based on the use of anti-K.
5. Frequencies given on page 262; based on the use of anti-Lu^a.
6. Frequencies given on page 352; based on the separate use of anti-Fy^a and anti-Fy^b.
7. Frequencies given on page 365; based on the separate use of anti-Jk^a and anti-Jk^b.

The combined exclusion at, for example, the Rh level is worked out thus: $[(1 - 0·3729) \times 0·2520] + 0·3729 = 0·5309$. The figures given in Table 83 would do for Western Europeans in general.

The mathematical aspects of the allied problems, doubtful identity, identical twins, doubtful parentage and disputed paternity, were standardized by Fisher[23], using MNSs as an example.

On rare occasions paternity could be proved beyond all reasonable doubt. If, for example, the accused man and the child were both B, NS, $C^w D''e/cde$, Lu(a+), K+ and the mother was of common groups, paternity would be proved, provided that the brothers of the accused had alibis. Outside the family of the accused there would not be another such man in ten million.

When the groups do not exclude a man being the true father we are sometimes asked whether he is more, or less, likely to be the true father than is a random man in the population being dealt with. We know there are other ways of treating the problem but this is how we look at it.

Taking a limited example in English people:

mother	child	putative father
O	A	AB
MSMs	MsNs	MsNs
rr	R_1r	R_1r
Fy(a+b−)	Fy(a+b−)	Fy(a+b+)

The chance that this putative father could supply the necessary sperm is, for each system, 0.5 and $(0.5)^4 = 0.0625$. The chance that a random man could do so is the multiple of the frequencies of the required genes, A, Ns, R_1 and Fy^a, which is 0.0172. This sounds impressive, the putative father is $3\frac{1}{2}$ times more likely to be the true father than is someone else! But it is of no biological significance: he would need to be at least 100 times more likely before any great weight should be given to this kind of argument.

There is a long history of the use of blood groups in affiliation cases in Europe and the United States. In Britain they have been used for many years as evidence, and their use was regularized, in England and Wales, by the passing of the Family Law Reform Act[24], 1969. An important change was that the Court can now ask for blood tests; previously this was left to one or the other side. A learned and very readable account of the legal state of the tests before the passing of the 1969 Act is given by Brownlie[25].

Concerning the Rh notation to be used in medico-legal reports in the United States there was an interesting episode. A supplementary report[26] of the Committee on Medicolegal Problems, American Medical Association, prepared by Subcommittee R.D. Owen, C. Stormont, I.B. Wexler and A.S. Wiener, Chairman, recommends that the 'Rh-Hr notations be kept as the standard and sole nomenclature for preparing approved medicolegal reports on the Rh-Hr types'. This prompted the following letter to *Science* signed by thirty-three distinguished workers in the U.S.A. and Canada[27].

'The undersigned object to the report in the *Journal of the American Medical Association* for 31 August 1957 on "Medicolegal applications of blood grouping tests." In our judgment this report is a highly biased document, and certain of us have already expressed contrary opinions during the course of the report's formulation, without much effect. The Subcommittee on Medicolegal Problems responsible for this report consisted of four members all of whom are from the United States and two of whom were the chief protagonists for one of the nomenclatures under dispute. Therefore we, the undersigned, do not intend to abide by the recommendations of the report, and we shall continue to use the C-D-E nomenclature until such time as a properly representative international body arrives at a definite nomenclature.' [Reprinted from *Science* by permission.]

We do not, in our Unit, do tests primarily for legal purposes though we are often involved when some discrepancy has been found which may be of scientific interest. We are, of course, doing affiliation tests when we test for the old groups any family included in the day's problems.

IDENTITY

All the blood group antibodies mentioned in this book if used in parallel would be capable of defining several million phenotypes; though many of the phenotypes would be so rare that they might not appear in a hundred years of steady work. Some of the possible genotypes must be so rare that they may never have formed the blood of an Englishman.

Phenotype differences within a race

The commonest blood group combination in England is O, Ms/Ns, P_1, CDe/cde, Lu(a–b+), K–k+, Le(a–b+), Fy(a+b+), Jk(a+b+), Yt(a+b–), Au(a+), Do(a+b+), Co(a+b–), Sc1,–2, and Xg(a+). Of females 1 in 1,000 belongs to this commonest combination and of males 1 in 1,429. A good example of a rare combination, unselected for any blood group oddity, is the third child in Figure 31 (page 512) the calculated frequency of whose combination is 1·6 in a hundred million.

Relative 'usefulness' of the systems

Fisher[23] suggested that a convenient way of comparing the 'usefulness' of the different systems of blood groups is to sum the squares of the phenotype frequencies. A figure is obtained which represents the percentage of failures to distinguish between two random samples of English blood. The systems fall into the following order of decreasing efficiency:

MNSs	16·4 per cent failures	
Rh	19·5	,,
A_1A_2BO	32·8	,,
Duffy	37·3	,,
Kidd	37·5	,,
Dombrock	38·2	,,
Xg, males	56·1	,,
Lewis	56·7	,,
P	66·6	,,
Xg, females	81·0	,,
Kell	83·7	,,
Colton	84·2	,,
Yt	85·1	,,
Lutheran	85·9	,,

The figures are based on the frequencies given in this book and assume the use of the following antisera: anti-A, -B, -A_1; anti-M, -N, -S, -s; anti-P_1; anti-C, -c, -C^w, -D, -E, -e; anti-Lu^a; anti-K; anti-Le^a, -Le^b; anti-Fy^a, -Fy^b; anti-Jk^a, -Jk^b; anti-Yt^b; anti-Do^a, -Do^b; anti-Co^b; anti-Xg^a. The use of anti-k, anti-Lu^b, anti-Yt^a and anti-Co^a make no difference to the calculations to one decimal place.

Differences between foetal and adult antigens

The most striking antigenic differences are (1) In cord cells the antigen I is very much weaker and the antigen i very much stronger than in adult cells (see page 449). (2) Cord cells are all of the phenotype Le(a–b–). (3) Rh negative cord cells are more strongly LW positive than are Rh negative adult cells (page 228).

Phenotypes that make racial distinctions

It is of course well known that different races of men have different frequencies of various blood group antigens and that blood groups are making an enormous contribution to physical anthropology. This aspect of the subject has been dealt with by Dr Mourant in his excellent book *The Distribution of the Human Blood Groups* (first edition 1950, second 1975).

The purpose of this section is to gather together certain antigenic distinctions that practically identify the racial origin of a single sample of blood.

The antigen V, the phenotype Fy(a–b–) and the antigen Js^a (pages 206, 354 and 288 respectively) are each of them almost diagnostic of the negro origin of a sample of blood (Table 83a). Twenty-seven per cent of New York negro samples disclose their origin by being V+; 68% of the remaining 73% of the samples disclose their origin by being Fy(a–b–); this leaves 23% of the samples not identified, but of these 20% will be recognized by anti-Js^a. So a total of about 82% of samples of blood from New York Negroes will unmistakably label themselves as such by these three phenotypes alone.

Table 83a. Some remarkable antigenic differences

	West African Negroes	American Negroes	Whites	Carib Indians
The antigen V	40%	27%	0·5%	
The phenotype Fy(a–b–)	90%	68%	0%	
The antigen Js^a		20%	0%	
The antigen Di^a	0%	0%	0%	36%

The less frequent phenotypes, Hu+, He+ and S–s–U– (S^uS^u), would also be diagnostic of negro blood.

The phenotype Di(a+) (page 372) nearly always indicates a Mongolian origin of a sample of blood. It is found in up to 10% of Japanese or Chinese samples. Though eagerly sought for it has, curiously, not been found in Eskimos.

The Gerbich antigen (page 411) provides another very dramatic example of racial differences in distribution: the antigen was found in all of 40,000 random Whites and 1,000 Negroes but in only 50% of the members of some New Guinea tribes.

REFERENCES

1 SCHATKIN S.B., SUSSMAN L.N. and YARBROUGH D.E. (1955) Blood test evidence to detect false claims of citizenship. *N.Y. Law J.*, **133**, 110–111 (cited by Sussman[38]).

2 PLATT R. and STRATTON F. (1956) Ovarian agenesis with male skin sex. Evidence against parthenogenesis. *Lancet*, **ii**, 120–121.

3 LINCOLN P.J. and DODD BARBARA E. (1973) An evaluation of factors affecting the elution of antibodies from bloodstains. *J. forens. Sci. Soc.*, **13**, 37–45.

4 LINCOLN P.J. (1973) A study of elution of blood group antibodies from red cells and its useful application to forensic serology. *Lond. Hosp. Gaz.*, **76**, No. 2 (Supp.), 1–11.

5 DODD BARBARA E. (1972) Some recent advances in forensic serology. *Med. Sci. Law*, **12**, 195–199.

6 HALDANE J.B.S. (1949) Mutation in Man. *Proc. 8th int. Congr. Genet., Hereditas*, Suppl., 267–273.

7 NEEL J.V. (1952) The study of human mutation rates. *Amer. Nat.*, **86**, 129–144.

8 STEVENSON A.C. and KERR C.B. (1967) On the distributions of frequencies of mutation to genes determining harmful traits in man. *Mutation Res.*, **4**, 339–352. (See p. 345.)

9 HENNINGSEN K. (1966) Exceptional MNSs- and Gm-types within a Danish family. Causal relationship or coincidence? *Acta genet.*, **16**, 239–241.

10 CONTRERAS MARCELA and TIPPETT PATRICIA (1974) The Lu(a–b–) syndrome and an apparent upset of P_1 inheritance. *Vox Sang.*, **27**, 369–371.

11 DUNSFORD I., LODGE T. and SPIELMANN W. (1961) The differentiation of CDe/cDE (R_1R_2) from CDE/cde (R_zr) in paternity testing. *Med. Sci. Law.*, **1**, 388–391.

12 HENNINGSEN K. (1957) Significance of $-D-$ chromosome in a legal paternity case. *Vox Sang.*, **2**, 399–405.

13 LAWLER SYLVIA D. and MARSHALL RUTH (1963) Apparent exclusions of parentage explained by $-D-$. *Proc. 2nd int. Congr. hum. Genet. Rome*, 1961, **2**, 852–854.

14 HEIKEN A. and GILES CAROLYN M. (1965) On the Rh gene complexes $D--$, $D(C)(e)$ and $d(c)(e)$. *Hereditas, Lund.*, **53**, 171–186.

15 HEIKEN A. and GILES CAROLYN M. (1966) A study of a family possessing the Rh gene complex $D--$ in the heterozygous state. *Acta genet.*, **15**, 155–161.

16 SHAPIRO M. (1960) Serology and genetics of a new blood factor: hrˢ. *J. forensic Med.*, **7**, 96–105.

17 ROSENFIELD R.E., HABER GLADYS V., SCHROEDER RUTH and BALLARD RACHEL (1960) Problems in Rh typing as revealed by a single Negro family. *Amer. J. hum. Genet.*, **12**, 147–159.

18 TIPPETT PATRICIA (1971) A case of suppressed Luᵃ and Luᵇ antigens. *Vox Sang.*, **20**, 378–380.

19 BOYD W.C. (1955) Chances of excluding paternity by the Rh blood groups. *Amer. J. hum. Genet.*, **7**, 229–235.

20 BOYD W.C. (1955) Compact tabular presentation of mother-child-alleged father combinations which establish non-paternity in the Rh blood group system. *Vox Sang.* (O.S.), **5**, 99–101.

21 BOYD W.C. (1955) The chances of excuding paternity by the MNS blood group system. *Amer. J. hum. Genet.*, **7**, 199–200.

22 SCHIFF F. and BOYD W.C. (1942) *Blood Grouping Technic*, Interscience Publishers, New York.

23 FISHER R.A. (1951) Standard calculations for evaluating a blood-group system. *Heredity*, **5**, 95–102.

24 *Family Law Reform Act* (1969) H.M. Stationery Office, chap. 46, pp. 15–18.

25 BROWNLIE A.R. (1965) Blood and the blood groups. A developing field for expert evidence. *J. forensic. Sci. Soc.*, **5**, 124–174.

26 OWEN R.D., STORMONT C., WEXLER I.B. and WIENER A.S. (1957) Medicolegal applications of blood-grouping tests. *J. Amer. med. Ass.*, **164**, 2036–2044.

27 ALLEN F.H., BEISER S.M., BOYD W.C., BROWN I.W., CEPPELLINI R., CHAPLIN H., CHOWN B., CROSBY W.H., DAMESHEK W., DAVIDSOHN I., DIAMOND L.K., DUNN L.C., GARN S.M., GIBLETT ELOISE R., GREENWALT T.J., GROVE-RASMUSSEN M., GUNSON H.H., HABERMAN S., HILL J.M., HOWE C., KABAT E.A., KREVANS J.R., LEVINE P., MCNEIL C., MOHN J.F., RAFFEL S., RICHARDSON-JONES A., ROSENFIELD R.E., ROSS J.B., SCUDDER J., STEINBERG A.G., STURGEON P. and WINTROBE M.M. (1958) Blood-group nomenclature. *Science*, **127**, 1255.
28 STURGEON P., METAXAS-BÜHLER M., METAXAS M.N., TIPPETT PATRICIA and IKIN E.W. (1970) An erroneous exclusion of paternity in a Chinese family exhibiting the rare MNSs gene complexes M^k and Ms^{III}. *Vox Sang.*, **18**, 395–406.

Chapter 26
Blood Groups in Twins and Chimeras

Interest in human twins was enlivened by the recognition that dizygotic pairs could, as a rarity, have a mixture of each others blood cells. Then the surprising observation was made in Paris that, as an extreme rarity, monozygotic pairs could be of different sex, an XY male and an XO Turner girl. Next followed the demonstration in Seattle that two sperm could, on occasion, fertilize two egg nuclei and the two zygotes grow into one body.

We cannot go into the mechanics of twinning but would suggest the following references: Edwards[102], 1968; Cameron[103], 1968; Corney, Robson and Strong[104], 1968.

DISTINCTION BETWEEN MONOZYGOTIC AND DIZYGOTIC TWINS

Blood groups are of practical importance in helping to decide whether twins are monozygotic or dizygotic. There are various reasons for making the distinction: they include, for example, the investigation of such rarities as those mentioned above, the study of the normal twinning processes and the choice of a donor for skin grafting. Blood groups are often applied when one of a supposedly monozygotic pair presents some abnormality.

If the blood groups or the sex be different (forgetting, for the moment the very rare XO:XY 'identical' pairs) the twins are dissimilar and the problem is solved; if the blood groups be the same, the problem is not solved but the chances of the twins being identical or dissimilar can be calculated. When the groups of the parents of the twins are known the calculation is relatively simple: when they are not known the calculation is extremely laborious but can be circumvented by the use of the tables of Dr Sheila Maynard Smith and the late Professor Penrose.

When parental groups are known

The approach to this problem which we have adopted was clearly stated by C.W. Cotterman[1]: 'Given one twin as found, and given the other relatives as found, what is the probability that the other twin should have been found to be

511

identical with the first twin in all phenotypes on the hypothesis of dizygous origin?'

There is a simple method suggested to us by Professor Penrose. Of all European twin pairs 65% are found to be like-sexed, and 35% unlike-sexed. If 35% are unlike-sexed and dizygotic the same percentage will be expected to be like-sexed and dizygotic. The remaining 30% will be like-sexed and monozygotic. These figures are the starting-point for the calculation of the chance of identity of like-sexed twins from their blood groups.

As an example, the calculation is applied to the family shown in Figure 31, which is taken from our records. Though it lacks some modern groups this is still

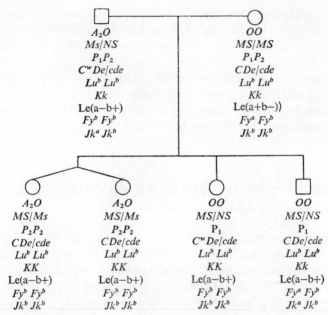

Fig. 31. A family with twins monozygotic for sure. (After Sanger and Race[3], 1952.) Antisera used: anti-A, $-A_1$, -B, anti-M, -N, -S, -s, anti-P_1, anti-C, $-C^w$, -c, -D, -E, anti-Lu^a, anti-K, -k, anti-Le^a, $-Le^b$, anti-Fy^a and anti-Jk^a.

the best example of proof of monozygosity by blood groups alone of all that we have tested. (This family was selected only for having more than two children: the blood samples were given to us by the late Dr Marshall Chalmers.)

The genotype of the father must be A_2O for he has O children. The MNSs tests on the father show only that he has M, N, S and s, but the group of the mother together with that of any of the children show that the father's genotype must be Ms/NS. The P_2P_2 twins show that both parents must be heterozygous P_1P_2.

The mating $A_2O \times OO$ will produce 50 A_2 and 50% O children. If one twin is A_2 then the chance that the other twin would also be A_2, if it were really dizygotic, is 0·5.

The mating $Kk \times Kk$, to take another example, will produce 50% Kk, 25% KK and 25% kk children. One of the twins is KK and the chance that the other would also be KK, if it were really dizygotic, is 0·25. The chances for and against identity of these remarkable twins can be stated thus:

estimated initial chance of dizygotic twins	0·70	initial chance of monozygotic twins	0·30
chance of dizygotic twins having the same sex	0·50	chance of monozygotic twins having the same sex	1·00
chance of dizygotic twins in this family having the same		chance of monozygotic twins having the same	
ABO groups	0·50	ABO groups	1·00
MNSs ,,	0·50	MNSs ,,	1·00
P ,,	0·25	P ,,	1·00
Rh ,,	0·25	Rh ,,	1·00
Kell ,,	0·25	Kell ,,	1·00
Duffy ,,	0·50	Duffy ,,	1·00
Kidd ,,	0·50	Kidd ,,	1·00
combined chance	0·00034	combined chance	0·30

relative chance of dizygotic : monozygotic in this family

$$= 0{\cdot}00034 : 0{\cdot}30$$

so that the probability that the twins in this family are monozygotic

$$= \frac{0{\cdot}30}{0{\cdot}30 + 0{\cdot}00034} = 0{\cdot}9989$$

and the probability that they are dizygotic

$$= \frac{0{\cdot}00034}{0{\cdot}30 + 0{\cdot}00034} = 0{\cdot}0011$$

The method was refined by Smith and Penrose[2]. If the two younger sibs in Figure 31 had not been tested then it would not be known whether the father were A_2O or A_2A_2. It takes time to calculate the relative chance that an $A_2 \times O$ mating should produce two A_2 children, but a simple method is to be found in Smith and Penrose[2]. We are including in Table 84 some information of this sort for Northern European twins, which we find useful.

When parental groups are not known

In a previous edition of this book we said: 'Tables showing the probability of twins being monozygotic when their parents have not been blood grouped would be quite useful. They would have to be compiled for all the systems, and for the variety of antisera that might be used within each system, and for the different

Table 84. Relative chances in favour of dizygosity of twin pairs; parental phenotypes known but genotype of at least one parent unknown. Some useful examples for Northern Europeans. (Calculated according to the method of Smith and Penrose[2])

Mating	Twins both	Relative chance of dizygosity	Mating	Twins both	Relative chance of dizygosity
$A_1 \times O$	A_1	0·6113	Fy(a+) × Fy(a+)	Fy(a+)	0·8815
$A_2 \times O$	A_2	0·5474	Fy(a+) × Fy(a−)	Fy(a+)	0·7072
B × O	B	0·5424			
$A_1 \times A_1$	A_1	0·8224	Jk(a+) × Jk(a+)	Jk(a+)	0·9102
$A_1 \times A_2$	A_1	0·6113	Jk(a+) × Jk(a−)	Jk(a+)	0·7571
$A_1 \times A_2$	A_2	0·3122			
			Do(a+) × Do(a+)	Do(a+)	0·8831
$P_1 \times P_1$	P_1	0·9034	Do(a+) × Do(a−)	Do(a+)	0·7100
$P_1 \times P_2$	P_1	0·7700			
Le(a−) × Le(a−) sec. sec.	Le(a−) sec. }	0·9123	Xg(a−) × Xg(a+) father mother	Xg(a+)	0·8303
Le(a+) × Le(a−) non-sec. sec.	Le(a−) sec. }	0·7634	Xg(a+) × Xg(a+) father mother	Xg(a+) sons	0·8303

races amongst which they might be used!' We should have said *very* useful, for so they have proved since Smith and Penrose[2] provided them for European populations. We were greatly indebted to the authors for permission to reprint five of their tables.

A general formula for calculating the relative chances of dizygosity in systems of two alleles is given in Table 85. The method was extended to other systems having a greater number of alleles, and Smith and Penrose's figures for ABO, MNSs and Rh are given in Tables 86, 87, and 88. The formulae in Table 85 have been applied to the 'newer' groups found since Smith and Penrose's paper appeared: the results are given in Table 89, and some 'short cuts' in Table 90.

Table 85. Relative chances in favour of dizygotic twin pairs in a system of two alleles (From Smith and Penrose[2], 1955)

Genotypic		Phenotypic	
Twin pair both	Relative chance in favour of dizygotic twins	Twin pair both	Relative chance in favour of dizygotic twins
AA	$\frac{1}{4}(1+p)^2$		
Aa	$\frac{1}{2}(1+pq)$ }	Ā	$1 - \frac{1}{4}q^2(3+q)/(1+q)$
aa	$\frac{1}{4}(1+q)^2$	ā	$\frac{1}{4}(1+q)^2$

A and a represent two alleles, with frequencies p and q.
Ā = phenotype representing the genotypes $AA + Aa$ and phenotype ā represents aa.

Table 86. Relative chances of dizygotic twin pairs when the ABO blood groups are the same. (From Smith and Penrose[2], 1955)

Twin pair both	Relative chance of dizygotic twins
O	0·6891
A_1 ⎫ A A_2 ⎭	0·6470 ⎫ 0·6945 0·4824 ⎭
B	0·4741
A_1B ⎫ AB A_2B ⎭	0·3239 ⎫ 0·3435 0·2849 ⎭

Table 87. Relative chances in favour of dizygotic twin pairs when the MNSs blood groups are the same. (From Smith and Penrose[2], 1955)

Anti-M, -N, -S, -s sera available		Anti-M, -N, -S sera available	
Twin pair both	Relative chance in favour of dizygotic twins	Twin pair both	Relative chance in favour of dizygotic twins
MMSS	0·3888	MS	0·5161
MMSs	0·4176		
MMss	0·4116	MsMs	0·4116
MNSS	0·3417	MNS	0·5044
MNSs	0·4556		
MNss	0·4733	MsNs	0·4733
NNSS	0·2915	NS	0·4138
NNSs	0·3831		
NNss	0·4827	NsNs	0·4827

As an example of the use of the tables we will take the twins of Figure 31. Without the information given by other members of the family the groups of the twins are:

A_2, MS/Ms, P_2, CDe/cde, Lu(a−), K+k−, Le(a−b+), Fy(a−), Jk(a−)

The chances in favour of the twins being dizygotic, when looked up in Tables 86–89, are those given in Table 91. The total relative chance of the twins being dizygotic, though so alike, is found by multiplying together the eleven entries.

Other references to calculations of probability of monozygosity are Fisher[17], Sutton, Clark and Schull[18] and Juel-Nielsen, Nielsen and Hauge[19].

Table 88. Relative chances in favour of dizygotic twin pairs when the Rhesus blood groups are the same. (From Smith and Penrose[2], 1955)

Twin pair both								Relative chance in favour of dizygotic pairs
Phenotype						Most likely genotype		
Reactions with anti-								
$C + C^w$	c	D	E	C^w	e			
−	+	−	−	−	+	cde/cde	rr	0·4821
−	+	+	−	−	+	cDe/cde	R^0r	0·3684
−	+	−	+	−	+	cdE/cde	$r''r$	0·3522
−	+	−	+	−	−	cdE/cdE	$r''r''$	0·2500
−	+	+	+	−	−	cDE/cDE	R^2R^2	0·3321
−	+	+	+	−	+	cDE/cde	R^2r	0·4179
+	+	−	−	−	+	Cde/cde	$r'r$	0·3512
+	+	+	−	−	+	CDe/cde	R^1r	0·5400
+	+	+	−	+	+	C^wDe/cde	$R^{1w}r$	0·3599
+	+	−	+	−	+	cdE/Cde	$r''r'$	0·2735
+	+	+	+	−	+	CDe/cDE	R^1R^2	0·4241
+	+	+	+	−	−	cDE/CDE	R^2R^z	0·2853
+	+	+	+	+	+	C^wDe/cDE	$R^{1w}R^2$	0·2943
+	−	−	−	−	+	Cde/Cde	$r'r'$	0·2500
+	−	+	−	−	+	CDe/CDe	R^1R^1	0·5021
+	−	+	−	+	+	C^wDe/CDe	$R^{1w}R^1$	0·3657
+	−	+	+	−	+	CDe/CDE	R^1R^z	0·3546
+	−	+	+	−	−	CDE/CDE	R^zR^z	0·2500
+	−	+	+	+	+	C^wDe/CDE	$R^{1w}R^z$	0·2500

We have modernized Smith and Penrose's shorthand Rh gene symbols.

Blood groups of twins

Details of blood groups are to be found in the following substantial series: Walsh and Kooptzoff[4], Simmons et al.[20] and Hauge[13]. But all previous surveys are likely to be eclipsed when a full account appears of a fast study of placentation with zygosity determination on over 700 pairs of twins in Birmingham[36,102,103]. Other precise studies of placentation were made at Oxford[104] and at Winnipeg[37].

For many years Mr James Shields of the Genetics Unit at the Maudsley Hospital has been sending us samples of blood from the twins. We find that the blood groups practically never contradict the opinion of such a skilled observer of twins.

Blood groups of triplets

The only large series is that reported by Hauge, Herrlin and Heiken[38] who give details of the groups of 54 sets of like-sexed triplets. The calculation of the probability of monozygosity is given by Herrlin and Hauge[39].

Stranc[40] describes three triplet sisters whose monozygotic origin was estab-

Table 89. Relative chances in favour of a dizygotic twin pair when the P, Lutheran, Kell, Secretor (or Lewis), Duffy, Kidd, Yt, Dombrock, Colton and Xg phenotypes are the same. (Derived from the formulae given in Table 85)

System	Twin pair both		Relative chance in favour of dizygotic twins	
P	P_1		0·8489	
	P_2		0·5699	
Lutheran	Lu(a+b−)	Lu(a+)	0·2699	0·5337
	Lu(a+b+)		0·5187	
	Lu(a−b+)	Lu(a−)	0·9614	
Kell	K+k−	K+	0·2734	0·5394
	K+k+		0·5218	
	K−k+	K−	0·9548	
Secretor (or Lewis)	Non-secretor [Le(a+)]		0·5425	
	Secretor [Le(a−)]		0·8681	
Duffy	Fy(a+b−)	Fy(a+)	0·5047	0·8099
	Fy(a+b+)		0·6219	
	Fy(a−b+)	Fy(a−)	0·6235	
Kidd	Jk(a+b−)	Jk(a+)	0·5732	0·8616
	Jk(a+b+)		0·6249	
	Jk(a−b+)	Jk(a−)	0·5519	
Yt	Yt(a+b−)	Yt(b−)	0·9591	
	Yt(a+b+)	Yt(b+)	0·5198	0·5356
	Yt(a−b+)		0·2711	
Dombrock	Do(a+b−)	Do(a+)	0·5041	0·8094
	Do(a+b+)		0·6218	
	Do(a−b+)	Do(a−)	0·6241	
Colton	Co(a+b−)	Co(b−)	0·9604	
	Co(a+b+)	Co(b+)	0·5192	0·5345
	Co(a−b+)		0·2504	
Xg	male Xg(a+)		0·8310	
	male Xg(a−)		0·6690	
	female Xg(a+)		0·9573	
	female Xg(a−)		0·6690	

lished in almost every way possible at the time: red cell and serum groups, biochemical dimorphisms, finger-prints, anatomical measurements etc. The final probability of monozygosity was 99·97%. One of the three had suffered burns involving 70% of her body. Skin grafts from her two sisters were life saving. (We were involved in the red cell grouping and found that the MN and Kidd reactions

Table 90. Relative chances in favour of dizygotic twin pairs given by four common combinations of the P, Lutheran, Kell, Lewis and Duffy blood groups. (From Smith and Penrose[2], 1955)

Groups the same for twin pairs	Relative chance in favour of dizygotic pairs
P+; Lu(a−); K−; Le(a−); Fy(a−)	0·4246
P+; Lu(a−); K−; Le(a−); Fy(a+)	0·5400
P+; Lu(a−); K−; Le(a+); Fy(a−)	0·2654
P+; Lu(a−); K−; Le(a+); Fy(a+)	0·3375

P+ = P_1 in our present notation.

Table 91. An example of the use of the tables of Smith and Penrose (See page 515)

Character	Relative chance of dizygosity
Initial odds	2·3333
Likeness in sex	0·5000
Likeness in ABO	0·4824
Likeness in MNSs	0·4176
Likeness in P	0·5699
Likeness in Rh	0·5400
Likeness in Lutheran	0·9614
Likeness in Kell	0·2734
Likeness in Lewis	0·8681
Likeness in Duffy	0·6235
Likeness in Kidd	0·5519
Total relative chance, pD	0·0057
Total chance, pD/(1 + pD)	0·0057

of the cells of the patient were apparently modified as a result of the burns. The reactions gradually returned to normal. We subsequently tested two other cases of severe burns without finding any comparable upset.)

Blood groups of quadruplets

The groups of a set of Australian quadruplets (Figure 32) very neatly demonstrated their four egg origin (Walsh[5]).

Blood groups of octuplets

In 1972 an East Berlin patient who had been treated for infertility was delivered of octuplets, none of whom survived. Prokop and Hermann[123] record blood

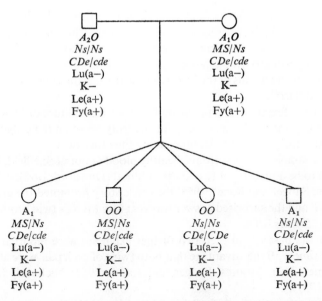

Fig. 32. Bellingen, New South Wales, quadruplets. (After Walsh[5], 1952.) That four different eggs were involved is shown by the mother's contribution to the first being A_1, *MS*, to the second being *O*, *MS* to the third being *O*, *Ns* and to the fourth being A_1, *Ns*.

groups and certain enzyme groups which demonstrate that seven were dissimilar while the relationship of one was not disclosed.

Blood groups of *foetus in foetu*

An example of this rare abnormality was investigated, from the zygosity point of view, by Boyce, Lockyer and Wood[82] (1972). A foetus-like tumour in a three-month-old male child was found, as expected, to be of the same phenotype groups as its host. The blood groups were determined from eluates from the powdered skin tissue of the tumour. An automated antibody detection method was used.

TWIN CHIMERAS

'In the current embryological (which is also the classical) sense, a "chimera" is an organism whose cells derive from two or more distinct zygote lineages, and this is the sense which the term "genetical chimera" is here intended to convey. "Gene tical mosaic" is less suitable, because a mosaic is formed of the cells of a single zygote lineage.' This definition, by Anderson, Billingham, Lampkin and Medawar[27] (1951) is still very useful.

In 1945, Owen[6] published his brilliant work on 'immunogenetic consequences of vascular anastomoses between bovine twins'. Anastomoses are usually present between dissimilar bovine twin embryos; primordial red cells belonging to one twin take root in the other twin and continue throughout the life of the host to produce red cells with genetically foreign antigens. Chorionic vascular anastomosis and transfer of endocrine secretions between bovine twins of different sex had been postulated as the cause of the freemartin condition by Lillie[7] as early as 1916. Interesting details of the history of the freemartin can be found in Moore, Graham and Barr[21].

A cow (of a female twin pair) or bull with such a mixture of blood transmits to the next generation the genes only for the truly begotten red cell antigens, not those for the antigens merely lent for life by the other twin.

When a sample of blood from a healthy blood donor at Sheffield, Mrs McK., was found to be a mixture of two kinds of blood (Dunsford, Bowley, Hutchison, Thompson, Sanger and Race[8], 1953) the cattle story prompted the question 'was she a twin?' and the surprised answer was yes: Mrs McK.'s twin brother had died in infancy 25 years before.

Four years passed and then two further examples were reported simultaneously, this time with the advantage that both twins of each pair were alive (Booth, Plaut, James, Ikin, Moores, Sanger and Race[9], 1957; Nicholas, Jenkins and Marsh[10], 1957).

The next propositus was found in Mexico[41]: to Dr Velez-Orozco's enquiry whether she were a twin she answered no; but Dr Velez-Orozco was then taken aside by her mother who said that there had indeed been twins but the boy was stillborn because of God's anger at the drunkenness of her husband.

We now know of 20 sets and some details are given in Table 92. We have very generously been given the opportunity to test half of them in our Unit.

Ascertainment

All but one of the examples in Table 92 presented themselves as ABO blood grouping problems by having a frank mixture of cells and by a missing agglutinin or, sometimes, in the first place by a missing agglutinin only. The exception (No. 17) came to be blood grouped because her lymphocytes had been found to be mosaic XX/XY.

The two populations of red cells may be separated by differential agglutination[9]. Mixtures of isozymes can be attributed to their rightful cell line if the tests are done on separated populations of red cells: mixtures in serum groups and white cell groups cannot be so assigned.

The true genotypes of the chimeras

Provided the pairs differ in their ABO groups the secretor results usually give the answer: for example Mrs McK. has in her saliva H but no A, therefore her true genetic group is O and her A cells are from her twin. The ABO and the other groups of the children of these chimeras have never contradicted the evidence of the saliva.

Measurement of the ABH transferases of the serum can also give the answer to the true genetic groups, again providing that the pairs differ in their ABO groups. Schachter *et al.*[88] found that Mrs De. (No. 11, Table 92), whose saliva had shown her A cells to be from her graft, had low A transferase activity. Professor Winifred Watkins and Dr Caroline Race demonstrated, in two sets of these twins (No. 15 and No. 16, Table 92) that the transferase corresponding to the true genetic groups was present in normal levels while that corresponding to the graft had low activity, and this was so even when the proportion of true genetic cells was minimal (Judy St., pair No. 15, Table 92). The transferase measurement is particularly useful when a twin is a non-secretor (Mr P.C., pair No. 16).

The Xg groups could on occasion show which are the true genetic groups of an unlike sex chimera pair. If the father is Xg(a+) and the twin's cells are mixtures of Xg(a+) and Xg(a−) then the Xg(a+) cell line truly belongs to the female twin and the Xg(a−) line to the male. Such a constellation has not yet turned up in twin chimera families but it has, twice, amongst the dispermic chimera families (London and Helsinki, Table 93).

Other significant observations

The inability of a chimera who is a secretor to secrete antigens provided by his twin has contributed to reasoning about the nature of the secretor process (see page 311).

The finding by Crookston, Tilley and Crookston[87] of the second known example of the antibody anti-A_1Le^b in one member of their chimera twin pair (Mrs De., No. 11) and the consequent brilliant deductions about the corresponding antigen are described on page 337.

In 1972 Mrs Crookston asked us a question which led to an investigation which showed that O cells grafted in an A chimera twin take up some of the host's A antigen as detected by some selected anti-A+B (group O) sera; this is described on page 40. A practical consequence of this observation is that, in counting the relative proportions of O and A cells in a mixture, anti-A and not anti-A+B should be used.

A pedigree of the family of the Wa. twins (No. 2) is given in the Xg chapter (page 584); it is placed there because the Xg groups are peculiar on two counts, neither of which is properly understood.

Also in the Xg chapter (page 586) is a note about the important part the Ko.-Heb. twins (No. 10) played in establishing that the *Xg* locus, when carried on a normal X, is not subject to inactivation.

Proportion of the mixtures as judged by the red cells

In the twins of Table 92 the proportion of cells of a particular group are:

different in 7 pairs	(No. 2, 3, 6, 8, 9, 10, 11)
about the same in 6 pairs	(No. 5, 7, 12, 15, 16, 19)
no information	(No. 1, 4, 13, 14, 17, 18, 20)

Table 92. Twin chimeras

Reference	Propositus and twin	Proportion of mixtures: and the groups in which they differ	Secretor and transferase	Karyotype (lymphocytes)
1. Dunsford, Bowley Hutchison, Thompson, Sanger and Race[8], 1953	Mrs McK.	61% O, K−, Jk(a+) 39% A_1, K+, Jk(a−)	sec. H	
	her brother died aged 3/12			
2. Booth, Plaut, James, Ikin, Moores, Sanger and Race[9], 1957	Miss Wa.	99% O, R^2r, Fy(a+), Jk(b−), Do(a−) 1% A, R^1r, Fy(a−)	sec. H	{ 98% XX 2% XY } ref. 47
	Mr Wa.	86% A_1, R^1r, Fy(a−), Jk(b+), Do(a+) 14% O, R^2r, Fy(a+), Do(a−)	sec. A, H	{ 91% XY 9% XX } ref. 47
3. Nicholas, Jenkins and Marsh[10], 1957	Mrs W.	49% O, Ms/Ns, R^2r, Le(a−b+) 51% A_1, Ns/Ns, R^2R^2, Le(a−b+)	sec. H	
	Mr G.	61% A_1, Ns/Ns, R^2R^2, Le(a+b−) 39% O, Ms/Ns, R^2r, Le(a+b−)	non-sec.	
4. Velez-Orozco[41], 1961	Sra F.	95% B, MS/Ms, R^1r, 5% A_1, MS/Ns, R^1R^z	sec. B	
	her brother stillborn			
5. Chown, Lewis and Bowman[42], 1963	baby boy*	15% A_2, MS/Ms, R^2r, K+Kp(a−), Jk(a+) 85% O, Ms/Ns, R^1r, K−Kp(a+), Jk(a−)	sec. A, H	{ 30% XY 70% XX } ref. 37
	baby girl*	85% O, Ms/Ns, R^1r, K−Kp(a+), Jk(a−) 15% A_2, MS/Ms, R^2r, K+Kp(a−), Jk(a+)	sec. H	{ 78% XX 22% XY } ref. 37
6. van der Hart and van Loghem[43], 1967	Mr Ba.	99·8% O, R^2r 0·2% B, R^1r	sec. H	{ 97% XY 3% XX }
	Miss Ba.	80% B, R^1r 20% O, R^2r	sec. B, H	{ 22% XX 78% XY }
7. van der Hart and van Loghem[43], 1967	Miss A.v.O.*	1% A 99% O	sec. A, H	
	Miss E.v.O.*	99% O 1% A	sec. H	

Table 92—*continued*

Reference	Propositus and twin	Proportion of mixtures: and the groups in which they differ	Secretor and transferase	Karyotype (lymphocytes)
8. Bias and Migeon[81], 1967	male Negro, mongol his brother, normal	95% A$_1$, Ns/Ns, Fy(a−) / 5% B, NS/Ns, Fy(a+) / all B, NS/Ns, Fy(a+)	sec. H	{ mostly 47, XY, G+ / some 46, XY / 46, XY
9. Gundolf[83], 1970; Gundolf and Hansen[84], 1972	Mr T.S.	73% O, R^1r {HL-A a/c / 27% B, R^1R^2 {HL-A b/c	sec. H	{ 87% XX / 13% XY
	Mrs M.R.	69% B, R^1R^2, Fy^aFy^a {HL-A b/c / 31% O, R^1r, Fy^aFy^b {HL-A a/c	sec. B, H	{ 34% XY / 66% XX
10. Ducos, Colombies, Marty, Blanc, Daver and Emond[85], 1970; Ducos et al.[86] 1971	Mme Ko.	90% O, MS/Ms, rr, Fy^bFy^b, Xg(a+) / 10% A$_1$,B, $MN.Ss$, R^1r, Fy^aFy^b, Xg(a−)	sec. H	
	M Heb.	65% A$_1$,B, $MN.Ss$, R^1r, Fy^aFy^b, Xg(a−) / 35% O, MS/Ms, rr, Fy^bFy^b, Xg(a+)	sec. A,B	
11. Crookston, Tilley and Crookston[87], 1970	Mrs De.	50% O, Fy^aFy^b, Jk^aJk^b, PGM$_1$ 1 / 50% A$_1$, Fy^bFy^b, Jk^aJk^a, PGM$_1$ 2-1	sec. H, weak A transf.[88]	{ 53% XX / 47% XY
12. Kaeser and Nennstiel[89], 1971	Mr Jo.	98% A$_1$, Fy^bFy^b, Jk^aJk^a, PGM$_1$ 2-1 / 2% O, Fy(a+)	sec. A,H	{ 99% XY / 1% XX
	Frau B.	few B, Ns/Ns, P$_1$ stronger, R^1R^2, Le(a+b−) / O, MS/Ns, P$_1$ weaker, R^1R^1, Le(a+b−)	non-sec.	
	Frau G.	O, MS/Ns, P$_1$ weaker, R^1R^1, Le(a−b+) / few B, Ns/Ns, P$_1$ stronger, R^1R^2, Le(a−b+)	(subtlety[89])	
13. Osińska and Woloszyn[90]; Schlesinger and Halasa[91], 1971	C.L. male aet. 23 male twin still-born	less A$_1$B, Ms/Ns, rr, Xg(a+), AcP$_1$ B / more O, MS/Ms, R^1r, Xg(a−), AcP$_1$, AB	sec. A, B, H	all XY
14. Carr and McDonald[92], 1974	Mrs Y. male twin, dead, Army report	30% A$_1$,B, MS/Ns, rr / 70% O, Ns/Ns, $R^{au}r$ / AB, Rh neg.	sec. A, B, H	lymphocytes XY fibroblasts XX

Table 92—*continued*

Reference	Propositus and twin	Proportion of mixtures: and the groups in which they differ	Secretor and transferase	Karyotype (lymphocytes)
15. Wrobel, McDonald, C. Race and Watkins[93], 1974	John St.	99% A₁, Ns/Ns, R¹r, Xg(a−) Gc 1 <1% B, Ms/Ns, R¹R¹, Xg(a+)	sec. A, H A transf.	{80% XY 20% XX
	Judy St.	<1% B, Ms/Ns, R¹R¹, Xg(a+) Gc 2 99% A₁, Ns/Ns, R¹r, Xg(a−)	sec. B, H B transf. (weak A)	{46% XX 54% XY
16. Lowes, Sullivan and Sabo[94], 1974	Mrs S.M.	10% B, R²r, Fyᵃfyᵇ, PGM₁ 1, GPT 2-1 90% A₁, rr, Fyᵇfyᵇ, PGM₁ 2-1, GPT 2	sec. B B transf. (weak A)	{XX XY
	Mr P.C.	90% A₁, rr, Fyᵇfyᵇ, PGM₁ 2-1, GPT 2 10% B, R²r, Fyᵃfyᵇ, PGM₁ 1, GPT 2-1	non-sec. A transf. (v. weak B)	XY
17. Robinson and Horsfield[95], 1973	female baby, A.K.	anti-s, mixed field Le(a+b−) {HL-A a/c	non-sec.	{XX 16 XY 29
	male baby, P.K.	anti-s, mixed field Le(a+b+) {HL-A b/d	sec. A, H	{XY 37 XX 11
18. Bowley et al.[96], 1974	Mrs U.T.	50% O, HL-A a/c 50% B, HL-A b/d	sec. H	{XX XY
	Twin brother	To be tested.		
19. Hosoi[97], 1973	Mr Y.F.*	89% A₁, Fyᵃfyᵃ, Jk(a+) 11% A₁B, Fyᵃfyᵇ, Jk(a−)	sec. A, H	
	Miss E.F.*	12% A₁B, Fyᵃfyᵇ, Jk(a−) 88% A₁, Fyᵃfyᵃ, Jk(a+)	sec. A, B, H	
20. Battey et al.[98], 1974	Mrs P.M.	7% A₁, NN, R¹r, Fy(a+) 93% O, MN, rr, Fy(a−)	sec. A, H	{4% XX 96% XY fibroblasts XX
	no known twin (page 530)			

* Both twins ascertained at the same time, during routine testing of twins. The other groups of the people in this table and the groups of further relatives may be found in the original papers or are available in our records.

The greater proportion of cells in the mixture need not indicate the true genetic group: notable examples are to be seen in pairs No. 7 and 15 where one member has only 1 % or less of cells genetically her own. Such a gross discrepancy suggests that in these cases one line of cells has enjoyed considerable selective advantage over the other, and in both environments.

Of the nature of the advantage little can be said about such small numbers. In seven informative members in whom the true genetic group appears to be at a disadvantage, O has not been dominated by A (No. 5, 7), by B (No. 12) or by AB (No. 14) and A has not been dominated by B (No. 15, 16) or by AB (No. 12). Putting this a different way, in twins with more grafted than genetic cells neither A nor B has yet won the day from O, nor has B won the day from A.

One wonders whether maternal antibodies, should they cross the placenta, might have an effect on the reception of the grafts. Again the figures are too small, and all we can extract is that there are only four instances in which the grafted cells are incompatible with the serum of the mother: in three of the four the grafts were minor (No. 2 Miss Wa., No. 8 mongol, No. 12 Frau G.) and in one major (No. 3 Mrs W.). On the other hand, there are 20 grafts compatible with the mothers' serum.

In appropriate male-female pairs, male red cells beat the female cells on three occasions and the female cells won once.

At first sight the major populations of karyotypes and of red cells appear to match very well, with the exception of No. 15. However, closer inspection shows that there are notable discrepancies, for example Miss Ba. (No. 6) and M Heb. (No. 10) each have a major population of their *own* red cells but a matching major population of *grafted* lymphocytes.

Changes in time

When retested three years later Mrs McK. (No. 1) who originally had 61 % O and 39 % A_1 was found[23] to have 70 % O and 30 % A_1: it was thought that this change was too great to be explained by the error of the technique.

The proportion in Mr Wa. (No. 2) is changing too, though that in his twin sister remains steady:

		1957	1959	1967	1972
Miss Wa.	O	99 %	98 %	99 %	99 %
	A_1	1 %	2 %	1 %	1 %
Mr Wa.	A_1	86 %	83 %	78 %	63 %
	O	14 %	17 %	22 %	37 %

All these counts were made by Professor Mollison and his colleagues.

In cattle the proportions of the mixtures are the same in each member of a pair, and the proportions of the mixtures change markedly in time[44]. Stone and his colleagues[44] report one most notable animal, the survivor of a pair. From the age of 1 month to 3 years its mixture was 90 % type I and 10 % type II: tested again

18

at the age of eight it had 2 % type I, 2 % type II and 96 % of its cells were type III (in type III the cells had the antigen combinations previously found only in either type I *or* type II cells). The authors conclude 'It is postulated that the "hybrid" cell type resulted from "mating" between the two hematopoietic tissues in the chimeric mixture and that the hybrid type had a distinct selective advantage.'

The karyotypes

In the early days a count of drumsticks in blood films from Mr Wa (No. 2) and Mr G. (No. 3) showed that they had some of their sisters' polymorphs in proportions compatible with their red cell mixtures (Davidson, Fowler and Smith[22]). Drumstick counts were also made[42] on the twin babies (No. 5).

Considering the hazards of grafting and perhaps selection, it is not surprising that the proportions in the lymphocyte mixtures of XX-XY pairs can sometmes disagree with the proportions of the red cell mixtures: notable examples are Miss Ba. (No. 6) and M Heb (No. 10).

In the few cases where fibroblast cells have been karyotyped, as expected, no mixtures were found: these cells were of the sex corresponding to that of the twin. The nuclear sexing of buccal smears, when done, also agreed with the sex of the twin.

Other polymorphic systems

In finding a mixture of platelet antigens, van der Hart and van Loghem[43] demonstrated that platelet precursors are amongst the cells that can be grafted in these twins.

The HL-A groups of the leucocytes are beginning to be used and have distinguished two populations (No. 9, No. 17 and No. 18).

Mixtures have also been detected in tests for the isozymes AcP_1, PGM_1 and GPT (No. 11, 13, 16).

The sex of the twins

In Table 92 there are 19 pairs of twins of known sex: 15 of them are of different sex and 4 of the same sex. Superficially this looks like a significant excess of XX-XY pairs, but problems of ascertainment are involved and we mention the count only that an eye may be kept on it in the future.

Acquired tolerance

Missing agglutinins

All the chimeras lack agglutinins for their grafted cells; for example a chimera genetically O but with grafted A cells has anti-B but not anti-A in the serum.

(Two examples[23, 43] were reported to have a weak anti-A_1 detectable only at low temperatures.)

This is an example of a general phenomenon outlined by Burnet and Fenner[12] and supported by the work of Owen[6]. According to the theory an animal does not produce antibody to an antigen to which it has been exposed in foetal life.

In whatever way the 10% or so of cattle twins who are not chimeras may be explained, the 90% who are suggest that the invading cells usually win the battle for tolerance. Though we have no clear ideas we cannot help wondering whether the outcome of the battle in man may have some bearing on the proportion of alien cells accepted. More information is needed, particularly about the ABO and HL-A groups of these people.

Incidentally, we must suppose that Nature has tried an experiment in the prevention of haemolytic disease due to anti-Rh. Madame Ko. (No. 10), for example, is genetically Rh negative but 10% of her cells are Rh positive: she presumably could not make anti-Rh however many Rh positive babies or transfusions she might have.

Skin grafts between chimera twins

Though they are of different genetical constitution reciprocal skin grafts between cattle chimera twins 'take'[27, 28], and this is thought to be an expression of tolerance acquired to tissue cells as well as to blood cells. Professor Woodruff[16], anticipating the same result in man, grafted skin between Miss Wa. and her brother in November 1957. The grafts did 'take' and a year later biopsy samples were examined (Woodruff and Lennox[29]). Surprisingly, in the brother, the nuclear sex of the skin in the area of the graft was found to be male, though there were islands of possibly female skin surviving: on the contrary, the sex of the grafted skin in the sister was clearly male. Woodruff and Lennox did not consider that the replacement in the brother of the female skin by male skin necessarily implied any lack of immunological tolerance, for autografts of bone may be replaced; but why the skin replacement happened only one way round remained a puzzle.

As we said above, only a few of the twin chimeras have been HL-A grouped but three showed two populations. Some years ago Professor Jon van Rood suggested to us that twin chimeras, who tolerate so well each other's tissues, should give some clues to secrets of success in transplantation in general.

The nine-banded armadillo is apparently born regularly in sets of monozygotic quadruplets. It was doubly surprising to learn[45] that skin grafts are not accepted between a set of quadruplets: the first surprise was to read that armadillos have skin.

Frequency of chimera twins

Though 90% of dizygotic twin calves have mixed blood the condition is extremely rare in man. Were it not so the transfusion services would have detected more

ABO mixtures, for, in England, about 34% of dizygotic twin pairs differ in their reactions with anti-A or with anti-B. (This figure is extracted from Smith and Penrose[2], Appendix Table 2, which gives phenotypic sib-sib ABO frequencies in England.) Furthermore, though a mixture such as that in Miss Wa. (No. 2), who had 99% O and 1% A cells, could easily have been missed when her cells were tested, the lack of anti-A in her serum would have precipitated further investigation. On the other hand, a converse mixture, 99% A and 1% O, would be missed.

This argument for the extreme rarity of twin chimerism seems to us so decisive that we are not giving, as we did in our fourth edition, some details of dizygotic twin investigation which had failed to show any evidence of chimerism: we have, however, kept the references[46, 20, 24, 25, 4, 37].

Chimeras that happen not to be mixed in their ABO groups may easily not be recognized unless the mixture approaches 50:50. However, several examples of mixtures, not chimerical, have been detected by Rh antibodies (see pages 236–238).

Turpin, Salmon and Cruveiller[26] found a double population of red cells in only one member of a pair of dizygotic twin babies. The mixture which was discovered when the twin was four months old had disappeared at six months. The 5% of invading cells, which could not have come from the mother, differed from those of the host in their MNS, Rh and Kidd groups. This interesting observation stimulated the full grouping of twins at birth in several centres, but the only subsequent newborn chimera pair found this way was that of Chown et al.[42] (No. 5, Table 92).

Fertility of chimera twins

It has long been known that the female of female-male cattle chimera twins are freemartins. Lillie's explanation, that the hormones of the male twin cross the chorionic anastomosis and disturb the proper development of the sex apparatus of the female twin, remained unshaken from 1916 for nearly half a century until the question was reopened by the work of Ohno and his collaborators[48, 49]. Primordial germ cells, as well as primordial marrow cells, can settle in the opposite twin (though not produce functional gametes). This has been shown also in the marmoset[51]. On the other hand, a hormonal cause of the cattle freemartin is learnedly supported by Anderson[61].

Five months after the publication of the first human chimera, mixed blood was reported in a pair of sheep twins[15]. The twins were of different sex and the female was found to be a freemartin. Several more examples are now known as described in the excellent paper by Dain and Tucker[99] (1970). In 1967, a goat XX-XY freemartin was reported[80]. In 1956, Billingham, Brent and Medawar[14] discovered that twin chicks (which, incidentally, seldom survive) are red cell chimeras—apparently all of them.

On the other hand human male-female chimera pairs are fertile, both the males and the females.

Artificial chimeras

The suppression, intentional or accidental, of marrow activity by irradiation and the subsequent injection of genetically foreign marrow is obviously a subject[30] which could be of immense importance to the species.

An outstandingly interesting account of a radiation chimera was given by Mathé and his colleagues[52, 53]. A man, aged 26, with acute lymphoblastic leukaemia was treated by total body irradiation followed by the injection of marrow cells from six close relatives. The patient lived for a year with blood groups not his own and he was apparently free of his leukaemia, but then he died of an infection.

Under this heading perhaps falls the extraordinary case reported by Beilby, Cade, Jelliffe, Parkin and Stewart[31]. A patient with Hodgkin's disease, who three and two years before had been treated with X-rays, suffered an acute marrow failure which was attributed to the chlorambucil with which she was being treated. She was given a transfusion of marrow from her sister (not a twin) which was apparently successful. The donor's cells contained the antigens D, E and N which had not been found in the patient's cells before the transfusion: after the transfusion they were found, the E with difficulty. After the transfusion, and for about two weeks, 6% of her cells reacted with anti-D, then fewer; but they rose again in six months' time to 24% and, 10 months after the transfusion, to 40%. The patient died about two years after the marrow transfusion.

A boy, group O, with acute lymphocytic leukaemia was transfused with white-cell-rich plasma from an AB patient with chronic myelogenous leukaemia. The red cells in the donor's plasma were estimated to account 'for no more than 10 per cent of the boy's calculated red cell mass', yet six weeks after the transfusion 56 per cent of his red cells were AB. Bronson and his colleagues[54] discuss other possibilities but favour the explanation of successful grafting of red cell precursors. The graft, however, had a short life, for AB cells could not be found six weeks later.

Swanson et al.[100] (1971) describe a boy with an immunological deficiency who at the age of five months was given a marrow transplant from his sister. Ten months later his red cells, as judged by their antigens, were those of his sister, but they had undergone one change: his sister, being O Le(b+), lacked the antigen A_1Le^b, but he, being genetically A_1 and Le(b+), had it and was able to stamp his sister's O Le(b+) cells circulating in him with the A_1Le^b label. This confirmed the coating power of A_1Le^b plasma molecules first recognized in the investigation of the chimera twin pair De. and Jo. (No. 11, Table 92) by Crookston et al.[87], and again in the St. twins[93] (No. 15, Table 92).

In a short but portentous letter to the Lancet, Naiman and his colleagues[55] described how a male child with haemolytic disease of the newborn transfused in utero rather earlier than was usual, turned out, when karyotyped 112 days after the transfusion, to be a mosaic for long and short Y chromosomes. The length of the Y chromosome is very strictly inherited: the father of the boy had a notably long Y while the Y of the donor was short. The child suffered from something like runt disease and the authors end with the warning 'To avert this complication of foetal transfusion we urge that efforts be made to render such blood free of leucocytes before administration.'

Other conditions simulating chimerism

A transient mixture of blood may suggest the possibility of a chimera: such mixtures may be caused by transfusion or by bleeding of a foetus into the mother's circulation. Several kinds of weak A, notably A_3, can look very like a mixture of A and O (see page 14). Leukaemia changes (page 29) and the change resulting from the acquisition of B (page 31) may also be mistaken for chimerical mixtures. and so may the Rh mosaicism associated particularly with myeloproliferative disease (page 237).

The transient T type of polyagglutinability has, when it was wearing off, been mistaken for chimerism (page 487) and so has the persistent mixed-field type of Tn polyagglutinability (page 490). The apparent mosaicism associated with old age (page 31) could also simulate chimerism. A more common source of error is the mixed field picture given by most anti-Sd[a] sera (page 395). The general subject of blood group mosaics was discussed by the authors[101] in 1972.

We do not know what to make of the case reported as a twin chimera by Ueno, Suzuki and Yamazawa[32]. Only one of the twins had an apparent mixture of blood (about 70% O and 30% A_1, on two occasions a year apart): her brother had only A_1 cells. As both the twins secrete A in their saliva we believe that both of them must be genetically A. Were it not that the separated 'A_1' and 'O' cells of the girl twin were reported to differ in their MN groups we would have guessed that she was an example of the curious 'A_1' and 'O' mixture found in several members of a Japanese family by Furuhata, Kitahama and Nozawa[33] (page 18).

Distinguishing between twin and dispermic chimerism

The diagnosis of twin chimerism is usually easy: the existence of a fellow twin who also has mixed blood settles it, and even the history of a fellow twin is helpful. When there is no twin or history of one the decision can be difficult for there remains the theoretical possibility of a resorbed twin or perhaps even of a graft *in utero* from the mother.

Dispermic chimerism would be established if fibroblast culture showed chromosomal mosaicism or if the skin were patchy in colour. If a chimera had an XX/XY karyotype he would probably not be fertile if he were of the dispermic type and he might be expected to have some abnormality of his external genitalia. An exception is the Detroit propositus (Table 93) who now has three children.

We have placed the chimera studied by Battey et al.[98] (No. 20) at the bottom of Table 92. She was outstanding in having no history of being a twin, nor was there any record of abnormal tissue born with her. Nevertheless, she is here

Table 93. Dispermic chimeras

References	Propositus and relatives	Characters demonstrating mosaicism in propositus			Double maternal contribution
		Markers	Lymphocytes	Others	
SEATTLE					
Gartler, Waxman and Giblett[62,63], 1962, 1963	girl aged 2	50% MS^u/MS, R^1R^2	$\{$ 50% XX $\atop$ 50% XY	one eye hazel, one brown; fibroblast XX/XY mosaicism: gonadal differences	
	father	MS^u/Ns, R^1r			
	mother	MS/Ns, R^2r MS^u/Ns, R^1R^2			
DETROIT					
Zuelzer, Beattie, Reisman, McGuire and Cohen[64,65], 1964	Mr D.W., aged 18	90% A,O,Jk^bJk^b, Hb AS, $Se\ se$	$\{$ 94% XY $\atop$ 6% XX	patchy skin (Negro-Amerindian-European ancestry); XX/XY mosaicism in dark skin only; slight gynaecomastia	Hb
		10% B,Jk^aJk^b, Hb A, $se\ se$			
	father	A,B,Jk^aJk^b, Hb A, $Se\ se$			
	mother	BO,Jk^aJk^b, Hb AS, $se\ se$			
PARIS I					
de Grouchy, Moullec, Salmon, Josso, Frézal, Lamy and others[66,67], 1964, 1965	male aged 20	Hp 2 − 2 + Hp 2 − 1	$\{$ 62% XX $\atop$ 38% XY	fibroblast XX/XY mosaicism; gonadal differences	
	father	Hp 2 − 1			
	mother	Hp 2 − 2			
VANCOUVER					
Miller, Dill, MacLean, Kaita, Lewis, Corey and Chown[68,69], 1964, 1967	C.G., boy aged 3	60% A,O,Lu^aLu^b,Fy^aFy^a $\{$ Hp 1 − 1 + Hp 2 − 1 $\atop$ PGM₁ mixture $\}$ 40% OO,Lu^bLu^b,Fy^aFy^b	$\{$ 60% XX $\atop$ 40% XY	extreme hypospadias	ABO Fy Hp
	father	OO,Lu^aLu^b,Fy^aFy^a, Hp 1 − 1, PGM₁ 2 − 1			
	mother	A_1O,Lu^bLu^b,Fy^aFy^b, Hp 2 − 1, PGM₁ 2 − 1			
WISCONSIN					
Myhre, Meyer, Opitz, Race, Sanger and Greenwalt[70], 1965	D.S., boy aged 12	85% OO,Jk^bJk^b	$\{$ 53% XX $\atop$ 47% XY	hypospadias	
		15% BO,Jk^aJk^b			
	father	BO,Jk^aJk^b			
	mother	A_2O,Jk^aJk^b			

Table 93—continued

References	Propositus and relatives	Markers	Lymphocytes	Others	Double maternal contribution
		Characters demonstrating mosaicism in propositus			
OSLO Brøgger and Gundersen[71], 1966	mongol boy aged 5	80% A_1B, P_1P_2 / 20% A_1O, P_2P_2	{80% normal / 20% trisomy G}		ABO P
	father	A_1, P_2P_2			
	mother	BO, P_1P_2			
GLASGOW Ferguson-Smith, Izatt, Renwick and Mack[72], 1966	F.B., male aged 15	97% OO, AcP BB, PGM_1 1–1 / 3% A_2O, AcP AC, PGM_1 2–1	{95% XY / 5% XX}	fibroblasts 73% XX; gonads both ovo-testes; hypospadias	AcP PGM_1
	father	A_2O, AcP BC, PGM_1 1–1			
	mother	OO, AcP AB, PGM_1 2–1			
DURBAN I Moores[79], 1966	Mrs T.R., aged 27	50% BO, Ms/Ns, R^1r, Sec / 50% A_1B, $MN.S$, rr, $se\ se$	all XX	extensive mottling of skin (Mrs T.R. is a Tamil.)	
	father	B, NN, R^1r $Se\ se$			
	mother	OO, NN, R^1R^1			
	husband	dead			
	children	two BO, MN, R^1r / one OO, MN, R^1r / one OO, NN, R^1r			
PARIS II Delarue, Liberge, Salmon and Lejeune[105], 1969	male aged 3 months	30% R^1r, Kk, Jk^aJk^b / 70% rr, kk, Jk^bJk^b	{5% XXY triploid / 95% XX}	liver, gonads and skin about 50% triploid	
	father	R_1r, Kk, Jk^aJk^b			
	mother	rr, kk, Jk^bJk^b			
TURIN Klinger, Miggiano, Tippett and Gavin[106], 1968. Ceppellini[107], 1972	Ilario G., male aged 20	75% MS/Ms, Fy^aFy^b, Xg(a−), HL–A, a/c / 25% Ms/Ns, Fy^aFy^a, Xg(a+), HL–A b/d	{40% XX / 60% XY}	hermaphrodite	HL–A

Table 93—*continued*

References	Propositus and relatives	Characters demonstrating mosaicism in propositus			Double maternal contribution
		Markers	Lymphocytes	Others	
BALTIMORE Park, Jones and Bias[108], 1970	L.B., female aged 13½ father mother	Ms/Ms, {Hp 2−1 Ms/Ns, {Hp 2−2 Ms/Ns, Hp 2−1 Ms/Ms, Hp 2−2	{46% XX 54% XY	true hermaphrodite	
DURBAN II Moores[109], 1969	Negro, female aged 6 weeks mother male twin	$BO, MS/NS, Fy^aFy^b$ $OO, MS/Ns, Fy^bFy^b$ $A_2O, NS/Ns, Fy^aFy^b$ $A_2O, MNSs, Fy^aFy^b$	all XX		MNSs
NEWCASTLE I Gray and Syrett[110], 1970	G.P., male aged 6 months father mother	40% $NS/Ns, Lu^bLu^b$ 60% $Ns/Ns, Lu^aLu^b$ $Ns/Ns, Lu^aLu^b$ $NS/Ns, Lu^aLu^b$	{20% XX 80% XY	hypospadias	MNSs
NEWCASTLE II Gray and Syrett[111], 1971	A.H., female aged 2 father mother	50% $A_1O, P_2P_2, rr, kk, Jk^aJk^b$ Sec 50% $OO, P_1P_2, R^2r, Kk, Jk^bJk^b$ se se $A_1O, P_1P_2, R^1r, Kk, Jk^aJk^b$ Se se $OO, P_2P_2, R^2r, kk, Jk^bJk^b$, Se se	{85% XX 15% XY	enlarged clitoris; gonads both ovotestes	Rh
GOTTINGEN Eberle, Gallasch and Truss[112], 1972	K.G., male aged 18 father mother	98% OO, kk 2% A_1, Kk A_1, kk A_1, Kk	{22% XX 78% XY	true hermaphrodite	K

Table 93—*continued*

References	Propositus and relatives	Markers	Lymphocytes	Others	Double maternal contribution
OXFORD Bobrow[113], 1971	G.M., male aged 4	more NS/Ns, {prob. Jk^aJk^a and Jk^aJk^b, less Ns/Ns, {prob. Do^aDo^b and Do^bDo^b, Hp 2−2, HL−A a/c Hp 2−1, HL−A b/c	52% XY 48% XX	hypospadias; fibroblasts 65% XY	Do probably
	father	NS/Ns, Jk^aJk^b, Do(a−), Hp2−1, HL−A a/b			
	mother	Ms/Ns, Jk^aJk^a, Do(a+), Hp2−2, HL−A c/d			
LONDON Polani[114], 1972	S.F.-B., girl aged 12	70% OO, MS/MS, kk, Fy^aFy^b, Jk^bJk^b, Xg(a−), AK 1 30% A_1, Ns/Ns, Kk, Fy^bFy^b, Jk^cJk^b, Xg(a+), AK 2−1	90% XY 10% XX	true hermaphrodite; fibroblasts XX and XY	MNSs, K, AK
	father	A_1O, MS/Ns, kk, Fy^aFy^b, Jk^cJk^c, Xg(a+), AK 1			
	mother	A_1O, MS/Ns, Kk, Fy^aFy^b, Jk^bJk^b, Xg(a−), AK 2−1			
LA JOLLA Benirschke et al.[115], 1972	O.S., female aged 20	50% Fy(a−), PGM₁ 2−1 50% Fy(a+), PGM₁ different	88% XX 12% XY	true hermaphrodite	
HELSINKI de la Chapelle, Schröder et al.[116], 1974	S, intersex, newborn	90% Ms/Ms, Jk^aJk^a, Xg(a−), ADA 2−1, HL−A b/d 10% MS/Ms, Jk^aJk^b, Xg(a+), ADA 1, HL−A a/c	92% XY 8% XX	true hermaphrodite; marker of No. 3 chromosome	ADA HL−A marked No. 3
	father	MS/Ms, Jk^aJk^b, Xg(a+), ADA 1, HL−A a/b			
	mother	Ms/Ns, Jk^aJk^b, Xg(a−), ADA 2−1, HL−A c/d			

Table 93—*continued*

References	Propositus and relatives	Characters demonstrating mosaicism in propositus			Double maternal contribution
		Markers	Lymphocytes	Others	
COLOGNE Pfeiffer[117], 1972	P.B. 'girl' aged 3 father mother	R^1r rr R^1r rr	{ 60% XY 40% XX	true hermaphrodite	
FRANKFURT Spielmann *et al.*[118], 1974	F.F. male blood donor father mother wife two daughters	85% O, *Ms/Ns* 15% A₁, *Ns/Ns* A₁, *Ms/Ns* O, *Ns/Ns* A₁, *MS/Ns* O, *Ns/Ns*	all XY		

The other groups of the people in this table and the groups of further relatives may be found in the original papers or are available in our records.

classified as a twin chimera because, though her lymphocytes are XY/XX, she is fertile; furthermore her fibroblast cultures were all XX and her buccal smear female. The theoretical possibility of a graft *in utero* from her mother is ruled out by her XY cells.

We presume we are right in listing as twin chimeras the three propositi whose twins are dead (Table 92). However, a lesson in jumping to conclusions is neatly, given by the Durban II dispermic chimera (Table 93). This baby girl might have been listed as a twin chimera had not Moores shown that the male twin did not have the same blood groups as either cell line of the propositus, whose lymphocytes, incidentally, were subsequently found to be all XX.

DISPERMIC CHIMERAS

This is another phenomenon of great interest disclosed by the fertile union of cytogenetics and blood grouping. The discovery was a Seattle triumph (Gartler, Waxman and Giblett[62, 63], 1962, 1963). A girl with a left eye hazel and a right eye brown was found to be mosaic in karyotype: about half her cultured lymphocytes were XX and about half XY. Further, she had two populations of red cells, as shown by the antigens E, N, S and s. At laparotomy a normal ovary was found on the left and an ovotestis on the right.

The only imaginable explanation was that two sperm had been involved in her engendering: the father, but not the mother, could have given brown *and* not-brown eye colour, X *and* Y, and the antigens E *and* e, and MS *and* Ns.

Since 1962 twenty further examples have been found, details of which are given in Table 93.

This type of chimerism is the result of the fertilization by two sperm of two maternal nuclei and the fusion of the two zygotes and their growth into one body. The state has been called generalized tissue mosaicism, whole body chimerism and tetragametic chimerism, but we prefer the shorter 'dispermic chimerism', for it is by the contribution of X and Y sperm that most of the cases listed in Table 93 were brought to light: a double contribution from the mother has, so far, been demonstrated in only about half the cases, but this proportion may grow with the increase of available markers.

In classifying chimeras in general, Ford[119] discusses which maternal cells may have been involved in the double fertilization, and there are several theoretical possibilities: 1, cells resulting from the suppression of the second meiotic division; 2, ovum and first polar body; 3, ovum and second polar body; 4, daughters of a divided ovum nucleus; and there is the possibility of the early fusion of two embryos such as can be made to happen in the mouse.

Table 93 would become unmanageable if we tried to give all the groups of the people there, and of further tested relatives; some are to be found in the original. papers and some are only in our records. It would be very difficult, if not impossible, to calculate from their markers whether and how often mothers contribute two egg cells which are genetically identical. Difficulties would arise if, for example, the chimera had a very small minor population. In that case certain of the antigens might not be detected, for purely serological reasons such as the strength of the antigen or the power of the available antisera, and this would confound observation for comparison with expectation based on the parental groups.

In the 21 examples of Table 93 the father can be seen to have contributed two different sperm to all but one (Oslo) whereas the mother can be seen to have contributed two genetically different germ nuclei to only 12 of the 21.

Ascertainment

The XX/XY propositi are usually detected at cytogenetic testing for reasons of a sex upset: two (Detroit and Wisconsin) were first found by a blood grouping laboratory. XX/XX and XY/XY cases will usually be found at blood grouping. That XX/XY cases select themselves is shown by the following count made from Table 93:

XX/XY	all XX	all XY
17	2	2

Other polymorphisms

HL-A typing is a very useful addition to these investigations, particularly in the detection of two maternal contributions, as illustrated by the Turin and Helsinki cases. The double maternal contribution in the Helsinki case was confirmed by the isozyme ADA and, in a most sophisticated way, by a No. 3 chromosome with a visible abnormality. Haptoglobins were useful in confirming a double maternal contribution in the Vancouver case.

Sibs of the chimeras

Seventeen brothers and twelve sisters have been blood grouped and none of them showed two populations of cells. Professor Polani asked us about this, for he was remembering a strain of mice with a high incidence of XX/XY intersexes believed to be due to the premature production of a lysin which removes the zona pellucida and allows two blastocysts to fuse. If something like this were happening in the mothers of human chimeras one would expect to find mixtures of blood groups in some of the sibs of propositi or perhaps amongst the offspring of their maternal aunts, but this has not yet been recognized.

Fertility of dispermic chimeras

Only one of the XX/XY members of Table 93 is known to be fertile: Mr D.W. (Detroit) has had three children since his chimera state was recognized (Beattie and Zuelzer, personal communication, 1974). One of the XXs was fertile, the other aged but 6 weeks; one of the XYs was fertile, the other a mongol. Fertile also was the XX/XY chimera No. 20, this we mention here only in case we were wrong to put her in Table 92 rather than 93.

Proportions of the mixtures

In Table 93 there are 12 XX/XY mixtures for which the proportion of XX and XY cells has been counted, and these proportions fit very closely those of the red cell mixtures in 6 but appear not to be related in 6. In all but two of the 12 we are guessing that the major line of the karyotype count is the major line of the red cell count, as it is in the two for which there is proof. The proof of which red cell line in fact represents XX and which XY can, at present, only be shown by the Xg constellation in the family. In the two successful cases (London and Helsinki) the Xg(a+) line must be the XX one, for the mothers of these two chimeras are Xg(a−) so the fathers must have contributed Xg^a, and therefore X to this line of their chimera offspring.

We are puzzled by this hint of two classes, the fitting and the non-fitting red and white cell proportions, and it serves as just one reason why these chimeras should continue to be investigated and published.

Secretion and the Lewis groups

The contribution of dispermic chimeras to the realization that secretion is controlled by the intracellular interaction of genetically independent loci is mentioned briefly on page 312.

The secretor and Lewis findings in the Detroit example were intricate and instructive. The propositus has nine sibs who make clear the secretor and Lewis genotypes of the parents: the father must be A_1B, *Se se*, *le le*, and the mother *BO*, *se se*, *Le Le*. The propositus, D.W., has approximately 90 % A_1, and 10 % B cells; he is most unusual in that his cells are Le(a+b−) yet he secretes A; furthermore, he does not secrete B. Apparently the sperm responsible for the greater amount of D.W.'s somatic cells carried A_1, *Se* and *le* and that responsible for the lesser amount carried *B* or *O*, *se*, *le*: so D.W. has a major population of A_1O, *Se se*, *Le le* cells which account for the secretion of A and a minor population of *BO* or *BB*, *se se*, *Le le*, which provides enough Le substance in the serum to make all the cells Le(a+). (There is less Le substance than in ordinary *se se*, *Le Le*, or *se se*, *Le le* people but more than in *Se se*, *Le* people.)

The secretor and Lewis groups of the Durban I case would be astonishing did they not exactly parallel those of the Detroit example. The cells of Mrs T.R. are Le(a+b−) and she secretes B and H but not A. (The other family members are all Le(a−) and, presumably, secretors.) The easiest explanation is that the mother of Mrs T.R. is *Sese* and that the father's contributions were A_1 and *se* in one sperm and *O* and *Se* in the other.

Excluding the baby (Durban II), two further propositi are Le(a+) yet secretors. Ilario G. (Turin) is A_1 Le(a+), sec A, H and Les: one cell line, we cannot tell which, must have A_1,Se, the other A_1, *sese*, *Le*. The Newcastle II propositus secretes A and H: she secretes markedly less A and H than expected of an A secretor but her saliva contains nearly as much Le substance as that from control Le(a+b−) people, so her A_1 cell line must represent *Se*, *Le* and her *O* cell line *sese*, *Le*.

Xg and X chromosome inactivation

The important contribution to the problem of Lyonization made by the Turin example, like that of the chimerical twin pair No. 10 (Table 92), in showing that Xg(a+) and Xg(a−) cells can coexist in one circulation is recorded in page 586. This has been further confirmed by the London and the Helsinki dispermics and by the twin chimera pairs No. 13 and 15.

XX/XY mosaicism without other evidence of dispermy

We were kindly given the opportunity to group the blood of nine other XX/XY mosaics but in whom we could find no evidence of red cell mosaicism. Three of them are published (Bain and Scott[73], Manuel, Allie and Jackson[74], Ribas-Mundó and Prats[75]).

The rare people who belong to this dispermic class can be thought of as a fusion of twins, dissimilar in their father's contribution and dissimilar or perhaps identical in that from their mother. The involvement of two sperm in the making of one offspring is known in other species—Bombyx, the silkworm, being especially gifted in this respect—but that it should happen in man came as a surprise. Since two sperm need not come from the same man it is a curious thought that in the long history of our species there must have been at least a few people born blessed with two fathers and one mother.

MONOZYGOTISME HÉTÉROCARYOTE

This is the name introduced by Turpin and Lejeune[56] in their admirable book *Les Chromosomes Humains* for a new class of twins discovered in France—twins who are monozygotic, as shown by blood groups, skin grafting etc., yet who do not have exactly the same complement of chromosomes. The accident is due to aneuploidy at some post-zygotic cell division preceding the laying down of the keels of the twins in their primitive streaks.

The first example was the consequence of aneuploidy in the subsequent divison of an XY zygote: at some division the Y was lost and one twin became a normal XY male and the other an XO Turner female (Turpin, Lejeune, Lafourcade, Chigot and Salmon[34, 35], 1961, 1963).

The second example followed aneuploidy of the autosome No. 21: one boy twin was normal and the other was trisomic for No. 21 and so had Down's syndrome (Lejeune, Lafourcade, Scharer, de Wolf, Salmon, Haines and Turpin[57], 1962).

Other examples followed: Edwards, Dent and Kahn[50] reported a monozygotic brother and sister of whom, surprisingly, the normal boy is XO and his sister, a mild example of Turner's syndrome, is an XO/XY mosaic. It was presumed that the boy has some Y chromosomes somewhere, though none was to be found in peripheral blood or skin cells. We cannot do justice to the brilliant analysis of this most complicated pair, it must be read in the original.

Both Edwards and his colleagues[50] and Mikkelsen, Frøland and Ellebjerg[58] describe pairs of monozygotic twin girls: both of each pair were mosaic XO/XX but one of each pair was seriously abnormal while the other was normal. A some-what similar case was reported by Benirschke and Sullivan[59]: by finding, as they anticipated, chromosome mosaicism in a surviving normal twin they were able to pin down, as XO, the chromosomal upset responsible for the gross malforma-tion of the other twin, who had died at birth seven years before.

At Oxford, Shine and Corney[120] encountered a remarkable monozygotic pair: an XO Turner with multiple deformities and a normal XX girl. The Xg groups were also interesting: Turner Xg(a−), normal twin Xg(a+), father Xg(a+). This combination shows that the missing X of the Turner was her father's.

A further monozygotic pair, one trisomic for 21 and the other normal, was reported by Bruins et al.[60]: and yet another was found by Macdonald and Polani (personal communication).

Two more monozygotic pairs, XO Turner girls with normal twin sisters, were investigated by Dr Mary Lucas and by Dr John Philip (personal communica-tions, 1973).

The chromosomal mosaicism present in the peripheral blood of both normal and abnormal members of some of these hétérocaryote pairs is often due, as Turpin and Lejeune[56] point out, to interchange *in utero* of marrow cells which 'take' in the opposite twin. (In our fourth edition we wrote 'In monozygotic twins, on the other hand, mixed blood must be very common—though impossible to demonstrate, at least by present methods.' We little thought how soon it was to become possible.)

PARTIAL TRIPLOIDY

Mention must be made of the remarkable case reported by Ellis, Marshall, Normand and Penrose[76] (1963). In attempting, on a previous occasion, to do justice to this notable observation one of us[77] wrote

'The daughter shown in Figure 33 has three sets of chromosomes, instead of the normal two, in about half of her skin cells. She was then found also to be very unusual indeed in her blood groups; for her red cells gave the reaction of group O but her saliva contained group B antigen.

Some of the epithelial cells of her mouth were found to have the B antigen also. Ellis and his colleagues[76] concluded that while the ABO genotype of the diploid cells must be *OO* that of the triploid cells must be *OOB*: that is to say the diploid line had been responsible for her blood while the triploid line had been responsible for her skin and for the antigen in her saliva. Since only the mother could have given both *B* and *O* genes the abnormality can be traced to the egg cell; and the interpretation is that the child began as an ordinary diploid zygote, the result of fusion of one sperm, carrying the blood group allele *O*, and one egg nucleus, also carrying an *O* allele. This normal zygote then divided into two daughter cells; but somehow the nucleus of the unextruded polar body, left over from the second meiotic division, managed to fuse with one of these two daughter cells, so contributing an extra haploid set of chromosomes marked by the presence of the blood group allele *B*. Here the female sex cells are seen to be just as enterprising to seize an unexpected opportunity as are spermatozoa.

'In this problem the blood groups advanced the understanding of the origin of the triploidy; but in return the triploidy has given information which will no doubt be useful in future attempts to learn more about the developmental background of the secretor phenomenon and the general sharing out of jobs at early post-zygotic cell divisions.'

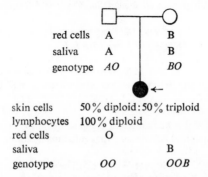

Fig. 33. A partially triploid female. (From the data of Ellis, Marshall, Normand and Penrose[76], 1963.)

Edwards and his colleagues[78] describe a triploid abortion whose blood groups, together with those of the parents, favoured a double maternal, rather than a double paternal contribution. Those wanting to learn about triploidy and about the many ways it may in theory arise should study this learned and thoughtful paper.

There is surely much more to be learnt from twin and dispermic chimeras and their existence ought to be recorded, possibly for future reinvestigation in the light of newer knowledge. Those in the position to find these cases are all very busy people who need not be called on to write a formal paper: all that is needed is a brief report, perhaps in telegrammatic form, giving such facts as time has allowed the gathering.

REFERENCES

1   COTTERMAN C.W. (1951) Personal communication.
2   SMITH SHEILA M. and PENROSE L.S. (1955) Monozygotic and dizygotic twin diagnosis. *Ann. hum. Genet.*, **19**, 273–289.

3 SANGER RUTH and RACE R.R. (1951) The MNSs blood group system. *Amer. J. hum. Genet.*, **3**, 332–343.

4 WALSH R.J. and KOOPTZOFF OLGA (1955) A study of twins. Blood groups and other data. *Aust. J. exp. Biol. med. Sci.*, **33**, 189–198.

5 WALSH R.J. (1952) The blood groups of quadruplets. *Australasian Annals of Medicine*, **1**, 140–141.

6 OWEN R.D. (1945) Immunogenetic consequences of vascular anastomoses between bovine twins. *Science*, **102**, 400–401.

7 LILLIE F.R. (1916) The theory of the free-martin. *Science*, **43**, 611–613.

8 DUNSFORD I., BOWLEY C.C., HUTCHISON ANN M., THOMPSON JOAN S., SANGER RUTH and RACE R.R. (1953) A human blood-group chimera. *Brit. med. J.*, **ii**, 81.

9 BOOTH P.B., PLAUT GERTRUDE, JAMES J.D., IKIN ELIZABETH W., MOORES PHYLLIS, SANGER RUTH and RACE R.R. (1957) Blood chimerism in a pair of twins. *Brit. med. J.*, **i**, 1456–1458.

10 NICHOLAS J.W., JENKINS W.J. and MARSH W.L. (1957) Human blood chimeras. A study of surviving twins. *Brit. med. J.*, **i**, 1458–1460.

11 IRWIN M.R. (1955) Chapter in *Biological Specificity and Growth*, Princeton University Press, p. 68.

12 BURNET F.M. and FENNER F. (1949) *The Production of Antibodies*, Macmillan, Melbourne.

13 HAUGE M. (1962) *Om blodtypernes anvendelse i den humane genetik.* Doctoral thesis, Copenhagen, pp. 203.

14 BILLINGHAM R.E., BRENT L. and MEDAWAR P.B. (1956) Quantitative studies on tissue transplantation immunity. III. Actively acquired tolerance. *Phil. Trans.*, **239**, 357–414.

15 STORMONT C., WEIR W.C. and LANE L.L. (1953) Erythrocyte mosaicism in a pair of sheep twins. *Science*, **118**, 695–696.

16 WOODRUFF M.F.A. (1953) A human blood group chimera. *Brit. med. J.*, **ii**, 1103.

17 FISHER R.A. (1951) Standard calculations for evaluating a blood-group system. *Heredity*, **5**, 95–102.

18 SUTTON H.E., CLARK P.J. and SCHULL W.J. (1955) The use of multi-allele genetic characters in the diagnosis of twin zygosity. *Amer. J. hum. Genet.*, **7**, 180–188.

19 JUEL-NIELSEN N., NIELSEN A. and HAUGE M. (1958) On the diagnosis of zygosity in twins and the value of blood groups. *Acta genet.*, **8**, 256–273.

20 SIMMONS R.T., GRAYDON J.J., JAKOBOWICZ RACHEL and DOIG R.K. (1960) A blood group genetical study made in a survey of illness in monozygotic and dizygotic twins. *Med. J. Aust.*, **ii**, 246–249.

21 MOORE K., GRAHAM MARGARET A. and BARR M.L. (1957) The sex chromatin of the bovine freemartin. *J. exp. Zool.*, **135**, 101–126.

22 DAVIDSON W.M., FOWLER J.F. and SMITH D.R. (1958) Sexing the neutrophil leucocytes in natural and artificial blood chimeras. *Brit. J. Haemat.*, **4**, 231–238.

23 DUNSFORD I. and STACEY S.M. (1957) Partial breakdown of acquired tolerance to the A antigen. *Vox Sang.*, **2**, 414–417.

24 OSBORNE R.H. and DE GEORGE FRANCES V. (1957) Selective survival in dizygotic twins in relation to the ABO groups. *Amer. J. hum. Genet.*, **9**, 321–330.

25 SUTTON H.E. (1958) Selective survival in dizygotic twins. *Amer. J. hum. Genet.*, **10**, 233–234.

26 TURPIN R., SALMON C. and CRUVEILLER J. (1959) A propos des chimères humaines présence temporaire d'une double population d'hématies chez l'un des jumeaux d'un couple dizygote. *Rev. franc. Études clin. biol.*, **4**, 809–811.

27 ANDERSON D., BILLINGHAM R.E., LAMPKIN G.H. and MEDAWAR P.B. (1951) The use of skin-grafting to distinguish between monozygotic and dizygotic twins in cattle. *Heredity*, **5**, 379–397.

28 BILLINGHAM R.E., LAMPKIN G.H., MEDAWAR P.B. and WILLIAMS H.LL. (1952) Tolerance to homografts, twin diagnosis, and the freemartin condition in cattle. *Heredity*, **6**, 201–212.

29   WOODRUFF M.F.A. and LENNOX B. (1959) Reciprocal skin grafts in a pair of twins showing
     blood chimerism. *Lancet*, ii, 476–478.
30   ILBERY P.L.T., KOLLER P.C. and LOUTIT J.F. (1958) Immunological characteristics of
     radiation chimeras. *J. nat. Cancer Inst.*, 20, 1051–1089.
31   BEILBY J.O.W., CADE IRENE S., JELLIFFE A.M., PARKIN DOROTHY M. and STEWART J.W.
     (1960) Prolonged survival of a bone-marrow graft resulting in a blood-group chimera.
     Brit. med. J., i, 96–99.
32   UENO S., SUZUKI K. and YAMAZAWA K. (1959) Human chimerism in one of a pair of twins.
     Acta genet., 8, 47–53.
33   FURUHATA T., KITAHAMA M. and NOZAWA T. (1959) A family study of the so-called blood
     group chimera. *Proc. imp. Acad. Japan*, 35, 55–57.
34   TURPIN R., LEJEUNE J., LAFOURCADE J., CHIGOT P.L. and SALMON C. (1961) Présomption de
     monozygotisme en dépit d'un dimorphisme sexuel: sujet masculin XY et sujet neutre
     haplo X. *C.R. Acad. Sci., Paris*, 252, 2945–2946.
35   LEJEUNE J. and TURPIN R. (1961) Détection chromosomique d'une mosaique artificielle
     humaine. *C.R. Acad. Sci., Paris*, 252, 3148–3150.
36   EDWARDS J.H. (1966) Twinning in man. Abstract in *Heredity*, 1967, 22, 161.
37   UCHIDA IRENE A., WANG H.C. and RAY M. (1964) Dizygotic twins with XX/XY chimerism.
     Nature, Lond., 204, 191.
38   HAUGE M., HERRLIN K.-M. and HEIKEN A. (1967) The distribution of blood groups in a
     series of triplets. *Acta genet.*, 17, 260–274.
39   HERRLIN K.-M. and HAUGE M. (1967) Determination of triplet zygosity. *Acta genet.*, 17,
     81–95.
40   STRANC M.F. (1966) Skin homograft survival in a severely burned triplet: study of triplet
     zygotic type. *Plastic reconstr. Surg.*, 37, 280–290.
41   VELEZ-OROZCO A.C. (1961) Estudio de una quimera. *Bol. Inst. Estud. méd. biol. Mex.*, 19,
     41–50.
42   CHOWN B., LEWIS MARION and BOWMAN J.M. (1963) A pair of newborn human blood
     chimeric twins. *Transfusion, Philad.*, 3, 494–495.
43   V.D., HART MIA and V. LOGHEM J.J. (1967) Blood group chimerism. *Vox Sang.*, 12, 161–172.
44   STONE W.H., FRIEDMAN JANIS and FREGIN AUDREY (1964) Possible somatic cell mating in
     twin cattle with erythrocyte mosaicism. *Proc. nat. Acad. Sci., Wash.*, 51, 1036–1044.
45   ANDERSON J.M. and BENIRSCHKE K. (1962) *Ann. N.Y. Acad. Sci.*, 99, 399 and (1963)
     Transplantation, 1, 306. Not seen, cited by BAKER L.N. (1964). Skin grafting in pigs:
     a search for monozygotic twins. *Transplantation*, 2, 434–435.
46   RACE R.R. and SANGER RUTH (1962) *Blood Groups in Man*, 4th ed. Blackwell Scientific
     Publications, p. 380.
47   WOODRUFF M.F.A., FOX M., BUCKTON KARIN A. and JACOBS PATRICIA A. (1962) The recog-
     nition of human blood chimaeras. *Lancet*, i, 192–194.
48   OHNO S., TRUJILLO J.M., STENIUS C., CHRISTIAN L.C. and TEPLITZ R.L. (1962) Possible
     germ cell chimeras among newborn dizygotic twin calves (*Bos taurus*). *Cytogenetics*, 1,
     258–265.
49   OHNO S. and GROPP A. (1965) Embryological basis for germ cell chimerism in mammals.
     Cytogenetics, 4, 251–261.
50   EDWARDS J.H., DENT TESSA and KAHN J. (1966) Monozygotic twins of different sex.
     J. med. Genet., 3, 117–123.
51   BENIRSCHKE K. and BROWNHILL LYDIA E. (1963) Heterosexual cells in testes of chimeric
     marmoset monkeys. *Cytogenetics*, 2, 331–341.
52   MATHÉ G., AMIEL J.L., SCHWARZENBERG L., CATTAN A. and SCHNEIDER M. (1963) Haemato-
     poietic chimera in man after allogenic (homologous) bone-marrow transplantation. *Brit.
     med. J.*, ii, 1633–1635.
53   MATHÉ G., AMIEL J.L., SCHWARZENBERG L., CATTAN A., SCHNEIDER M., DE VRIES M.J.,
     TUBIANA M., LALANNE C., BINET J.L., PAPIERNIK M., SEMAN G., MATSUKURA M.,

MERY A.M., SCHWARZMANN V. and FLAISLER A. (1965) Successful allogenic bone marrow transplantation in man: chimerism, induced specific tolerance and possible anti-leukemic effects. *Blood*, **25**, 179–196.

[54] BRONSON W.R., McGINNISS MARY H. and MORSE E.E. (1964) Hematopoietic graft detected by a change in ABO group. *Blood*, **23**, 239–249.

[55] NAIMAN J.L., PUNNETT HOPE H., DESTINÉ MARIE L. and LISCHNER H.W. (1966) Yy chromosomal chimerism. *Lancet*, **ii**, 590.

[56] TURPIN R. and LEJEUNE J. (1965) *Les Chromosomes Humains*. Gauthier-Villars, Paris, pp. 535.

[57] LEJEUNE J., LAFOURCADE J., SCHARER K., DE WOLFF E., SALMON C., HAINES M. and TURPIN R. (1962) Monozygotisme hétérocaryote: jumeau normal et jumeau trisomique 21. *C.R. Acad. Sci.*, Paris, **254**, 4404–4406.

[58] MIKKELSEN MARGARETA, FRØLAND A. and ELLEBJERG J. (1963) XO/XX mosaicism in a pair of presumably monozygotic twins with different phenotypes. *Cytogenetics*, **2**, 86–98.

[59] BENIRSCHKE K. and SULLIVAN M.M. (1965) Chromosomally discordant monozygous twins. *Hum. Chromos. Newsl.*, No. **15**, 3.

[60] BRUINS J.W., BOLHUIS J. VAN, BIJLSMA J.B. and NIJENHUIS L.E. (1963) Discordant mongolism in monozygotic twins. *Proc. 11th int. Congr. Genet.*, The Hague (not seen).

[61] ANDERSON J.M. (1965) Chimaeras and mosaics. *Lancet*, **i**, 1337–1338.

[62] GARTLER S.M., WAXMAN S.H. and GIBLETT ELOISE (1962) An XX/XY human hermaphrodite resulting from double fertilization. *Proc. nat. Acad. Sci.*, **48**, 332–335.

[63] GIBLETT ELOISE R., GARTLER S.M. and WAXMAN S.H. (1963) Blood group studies on the family of an XX/XY hermaphrodite with generalized tissue mosaicism. *Amer. J. hum. Genet.*, **15**, 62–68.

[64] ZUELZER W.W., BEATTIE KATHRYN M. and REISMAN L.E. (1964) Generalized unbalanced mosaicism attributable to dispermy and probable fertilization of a polar body. *Amer. J. hum. Genet.*, **16**, 38–51.

[65] BEATTIE KATHYRYN M., ZUELZER W.W., McGUIRE DELORES A. and COHEN FLOSSIE (1964) Blood group chimerism as a clue to generalized tissue mosaicism. *Transfusion, Philad.*, **4**, 77–86.

[66] DE GROUCHY J., MOULLEC J., SALMON C., JOSSO N., FRÉZAL J. and LAMY M. (1964) Hermaphrodisme avec caryotype XX/XY étude génétique d'un cas. *Annls Génét.*, **7**, 25–30.

[67] JOSSO NATHALIE, DE GROUCHY J., AUVERT J., NEZELOF C., JAYLE M.F., MOULLEC J., FRÉZAL J., DE CASAUBON A. and LAMY M. (1965) True hermaphroditism with XX/XY mosaicism, probably due to double fertilization of the ovum. *J. clin. Endocr. Metab.*, **25**, 114–126.

[68] MILLER J.R., DILL F.J., MACLEAN R., KAITA HIROKO and LEWIS MARION (1964) XX/XY and blood group mosaicism resulting from a double fertilization. Meeting Amer. Soc. hum. Genet., Boulder, Colorado. *Abstracts*, p. 18.

[69] COREY MARGARET J., MILLER J.R., MACLEAN J.R. and CHOWN B. (1967) A case of XX/XY mosaicism. *Amer. J. hum. Genet.*, **19**, 378–387.

[70] MYHRE B.A., MEYER T., OPITZ J.M., RACE R.R., SANGER RUTH and GREENWALT T.J. (1965) Two populations of erythrocytes associated with XX/XY mosaicism. *Transfusion, Philad.*, **5**, 501–505.

[71] BRØGGER A. and GUNDERSEN S.K. (1966) Double fertilization in Down's syndrome. *Lancet*, **i**, 1270–1271.

[72] FERGUSON-SMITH M.A., IZATT MARION, RENWICK J.H. and MACK W.S. (1966) Unpublished observations.

[73] BAIN A.D. and SCOTT J.S. (1965) Mixed gonadal dysgenesis with XX/XY mosaicism. The evidence for the occurrence of fertilization by two spermatozoa in man. *Lancet*, **i**, 1035–1039.

[74] MANUEL M.A., ALLIE A. and JACKSON W.P.U. (1965) A true hermaphrodite with XX/XY chromosome mosaicism. *S. Afr. med. J.*, **39**, 411–414.

75 RIBAS-MUNDÓ M. and PRATS J. (1965) Hermaphrodite with mosaic XX/XY/XXY. *Lancet*, **ii**, 494.

76 ELLIS J.R., MARSHALL RUTH, NORMAND I.C.S. and PENROSE L.S. (1963) A girl with triploid cells. *Nature, Lond.*, **198**, 411.

77 RACE R.R. (1965) Contributions of blood groups to human genetics. *Proc. Roy. Soc.*, B, **163**, 151–168.

78 EDWARDS J.H., YUNCKEN CATHERINE, RUSHTON D.I., RICHARDS SUSAN and MITTWOCH URSULA (1967) Three cases of triploidy in man. *Cytogenetics*, **6**, 81–104.

79 MOORES PHYLLIS P. (1966) An Asiatic blood group chimera. Paper read at Blood Trans. Congr., Port Elizabeth.

80 ILBERY P.L.T. and WILLIAMS D. (1967) Evidence of the freemartin condition in the goat. *Cytogenetics*, **6**, 276–285.

81 BIAS WILMA B. and MIGEON BARBARA R. (1967) Blood-group chimaerism with Down's syndrome. *Lancet*, **ii**, 257.

82 BOYCE M.J., LOCKYER J.W. and WOOD C.B.S. (1972) Foetus in foetu: serological assessment of monozygotic origin by automated analysis. *J. clin. Path.*, **25**, 793–798.

83 GUNDOLF F. (1970) Blood group chimerism in a Danish pair of twins. *Acta path. microbiol. Scand.*, **78**, 98–100.

84 GUNDOLF F. and HANSEN H.E. (1972) Lymphocyte and HL-A chimerism in a pair of blood group chimeric twins. *Acta path. microbiol. Scand.*, **80**, 152–154.

85 DUCOS J., COLOMBIES P., MARTY Y., BLANC M., DAVER J. and EMOND J. (1970) Double population cellulaire chez deux jumeaux hétéro-caryotes. *Rev. fr. Transf.*, **13**, 261–266.

86 DUCOS J., MARTY YVONNE, SANGER RUTH and RACE R.R. (1971) Xg and X chromosome inactivation. *Lancet*, **ii**, 219–220.

87 CROOKSTON MARIE C., TILLEY CHRISTINE A. and CROOKSTON J.H. (1970) Human blood chimaera with seeming breakdown of immune tolerance. *Lancet*, **ii**, 1110–1112.

88 SCHACHTER H., MICHAELS M.A., CROOKSTON MARIE C., TILLEY CHRISTINE A. and CROOKSTON J.H. (1971) A quantitative difference in the activity of blood group A-specific N-acetylgalactosaminyltransferase in serum from A_1 and A_2 human subjects. *Biochem. Biophys. res. Commun.*, **45**, 1011–1018.

89 KAESER A. and NENNSTIEL H.J. (1971) Chimärismus vom Typ O/B in zwei neuentdeckten Fällen mit Differenz der Lewis-Gruppen und der Antigenstärken von H und P_1. *Blut*, **22**, 229–236.

90 OSINSKA MARIA and WOLOSZYN TERESA (1971) A rare case of embryonic chimerism in human twins. *Arch. Immunol. Ther. Exp.*, **19**, 657–665.

91 SCHLESINGER DANUTA and HALASA JOLANTA (1971) A case of chimerism in an erythrocytic enzyme group system. *Arch. Immunol. Ther. Exp.*, **19**, 675–678.

92 CARR E.O. and MCDONALD L.A. (1974) Another example of human chimerism. *Transfusion, Philad.*, **14**, 475–476.

93 WROBEL DAMIANA M., MCDONALD IONE, RACE CAROLINE and WATKINS WINIFRED M. (1974) 'True' genotype of chimeric twins revealed by blood-group gene products in plasma. *Vox Sang.*, **27**, 395–402.

94 LOWES B.C.R., SULLIVAN J.P. and SABO BERNICE H. (1974) Unpublished observations.

95 ROBINSON E.A.E. and HORSFIELD I. (1973) In preparation.

96 BOWLEY C.C., GELSTHORPE K. and STAPLETON R.R. (1974) Personal communication: investigation continuing.

97 HOSOI T. (1973) Unpublished observations.

98 BATTEY DIANA A., BIRD G.W.G., MCDERMOTT A., MORTIMER C.W., MUTCHINICK O.M. and WINGHAM JUNE (1974) Another human chimaera. *J. Med. Genet.*, **11**, 283–287.

99 DAIN ANNE R. and TUCKER ELIZABETH M. (1970) Cytogenetic, anatomical and blood group studies of sheep twin chimaeras. *Proc. Roy. Soc.*, **175**, 183–200.

100 SWANSON JANE, CROOKSTON MARIE C., YUNIS E., AZAR M., GATTI R.A. and GOOD R.A. (1971) Lewis substances in a human marrow-transplantation chimaera. *Lancet*, **i**, 396.

[101] RACE R.R. and SANGER RUTH (1972) Blood group mosaics. *Haematologia*, **6**, 63–71.

[102] EDWARDS J.H. (1968) The value of twins in genetic studies. *Proc. Roy. Soc. Med.*, **61**, 227–229.

[103] CAMERON A.H. (1968) The Birmingham twin survey. *Proc. Roy. Soc. Med.*, **61**, 229–234.

[104] CORNEY G., ROBSON ELIZABETH B. and STRONG S.J. (1968) Twin zygosity and placentation. *Ann. Hum. Genet.*, **32**, 89–96.

[105] DELARUE FRANÇOISE, LIBERGE GENÈVIEVE, SALMON C. and LEJEUNE J. (1969) Une chimère avec une population triploide décelable par trois systèmes de groupes sanguins. *Rev. fr. Transf.*, **13**, 129–134.

[106] KLINGER R., MIGGIANO V.C., TIPPETT P. and GAVIN J. (1968) Diabete mellito e nanismo ipofisario in chimera XX, XY. *Atti Accad. med. Lomb.*, **23**, 1392–1396.

[107] CEPPELLINI R. (1972) Old and new facts and speculations about transplantation antigens of man. In *Progress in Immunology*: 1*st Int. Congr. Immunol.*, Washington, 1971. Ed. B. Amon, Academic Press, N.Y., pp. 46–48.

[108] PARK I.-J., JONES H.W. and BIAS WILMA B. (1970) True hermaphroditism with 46,XX/46,XY chromosome complement. *Obst. Gynec.*, *N.Y.*, **36**, 377–387.

[109] MOORES PHYLLIS P. (1969) Personal communication.

[110] GRAY J.E. and SYRETT J.E. (1970) Personal communication.

[111] GRAY J.E. and SYRETT J.E. (1971) Personal communication.

[112] EBERLE P., GALLASCH E. and TRUSS F. (1972) XX/XY-Hermaphroditismus verus mit Blutchimäre. *Blut* **25**, 255–264.

[113] BORROW M. (1971) Personal communication.

[114] POLANI P.E. (1972) Personal communication.

[115] BENIRSCHKE, K., NAFTOLIN F., GITTES, R., KHUDR G., YEN S.S.C. and ALLEN F.H. (1972) True hermaphroditism and chimerism. *Am. J. Obst. Gynec.*, **113**, 449–458.

[116] DE LA CHAPELLE A., SCHRÖDER J., RANTANEN P., THOMASSON B., NIEMI M., TIILIKAINEN ANJA, SANGER RUTH and ROBSON ELIZABETH (1974) Early fusion of two human embryos. *Ann. hum. Genet.*, **38**, 63–75.

[117] PFEIFFER R.A. (1972) Unpublished observations.

[118] SPIELMANN W. (1974) Personal communication.

[119] FORD C.E. (1969) Mosaics and chimaeras. *Brit. med. Bull.*, **25**, 104–109.

[120] SHINE I.B. and CORNEY G. (1966) Turner's syndrome in monozygotic twins. *J. med. Genet.*, **3**, 124–128.

[121] GOTTESMAN I.I. and SHIELDS J. (1972) *Schizophrenia and genetics: a twin study vantage point.* Academic Press, New York and London, pp. 433.

[122] MOORES PHYLLIS (1973) Blood group and tissue mosaicism in a Natal Indian woman. *Acta Haemat.*, **50**, 299–304.

[123] PROKOP O. and HERRMANN U. (1973) Blutgruppenbefunde bei Achtlingen. *Zbl. Gynäk.*, **95**, 1497.

Chapter 27
Blood Groups and Mapping of the Autosomes

For over 40 years people have been trying to find examples in man of the pheno-menon of linkage, known in other species since 1911.

The first success came in 1937 when Bell and Haldane demonstrated that the loci for colour blindness and for haemophilia, both known to be carried on the X chromosome, were within measurable distance of each other—were linked.

But autosomal linkage, linkage on the non-sex chromosomes, was a more difficult problem and in the early days the chances of showing it in man were pretty forlorn because of the shortage of marker characters. The earlier attempts had to be confined practically to the ABO and MN groups. But as the list of blood groups grew, the result of work in blood transfusion laboratories, the search became more hopeful and was first rewarded in 1951 when Jan Mohr found the *Lutheran* and *Secretor* loci to be quite close to each other on the same chromo-some. Thus blood groups provided the first example in man of autosomal linkage and consequently the first examples of autosomal crossing-over.

Study of the *Lutheran-Secretor* linkage, and of other blood group linkages which quickly followed it, led in 1965 to the recognition that in humans, as in some other species, the rate of crossing-over at meiosis can be higher in females than in males—an observation which was to affect all subsequent work on the detection and measurement of human linkages.

The next big step was the placing for the first time of a human locus on a numbered autosome: this happened in 1968 when the *Duffy* locus was shown to be on autosome No. 1.

In the last ten years the finding of many new markers in addition to blood groups, the great advance in methods of making chromosomal detail visible, and the invention of hybrid cell culture techniques have resulted in tremendous progress in human chromosome mapping. So far has this subject now ranged that all we can do is to confine ourselves to contributions made by the blood groups.

General treatment of the problems involved in linkage detection and chromo-some mapping may be found in Renwick[39, 40], Weitkamp[41], Robson[42], Bodmer[43] and Ruddle *et al.*[44]. How rapidly the subject is moving forwards (and only occa-sionally backwards) may be seen from the bi-annual Human Chromosome Mapping Newsletter issued from Johns Hopkins by Dr McKusick, and from the

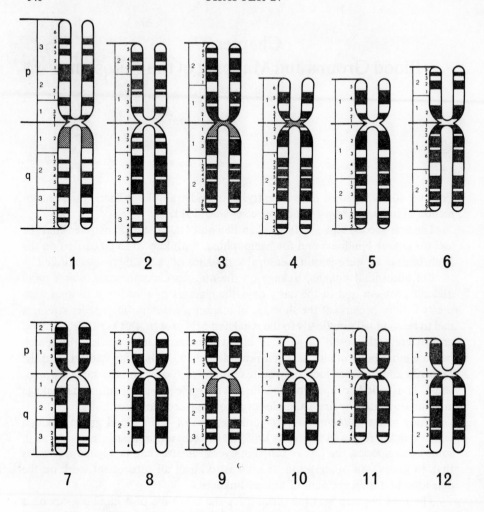

Fig. 34. Diagrammatic representation of chromosome bands as observed with the Q-, G-, and R-staining methods; centromere representative of Q- staining method only. (From *Paris Conference* (1971): *Standardization in Human Cytogenetics*. In *Birth Defects: Orig. Art. Ser.*, ed. D. Bergsma. Published by The National Foundation—March of Dimes, White Plains, N.Y. Vol. VIII (7), 1972.)

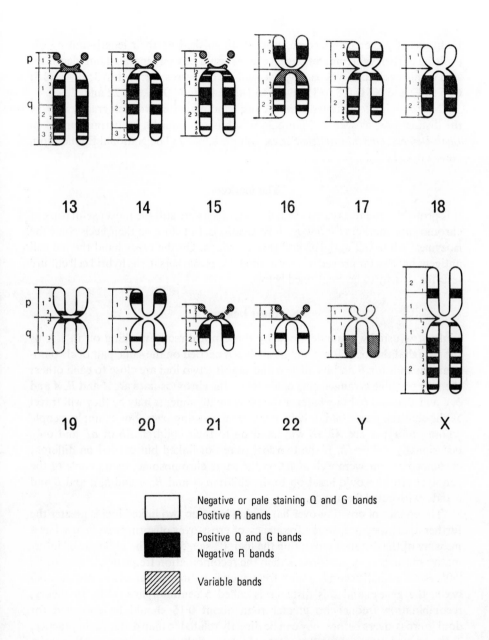

13   14   15   16   17   18

19   20   21   22   Y   X

☐ Negative or pale staining Q and G bands
Positive R bands

■ Positive Q and G bands
Negative R bands

▨ Variable bands

yearly international meetings on human gene mapping sponsored by the National Foundation, March of Dimes.

The chromosomes

Until recently the chromosomes were distinguished by their length and by the position of their centromeres. Seven classes could be well separated but identification within each class was usually uncertain. The classes are: A, 1 to 3; B, 4 and 5; C, 6 to 12 and X; D, 13 to 15; E, 16 to 18; F, 19 and 20; G, 21, 22 and Y.

New staining techniques now disclose banding patterns which greatly narrow the distinctions, as seen in Figure 34 which is reproduced, by permission, from *Birth Defects, Original Article Series*, volume 8, no. 7 (The National Foundation, New York, 1972).

The markers

It is probably true to say that the red cell antigens are still the most useful class of chromosome markers for *linkage* investigations, but close on their heels come the isozymes, white cell antigens and serum groups. On the other hand the red cell antigens have so far proved of very limited use as markers in the hybrid cell culture tests for *synteny* to be mentioned below.

About linkage

Linkage is usually misunderstood by those not directly working on it. Let us suppose that the locus for *A* and its allele *a* is carried on the same pair of chromosomes as that for *B* and its allele *b* and that the two loci are close to each other; then the possible arrangements of alleles on the chromosomes are *A* and *B*, *A* and *b*, *a* and *B*, *a* and *b*, but whatever the parental alignments may be they will travel to the children reassorted only by occasional crossing-over. For example, people whose genotypes are *Ab/aB* will hand on to their children *Ab* or *aB* and only occasionally *AB* or *ab*. If the two loci were not linked but carried on different chromosomes, or were well apart on the same chromosome, then people of the genotype *Aa Bb* would hand on to the children *A* and *B*, *A* and *b*, *a* and *B* and *a* and *b* with equal frequency.

The chance of crossing-over happening between two linked loci is greater the further apart they are, so the frequency of cross-over offspring can be used as a measure of the distance separating the loci. If, say, 5% of the children of informative matings were cross-overs then the recombination frequency is said to be 0·05. Such a small recombination frequency is a direct index of the distance between the genes; and this distance is called 5 centimorgans (cM). In theory, recombination frequencies greater than about 0·15 should be corrected for double cross-overs before they can be directly related to map distance: in practice, in the present rather elementary state of human linkage measurement the correction is seldom applied (see page 595).

The introduction of the hybrid cell culture technique into chromosome mapping affected nomenclature, so something needs to be said about this brilliant new approach even though blood groups are, so far, but little involved. Here is our account, which, as may be noticed, skates over all the difficult parts: human fibroblasts and mouse or hamster fibroblasts are put together and treated with a virus which makes them fuse. The hybrid nuclei continue to divide but, as the divisions go on, one after another of the human chromosomes is expelled from the nucleus and the departure of a certain chromosome may be seen to coincide with the departure from the line of a certain character, say one of the isozymes. In general, the hybrid cell culture technique cannot show linkage, that is measure the distance between two loci, but it can show which chromosome the locus for a character is on. The coincident departure of a chromosome and *two* marker characters can show that the two markers are on the same chromosome but gives no linkage information about the distance between them. Characters to be used in the cell culture tests must be expressed in fibroblasts and detectable by chemical or occasionally by micro-serological methods.

When the hybrid cell method began to show that the loci for two characters were carried on the same autosome, two characters between which no linkage had been demonstrated by pedigree methods, Dr J.H. Renwick decided that the time had come for the tightening up of the use of the word linkage and for the introduction of a new word for one or more loci being on a chromosome but with or without linkage information. The word he chose was synteny, and here is his definition[40] of the two states:

'*Linkage*. Linkage between two loci will be said to exist when the true recombination fraction is less than 0·5 in one or both sexes. Linked loci are then loci possessing a true relationship of linkage, either directly or through mutual linkage to an intermediate locus. A set of linked loci constitutes a linkage group.

'*Synteny* (Gk: *syn* = together; *taenia* = ribbon). Two loci may be so far apart on the same chromosome that linkage cannot be demonstrated. It is, therefore, useful to have the word "synteny" to indicate presence together on the same chromosome, whether or not the loci have been shown to be linked. All sex-linked loci in a diploid species are known to be syntenic but are not necessarily demonstrably linked even through an intermediary.'

DETECTION OF LINKAGE

Mathematical methods for the detection and measurement of linkage in man were polished and waiting for the data they deserved. Those developed by Bernstein, Wiener, Hogben, Haldane, Fisher, Finney, Bailey, C.A.B. Smith and Morton were designed for the analysis of families, but a method of detecting linkage by means of sib pairs was introduced by Penrose. References to most of these works will be found in Smith[2, 3].

Fortunately for the non-mathematicians it is not necessary to understand the tests to apply at any rate some of them. A great service was done for us innumerates

by Finney[5] and by Maynard Smith, Penrose and Smith[6] who gave recipes
for the application of the u statistics on the one hand and the lod scores on the
other. It seems a pity that blood groupers should not have the pleasure of
recognizing a close linkage should they meet one and to this end in previous
editions we gave elementary instructions for applying the u statistics of Fisher[7, 8]
and Finney[5] and, in the last edition, both the u statistics and the lod score method.
Lod scores are now so generally used that this time we shall confine our attempted
description to this method alone.

The lod scores

The main advantage of the lod scores over the u statistics, at the rough but ready
level of reckoning that we are describing, is that the evidence ('phase known') of
the valuable three generation families can be pooled with that of the less valuable
but more available two generation families.

The lod scores ('lod' means 'log odds', i.e. 'log probability ratio') are based on
the work of Haldane and Smith[1] and of Morton[9, 10]. Maynard Smith, Penrose
and Smith[6] in *Mathematical Tables for Research Workers in Human Genetics*
give an admirable section which 'describes the simplest method of using lod
scores'. The contents of this short book may at first look formidable, but from it
is to be acquired the power to cope with linkage problems without computer help
and, incidentally, much pleasure from the clear brilliance of the presentation.

The 'main character', say a rare 'dominant' disease or a new blood group
antigen, is called G and its absence g. More complicated situations produced by
other alleles G_1, G_2 etc. can be coped with. The 'test character' is one of the
routine markers for which the family has been tested: it is called T and its absence
t (and T_1, T_2 etc. in certain matings involving more complicated markers).

The lod scores represent the weight of the evidence given by a family for or
against linkage at recombination fractions (θ) ranging from 0·00 to 0·45. Autosomal linkage can be considered established when in a collection of families the
sum of the lod scores at any value of θ reaches +3. If the sum of the lod scores at a
given value of θ is less than −2 then linkage at that value is ruled out[6].

In presenting the sum of lod scores for a series of families it is necessary to
divide them for:
1   those in which the male is the doubly heterozygous parent;
2   those in which the female is the doubly heterozygous parent.
This is because in all the proved autosomal linkages in man the recombination
rate is higher in the female.

Mrs Maynard Smith, the late Professor Penrose and Professor C.A.B. Smith
kindly allowed us to compile the table of lod scores (Table 94) from Tables 44,
45 and 51a of their book[6], with the addition of some intervening scores provided
by Professor Smith. Shortly after Table 94 was assembled, Professor Smith
published tables[45, 46] with further intervening scores particularly useful for
recombination fractions less than 0·05.

We have found Table 94 very useful and we hope that other blood groupers may find it so too. However, it should not be forgotten that if anything but the simplest of main and test characters are being used, the rules and further tables should be consulted in the original[6,45,46].

We shall confine ourselves to the simpler, and most informative, situations: the scoring of three generation families through 'phase known' parents, and of two generation families in which the phase of the heterozygous parent is not known. In the two generation families a z_1 score is applied, sometimes with an e_1 correction.

We shall take as an example the scoring of the imaginary family in Figure 35 to illustrate both the treatment of a three generation and a two generation family.

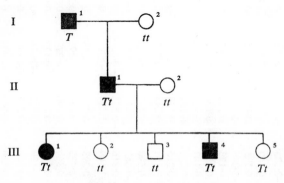

Fig. 35. An imaginary family. Black = a dominant character, G: T and t = alleles of a marker system.

Three generation families

If three generation families are available a fairly close linkage could be seen and the recombination fraction arrived at without resort to mathematics. Take the imaginary family in Figure 35. Black represents some character controlled by a gene active in single dose (the 'main' character) and T represents some marker character such as a blood group. II-1 has received *black* with T from his father (and is therefore 'phase known') and he has handed on *black* with T to III-1 and III-4 (two non-recombinants): II-1 has received *not-black* with t from his mother and he has handed on *not-black* with t to III-2 and III-3 (two more non-recombinants). But II-1 has handed on *not-black*, which came to him on a maternal chromosome, with T, which came to him on a paternal chromosome, to III-5 (one recombinant). If more families showed approximately this ratio of four non-recombinants to one recombinant then the two loci are linked and their recombination fraction is about 0·2.

But the lod scores help in two ways: they show when the evidence collected is enough to establish the linkage and, as mentioned above, they enable the three generation evidence to be pooled with that given by two generation families.

Table 94. The lod scores for families with up to seven children: parents phase known and phase unknown. (The z_1 and e_1 values are from Maynard Smith, Penrose and Smith[6] (1961), with some intervening values provided by Professor C.A.B. Smith)

No.	Scored children Count		θ, the recombination fraction									
			0·00	0·05	0·1	0·15	0·2	0·25	0·3	0·35	0·4	0·45
1.	1 n-r	0 r	0·301	0·279	0·255	0·230	0·204	0·176	0·146	0·114	0·079	0·041
	0 n-r	1 r	$-\infty$	$-1\cdot000$	$-0\cdot699$	$-0\cdot523$	$-0\cdot398$	$-0\cdot301$	$-0\cdot222$	$-0\cdot155$	$-0\cdot097$	$-0\cdot046$
2.	2 n-r	0 r	0·602	0·558	0·510	0·460	0·408	0·352	0·292	0·228	0·158	0·082
	1 n-r	1 r	$-\infty$	$-0\cdot721$	$-0\cdot444$	$-0\cdot293$	$-0\cdot194$	$-0\cdot125$	$-0\cdot076$	$-0\cdot041$	$-0\cdot018$	$-0\cdot005$
	0 n-r	2 r	$-\infty$	$-2\cdot000$	$-1\cdot398$	$-1\cdot046$	$-0\cdot796$	$-0\cdot602$	$-0\cdot444$	$-0\cdot310$	$-0\cdot194$	$-0\cdot092$
	z_1 2:0		0·301	0·258	0·215	0·173	0·134	0·097	0·064	0·037	0·017	0·004
	z_1 2:0	e_1 2:0	0·477	0·395	0·319	0·250	0·190	0·135	0·088	0·050	0·023	0·005
	z_1 2:0	e_1 1:1	0·176	0·154	0·131	0·107	0·085	0·062	0·041	0·024	0·011	0·003
	z_1 1:1		$-\infty$	$-0\cdot721$	$-0\cdot444$	$-0\cdot292$	$-0\cdot194$	$-0\cdot125$	$-0\cdot076$	$-0\cdot041$	$-0\cdot018$	$-0\cdot004$
	z_1 1:1	e_1 2:0	$-\infty$	$-0\cdot584$	$-0\cdot340$	$-0\cdot215$	$-0\cdot138$	$-0\cdot087$	$-0\cdot052$	$-0\cdot028$	$-0\cdot012$	$-0\cdot003$
	z_1 1:1	e_1 1:1	$-\infty$	$-0\cdot825$	$-0\cdot528$	$-0\cdot358$	$-0\cdot243$	$-0\cdot160$	$-0\cdot099$	$-0\cdot054$	$-0\cdot024$	$-0\cdot005$
3.	3 n-r	0 r	0·903	0·837	0·765	0·690	0·612	0·528	0·438	0·342	0·237	0·123
	2 n-r	1 r	$-\infty$	$-0\cdot442$	$-0\cdot189$	$-0\cdot063$	0·010	0·051	0·070	0·073	0·061	0·036
	1 n-r	2 r	$-\infty$	$-1\cdot721$	$-1\cdot143$	$-0\cdot816$	$-0\cdot592$	$-0\cdot426$	$-0\cdot298$	$-0\cdot196$	$-0\cdot115$	$-0\cdot051$
	0 n-r	3 r	$-\infty$	$-3\cdot000$	$-2\cdot097$	$-1\cdot569$	$-1\cdot194$	$-0\cdot903$	$-0\cdot666$	$-0\cdot465$	$-0\cdot291$	$-0\cdot138$
	z_1 3:0		0·602	0·533	0·465	0·393	0·318	0·243	0·170	0·104	0·049	0·013
	z_1 3:0	e_1 3:0	0·845	0·718	0·604	0·495	0·391	0·292	0·201	0·121	0·057	0·015
	z_1 3:0	e_1 2:1	0·544	0·485	0·427	0·364	0·296	0·228	0·160	0·098	0·047	0·012
	z_1 2:1		$-\infty$	$-0\cdot721$	$-0\cdot444$	$-0\cdot292$	$-0\cdot194$	$-0\cdot125$	$-0\cdot076$	$-0\cdot041$	$-0\cdot018$	$-0\cdot004$
	z_1 2:1	e_1 3:0	$-\infty$	$-0\cdot536$	$-0\cdot305$	$-0\cdot190$	$-0\cdot121$	$-0\cdot076$	$-0\cdot045$	$-0\cdot024$	$-0\cdot010$	$-0\cdot002$
	z_1 2:1	e_1 2:1	$-\infty$	$-0\cdot769$	$-0\cdot482$	$-0\cdot321$	$-0\cdot216$	$-0\cdot140$	$-0\cdot086$	$-0\cdot047$	$-0\cdot020$	$-0\cdot005$
4.	4 n-r	0 r	1·204	1·116	1·020	0·920	0·816	0·704	0·584	0·456	0·316	0·164
	3 n-r	1 r	$-\infty$	$-0\cdot163$	0·066	0·167	0·214	0·227	0·216	0·187	0·140	0·077
	2 n-r	2 r	$-\infty$	$-1\cdot442$	$-0\cdot888$	$-0\cdot586$	$-0\cdot388$	$-0\cdot250$	$-0\cdot152$	$-0\cdot082$	$-0\cdot036$	$-0\cdot010$
	1 n-r	3 r	$-\infty$	$-2\cdot721$	$-1\cdot842$	$-1\cdot339$	$-0\cdot990$	$-0\cdot727$	$-0\cdot520$	$-0\cdot351$	$-0\cdot212$	$-0\cdot097$
	0 n-r	4 r	$-\infty$	$-4\cdot000$	$-2\cdot796$	$-2\cdot092$	$-1\cdot592$	$-1\cdot204$	$-0\cdot888$	$-0\cdot620$	$-0\cdot388$	$-0\cdot184$
	z_1 4:0		0·903	0·814	0·720	0·621	0·517	0·409	0·298	0·190	0·094	0·025
	z_1 4:0	e_1 4:0	1·176	1·013	0·865	0·724	0·589	0·457	0·328	0·206	0·101	0·027

Table 94—continued

No.	Scored children Count		0·00	0·05	0·1	0·15	0·2	0·25	0·3	0·35	0·4	0·45
								θ, the recombination fraction				
	z₁ 4:0	e₁ 3:1	0·875	0·795	0·708	0·614	0·513	0·407	0·297	0·190	0·094	0·025
	z₁ 4:0	e₁ 2:2	0·875	0·787	0·696	0·600	0·500	0·397	0·290	0·185	0·092	0·024
	z₁ 3:1		−∞	−0·464	−0·229	−0·119	−0·060	−0·028	−0·011	−0·003	−0·001	−0·000
	z₁ 3:1	e₁ 4:0	−∞	−0·266	−0·084	−0·016	0·012	0·020	0·019	0·013	0·006	0·002
	z₁ 3:1	e₁ 3:1	−∞	−0·483	−0·241	−0·126	−0·064	−0·030	−0·012	−0·003	−0·001	0·000
	z₁ 3:1	e₁ 2:2	−∞	−0·491	−0·253	−0·140	−0·077	−0·040	−0·019	−0·008	−0·003	−0·001
	z₁ 2:2		−∞	−1·442	−0·887	−0·585	−0·388	−0·250	−0·151	−0·082	−0·035	−0·009
	z₁ 2:2	e₁ 4:0	−∞	−1·243	−0·742	−0·482	−0·316	−0·202	−0·121	−0·066	−0·028	−0·007
	z₁ 2:2	e₁ 3:1	−∞	−1·461	−0·899	−0·592	−0·392	−0·252	−0·152	−0·082	−0·035	−0·009
	z₁ 2:2	e₁ 2:2	−∞	−1·469	−0·911	−0·606	−0·405	−0·262	−0·159	−0·087	−0·037	−0·010
5.	5 n-r	0 r	1·505	1·395	1·275	1·150	1·020	0·880	0·730	0·570	0·395	0·205
	4 n-r	1 r	−∞	0·116	0·321	0·397	0·418	0·403	0·362	0·301	0·219	0·118
	3 n-r	2 r	−∞	−1·163	−0·633	−0·356	−0·184	−0·074	−0·006	0·032	0·043	0·031
	2 n-r	3 r	−∞	−2·442	−1·587	−1·109	−0·786	−0·551	−0·374	−0·237	−0·133	−0·056
	1 n-r	4 r	−∞	−3·721	−2·541	−1·862	−1·388	−1·028	−0·742	−0·506	−0·309	−0·143
	0 n-r	5 r	−∞	−5·000	−3·495	−2·615	−1·990	−1·505	−1·110	−0·775	−0·485	−0·230
	z₁ 5:0		1·204	1·093	0·975	0·851	0·720	0·581	0·436	0·288	0·149	0·042
	z₁ 5:0	e₁ 5:0	1·491	1·292	1·113	0·946	0·784	0·622	0·461	0·301	0·155	0·043
	z₁ 5:0	e₁ 4:1	1·190	1·088	0·976	0·855	0·725	0·585	0·439	0·290	0·150	0·042
	z₁ 5:0	e₁ 3:2	1·190	1·080	0·963	0·841	0·712	0·575	0·432	0·286	0·148	0·042
	z₁ 4:1		−∞	−0·186	0·022	0·099	0·124	0·118	0·095	0·063	0·031	0·008
	z₁ 4:1	e₁ 5:0	−∞	0·013	0·160	0·194	0·188	0·159	0·120	0·076	0·037	0·009
	z₁ 4:1	e₁ 4:1	−∞	−0·191	0·023	0·103	0·129	0·122	0·098	0·065	0·032	0·008
	z₁ 4:1	e₁ 3:2	−∞	−0·199	0·010	0·089	0·116	0·112	0·091	0·061	0·030	0·008
	z₁ 3:2		−∞	−1·442	−0·887	−0·585	−0·388	−0·250	−0·151	−0·082	−0·035	−0·009
	z₁ 3:2	e₁ 5:0	−∞	−1·243	−0·749	−0·490	−0·324	−0·209	−0·126	−0·069	−0·029	−0·008
	z₁ 3:2	e₁ 4:1	−∞	−1·447	−0·886	−0·581	−0·383	−0·246	−0·148	−0·080	−0·034	−0·009
	z₁ 3:2	e₁ 3:2	−∞	−1·455	−0·899	−0·595	−0·396	−0·256	−0·155	−0·084	−0·036	−0·009
6.	6 n-r	0 r	1·806	1·674	1·530	1·380	1·224	1·056	0·876	0·684	0·474	0·246
	5 n-r	1 r	−∞	0·395	0·576	0·627	0·622	0·579	0·508	0·415	0·298	0·159
	4 n-r	2 r	−∞	−0·884	−0·378	−0·126	0·020	0·102	0·140	0·146	0·122	0·072
	3 n-r	3 r	−∞	−2·163	−1·332	−0·879	−0·582	−0·375	−0·228	−0·123	−0·054	−0·015

Table 94—*continued*

No.	Scored children	Count	\u03b8, the recombination fraction									
			0·00	0·05	0·1	0·15	0·2	0·25	0·3	0·35	0·4	0·45
	2 n-r	4 r	−∞	−3·442	−2·286	−1·632	−1·184	−0·852	−0·596	−0·392	−0·230	−0·102
	1 n-r	5 r	−∞	−4·721	−3·240	−2·385	−1·786	−1·329	−0·964	−0·661	−0·406	−0·189
	0 n-r	6 r	−∞	−6·000	−4·194	−3·138	−2·388	−1·806	−1·332	−0·930	−0·582	−0·276
	z_1 6:0		1·505	1·371	1·231	1·082	0·924	0·756	0·578	0·393	0·211	0·061
	z_1 6:0	e_1 6:0	1·799	1·563	1·358	1·166	0·978	0·790	0·598	0·403	0·215	0·062
	z_1 6:0	e_1 5:1	1·498	1·373	1·237	1·090	0·932	0·762	0·583	0·396	0·212	0·061
	z_1 6:0	e_1 4:2	1·498	1·365	1·226	1·078	0·921	0·754	0·577	0·393	0·211	0·061
	z_1 6:0	e_1 3:3	1·498	1·364	1·224	1·076	0·919	0·752	0·575	0·391	0·210	0·061
	z_1 5:1		−∞	0·093	0·276	0·329	0·323	0·284	0·222	0·149	0·076	0·021
	z_1 5:1	e_1 6:0	−∞	0·285	0·403	0·413	0·377	0·318	0·242	0·159	0·080	0·022
	z_1 5:1	e_1 5:1	−∞	0·095	0·282	0·337	0·331	0·290	0·227	0·152	0·077	0·021
	z_1 5:1	e_1 4:2	−∞	0·087	0·271	0·325	0·320	0·282	0·221	0·149	0·076	0·021
	z_1 5:1	e_1 3:3	−∞	0·086	0·269	0·323	0·318	0·280	0·219	0·147	0·075	0·021
	z_1 4:2		−∞	−1·185	−0·673	−0·412	−0·254	−0·153	−0·087	−0·044	−0·018	−0·004
	z_1 4:2	e_1 6:0	−∞	−0·993	−0·546	−0·328	−0·200	−0·119	−0·067	−0·034	−0·014	−0·003
	z_1 4:2	e_1 5:1	−∞	−1·183	−0·667	−0·404	−0·246	−0·147	−0·082	−0·041	−0·017	−0·004
	z_1 4:2	e_1 4:2	−∞	−1·191	−0·678	−0·416	−0·257	−0·155	−0·088	−0·044	−0·018	−0·004
	z_1 4:2	e_1 3:3	−∞	−1·192	−0·680	−0·418	−0·259	−0·157	−0·090	−0·046	−0·019	−0·004
	z_1 3:3		−∞	−2·164	−1·331	−0·877	−0·582	−0·375	−0·227	−0·123	−0·053	−0·013
	z_1 3:3	e_1 6:0	−∞	−1·972	−1·204	−0·793	−0·528	−0·341	−0·207	−0·113	−0·049	−0·012
	z_1 3:3	e_1 5:1	−∞	−2·162	−1·325	−0·869	−0·574	−0·369	−0·222	−0·120	−0·052	−0·013
	z_1 3:3	e_1 4:2	−∞	−2·170	−1·336	−0·881	−0·585	−0·377	−0·228	−0·123	−0·053	−0·013
	z_1 3:3	e_1 3:3	−∞	−2·171	−1·338	−0·883	−0·587	−0·379	−0·230	−0·125	−0·054	−0·013
7.	7 n-r	0 r	2·107	1·953	1·785	1·610	1·428	1·232	1·022	0·798	0·553	0·287
	6 n-r	1 r	−∞	0·674	0·831	0·857	0·826	0·755	0·654	0·529	0·377	0·200
	5 n-r	2 r	−∞	−0·605	−0·123	0·104	0·224	0·278	0·286	0·260	0·201	0·113
	4 n-r	3 r	−∞	−1·884	−1·077	−0·649	−0·378	−0·199	−0·082	−0·009	0·025	0·026
	3 n-r	4 r	−∞	−3·163	−2·031	−1·402	−0·980	−0·676	−0·450	−0·278	−0·151	−0·061
	2 n-r	5 r	−∞	−4·442	−2·985	−2·155	−1·582	−1·153	−0·818	−0·547	−0·327	−0·148
	1 n-r	6 r	−∞	−5·721	−3·939	−2·908	−2·184	−1·630	−1·186	−0·816	−0·503	−0·235
	0 n-r	7 r	−∞	−7·000	−4·893	−3·661	−2·786	−2·107	−1·554	−1·085	−0·679	−0·322

Table 94—*continued*

No.	Count z_1	Count e_1	θ, the recombination fraction									
			0·00	0·05	0·1	0·15	0·2	0·25	0·3	0·35	0·4	0·45
	7:0		1·806	1·650	1·486	1·312	1·128	0·932	0·723	0·502	0·278	0·084
	7:0	7:0	2·104	1·833	1·601	1·384	1·173	0·959	0·738	0·510	0·281	0·085
	7:0	6:1	1·803	1·655	1·494	1·321	1·136	0·938	0·727	0·505	0·279	0·084
	7:0	5:2	1·803	1·647	1·484	1·311	1·127	0·932	0·723	0·502	0·278	0·084
	7:0	4:3	1·803	1·647	1·483	1·309	1·125	0·930	0·722	0·501	0·278	0·084
	6:1		$-\infty$	0·371	0·532	0·559	0·526	0·456	0·360	0·247	0·131	0·037
	6:1	7:0	$-\infty$	0·554	0·601	0·631	0·571	0·483	0·375	0·255	0·134	0·038
	6:1	6:1	$-\infty$	0·376	0·540	0·568	0·534	0·462	0·364	0·250	0·132	0·037
	6:1	5:2	$-\infty$	0·368	0·530	0·558	0·525	0·456	0·360	0·247	0·131	0·037
	6:1	4:3	$-\infty$	0·368	0·529	0·556	0·523	0·454	0·359	0·246	0·131	0·037
	5:2		$-\infty$	−0·907	−0·422	−0·192	−0·070	−0·007	0·019	0·022	0·014	0·004
	5:2	7:0	$-\infty$	−0·724	−0·307	−0·120	−0·025	0·020	0·034	0·030	0·017	0·005
	5:2	6:1	$-\infty$	−0·902	−0·414	−0·183	−0·062	−0·001	0·023	0·025	0·015	0·004
	5:2	5:2	$-\infty$	−0·910	−0·424	−0·193	−0·071	−0·007	0·019	0·022	0·014	0·004
	5:2	4:3	$-\infty$	−0·910	−0·425	−0·195	−0·073	−0·009	0·018	0·021	0·014	0·004
	4:3		$-\infty$	−2·164	−1·331	−0·877	−0·582	−0·375	−0·227	−0·123	−0·053	−0·013
	4:3	7:0	$-\infty$	−1·981	−1·216	−0·805	−0·537	−0·348	−0·212	−0·115	−0·050	−0·012
	4:3	6:1	$-\infty$	−2·159	−1·323	−0·868	−0·574	−0·369	−0·223	−0·120	−0·052	−0·013
	4:3	5:2	$-\infty$	−2·167	−1·333	−0·878	−0·583	−0·375	−0·227	−0·123	−0·053	−0·013
	4:3	4:3	$-\infty$	−2·167	−1·334	−0·880	−0·585	−0·377	−0·228	−0·124	−0·053	−0·013

n-r = non-recombinant;   r = recombinant.

Families with more than seven informative children. The scores for larger 'phase-known' families can easily be calculated by multiplying the score for 1 n-r and that for 1 r (top of table) by the number of non-recombinants and recombinants observed. For larger two generation families the formulae for working out z_1 and e_1 scores are given by Maynard-Smith, Penrose and Smith[6]. However, we have discovered a simple trick for obtaining the lod scores provided the count is not 8:0, 9:0 etc. Say the count for z_1 is 6:2 then very nearly the right answer for z_1 may be obtained by adding the z_1 scores for 2:2 to those for 4:0, or those for 1:1 to those for 5:1 (1:1, 2:2, 3:3 etc. must be used) and we forget about e_1 in such large families as it makes very little difference.

Further intervening values of θ. Smith[45], 1968, provides scores also for θ 0·01, 0·02, 0·03, 0·04, 0·075, 0·125 and 0·175 for both phase-known and phase unknown families.

19

The lod scores contributed by this family are found by looking up 4 non-recombinants: 1 recombinant in Table 94.

Two generation families

Consider that the grandparents in Figure 35 had not been tested and that the family consists of only the parents (generation II) and their five children. Black is the main character; T the test character. The father II-1 is the doubly heterozygous parent but his phase, coupling or repulsion, is unknown so the z_1 scores must be applied and the count for the children is 4:1, derived from the numbers on the left and right in the following scheme:

	not		not
black	black	black	black
T	t	t	T
2	2		1

It is convenient to write the larger number first, 4:1 rather 1:4.

A correction e_1 is needed only when the test character genotype of a parent has to be derived from an offspring involved in the count for z_1 scoring: for example, when an A_1 parent is shown to be A_1O by one of the children used in the linkage count, or when an Xg(a+) mother is shown to be Xg^aXg by an Xg(a−) child used in the count.

The count for e_1 scoring in this family, that is the number of children with and without the main character, is 3:2 (the larger number is again written first). The scores for the count z_1 4:1, e_1 3:2 are then looked up in Table 94, and the lod scores for the various values of θ, the recombination fraction, are added to those for other families tested for the same two characters.

When z_1 4:1 e_1 3:2 is looked up in Table 94 it is seen to give much lower lod scores than the 4 non-recombinants:1 recombinant of the family when the grandparents were included—an illustration of the great superiority of three over two generation families (and this is true whether the information is in favour of linkage or against it).

In this generalized example of a two generation family the effect of t is, strictly speaking, recessive like that of O or P_2, but in most blood groups the genotype of the heterozygous parent is usually known from serological tests without calling on information drawn from other family members and therefore no e_1 scores are needed. In practice, some experts and their computers ignore e_1 scores altogether, but it is not for us to judge whether this is a good thing; it doesn't make very much difference either way.

A practical example

The pedigree in Figure 36 is taken from our records: it is part of a large Finnish kindred in which a 'new' rare antigen (main character) is segregating[47].

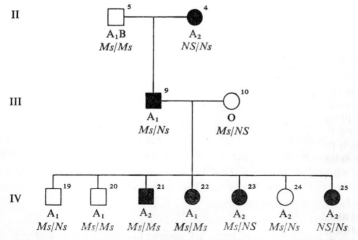

Fig. 36. Pedigree used to illustrate the scoring for linkage of two and three generation families. Black = An(a+); hollow = An(a−).

In order to emphasize the advantage of three generation families this one will be scored without and with the information given by the grandparents. The counts are:

	2 generation	3 generation
ABO	z_1 5:2, e_1 4:3	5 non-rec.: 2 rec.
MNSs	z_1 5:2	2 non-rec.: 5 rec.

In the 2 generation count for ABO the e_1 score is added because the genotype of the father, III-9, can be recognized only by the presence of A_2 in his children. Reference to Table 94 shows how much more information for or against linkage is provided by the testing of the grandparents. Incidentally, the combined evidence of this and other families showed that the locus for the main character is not within direct measurable distance of the *ABO* or *MNSs* loci.

As a further exercise it may be worth pointing out that had III-10 been *Ms/Ns* rather than *Ms/NS* (and consequently passed on *Ns* to IV-23 and IV-25) then only the *Ms/Ms* and *Ns/Ns* children could have been used in the count: the *Ms/Ns* children would have to be ignored because it would not be known whether their *Ms* or their *Ns* had come from the father.

The lod scores as we have attempted to describe them will cope with most of the situations met in blood grouping laboratories where the main character is usually a disease or a 'new' antigen of low frequency. If, however, the main character is of a higher frequency, such as the antigen Do[a] (before the finding of anti-Do[b]), it is a pity to ignore the information given by Do(a+) × Do(a+) matings with some Do(a−) children which can score through both parents. In order to extract the maximum information from such two generation families z_2 or z_3 scores should, strictly, be used and these are clearly described by Maynard-Smith, Penrose and Smith[6], and by Smith[45, 46].

Relating lod scores to probability of linkage

We have already said that autosomal linkage may be considered established if the sum of lod scores at any value of θ reaches +3, and excluded at any value of θ

at which it is less than −2. Unless linkage is close it takes a lot of families to reach 3, and we are impatient to know how we are getting on in the meantime: the following is a guide to the correct pitching of excitement.

The antilog of the sum of the lod scores for the various values of θ gives the relative probability of linkage at each value. Drawing successive graphs (values of θ along the bottom and relative probabilities up the side) as families roll in gives great pleasure, especially when a mere molehill grows into a mountain. The *average height*, say H, of the antilog graph indicates the odds on linkage being present, which are approximately H:20. Thus if H is less than 20, the odds are that the loci are unlinked; if H is 1,000, there are odds on linkage of 1,000 to 20, or 50 to 1. The detection of linkage between two loci known to be X-borne is less rigorous and the ratio H:1 may be taken as the odds on the two loci being within measurable distance of each other.

Having been given this extremely useful higher mathematical advice by Professor C.A.B. Smith we were shy to ask how to find the average height of a curve, so enquired of our very young colleagues: there seemed to be general agreement that if you measure equal intervals along the base line (the more the intervals the greater the accuracy), raise perpendiculars therefrom to meet the curve, measure their heights, sum these heights and divide the sum by the number of perpendiculars, you descend to the average height. If the lod scores for nine values of θ, as set out in Table 94, have been used to construct the relative probability curve then a sufficiently accurate fixing of the average height is given by dividing the sum of the antilogs of the lod scores by 9, unless we are much mistaken.

The 90% probability limits we obtain by the method, suggested to us by Professor C.A.B. Smith, of counting the graph paper squares below the curve and cutting off from each tail one twentieth of their number.

AUTOSOMAL LINKAGES INVOLVING BLOOD GROUPS

Because of their good start, it is not surprising that blood group markers provided all the autosomal linkages known up to 1966. A list of linkages brought to light by blood group markers is given in Table 95. We have divided them into established, probable or possible, according to the evidence available by February 1974.

Lutheran (*Lu*) and Secretor (*Se*)

In 1951 the first example of autosomal linkage in man was discovered by Mohr[11-13] when he made an almost certain case for linkage between the *Lutheran* and what then seemed to be the *Lewis* genes, but which later emerged as the related *secretor* genes.

Table 95. Autosomal blood group loci and their linkages

Blood group locus	Linked locus	Recombi- nation % male	Year first proposed	References	State
Lu	Se (secretor)	10	1951	11–13, 79, 4, 16–18, 48–50	established
	Dm (myotonic dystrophy)	13*	1954	13, 49, 50	established
Se	Dm (myotonic dystrophy)	8*	1954	13, 49, 50	established
Rh	El₁ (elliptocytosis)	<3	1953	20–27, 77	established
	PGD (6-phosphogluconate dehydrogenase)	13	1971	52, 53	established
	PGM₁ (phosphoglucomutase)	26	1971	56, 81, 53	established
	PPH (phosphopyruvate hydratase, or enolase)	0	1973	86, 90	possible
Fy	Cae (zonular cataract)	0	1963	35	probable
	Iqh (uncoiler-1)	10	1968	88, 89, 93	established
	AmS (salivary amylase)	17	1972	95, 97	established
	AmP (pancreatic amylase)	17	1972	94, 95, 97	established
ABO	Np (nail-patella)	10	1955	28–34, 19, 98	established
	AK (adenylate kinase)	10	1968	80, 99–101	established
MNSs	Tys (sclerotylosis)	4*	1967	76, 83	established
	Do (Dombrock blood group)	35	1972	136	possible
Le	AcP₁ (red cell acid phosphatase)	15*	1971	104	possible
	C'3 (complement C3)	7	1974	133	established
P	ADA (adenosine deaminase)	20	1970	108, 109, 107	probable
	HL-A (white cell groups)	30	1972	107	possible
Wr	Sdᵃ (strong Sdᵃ antigen)	0	1973	110	possible
i	congenital cataract	0	1972	111	possible
Ch	HL-A LA / Four	4.5* / 1·5*	1974	132	established

* Recombination fraction not divided for sex.

The linkage was first detected by Penrose's[14,15] sib pair method and later confirmed in families by the u statistics of Fisher[5,7,8].

The linkage is between the *Lutheran* and *secretor* loci (Sanger and Race[79], 1958; Lawler and Renwick[4], 1959; Metaxas, Metaxas-Bühler, Dunsford and Holländer[16], 1959; Greenwalt[17], 1961). The recombination frequency was estimated[17] as about 0·15. The appearance of linkage with the *Lewis* genes was due to their phenotypic expression on red cells being controlled by the *secretor* genes. It is now known that the *Lewis* genes, *Lele*, are not linked to the *secretor* or to the *Lutheran* genes (see page 333).

Recombination rate in males and females

In 1962, P.J.L. Cook, then a medical student, applied for the first time the lod score method to the published Lutheran-secretor linkage data: he was also given the details of five more informative families tested by Dr Cleghorn and four more from other sources. As expected the lod scores gave about the same recombination fraction as had the u scores. But in the setting out of the scores Cook divided the families into those in which the mother was the double heterozygote and those in which the father was. The results suggested a higher recombination rate in the mother than in the father. Such a difference in frequency of crossing-over in the two sexes is known in other species, the limit being reached in Drosophila in which there is no crossing-over in the male.

At about the same time, and independently, Renwick was studying in the same way the ABO:nail-patella data (see below) and came up against the same hint. The two papers, Cook[18] and Renwick and Schulze[19] came out in 1965 and the conclusion was that recombination in the female was probably 1·7 times that in the male.

This observation fundamentally affected future searches for autosomal linkage and its measurement: the detection of a linkage which is not a close one may be prevented by including the lod scores derived from the offspring of doubly heterozygous females.

Myotonic dystrophy (*Dm*)

In 1954 Mohr[13] found a hint of linkage between *Dm* and *Lu* and between *Dm* and *Se*. After a gap of 17 years these hints of linkages, which could have practical implications in genetic counselling, were looked at again.

In 1971 Renwick and his colleagues[49] submitted the results of British families, together with Mohr's original data[13], to a 'three-locus computer analysis': practically all the families involved were of a kind which could not be coped with by the lod score methods as described in this chapter. In 1972 Harper *et al.*[50] analysed American families on the computer. Together the three investigations established linkage between both *Dm* and *Lu* and between *Dm* and *Se*: the recombination fractions in our Table 95 are not divided for sex. The order of the loci is not yet known: it seems[50] that 'the orders *Lu-Se-Dm* and *Dm-Lu-Se* are, respectively, only 1·7 and 1·4 times more likely than the order *Se-Dm-Lu*'.

Rh and other loci

Elliptocytosis (*El₁*)

Lawler's searches, at the Galton Laboratory, were crowned with success when, in 1953, she and her collaborators demonstrated linkage between the genes for Rh and for oval red cells (Chalmers and Lawler[20]; Goodall, Hendry, Lawler and Stephen[21, 22]: Lawler and Sandler[23]).

In a very impressive statistical analysis of the 14 pedigrees published up to 1955 Morton[24] concluded, as had Lawler and her colleagues, that the evidence for linkage is overwhelming. But he further observed that while in some of the families capable of giving information the linkage is obviously close, in others there is no sign of linkage. Morton said: 'It is suggested that elliptocytosis is not a single genetic entity in different pedigrees, but depends on either of two dominant factors, one of which [now called El_1] is linked to the Rh locus. Linkage studies have great value in the detection and analysis of genetic heterogeneity, the recognition of which may help to resolve biochemical and clinical heterogeneity.'

Morton calculated that the elliptocytosis gene which *is* linked to *Rh* is closely linked: the recombination frequency being 0.033 ± 0.023. Clarke and his colleagues[25] (1960) reported two more informative families with no example of crossing-over and, using Morton's method, they recalculated the total recombination frequency to be 0.029 ± 0.020.

The possibility was considered[26] that a haemolytic form of elliptocytosis might be controlled by the locus not linked to *Rh*, but this was called in question by an Australian family in which several members had elliptocytosis (*Rh*-linked) one of whom had haemolytic attacks[27].

An investigation in Holland, involving 400 members of six families, was reported by Geerdink and his colleagues[77]. One large family showed close linkage with *Rh*, three families ruled out linkage and two were not informative. Thus the investigation confirmed the existence of two alternative genetic backgrounds for elliptocytosis.

6-phosphogluconate dehydrogenase (*PGD*)

Weitkamp and his colleagues[51, 52] noted some evidence in favour of this linkage in 1970, and confirmed it in 1971. In 1973 Robson and her colleagues[53] provided more data and the present view of the recombination fraction is 0.13 in males. Further supporting data were assembled[141] in 1974.

In 1972 Fialkow and his colleagues[54] described a patient with chronic myelocytic leukaemia who could only be interpreted as hemizygous for *Rh and* hemizygous for *PGD* thus supporting the linkage or, more strictly, the synteny of the two loci.

Phosphoglucomutase (*PGM₁*)

In 1971 Westerveld and his colleagues[55], by the hamster-man hybrid method, demonstrated synteny between PGM_1 and *PGD*. Immediately following this, linkage was recognized between *Rh* and PGM_1 (Renwick[56], Cook et al.[81]). The massive data resulting from the work of the Galton Laboratory were analysed by Robson et al.[53] and the recombination fraction in the male shown to be 0.26. Further supporting data were assembled[141] in 1974.

Phosphopyruvate hydratase (*PPH*)

Linkage with *Rh* looked very likely when Giblett *et al.*[86] found a Cree family in which a variant of *PPH* was segregating, from the father, so informatively that the family gave a z_1 count of $8:0$ and therefore a lod score of $2 \cdot 107$ at $\theta' = 0 \cdot 00$. (While θ is used for the recombination fraction calculated from male and female parents, θ' is often used to specify that it has been calculated from the male parent.) Linkage seemed established until a Winnipeg family, in which the mother was phase known, showed 1 non-recombinant to 4 recombinants; this made Lewis and her colleagues[90] (1973) wonder whether a small inversion in one or the other family might explain the discrepancy.

Hybrid cultures showed the *PPH* locus to be syntenic on No. 1 (Burgerhout *et al.*[84], 1974). The rarity of PPH variants rather limits its use in mapping.

Duffy (*Fy*) and other loci

A congenital cataract (*Cae*)

A large English family first described by Nettleship in 1909 was reinvestigated by Renwick and Lawler[35] (1963). The condition is described as 'congenital, zonular, pulverulent cataract'. The linkage between the cataract locus and the *Duffy* locus is not obvious in the large pedigree, but was disclosed by higher mathematics and by computer analysis. The linkage is very close: no definite recombinants were found in the family.

Uncoiler-1 (*1qh*)

Uncoiler-1 is an inherited visible deformity of the long arm of No. 1 autosome, close to the centromere. When, in 1968, Donahue, Renwick, de los Cobos Borgaonkar, Bias and McKusick[88, 89] found linkage between the Duffy groups and the abnormality, they were, microcosmonauts all, plotting for the first time a human marker locus on its right *autosome*.

References to later work supporting this linkage are to be found in the masterly paper by Cook, Robson, Buckton, Jacobs and Polani[93] on the relative position of loci on autosome No. 1.

Amylase, pancreatic (*AmP*) and salivary (*AmS*)

Linkage between *Fy* and *AmP* was convincingly established by Hill, Rowe and Lovrien[94] early in 1972. A recent estimate[95] of the male recombination fraction is about $0 \cdot 17$. Further supporting data were assembled[141] in 1974.

AmP and *AmS* are thought to represent separate loci but must be very close, for Rivas and his colleagues[97] report no recombination on 21 occasions when it might have been observed.

In 1971 Kamarýt and his colleagues[96] in Brno had made a strong case for linkage between *AmP* and *Iqh*, and this assignation to chromosome 1 was confirmed by the linkage between *AmP* and *AmS* and *Fy*.

ABO and other loci

Nail-patella (*Np*)

Another search for linkage, made by the Galton Laboratory, was brilliantly successful. Renwick and Lawler[28] (1955) discovered that the allele responsible for the rare dominant condition called 'nail-patella syndrome' or 'hereditary onychoosteodysplasia' is within measurable distance of the *ABO* locus. Six large families were investigated, and the linkage beautifully demonstrated.

Lawler, Renwick and their colleagues[29-32] tested 17 families and the estimate of the recombination fraction was $0·096 \pm 0·024$.

Renwick and Izatt[33], in 1965, collected all the data—25 informative families (and there is a good one since[34]). These families confirmed the previous recombination fraction, but when divided for the two sexes the fractions become, 0·084 for the male, and 0·146 for the female[19]. Schleutermann et al.[98] added some more families and the recombination rate (together with 95% probability limits) then became 0·10 (0·05–0·14) in males and 0·15 (0·08–0·22) in females.

Adenylate kinase (*AK*)

From the start the evidence for this linkage was strong (Rapley, Robson, Harris and Maynard Smith[80], 1968). Confirmation quickly followed[99-101]. Dr Bette Robson kindly allowed us to quote the vast data accumulated in the Galton Laboratory up to September 1973: the recombination rate (together with the 95% probability limits) is 0·10 (0·07 to 0·16) in males and 0·20 (0·14 to 0·29) in females.

These recombination rates are very close to those for the *ABO*:*Np* linkage which is to be expected for *Np* and *AK* are very closely linked: indeed Schleutermann et al.[98] found no recombination on 53 occasions when it could have been observed, nor did Sobel et al.[102] on 8 occasions.

Xeroderma pigmentosum

El-Hafnawi, Maynard Smith and Penrose[36] (1965) studied 34 Egyptian families with this recessive complaint. The evidence of linkage between the locus responsible and the *ABO* locus is overwhelming and the recombination fraction is about 0·18.

However, this straightforward story was shown, by further penetrating analysis, perhaps not to be the whole truth: a highly significant excess of group O, and deficit of groups A, B and AB, was noticed amongst the affected members of

19*

the families. So the possibility that the manifestation of the disease was perhaps suppressed by the presence of A or B antigens had to be thought of, and the authors ended their paper thus: 'Further work must be undertaken to determine whether there is such a direct association between x.d.p. and blood group O, with or without genetic linkage.' We know of only one publication[103] since and it brings some slight support for a preponderance of group O sufferers.

MNSs and other loci

Sclerotylosis (*Tys*)

Dr Mennecier in his thesis[76] (Lille, 1967) established the existence of close linkage between the *MNSs* locus and the locus for a newly described dominant condition 'génodermatose scléro-atrophiante et kératodermique des extrémités' (Huriez *et al.*[82]). Dr Mennecier discovered the linkage as a result of applying the *u* statistics. However, the evidence was seen to be much more overwhelming when the phase-known recombinants and non-recombinants in the large three generation family were simply counted: 12 non-recombinants to O recombinants. In the second generation there is one recombinant (z_1 8:1). The lod score analysis (Deminatti *et al.*[83]) gives a most likely recombination fraction of about 0·04, with fairly narrow probability limits, and the height of the curve is more than 21,000, an altitude almost beyond the reach of doubt (odds on linkage about 300 to 1).

The condition is now referred to as sclerotylosis and given the symbol *Tys*.

Dombrock blood groups (*Do*)

A slight hint of linkage between *MNSs* and *Do* was to be seen in an early report from our Unit, and a second series of families gave support (Tippett *et al.*[135, 136], 1967, 1972). Subsequent families tested in the Unit have reduced the height of the curve, but a hint of linkage still remains: θ' being about 0·35. At such a high recombination rate it will probably take years to find enough informative three generation families to decide for or against linkage.

Other hints of linkage with *MNSs* are: red cell acid phosphatase (AcP_1) (Mace and Robson[137], 1974) and the β-haemoglobin locus (Weitkamp *et al.*[138], 1972).

Lewis and other loci

Red cell acid phosphatase (AcP_1)

This seemed a good probable (van Cong and Moullec[104], 1971): the sum of the lod scores at $\theta = 0\cdot2$ was 2·067; the doubly heterozygous parents were not divided for sex. However, Weitkamp *et al.*[133] say 'Our data do not support the possibility of close linkage' and that details will be published.

Complement C3 (*C'3*)

This looks established (Weitkamp *et al.*[133], 1974). The sum of lod scores at $\theta = 0.1$ was 3.05 and, when divided by sex, recombination was more frequent in the female.

P and other loci

It seems that not both of the adumbrated linkages of *P* with *ADA* and *P* with *HL-A* can be correct, if correct are the claims that *ADA* is on No. 20 (Tischfield *et al.*[134]) and *HL-A* on No. 6 (Lamm *et al.*[116], Pearson[130] and other since).

Adenosine deaminase (*ADA*)

There is moderate evidence for linkage with *P* at $\theta = 0.2$ (Cook *et al.*[108]; Weit kamp[109]; Edwards *et al.*[107]).

HL-A

A case has been made by Fellous and his colleagues[105, 106] for synteny with *P* and there is suggestive evidence of linkage, at $\theta = 0.3$ (Edwards *et al.*[107], 1972), but linkage at such a distance is hard to establish.

Wright (*Wr^a*) and strong Sd^a antigen (*Sd^a*)

On page 398 we described a family in which two rare antigens were segregating, Wr^a and the very rare strong form of Sd^a: the lod scores were tantalizingly suggestive of linkage, 1.806 at $\theta = 0.00$ (Lewis *et al.*[110], 1973).

The antigen i and congenital cataract

In 1972, Yamaguchi, Okubo and Tanaka[111] reported the finding of four i propositi in routine testing of blood donors. The i condition being recessive and extremely rare in adults (page 449), the families of the propositi were also tested. The 4 propositi had between them 11 sibs of whom 4 were *ii*: all 8 *ii* sibs complained of poor vision 'due to a congenital cataract' whereas the vision of the 7 non-*ii* sibs was normal. The four families were not related to each other.

The lod scores show that the linkage is established (sum lods at $\theta = 0.00$ is + 3.4)—if it is a case of linkage rather than pleiotropy.

Chido (*Ch*) and *HL-A*

This linkage is described in Chapter 23 (page 477).

Linkage or pleiotropy?

Before recombination is observed between two characters which appear to be linked (that is with a suggestive lod score highest at $\theta = 0.00$) it cannot be certain whether they are controlled by two linked loci or by one locus having diverse effects (pleiotropy). In this category still falls the relation of *Fy* to *Cae*, of *Wr^a* to Sd(a++) and of *i* to the congenital cataract.

On rare occasion a false appearance of linkage might result from the presence in a family of an inhibitor gene capable of inhibiting the activity of several genetically unrelated loci. An example is *In(Lu)* (page 267) which inhibits the expression of the Lutheran and Auberger antigens and at least depresses P$_1$ and i.

Searches for linkages between the blood group loci

The only positive linkage is that between *Lutheran* and *secretor*. Although *Rh* and *Duffy* are syntenic, both residing on No. 1 chromosome, they are not linked: vast data from our own Unit[112] and from the Galton Laboratory[53] give such big negative lod scores that linkage is excluded even at a recombination fraction as high as 0·40. A linkage between *MNSs* and *Dombrock* is, so far, in the 'possible' class. The relationship of *Wright* and *Sid* is unsure.

These apart, no linkages have been found between the blood group markers although many thousands of families have been analysed, and references were given in our earlier editions.

It is a good thing that linkages between the blood group marker loci are so few: it suggests that they are well spread out over the chromosomes and the readier to catch other linkages.

A list of linkages not involving blood groups

It may be useful to give references to the established linkages we know of which involve markers other than blood groups. The list, which does not include syntenies, is surprisingly short, though we may have missed some:

> Transferrins (*Tf*) and serum cholinesterase (*E$_1$*)[37]
> *Gc* and albumin (*Alb*)[38, 90, 91, 113, 114]
> *Gm* and *Pi*[115]
> *HL-A* and *PGM$_3$*[116]
> *HL-A* and *GBG*[149]
> *Hbβ* and *Hbδ*, summary[117]
> *AmP* and *AmS*[95, 97] and see Table 95.

WHERE ARE THE BLOOD GROUP LOCI?

Fy and *Rh*

The first blood group locus to be assigned to its chromosome was *Xg* to the X in 1962, but this will be dealt with in Chapter 28. *Duffy* (*Fy*) was the first locus to be assigned to a human autosome: this happened as recently as 1968.

The story of the progressive mapping of No. 1 chromosome is rather dramatic and worth telling as a whole, not just as far as it involves Duffy and Rh.

First[35] *Fy* was known to be linked to *Cae*, then[89] *Fy* was found to be linked to uncoiler-1 (*1qh*) so this put *Fy* and *Cae* on No. 1. Then[96] *AmP* was found to be linked to *1qh*, and *AmP* was known[97] to be linked to *AmS*. So much for the Duffy linkage group.

The first *Rh* linkage[20] was with El_1, then *Rh* was found[52] to be linked to *PGD*. The next step was the demonstration[55] by means of a hamster-man hybrid cell culture that *PGD* was syntenic with PGM_1 and tests on families immediately confirmed this[53, 56] by showing linkage between *Rh* and PGM_1.

Then peptidase C (*Pep C*) was brought[118] into the picture when it was found to be syntenic with PGM_1, so *Pep C* therefore must be on the Rh chromosome. The last dramatic step was the finding[119] that *Pep C* is syntenic with No. 1 chromosome. So the Rh linkage group, led by *Pep C* trooped on to No. 1.

Conjecture about the order of loci on No. 1 has been lively. Cook *et al.*[93] favour the following: PGD–Rh–PGM_1–Fy–AmP–$Pep\ C$. As noted above, it is certain that *Rh* and *Fy* are too far apart for linkage between them to be directly measurable.

In 1968 Aarskog[131] recorded a child with a deletion involving half of one arm of No. 1. Since No. 1 is mediocentric it could not at the time be said whether the deletion was of the short or the long arm, and the child died, at 5 months. He was R_2r and Fy(a+b+), so neither *Rh* nor *Fy* is sited on the missing bit.

The regional location of *Rh*, PGM_1, *PGD* and *Fy* on chromosome 1 is becoming more precise[142-144] and summaries of the current situation appear from time to time[141].

Other blood group loci

There is some evidence concerning *MNSs*, *P*, *Lewis* and *Kidd* but none of these assignments can yet be considered established.

MNSs. German, Walker, Stiefel and Allen[139] (1969) described a boy with a reciprocal translocation between the long arm of No. 2 and the long arm of No. 4. The boy was M, though his father was N, and the possibility that the *MN* locus might be one of these two chromosomes was considered. With the development of banding techniques, the boy was reinvestigated in 1973 by German and Chaganti[140] who found that in the translocation a segment of the long arm of No. 2 had been lost. This demonstration that part of No. 2 was missing supported the tentative assignment of the *MN* locus to this chromosome.

P. By the cell hybrid method Fellous *et al.*[105, 106] found *HL-A* and *P* to be syntenic. *HL-A* and PGM_3 are linked (Lamm *et al.*[116]) and seem settled on chromosome 6 (Pearson[130] and other references in Bootsma and Giblett[147]), so it seems reasonable to suppose *P* to be on No. 6 also. But, the snag is that there is moderately good evidence (see above) for *P* being linked to *ADA*, and *ADA* is tentatively assigned to chromosome 20.

Le. If the assigning of AcP_1 to the short arm of chromosome 2 (Ferguson-Smith *et al.*[120], 1973) be confirmed, and if the possible linkage of *Le* and AcP_1 also be confirmed, then *Lewis* would become another blood group locus to find its chromosome.

Jk. In 1966 Hultén *et al.*[145] found slight evidence of linkage between *Jk* and a reciprocal translocation between No. 2 and one of the 6 to 12 group, and in 1973 Shokeir *et al.*[146], by the deletion mapping method, made a provisional case for *Jk* being on No. 7, though few blood group details were given.

Negative evidence

Negative evidence of location is provided if a person who lacks part of one of a pair of autosomes can be proved to be heterozygous at a marker locus. If, for

Table 96. Blood group loci not yet certainly assigned to a particular autosome: evidence of where they are not cited

Marker system	Marker locus not on	References	Marker system	Marker locus not on	References
ABO	5p	57	Kell	5p	73
	11, distal q	148		11, distal q	148
	13p	87		16, extremities of	126
	18p	121		18, part of q	78
	18q	122		18, extremities of	71
				Dq	74
MNSs	1, extremities of	58			
	5p	57, 59, 60, 61	Kidd	1, extremities of	58
	11, distal q	148		5p	57, 59, 75
	13p	62,87		13p	62, 87
	Dp	57, 59		18p	57, 69, 59
	D 1/3 q	63, 59		17 or 18p	125
	13q	123		18, part of q	78,92
	14, extremities of	85		18, extremities of	57
	Ep	59		22 or 22, extremities of	72
	18p	64–66, 57, 121, 124		G (monosomy)	127
	18, part of q	57, 78		Dq	74
	18, extremities of	57, 67		22, distal q	129
	18q	68			
	G (monosomy)	127	Dombrock	5p	59
	21 (? monosomy)	70, 128			
	Dq	59, 74			
	22, distal q	129	Colton	5p	59

Letters are used when the autosome number was not precisely identified: D = 13, 14 or 15; E = 16, 17 or 18; G = 21 or 22. p = short arm, q = long arm.

example, such a person were group AB, MN then the *ABO* and *MN* loci could not be sited on the missing bit of autosome. There is a good deal of negative evidence of this kind, as will be seen in Table 96: only markers with two or more positively detectable alleles can contribute.

There is a limit to this kind of information if the marker tests are confined to children born alive: most major deletions and monosomies are aborted and it is to the testing of abortions that we shall have to look for much further progress along this line.

The exploration of the human chromosomes now so feverishly active has something of the excitement of geographical cartography, and quite a lot of people deserve a doublet of velvet such as Columbus offered to the first man to see land.

REFERENCES

[1] HALDANE J.B.S. and SMITH C.A.B. (1947) A new estimate of the linkage between the genes for colour-blindness and haemophilia in man. *Ann. Eugen., Lond.*, 14, 10–31.

[2] SMITH C.A.B. (1953) The detection of linkage in human genetics. *J. Roy. stat. Soc., B.*, 15, 153–192.

[3] SMITH C.A.B. (1959) Some comment on the statistical methods used in linkage investigations. *Amer. J. hum. Genet.*, 11, 289–304.

[4] LAWLER SYLVIA D. and RENWICK J.H. (1959) Blood groups and genetic linkage. *Brit. med. Bull.*, 15, 145–149.

[5] FINNEY D.J. (1940) The detection of linkage. *Ann. Eugen., Lond.*, 10, 171–214.

[6] MAYNARD SMITH SHEILA, PENROSE L.S. and SMITH C.A.B. (1961) *Mathematical Tables for Research Workers in Human Genetics*, Churchill, London, pp. 74.

[7] FISHER R.A. (1935) The detection of linkage with 'dominant' abnormalities. *Ann. Eugen., Lond.*, 6, 187–201.

[8] FISHER R.A. (1935) The detection of linkage with recessive abnormalities. *Ann. Eugen., Lond.*, 6, 339–351.

[9] MORTON N.E. (1955) Sequential tests for the detection of linkage. *Amer. J. hum. Genet.*, 7, 277–318.

[10] MORTON N.E. (1957) Further scoring types in sequential linkage tests, with a critical review of autosomal and partial sex linkage in man. *Amer. J. hum. Genet.*, 9, 55–75.

[11] MOHR J. (1951) A search for linkage between the Lutheran blood group and other hereditary characters. *Acta path. microbiol. scand.*, 28, 207–210.

[12] MOHR J. (1951) Estimation of linkage between the Lutheran and the Lewis blood groups. *Acta path. microbiol. scand.*, 29, 339–344.

[13] MOHR J. (1954) *A Study of Linkage in Man*, pp. 119, Munksgaard, Copenhagen.

[14] PENROSE L.S. (1935) The detection of autosomal linkage in data which consist of pairs of brothers and sisters of unspecified parentage. *Ann. Eugen., Lond.*, 6, 133–138.

[15] PENROSE L.S. (1946) A further note on the sib-pair linkage method. *Ann. Eugen., Lond.*, 13, 25–29.

[16] METAXAS M.N., METAXAS-BÜHLER MARGRIT, DUNSFORD I. and HOLLÄNDER L. (1959) A further example of anti-Lu^b together with data in support of the Lutheran-secretor linkage in man. *Vox Sang.*, 4, 298–307.

[17] GREENWALT T.J. (1961) Confirmation of linkage between the Lutheran and secretor genes. *Amer. J. hum. Genet.*, 13, 69–88.

[18] COOK P.J.L. (1965) The Lutheran-secretor recombination fraction in man: a possible sex difference. *Ann. hum. Genet.*, **28**, 393–401.

[19] RENWICK J.H. and SCHULZE JANE (1965) Male and female recombination fractions for the nail-patella: ABO linkage in man. *Ann. hum. Genet.*, **28**, 379–392.

[20] CHALMERS J.N.M. and LAWLER SYLVIA D. (1953) Data on linkage in man: elliptocytosis and blood groups. I. Families 1 and 2. *Ann. Eugen., Lond.*, **17**, 267–271.

[21] GOODALL H.B., HENDRY D.W.W., LAWLER SYLVIA D. and STEPHEN S.A. (1953) Data on linkage in man: elliptocytosis and blood groups. II. Family 3. *Ann. Eugen., Lond.*, **17**, 272–278.

[22] GOODALL H.B., HENDRY D.W.W., LAWLER SYLVIA D. and STEPHEN S.A. (1954) Data on linkage in man: elliptocytosis and blood groups. III. Family 4. *Ann. Eugen. Lond.*, **18**, 325–327.

[23] LAWLER SYLVIA D. and SANDLER M. (1954) Data on linkage in man: elliptocytosis and blood groups. IV. Families 5, 6 and 7. *Ann. Eugen., Lond.*, **18**, 328–334.

[24] MORTON N.E. (1956) The detection and estimation of linkage between the genes for elliptocytosis and the Rh blood type. *Amer. J. hum. Genet.*, **8**, 80–96.

[25] CLARKE C.A., DONOHOE W.T.A., FINN R., McCONNELL R.B., SHEPPARD P.M. and NICHOL D.S.H. (1960) Data on linkage in man: ovalocytosis, sickling and the Rhesus blood group complex. *Ann. hum. Genet., Lond.*, **24**, 283–287.

[26] BANNERMAN R.M. and RENWICK J.H. (1962) The hereditary elliptocytosis: clinical and linkage data. *Ann. hum. Genet., Lond.*, **26**, 23–38.

[27] LOVRIC V.A., WALSH R.J. and BRADLEY MARGARET A. (1965) Hereditary elliptocytosis: genetic linkage with the Rh chromosome. *Aust. Ann. Med.*, **14**, 162–166.

[28] RENWICK J.H. and LAWLER SYLVIA D. (1955) Linkage between the ABO and nail-patella loci. *Ann. hum. Genet., Lond.*, **19**, 312–331.

[29] JAMESON R.J., LAWLER SYLVIA D. and RENWICK J.H. (1956) Nail-patella syndrome: clinical and linkage data on family G. *Ann. hum. Genet.*, **20**, 348–360.

[30] RENWICK J.H. (1956) Nail-patella syndrome: evidence for modification by alleles at the main locus. *Ann. hum. Genet.*, **21**, 159–169.

[31] LAWLER SYLVIA D., RENWICK J.H. and WILDERVANCK L.S. (1957) Further families showing linkage between the ABO and nail-patella loci, with no evidence of heterogeneity. *Ann. hum. Genet.*, **21**, 410–419.

[32] LAWLER SYLVIA D., RENWICK J.H., HAUGE M., MOSBECH J. and WILDERVANCK L.S. (1958) Linkage tests involving the P blood group locus and further data on the ABO: nail-patella linkage. *Ann. hum. Genet.*, **22**, 342–355.

[33] RENWICK J.H. and IZATT MARIAN M. (1965) Some genetical parameters of the nail-patella locus. *Ann. hum. Genet.*, **28**, 369–378.

[34] SHARMA J.C. (1966) Nail-patella syndrome in an Indian family: clinical and linkage data. *Ann. hum. Genet.*, **30**, 193–195.

[35] RENWICK J.H. and LAWLER SYLVIA D. (1963) Probable linkage between a congenital cataract locus and the Duffy blood group locus. *Ann. hum. Genet.*, **27**, 67–84.

[36] EL-HEFNAWI H., MAYNARD SMITH SHEILA and PENROSE L.S. (1965) Xeroderma pigmentosum—its inheritance and relationship to the ABO blood-group system. *Ann. hum. Genet.*, **28**, 273–290.

[37] ROBSON ELIZABETH B., SUTHERLAND I. and HARRIS H. (1966) Evidence for linkage between the transferrin locus (Tf) and the serum cholinesterase locus (E_1) in man. *Ann. hum. Genet.*, **29**, 325–336.

[38] WEITKAMP L.R., RUCKNAGEL D.L. and GERSHOWITZ H. (1966) Genetic linkage between, structural loci for albumin and group specific component (Gc). *Amer J. hum. Genet.*, **18** 559–571.

[39] RENWICK J.H. (1969) Progress in mapping human autosomes. *Brit. med. Bull.*, **25**, 65–73.

[40] RENWICK J.H. (1971) The mapping of human chromosomes. *A. Rev. Genet.*, **5**, 81–120.

41 WEITKAMP L.R. (1972) Human autosomal linkage groups. In *Human Genetics*, Excerpta Medica, Amsterdam, 445–460.

42 ROBSON ELIZABETH B. (1972) Gene assignment. In *Human Genetics*, Excerpta Medica, Amsterdam, 461–467.

43 BODMER W.F. (1972) Linkage analysis using human-mouse hybrid cells. In *Human Genetics* Excerpta Medica, Amsterdam, 365–373.

44 RUDDLE F.H., CHEN T.R. and BOONE C.M. (1972) Assignment of genes to chromosomes using somatic cell hybrids (TK:E17; LDH-A:C-11). In *Human Genetics*, Excerpta Medica, Amsterdam, 374–380.

45 SMITH C.A.B. (1968) Linkage scores and corrections in simple two- and three-generation families. *Ann. hum. Genet.*, 32, 127–150.

46 SMITH C.A.B. (1969) Further linkage scores and corrections in two- and three-generation families. *Ann. hum. Genet.*, 33, 207–223.

47 FURUHJELM U., NEVANLINNA H.R., GAVIN JUNE and SANGER RUTH (1972) A rare blood group antigen An^a (Ahonen). *J. med. Genet.*, 9, 385–391.

48 RENWICK J.H. (1968) Ratio of female to male recombination fractions in man. *Bull. Europ. Soc, Hum. Genet.*, 2, 7–14.

49 RENWICK J.H., BUNDEY SARAH E., FERGUSON-SMITH M.A. and IZATT MARIAN M. (1971) Confirmation of linkage of the loci for myotonic dystrophy and ABH secretion. *J. med. Genet.*, 8, 407–416.

50 HARPER P.S., RIVAS MARIAN L., BIAS WILMA B., HUTCHINSON JUDITH R., DYKEN P.R. and McKUSICK V.A. (1972) Genetic linkage confirmed between the locus for myotonic dystrophy and the ABH-secretion and Lutheran blood group loci. *Amer. J. Hum. Genet.*, 24, 310–316.

51 WEITKAMP L.R., GUTTORMSEN S.A., SHREFFLER D.C., SING C.F. and NAPIER J.A. (1970) Genetic linkage relations of the loci for 6-phosphogluconate dehydrogenase and adenosine deaminase in man. *Amer. J. Hum. Genet.*, 22, 216–220.

52 WEITKAMP L.R., GUTTORMSEN S.A. and GREENDYKE R.M. (1971) Genetic linkage between a locus for 6-PGD and the Rh locus: evaluation of possible heterogeneity in the recombination fraction between sexes and among families. *Amer. J. Hum. Genet.*, 23, 462–470.

53 ROBSON E.B., COOK P.J.L., CORNEY G., HOPKINSON D.A., NOADES J. and CLEGHORN T.E. (1973) Linkage data on *Rh*, *PGM*₁, *PGD*, *Peptidase C* and *Fy* from family studies. *Ann. Hum. Genet.*, 36, 393–399.

54 FIALKOW P.J., LISKER R., GIBLETT ELOISE R., ZAVALA C., COBO AZEYDÉH and DETTER J. (1972) Genetic markers in chronic myelocytic leukaemia: evidence opposing autosomal inactivation and favouring 6-PGD-Rh linkage. *Ann. Hum. Genet.*, 35, 321–326.

55 WESTERVELD A., VISSER R.P.L.S., MEERA KHAN P. and BOOTSMA D. (1971) Loss of human genetic markers in man-Chinese hamster somatic cell hybrids. *Nature New Biol.*, 234, 20–24.

56 RENWICK J.H. (1971) The Rhesus syntenic group in man. *Nature*, Lond., 234, 475.

57 SALMON C., ROPARTZ C., DE GROUCHY J., LEJEUNE J., SALMON D., RIVAT L., ROUSSEAU P.-Y., LIBERGE G. and DELARUE F. (1966) Exclusion de certaines localisations autosomiques des gènes de groupes sanguins et sériques. *Annls. Genet.*, 9, 9–11.

58 GORDON R.R. and COOKE P. (1964) Ring-1 chromosome and microcephalic dwarfism. *Lancet*, ii, 1212–1213. Blood groups subsequently done by I. Dunsford.

59 Blood Group Research Unit. Unpublished observations, samples sent by Penrose L.S., Ceppellini R., Polani P.E., Opitz J., Edwards J.H. and Richards B.W.

60 HUSTINX T.W.J. and WIJFFELS J.C.H.M. (1965) Cri du chat syndrome. Partial deletion of the short arm of a chromosome No. 5. *Maandschr. Kindergeneesk.*, 33, 286–298.

61 WOLF U., REINWEIN H., GEY W. and KLOSE J. (1966) Cri-du-chat syndrom mit Translokation 5/D₂. *Humangenetik*, 2, 63–77.

62 BUCHANAN J.G., PEARCE LORNA and WETHERLEY-MEIN G. (1964) The May-Hegglin anomaly. A family report and chromosome study. *Brit. J. Haemat.*, 10, 508–512. Subsequently

tested at the Blood Group Research Unit and the Human Biochemical Genetics Research Unit.

63 LELE KUSUM P., PENROSE L.S. and STALLARD H.B. (1963) Chromosome deletion in a case of retinoblastoma. *Ann. hum. Genet.*, **27**, 171–174.

64 LAWLER SYLVIA D. (1964) Localisation of autosomal genes in man. *Hum. Biol.*, **36**, 146–156.

65 DYKE H.E. VAN, VALDMANIS AINA and MANN J.D. (1964) Probable deletion of the short arm of chromosome 18. *Amer. J. hum. Genet.*, **16**, 364–374.

66 SUMMITT R.L. (1964) Deletion of the short arm of chromosome 18. *Cytogenetics*, **3**, 201–206.

67 LUCAS MARY, KEMP N.H., ELLIS J.R. and MARSHALL RUTH (1963) A small autosomal ring chromosome in a female infant with congenital malformations. *Ann. hum. Genet.*, **27**, 189–195.

68 WOLF U., REINWEIN H., GORMAN LINDA Z. and KÜNZER W. (1967) Deletion on long arm of a chromosome 18 (46,XX,18q−). *Humangenetik*, **5**, 70–71.

69 REINWEIN H., RITTER H. and WOLF U. (1967) Deletion of short arm of a chromosome 18 (46,XX,18p−). *Humangenetik*, **5**, 72–73.

70 GRIPENBERG ULLA, ELFVING J. and GRIPENBERG L. (1972) A 45,XX,21− child: attempt at a cytological and clinical interpretation of the karyotype. *J. Med. Genet.*, **9**, 110–115.

71 RICHARDS B.W., RUNDLE A.T., ZAREMBA J. and STEWART A. (1970) Ring chromosome 18 in a mentally retarded boy. *J. ment. Defic. Res.*, **14**, 174–186.

72 HECHT F., WELEBER R.G. and GIBLETT ELOISE R. (1967) Chromosome anomalies. *Lancet*, **i**, 848.

73 MACINTYRE M.N., STAPLES W.I., LAPOLLA J. and HEMPEL JOANNE M. (1964) The 'cat cry' syndrome. *Am. J. Dis. Child.*, **108**, 538–542.

74 LAURENT C., COTTON J-B., NIVELON A. and FREYCON M.-TH. (1967) Deletion partielle du bras long d'un chromosome du group D (13–15):Dq−. *Annls. Génét.*, **10**, 25–31

75 STEELE M.W., BREG W.R., EIDELMAN A.I., LION D.T. and TERZAKIS T.A. (1966) A B-group ring chromosome with mosaicism in a newborn with cri du chat syndrome. *Cytogenetics*, **5**, 419–429.

76 MENNECIER M. (1967) *Individualisation d'une Nouvelle Entité: la Génodermatose Scléro-Atrophiante et Kératodermique des Extrémités Fréquemment Dégénerative. Etude Clinique et Génétique (Possibilité de Linkage avec le Systeme MNSs)*. M.D. Thesis, University of Lille, pp. 163.

77 GEERDINK R.A., NIJENHUIS L.E. and HUIZINGA J. (1967) Hereditary elliptocytosis: linkage data in man. *Ann. hum. Genet.*, **30**, 363–378.

78 INSLEY J. (1967) Syndrome associated with a deficiency of part of the long arm of chromosome no. 18, *Archs. Dis. Childh.*, **42**, 140–146.

79 SANGER RUTH and RACE R.R. (1958) The Lutheran-secretor linkage in Man: support for Mohr's findings. *Heredity*, **12**, 513–520.

80 RAPLEY SANDRA E., ROBSON ELIZABETH B., HARRIS H. and MAYNARD SMITH SHEILA (1968) Data on the incidence, segregation and linkage relations of the adenylate kinase (AK) polymorphism. *Ann. hum. Genet.*, **31**, 237–242.

81 COOK P.J.L., NOADES JEAN, HOPKINSON D.A. and ROBSON E.B. (1972) Demonstration of a sex difference in recombination fraction in the loose linkage, *Rh* and *PGM*$_1$. *Ann. Hum. Genet.*, **35**, 239–242.

82 HURIEZ C., DEMINATTI M., AGACHE P. and MENNECIER M. (1968) Une dénodysplasie non encore individualisée: la génodermatose scléro-atrophiante et kératodermique des extrémitiés fréquemment dégénérative. *Sem. Hôp.*, *Paris*, **44**, 481 (Not seen).

83 DEMINATTI M., DELMAS-MARSALET Y., MENNECIER M., MARQUET S., AGACHE P. and HURIEZ C. (1968) Étude du linkage probable entre une génodermatose a transmission autosomale dominante et le système de groupe sanguin MNSs. *Annls. Génét.*, **11**, 217–224.

84 BURGERHOUT W.G., JONGSMA A.P.M. and MEERA KHAN P. (1974) Regional assignments of seven enzyme loci on chromosome 1 of man. *Cytogenet. Cell Genet.*, **13**, 73–75.

[85] SPARKES R.S., CARREL R.E. and WRIGHT S.W. (1967) Absent thumbs with a ring D2 chromosome: a new deletion syndrome. *Amer. J. hum. Genet.*, **19**, 644–659.

[86] GIBLETT E.R., CHEN S.-H., ANDERSON J.E. and LEWIS M. (1974) A family study suggesting genetic linkage of phosphopyruvate hydratase (enolase) to the Rh blood group system *Cytogenet. Cell Genet.* **13**, 91–92.

[87] BIAS WILMA B. and MIGEON BARBARA R. (1967) Haptoglobin: a locus on the D_1 chromosome? *Amer. J. hum. Genet.*, **19**, 393–398.

[88] DONAHUE R.P., RENWICK J.H., COBOS L. DE LOS, BORGAONKAR D.S., BIAS W.B. and McKUSICK V.A. (1968) Karyotypic and linkage analysis in two pedigrees with marker chromosomes. *Clin. Res. Abstracts*, **16**, 296.

[89] DONAHUE R.P., BIAS WILMA B., RENWICK J.H. and McKUSICK V.A. (1968) Probable assignment of the Duffy blood group locus to chromosome 1 in man. *Proc. nat. acad. Sci.*, **61**, 949–955.

[90] LEWIS MARION (1973) Personal communication.

[91] KAARSALO E., MELARTIN L. and BLUMBERG B.S. (1967) Autosomal linkage between the albumin and Gc loci in humans. *Science*, **158**, 123–125.

[92] NANCE W.E., HIGDON SARAH H., CHOWN B. and ENGEL E. (1968) Partial E-18 long-arm deletion. *Lancet*, **i**, 303.

[93] COOK P.J.L., ROBSON ELIZABETH B., BUCKTON KARIN E., JACOBS PATRICIA A. and POLANI P.E. (1973) Segregation of genetic markers in families with chromosome polymorphisms and structural rearrangements involving chromosome 1. *Ann. Hum. Genet.*, **37**, 261–274.

[94] HILL CINDA J., ROWE SHIRLEY I. and LOVRIEN E.W. (1972) Probable genetic linkage between human serum amylase (Amy_2) and Duffy blood group. *Nature, Lond.*, **235**, 162–163.

[95] MERRITT A.D., LOVRIEN E.W., RIVAS MARIAN L. and CONNEALLY P.M. (1973) Human amylase loci: genetic linkage with the Duffy blood group locus and assignment to linkage group 1. *Am. J. Hum. Genet.*, **25**, 523–538.

[96] KAMARÝT J., ADÁMEK R. and VRBA M. (1971) Possible linkage between uncoiler chromosome Un 1 and amylase polymorphism Amy 2 loci. *Humangenetik*, **11**, 213–220.

[97] RIVAS M.L., MERRITT A.D., LOVRIEN E.W. and CONNEALLY P.M. (1972) The amylase (Amy_1, Amy_2) and Duffy linkage group. *Am. J. Hum. Genet.*, **24**, 40a.

[98] SCHLEUTERMANN DONNA A., BIAS WILMA B., MURDOCH J.L. and McKUSICK V.A. (1969) Linkage of the loci for the nail-patella syndrome and adenylate kinase. *Am. J. Hum. Genet.*, **21**, 606–630.

[99] WEITKAMP L.R., SING C.F., SHREFFLER D.C. and GUTTORMSEN S.A. (1969) The genetic linkage relations of adenylate kinase: further data on the *ABO-AK* linkage group. *Am. J. Hum. Genet.*, **21**, 600–605.

[100] WILLE B. and RITTER H. (1969) Zur formalen Genetik der Adenylatkinasen (EC: 2.7.4.3). Hinweis auf Kopplung der loci für AK und ABO. *Humangenetik*, **7**, 263.

[101] WENDT G.G., RITTER H., ZILCH I., TARIVERDIAN G., KINDERMANN I. and KIRCHBERG G. (1971) Genetics and linkage analysis on adenylate kinase. *Humangenetik*, **13**, 347–349.

[102] SOBEL R.S., TIGER A. and GERALD P.S. (1971) A second family with the nail-patella allele and the adenylate kinase allele in coupling. *Amer. J. hum. Genet.*, **23**, 146–149.

[103] PISANI M., DELUCA M. and ROSSI A. (1970) Xeroderma pigmentosum and blood groups (In Italian) *G. Ital. Derm.* **45**-III(1):28-34. Original not seen, abstract in Birth Defects, July 1970, 7, No. 7, 22.

[104] VAN CONG N. and MOULLEC J. (1971) Linkage probable entre les groupes de phosphatase acide des globules rouges et le système Lewis. *Annls. Génét.*, **14**, 121–125.

[105] FELLOUS M., BILLARDON C., DAUSSET J. and FRÉZAL J. (1971) Linkage probable entre les locus 'HLA' et 'P'. *C.R. Acad. Sc.*, Paris, **272**, 3356–3359.

[106] FELLOUS M., COUILLIN P., NEAUPORT-SAUTES C., FREZAL J., BILLARDON C. and DAUSSET J. (1973) Studies of human alloantigens on man-mouse hybrids: possible synteny between HL-A and P systems. *Eur. J. Immunol.*, **3**, 543–548.

107 EDWARDS J.H., ALLEN F.H., GLENN K.P., LAMM L.U. and ROBSON E.B. (1972) The linkage
     relationships of HL-A. In: *Histocompatibility Testing*, Munksgaard, Copenhagen,
     745–751.

108 COOK P.J.L., HOPKINSON D.A. and ROBSON ELIZABETH B. (1970) The linkage relationships
     of adenosine deaminase. *Ann. hum. Genet.*, **34**, 187–188.

109 WEITKAMP L.R. (1971) Further data on the genetic linkage relations of the adenosine de-
     aminase locus. *Human Hered.*, **21**, 351–356.

110 LEWIS MARION, KAITA HIROKO, CHOWN B., TIPPETT PATRICIA, GAVIN JUNE, SANGER
     RUTH, GIBLETT ELOISE and STEINBERG A.G. (1973) A family with the rare red cell antigens
     Wr^a and 'super' Sd^a. *Vox Sang.*, **25**, 336–340.

111 YAMAGUCHI H., OKUBO Y. and TANAKA M. (1972) A note on possible close linkage between
     the Ii blood locus and a congenital cataract locus. *Proc. Jap. Acad.*, **48**, 625–628.

112 SANGER RUTH, TIPPETT PATRICIA, GAVIN JUNE and RACE R.R. (1973) Failure to demon-
     strate linkage between the loci for the Rh and Duffy blood groups. *Ann. hum. Genet.*,
     36, 353–354.

113 KUEPPERS F., HOLLAND P.V. and WEITKAMP L.R. (1969) Albumin Santa Ana: a new in-
     herited variant. *Human Hered.*, **19**, 378–384.

114 WEITKAMP L.R., RENWICK J.H., BERGER J., SHREFFLER D.C., DRACHMANN O., WUHRMANN
     F., BRAEND M. and FRANGLEN G. (1970) Additional data and summary for albumin-Gc
     linkage in man. *Human Hered.*, **20**, 1–7.

115 GEDDE-DAHL T., FAGERHOL M.K., COOK P.J.L. and NOADES JEAN (1972) Autosomal linkage
     between the *Gm* and *Pi* loci in man. *Ann. hum. Genet.*, **35**, 393–399.

116 LAMM L.U., SVEJGAARD A. and KISSMEYER-NIELSEN F. (1971) PGM$_3$: HL-A is another
     linkage in man. *Nature, Lond.*, **231**, 109–110.

117 MISHU MONA K. and NANCE W.E. (1969) Further evidence for close linkage of the *Hbβ*
     and *Hbδ* loci in man. *J. med. Genet.*, **6**, 190–192.

118 VAN CONG N., BILLARDON C., PICARD J.-Y., FEINGOLD J. and FRÉZAL J. (1971) Liaison
     probable (linkage) entre les locus *PGM$_1$* et peptidase C chez l'homme. *C.R. Acad. Sc..
     Paris*, **272**, 485–487.

119 RUDDLE F., RICCIUTI F., MCMORRIS F.A., TISCHFIELD J., CREAGAN R., DARLINGTON G.
     and CHEN T. (1972) Somatic cell genetic assignment of peptidase C and the Rh linkage
     group to chromosome A-1 in man. *Science*, **176**, 1429–1431.

120 FERGUSON-SMITH M.A., NEWMAN B.F., ELLIS P.M., THOMSON D.M.G. and RILEY I.D,
     (1973) Assignment by deletion of human red cell acid phosphatase gene locus to the
     short arm of chromosome 2. *Nature New Biol.* **243**, 271–274.

121 WEISS L. and MAYEDA K. (1969) A patient with a short arm deletion of chromosome 18
     (46,XY,18p–). *J. med. Genet.*, **6**, 216–219.

122 STEWART JANET M., GO S., ELLIS E. and ROBINSON A. (1970) Absent IgA and deletions of
     chromosome 18. *J. med. Genet.*, **7**, 11–19.

123 ALLDERDICE P.W., DAVIS J.G., MILLER O.J., KLINGER H.P., WARBURTON D., MILLER D.A.,
     ALLEN F.H., ABRAMS C.A.L. and MCGILVRAY E. (1969) The 13q– deletion syndrome.
     Amer. J. hum. Genet., **21**, 499–512.

124 DE GROUCHY J., BONNETTE J. and SALMON C. (1966) Délétion du bras court du chromosome
     18. *Annls Génét.*, **9**, 19–26.

125 DE GROUCHY J., LAMY M., THIEFFRY S., ARTHUIS M. and SALMON C. (1963) Dysmorphie
     complexe avec oligophrénie: délétion des bras courts d'un chromosome 17-18. *C.R.
     Acad. Sc., Paris*, **256**, 1028–1029.

126 PERGAMENT E., PIETRA G.C., KADOTANI T., SATO H. and BERLOW S. (1970) A ring chromo-
     some No. 16 in an infant with primary hypoparathyroidism. *J. Pediat.*, **76**, 745–
     751.

127 AL-AISH M.S., DE LA CRUZ F., GOLDSMITH L.A., VOLPE J., MELLA G. and ROBINSON J.C.
     (1967) Autosomal monosomy in man. Complete monosomy G (21-22) in a four and one
     half year old mentally retarded girl. *New Engl. J. Med.*, **277**, 777–784.

[128] RICHMOND H.G., MACARTHUR P. and HUNTER D. (1973) A 'G' deletion syndrome anti-mongolism. *Acta Paediat. Scand.*, **62**, 216–220.

[129] BÜHLER ERICA and METAXAS M.N. (1972) Personal communication.

[130] PEARSON P.L. (1972) The identification of chromosomes in hybrid cells. *Bull. Eur. Soc. Hum. Genet.*, November, 54–61.

[131] AARSKOG D. (1968) A large deletion of chromosome No. 1 (46,XY,1?–). *J. med. Genet.*, **5**, 322–325.

[132] MIDDLETON JANICE, CROOKSTON MARIE C., FALK JUDITH A., ROBSON ELIZABETH B., COOK P.J.L., BATCHELOR J.R., BODMER JULIA, FERRARA G.B., FESTENSTEIN H., HARRIS R., KISSMEYER-NIELSEN F., LAWLER SYLVIA D., SACHS J.A. and WOLF EVA (1974) Linkage of Chido and HL-A. *Tissue Antigens*, **4**, 366–373.

[133] WEITKAMP L.R., JOHNSTON E. and GUTTORMSEN S.A. (1974) Probable genetic linkage between the loci for the Lewis blood group and complement C3. *Cytogenet. Cell Genet.*, **13**, 183–184.

[134] TISCHFIELD J.A., CREAGAN R.P., NICHOLS E. and RUDDLE F.H. (1974) Assignment of adenosine deaminase to chromosome 20. *Cytogenet. Cell Genet.*, **13**, 160–163.

[135] TIPPETT P. (1967) Genetics of the Dombrock blood group system. *J. Med. Genet.*, **4**, 7–11.

[136] TIPPETT PATRICIA, GAVIN JUNE and SANGER RUTH (1972) The Dombrock system: linkage relations with other blood group loci. *J. Med. Genet.*, **9**, 392–395.

[137] MACE M. and ROBSON E.B. (1974) Linkage data on AcP_1 and *MNSs*. *Cytogenet. Cell Genet.*, **13**, 123–125.

[138] WEITKAMP L.R., ADAMS M.S. and ROWLEY P.T. (1972) Linkage between the MN- and Hb β-loci? *Human Hered.*, **22**, 566–572.

[139] GERMAN J.L., WALKER M.E., STIEFEL F.H. and ALLEN F.H. (1969) Autoradiographic studies of human chromosomes. II. Data concerning the position of the *MN* locus. *Vox Sang.*, **16**, 130–145.

[140] GERMAN J. and CHAGANTI R.S.K. (1973) Mapping human autosomes: assignment of the MN locus to a specific segment in the long arm of chromosome No. 2. *Science*, **182**, 1261–1262.

[141] HAMERTON J.L. and COOK P.J.L. (1974) Report of the committee on the genetic constitution of chromosome 1. *Cytogenet. Cell Genet.*, **13**, 13–20.

[142] DOUGLAS G.R., McALPINE PHYLLIS J. and HAMERTON J.L. (1973) Regional localization of loci for human PGM_1 and *6PGD* on human chromosome one by use of hybrids of Chinese hamster-human somatic cells. *Proc. Nat. Acad. Sci.*, **70**, 2737–2740.

[143] LEE CATHERINE S.N., YING K.L. and BOWEN P. (1974) Position of the Duffy locus on chromosome 1 in relation to breakpoints for structural rearrangements. *Amer. J. Hum. Genet.*, **26**, 93–102.

[144] MARSH W.L., CHAGANTI R.S.K., GARDNER F.H., MAYER K., NOWELL P.C. and GERMAN J. (1974) Mapping human autosomes: evidence supporting assignment of Rhesus to the short arm of chromosome No. 1. *Science*, **183**, 966–968.

[145] HULTÉN MAJ, LINDSTEN J., PEN-MING L.M., FRACCARO M., MANNINI ANNA, TIEPOLO L., ROBSON E.R., HEIKEN A. and TILLINGER K.-G. (1966) Possible localization of the genes for the Kidd blood group on an autosome involved in a reciprocal translocation. *Nature, Lond.*, **211**, 1067–1068.

[146] SHOKEIR M.H.K., YING K.L. and PABELLO P. (1973) Deletion of the long arm of chromosome no. 7: tentative assignment of the Kidd (Jk) locus. *Clin. Genet.*, **4**, 360–368.

[147] BOOTSMA D. and GIBLETT E.R. (1974) Report of the committee on the genetic constitution of autosomes other than chromosome 1. *Cytogenet. Cell Genet.*, **13**, 21–28.

[148] JACOBSEN PETREA, HAUGE M., HENNINGSEN K., HOBOLTH N., MIKKELSEN MARGARETA and PHILIP J. (1973) An (11;21) translocation in four generations with chromosome 11 abnormalities in the offspring: a clinical, cytogenetical and gene marker study. *Hum. Hered.*, **23**, 568–585.

[149] ALLEN F.H. (1974) Linkage of HL-A and GBG. *Vox Sang.*, **27**, 382–384.

Chapter 28
The Xg Blood Groups

The sudden recognition during the investigation of a 'new' antibody that the corresponding antigen must be controlled by an X-borne locus (Mann, Cahan, Gelb, Fisher, Hamper, Tippett, Sanger and Race[1], 1962) opened fresh possibilities in the application of blood groups to human genetics, possibilities which have been realized richly, though more slowly than was hoped in the first enthusiasm.

The antibody which defined the new antigen was met during cross-matching tests on a patient, Mr And., attending the Butterworth Hospital, Grand Rapids; Mr And. had been transfused many times for severe nose bleeds due to familial telangiectasia.

The first clue to the X-linkage was given when families were found which excluded the antigen, a dominant character, from being part of the ABO, MNSs or Rh systems but did not exclude an association with sex. Our experience with other antigens had been that sex is about as efficient at demonstrating genetical independence as are ABO, MNSs or Rh, and this led within minutes to the recognition of a different distribution of the new antigen in the two sexes. Blood samples from more families were rapidly collected and, one after the other, were found to obey the quite complicated rules which can be worked out for the inheritance of a dominant antigen which is X-borne.

An X-borne red cell antigen was immediately seen to have possible use in X-mapping, X-chromosome abnormalities and aneuploidies and in the problem, not at that time so triumphantly settled, of X-chromosome inactivation.

The antigen was called Xg[a], the antibody anti-Xg[a], the phenotypes Xg(a+) and Xg(a−), the allele responsible for the antigen, Xg^a, and that for its so far silent allele, Xg.

FREQUENCIES

The incidence of the antigen Xg[a] in the two normal sexes of unrelated people of Northern European stock was reported in several papers[1-4, 32], in the last of which (Sanger, Tippett and Gavin[32], 1971) all our results were given separately according to the countries of origin of the samples, but here the 6,784 unrelated Northern Europeans are simply summed:

	Xg(a+)	Xg(a−)	Total
males	2,304	1,209	3,513
	65·6%	34·4%	
females	2,900	371	3,271
	88·7%	11·3%	

The gene frequencies are calculated by the formula of Haldane[6] (1963)

$$\text{frequency of gene } Xg = \frac{[4(2f+m)(b+2d)+a^2]^{\frac{1}{2}} - a}{2(2f+m)}$$

frequency of gene $Xg^a = 1 -$ frequency of Xg.

where the letters represent the absolute numbers observed in the following categories:

	Xg(a+)	Xg(a−)	Total
males	a	b	m
females	c	d	f

The gene frequencies are found to be

$$Xg^a \quad 0·659$$
$$Xg \quad 0·341$$

and the frequencies thus calculated from the male and female absolute numbers can be recombined to give the expected genotype and phenotype frequencies:

males		females	
Xg^a	0·659	Xg^aXg^a	0·434
Xg	0·341	Xg^aXg	0·450 } 0·884
		$XgXg$	0·116

In addition to progressive publications from this Unit summed above, substantial series of tests on unrelated people of Northern European origin have been reported: 588 Canadians[5], 1,382 U.S.A. Whites[10], 558 Swiss[33] and 2,404 Viennese[34,35] all agreeing pretty well with each other. Some smaller collections from other peoples are noted at the end of this chapter.

INHERITANCE

The following paragraphs and Figure 37 are taken, by permission, from the *Canadian Journal of Genetics and Cytology* (Sanger[7], 1966).

'The pattern of inheritance of X-linked characters is the more or the less obvious depending whether the character is recessive, intermediate or dominant.

Figure 37 shows one of a number of Sardinian families which illustrate, at the same time, the inheritance of recessive, intermediate and dominant X-linked characters.

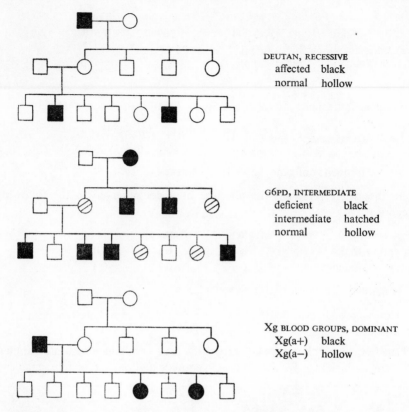

Fig. 37. A Sardinian family, investigated by Professor M. Siniscalco and Dr G. Filippi, illustrating the inheritance of recessive, intermediate and dominant X-linked characters. (From Sanger[7], 1966.)

(a)   Recessives, like deutan colour-blindness, are easy to recognize as such: none of the children of an affected man show the condition [provided his wife lacks the deutan allele] but his daughters are all carriers and transmit it, on the average, to half their sons.

(b)   G6PD is a good example of an intermediate X-linked character. Carrier females can usually be spotted and distinguished from homozygous affected females. The grandmother in the middle pedigree is homozygous and, as expected, both her sons are deficient and, since her husband is normal, both her daughters are intermediate. The issue of the married intermediate daughter fit well enough with expectation, which is that half her sons should be deficient and half normal and half her daughters should be intermediate and half normal.

(c)   The blood group antigen Xg^a is a dominant character. This family illustrates two points: the mating father Xg(a+) by mother Xg(a−), in the second generation on the left, can produce only Xg(a−) sons, for their single X comes from their mother: and all the daughters from this mating must be Xg(a+), for the girls must have their father's X which carries the gene for the antigen. The pedigree also illustrates that Xg(a−) daughters must have Xg(a−) fathers.'

A rather neat confirmation of the X-linkage of a character such as Xg is provided by XO Turner females having the male distribution of the antigen (Chapter 30).

The families

From the frequencies given above may be calculated the expected frequencies of the four mating types in the population being dealt with, and also the expected incidence of the Xg groups in their offspring. Table 97 gives the formulae for families in which both parents were tested and for families in which only one parent was tested.

These formulae have been applied in Table 98 to 1,348 Northern European families with 3,272 children tested in our Unit[32] and to 294 White Canadian families with 797 children (Chown, Lewis and Kaita[5]). The agreement between the observed and the expected incidence of mating types and proportion of Xg(a+) and Xg(a−) amongst the offspring is very good.

The Xg groups of a further 1,192 Northern European families, but lacking one parent, with 2,552 children were reported from our Unit[32]: these and a great many Sardinian, Israeli, Negro, Chinese and other families have all contributed to the overwhelming evidence that the locus for Xg is on the X chromosome.

Exceptional children

In Table 98 there are 12 children who appear to break the rules of X-linked inheritance. No exceptions were disclosed in the further 1,192 families lacking one parent. Exceptions could be explained by illegitimacy, but all the families were tested for a variety of other groups besides Xg and any members shown to be illegitimate by these other groups were omitted from the counts. Of course, XO daughters of Xg(a+) fathers are often Xg(a−), and XXY sons of Xg(a−) mothers are sometimes Xg(a+), but families with such X chromosome abnormalities are excluded from this table and are dealt with in Chapter 30.

Xg(a−) daughters of Xg(a+) fathers

The four such exceptional girls in Table 98 were discussed at some length by Sanger et al.[32], who considered that the exceptions did not carry much weight: two of them were trisomic babies (see page 588); to fit the third into her family required the postulation of a rare autosomal blood group genotype and the sample from the fourth was too small to allow enough grouping to check her parentage adequately.

Table 97. Expected distribution of Xg groups in parents and offspring (From Noades, Gavin, Tippett, Sanger and Race[4], 1966)

Total	Mating Type Father	Mating Type Mother	Frequency	In sons Obs. total	In sons Xg(a+)	In sons Xg(a−)	In daughters Obs. total	In daughters Xg(a+)	In daughters Xg(a−)
p_n	Xg(a+)	Xg(a+)	$p_n \times Xg^a \times ♀Xg(a+)$	s_1	$s_1 \times (a)$	$s_1 \times (b)$	d_1	all	none
	Xg(a+)	Xg(a−)	$p_n \times Xg^a \times ♀Xg(a-)$	s_2	none	all	d_2	all	none
	Xg(a−)	Xg(a+)	$p_n \times Xg \times ♀Xg(a+)$	s_3	$s_3 \times (a)$	$s_3 \times (b)$	d_3	$d_3 \times (a)$	$d_3 \times (b)$
	Xg(a−)	Xg(a−)	$p_n \times Xg \times ♀Xg(a-)$	s_4	none	all	d_4	none	all
p_1	Xg(a+)	?	$p_1 \times Xg^a$	s_5	$s_5 \times Xg^a$	$s_5 \times Xg$	d_5	all	none
	Xg(a−)	?	$p_1 \times Xg$	s_6	$s_6 \times Xg^a$	$s_6 \times Xg$	d_6	$d_6 \times Xg^a$	$d_6 \times Xg$
p_2	?	Xg(a+)	$p_2 \times ♀Xg(a+)$	s_7	$s_7 \times (a)$	$s_7 \times (b)$	d_7	$d_7 \times (c)$	$d_7 \times (d)$
	?	Xg(a−)	$p_2 \times ♀Xg(a-)$	s_8	none	all	d_8	$d_8 \times Xg^a$	$d_8 \times Xg$

$$(a) = \frac{Xg^a}{♀Xg(a+)} \quad (b) = 1 - (a) \quad (c) = Xg^a + (b) \quad (d) = 1 - (c)$$

Xg^a and Xg = the gene frequencies in the appropriate population. ♀Xg(a+) and ♀Xg(a−) = the calculated frequency of the two phenotypes in the females of the appropriate population.

p_n = total number of families with both parents grouped; p_1 = mother not grouped, p_2 = father not grouped.

Table 98. Xg groups of 1,642 families of Northern European extraction and their 4,069 children. (From Sanger, Tippett and Gavin[32] and Chown, Lewis and Kaita[5])

Mating Type		Number	Offspring						Total offspring
			Sons			Daughters			
Father	Mother		Total	Xg(a+)	Xg(a−)	Total	Xg(a+)	Xg(a−)	
Xg(a+)	Xg(a+)	959 (956·5)	1,281	966 (954·3)	315 (326·7)	1,100	1,097 (1100·0)	3*	2,381
Xg(a+)	Xg(a−)	133 (125·5)	183	8*	175 (183·0)	156	155 (156·0)	1*	339
Xg(a−)	Xg(a+)	479 (495·0)	611	448 (455·2)	163 (155·8)	549	405 (409·0)	144 (140·0)	1,160
Xg(a−)	Xg(a−)	71 (65·0)	103	0	103 (103·0)	86	0	86 (86·0)	189
		1,642	2,178			1,891			4,069

No family is included in this table if a member has any form of sex chromosome aneuploidy.
* Exceptional children; see text. Expected numbers are in brackets.

Xg(a+) sons of Xg(a−) mothers

These are very rare and very important. The eight such exceptional sons of Table 98 belong to three English families and one Canadian.

Je. family[8]:   father Xg(a+), mother Xg(a−), both of two sons Xg(a+)
Bu. family[8]:   father Xg(a+), mother Xg(a−), all three sons Xg(a+)
Fe. family[5]:   father Xg(a+), mother Xg(a−), the only son Xg(a+)
Wa. family[48]: father Xg(a+), mother Xg(a−), both of two sons Xg(a+)

A possible explanation which we had come to favour was that in the ancestry of the fathers of the Xg(a+) boys a small portion of an X, involving the Xg locus (occupied by the allele Xg^a), had become translocated on to a Y, or even on to an autosome. However, when family Wa. was tested the groups of three generations excluded, in their case at any rate, a translocation on to a Y.

As the Xg groups of this family have not been published in full we thought they should be recorded (Figure 38) here rather than in the chapter dealing with chimeras: they are very surprising and lacked explanation when retested in 1967 (unpublished work with Dr T.E. Cleghorn and Dr K.L. Rogers). A sister, II-3, and brother, II-4, are chimerical twins (page 522). II-3 has 99% of her own O, Xg(a+) cells and 1% of her brother's A, Xg(a+) cells. II-4 has 78% of his own cells and 22% of his sister's. The first strange thing is that his own cells are Xg(a+) though his mother, I-2 ,is Xg(a−): he cannot be a rare but perhaps possible person with Xg^a on his Y because his son, III-3 ,to whom he must have given his Y, is Xg(a−).

The next strange thing is that II-1 is also Xg(a+) and he is not XXY because he has children. It was not until 4 years later that the work of Buckton *et al.*[49], mentioned in the next paragraph, provided a possible explanation and we were driven to believe that I-2 though phenotypically Xg(a−) as judged by her red cells

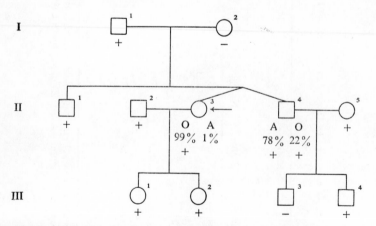

Fig. 38. The family Wa. showing exceptional inheritance of the Xg groups. II-3 and II-4 are twin chimeras. + = Xg(a+), − = Xg(a−), arrow = propositus.

is genotypically Xg^aXg as judged by her offspring. Of course it would be fine if a marrow culture of I-2 showed that she was mainly XO and a fibroblast culture showed that these cells were Xg(a+), but we had not the heart to trouble further a person who had already been very helpful on several occasions.

A complete explanation of a fifth exceptional family was provided by Buckton et al.[49] (1971) and, for all we know, could have served for the four exceptional families in this section. The family was tested after Table 98 was closed, but it would not have been admitted in any case for sex-chromosome aneuploidy was involved. The propositus is, however, a phenotypically normal mother who was caught in a survey: her peripheral blood was found to be mosaic XO/XX, the two cells lines being in the approximate proportion of 1 to 2. The mother and her husband were phenotypically Xg(a−) but one son and one daughter were Xg(a+). It was assumed, because of her fertility, that her gonads were, at least in part, XX and, because of the exceptional Xg inheritance, that her genotype must be Xg^aXg but that her red cells were derived from a predominantly XO line carrying only Xg; the latter presumption was supported when the karyotype of her marrow showed about 90% of the cells to be XO—and we know we cannot usually detect the Xg^a antigen in an artificial mixture of 90% Xg(a−) and 10% Xg(a+) cells.

The existence of these Xg(a+) sons of Xg(a−) mothers could be attributed to Lyonization, provided the Xg locus when carried on a structurally normal X is subject to inactivation but this, as will be seen in the next section, it is not.

OTHER NOTES ABOUT Xg

Xg and the Lyon hypothesis

According to the theory of Lyon[11–14], one of the two X chromosomes in each somatic cell of the female is inactivated at a very early stage in embryonic development and it is a matter of chance which X, the paternal or the maternal, is inactivated in any one cell; but once an X is inactivated this same X, paternal or maternal, remains inactive in all the descendants of that cell.

The truth of the theory is now triumphantly established by means of clonal studies involving the X-borne enzymes glucose-6-phosphate dehydrogenase (G6PD), hypoxanthine guanine phosphoribosyl transferase (HGPRT), those causing Hunter's syndrome and Fabry's disease, and phosphoglycerate kinase (PGK). The first, G6PD, was by Davidson et al.[50] and it happened in 1963: the other references may be found in Gartler et al.[51]. More recently, inactivation (lyonization as it has come to be called) was further demonstrated in hypohidrotic ectodermal dysplasia[62]. But in 1962 at the time of the recognition of Xg there was doubt whether the inactivation applied to man and it was hoped that Xg would settle the question.

The following account of the course of events is largely cribbed from a report given by one of us[58] to the International Congress of Human Genetics in 1971.

A consequence of the theory was that in the average Xg^aXg female half the red cells should be Xg(a+) and half Xg(a−): but anti-Xg^a did not give a crisp answer, because many unagglutinated cells were always to be seen[2] in the reactions of hemizygous Xg(a+) males. As the truth of the theory became more and more firmly established, the contribution of Xg became limited to the question whether inactivation involves all the loci on the X. Each successive piece of evidence from Xg had, however, to be qualified because of the theoretical possibility that the antigen Xg^a, unlike nearly all other red cell antigens, might be merely adsorbed on the red cell surface.

If the antigen Xg^a were not made by the ancestors of the red cells but were made elsewhere and secondarily taken up by the red cells, then Xg could give no information about lyonization because random inactivation of Xs in an Xg^a heterozygote would presumably allow sufficient antigen to be made to supply all the red cells. There was never any evidence for such a theoretical Xg^a factory separated from the red cell line, but its non-existence took a long time to prove. The factory idea would be disproved if two populations of red cells, Xg(a+) and Xg(a−), could be found in one circulation—the two kinds of cells launched from one marrow. This we had sought, for some years, in twin chimeras and cases of dispermy but without success until 1968 (Klinger et al.[52]) and, even more convincingly, in 1971 (Ducos et al.[53]), when separable mixtures of Xg(a+) and Xg(a−) cells were found in one and the same circulation; and other examples were found later.

The evidence that Xg is in fact not involved in inactivation began to be collected in 1963 when Gorman, di Re, Treacy and Cahan[15] devised a technique which failed to show a mixture of Xg(a+) and Xg(a−) cells in known Xg^aXg females even though the technique easily detected artificial 50:50 mixtures of hemizygous Xg(a+) and Xg(a−) cells: this we were able to confirm.

Gorman and his colleagues made the further important observation:

'When the sparse number of free cells shaken off Xg(a+) hemizygote and heterozygote buttons [the deposit after centrifuging] were Xg^a typed again they were Xg(a+). Free cells shaken off buttons from artificial mosaics were Xg(a−) on retyping except on one occasion when they were weakly Xg(a+). This is further evidence that female heterozygotes do not have appreciable numbers of Xg(a−) cells as do artificial mosaics.'

Another approach involved the number of cells present in the embryo at the time of inactivation. Gandini and his collaborators[54] (1968), from a study of women known to be heterozygous at the locus for G6PD, estimated that at the time of inactivation the primordial cells destined to form the erythroid series number '8 or less'. If the Xg locus were subject to inactivation then there should be a slight excess of Xg(a−) females in adequately large random series when analysed by the gene frequencies derived from the males of that series, because some heterozygotes would be grouped as negative. In a sample of over 3,000 unrelated females tested in our Unit[32] there was, on the contrary, a slight shortage of Xg(a−). This was somewhat incompatible with inactivation at an 8-cell stage and completely incompatible with it happening at, for example, a 4-cell stage. So here was some further evidence against the inactivation of *Xg*.

Further evidence against the inactivation of *Xg* came, in 1970, from the Xg grouping of two series of women with chronic myeloid leukaemia carried out by Fialkow and his colleagues[55] in Seattle and Mexico City and by Lawler and Sanger[56] in London. It appears to be accepted that the marrow cells of these patients are clonal, being descended from a single stem cell as demonstrated by G6PD tests[57]. Assuming that this is correct then, if *Xg* were subject to inactivation, females with the disease should have the male distribution of the Xg groups because they would each have, in all their red cells, the product of one and the same functional *Xg* locus. But in both series the Xg distribution was female and differed significantly from that of the male. This we consider very powerful evidence against the inactivation of the *Xg* locus.

Another piece of evidence against the inactivation of *Xg* was gathered by Fialkow[59] from the literature about the Lesch-Nyhan X-borne disease. Hetero-zygous carriers can be detected by an intermediate amount of the enzyme HGPRT in their fibroblasts, but their red cells have the normal enzyme activity. It is thought that there is selective inactivation in the marrow of the X carrying the abnormal gene for the lack of the enzyme. Three *Xg* heterozygotes were found who by pedigree evidence had *Xg^a* only on the inactivated chromosome; never-theless they had Xg^a antigen on their red cells.

Further but more direct evidence is illustrated by a remarkable family investi-gated by Buckton and her colleagues[60] which almost certainly gives direct evidence that the allele *Xg^a* when carried on an inactive late-labelling X can nevertheless produce its antigen. A mother and daughter have a balanced trans-location t(Xp−; 14q+), the short arm of one X being translocated on to the long arm of a No. 14. In both these female members of the family who have the trans-location balanced it is the normal X which is late-labelling. The mother is Xg(a−); the father is Xg(a+) and his X is late-labelling in his daughter—yet it has made her Xg(a+).

There remains the evidence from Salt Lake City[16] which received a lot of attention in 1968. It seemed to show that the *Xg* locus was subject to inactivation. The evidence was based on the Xg groups of the separated parts of two morpho-logically distinct populations of cells in two sisters heterozygous for X-linked sideroachrestic anaemia. However, in 1970 Weatherall and his colleagues[61] test-ing a similar English family found no evidence for inactivation. Furthermore, thanks to the kindness of Dr Lee we were sent samples from members of the Salt Lake City family, but in our hands the original results could not be confirmed.

So, in company with the Seattle workers, we are convinced that the *Xg* locus escapes inactivation when carried on a normal X—the first and so far only demon-stration, at any rate in man, that inactivation does not involve the whole of the 'inactive' X. This absence of inactivation applies to erythropoietic tissue, that it almost certainly applies also to the *Xg* locus of fibroblasts will be seen from the section below on 'Xg^a outside the red cells'.

What happens when the *Xg* locus is on a structurally abnormal X will be discussed in the chapter on sex-chromosome aneuploidy.

Further examples of anti-Xg^a

The antigen Xg^a is obviously not a good stimulator of antibody because about 20% of transfusions are of the kind to give the recipient a chance to make the antibody. A year passed before a second example was found, this time in Inverness (Cook, Polley and Mollison[17], 1963). This antibody was a useful one. Three further examples were identified[18-20], one of them[19,36] being 'auto', and one[20] apparently of 'natural occurrence'. These three, however, were not strong enough to be of practical use. The sixth example[21], on the other hand, is a powerful one, as good as that of Mr And., the original maker: it was the triumphant result of the immunization of a volunteer at Hyland Laboratories, Los Angeles. The seventh example[31] was found at the New York Blood Center and is another good one: it was made by a much transfused man. The eighth, ninth and tenth examples, found in Dunedin N.Z., Zürich[33] and Amsterdam, were each capable of agglutinating Xg(a+) cells suspended in saline. We know of four more examples, found in St John, N.B., Miami, Boston and Cincinnati.

All save 2 of the 14 examples of anti-Xg^a were found in males, which is not surprising considering their higher proportion of Xg(a−). The first anti-Xg^a to be found in a woman was the auto example noted above[19,36]: she was pregnant and suffered from severe anaemia. The second was from a Japanese Xg(a−) woman in Boston[63].

It is perhaps worth recording that, as far as we know, only 3 of the 14 anti-Xg^a sera contain other antibodies (all three Rh). This is convenient and rather strikingly different from other recently discovered antibodies which tend to be accompanied by a number of long recognized immune antibodies.

All the useful examples of anti-Xg^a have shown, in our hands, the same nicety of palate for antiglobulin sera.

Development

The antigen is well developed at birth, though perhaps not fully so: we have had trouble in grouping an occasional cord sample. We have evidence that the Xg^a antigen of babies with the trisomies of Down, Edwards and Patau tends to be weaker than that of normal babies.

Toivanen and Hirvonen[44] tested 54 foetuses of ages ranging from 6 to 20 weeks and 36 gave the Xg(a−) reaction. Seven foetuses were 12 weeks old or less and of these 6 were negative and 1 very weakly positive: clearly the Xg^a antigen is not well developed until late in foetal life. The same authors[45] observe 'Forty-four full-term newborns were tested for Xg^a resulting in frequencies very close to those found in adults, but with clearly lower scores'.

Dosage

Hemizygotes react as strongly as homozygotes: heterozygotes may or may not give a distinctly weaker reaction. Between 5 and 10% of Xg(a+) females give notably weak reactions (though, fortunately, strong enough to avoid confusion with the negatives); these weak reactors, when their family groups are informative, are all seen to be heterozygotes. However, the weakness is not a practical test for heterozygosis for most heterozygotes give good strong positive reactions. The weakness is, in our experience, an inherited character, perhaps adumbrating a third allele similar to A_2. Males giving weaker reactions are very rare: XO females giving weaker reactions are less rare.

The antigen Xg^a outside the red cells

We could find no trace of the antigen in serum or saliva: it was looked for (Edwards, Ferguson and Coombs[22]), but not found, on spermatozoa.

Late in 1973 came from Oxford the very welcome news that Xg^a could be detected on cultured fibroblasts, even up to at least the twelfth passage (Fellous, Bengtsson, Finnegan and Bodmer[46], 1974) and also in man-man, man-mouse and man-hamster hybrid lines. The antigen could also be detected on some cultured lymphoid cell lines, though not on fresh peripheral blood lymphocytes. The antigen is detected in these cell cultures by a micro complement-fixation method developed by Colombani and his colleagues[47] for platelets.

The recognition of Xg^a on fibroblast cultures has already been used by the Oxford workers to show that the *Xg* locus of fibroblasts, like that of erythroblasts, is not subject to inactivation: eleven clones were isolated from the fibroblast culture of a donor known to be heterozygous *Xg^{a}Xg* and all these clones gave the reaction Xg(a+). This aspect of the work continues, as does an attempt to use cell fusion methods to fix the precise position of *Xg* on the X.

The antigen Xg^a in gibbons

Xg^a, or an antigen indistinguishable from it, is found in gibbons, *Hylobates lar lar* (Gavin et al.[23]). Furthermore the antigen appears, from its different distribution in the two sexes ($\chi^2 = 4.2$ for 1 d.f., P = 0.04) to be inherited as an X-linked dominant character as it is in man. So far we have tested 42:

	Xg(a+)	Xg(a−)
males	7 (8·2)	21 (19·8)
females	8 (7·0)	6 (7·0)

the figures in brackets represent the expected distribution using Haldane's formula given on page 579.

Samples from 5 *Hylobates pileatus* all lacked the antigen as did samples from 67 chimpanzees, 2 gorillas, 20 orangutans, 60 baboons, 31 Celebes black apes and various monkeys, mice and dogs and, also[37], one coelacanth.

20

That Xg is X-linked[4] in the gibbon is the less surprising considering that haemophilia is X-linked in the dog and the horse, Christmas disease in the dog, G6PD in the horse, the donkey, the hare and drosophila, and anhidrotic ecto-dermal dysplasia in cattle. There must be some powerful evolutionary reason why the loci for these characters are X-borne and Dr S. Ohno has put forward[30] the startling and very satisfying theory that the X chromosome has kept more or less the same complement of loci throughout the whole of mammalian history.

Anthropological differences

The supply of anti-Xg[a] has seldom allowed samples to be tested purely to establish the frequencies in different people, but this is gradually being overcome. Most of the substantial figures in Table 99 were gathered from the results of tests primarily connected with X-mapping investigations.

Table 99. Xg gene frequencies in different people

	Total (unrelated) tested	Gene frequency Xg^a	Xg
Of N. European extraction, see test		0·66	0·34
Sardinians[24]	322	0·76	0·24
Israelis[25], non-Ashkenazi	201	0·68	0·32
Indians, Bombay[26]	100	0·65	0·35
Chinese, Singapore[27]	64	0·46	0·54
Chinese, Mainland[10]	171	0·60	0·40
Chinese, Taiwan[10]	178	0·53	0·47
Chinese, Hakka[10]	136	0·53	0·47
Taiwan aborigines[10]	164	0·38	0·62
Mariana Islands, Chamorros[28]	109	0·65	0·35
Negroes, New York and Jamaica[29]	219	0·55	0·45
Navajo Indians[10]	308	0·77	0·23
Australian Aborigines[38]	352	0·79	0·21
New Guineans[38]	263	0·85	0·15
Greeks[39]	638	0·55	0·45
Thais[40]	181	0·57	0·43
Japanese[41]	98	0·64	0·36
Spaniards in Barcelona[42]	636	0·59	0·41
Singapore Chinese[43]	101	0·45	0·55
Singapore Malays[43]	72	0·54	0·46
Singapore Indians[43]	91	0·57	0·43

It can be seen that of the people tested the Chinese have the lowest frequency of Xg^a and the New Guineans the highest. If the gibbons were admitted, as honorary members, to Table 99 they would be outstanding: Xg^a 0·29, Xg 0·71, but these figures must be very approximate, for only 42 gibbons were tested.

Serologically the Xg system was just one more addition to the lengthening list of blood group markers; but, simply because it happened to be X-linked, it cascaded a Niagara of a correspondence, largely over the subjects of the next two chapters.

REFERENCES

1   MANN J.D., CAHAN A., GELB A.G., FISHER NATHALIE, HAMPER JEAN, TIPPETT PATRICIA, SANGER RUTH and RACE R.R. (1962) A sex-linked blood group. *Lancet*, i, 8–10.
2   SANGER RUTH, RACE R.R., TIPPETT PATRICIA, HAMPER JEAN, GAVIN JUNE and CLEGHORN T.E. (1962) The X-linked blood group system Xg: more tests on unrelated people and on families. *Vox Sang.*, 7, 571–578.
3   GAVIN JUNE, TIPPETT PATRICIA, SANGER RUTH and RACE R.R. (1964) The X-linked blood group system Xg: II. Still more tests on unrelated people and on families. *Vox Sang.*, 9, 146–152.
4   NOADES JEAN, GAVIN JUNE, TIPPETT PATRICIA, SANGER RUTH and RACE R.R. (1966) The X-linked blood group system Xg. Tests on British, Northern American and Northern European unrelated people and families. *J. med. Genet.*, 3, 162–168.
5   CHOWN B., LEWIS MARION and KAITA HIROKO (1964) The Xg blood group system: data on 294 white families, mainly Canadian. *Can. J. Genet. Cytol.*, 6, 431–434.
6   HALDANE J.B.S. (1963) Tests for sex-linked inheritance on population samples. *Ann. hum. Genet.*, 27, 107–111.
7   SANGER RUTH (1965) Genes on the X chromosome. *Can. J. Genet., Cytol.*, 7, 179–188.
8   SANGER RUTH, RACE R.R., TIPPETT PATRICIA, GAVIN JUNE, HARDISTY R.M. and DUBOWITZ V. (1964) Unexplained inheritance of the Xg groups in two families. *Lancet*, i, 955–956.
9   FERGUSON-SMITH M.A. (1966) X-Y chromosomal interchange in the aetiology of true hermaphroditism and of XX Klinefelter's syndrome. *Lancet*, ii, 475–476.
10   DEWEY W.J. and MANN J.D. (1967) Xg blood group frequencies in some further populations. *J. med. Genet.*, 4, 12–15.
11   LYON MARY F. (1961) Gene action in the X-chromosome of the mouse (*Mus musculus* L.) *Nature, Lond.*, 190, 372–373.
12   LYON MARY F. (1961) Genetic factors on the X chromosome. *Lancet*, ii, 434.
13   LYON MARY F. (1962) Sex chromatin and gene action in the mammalian X-chromosome. *Amer. J. hum. Genet.*, 14, 135–148.
14   LYON MARY F. (1972) *X*-chromosome inactivation and developmental patterns in mammals. *Biol. Rev.*, 47, 1–35.
15   GORMAN J.G., DI RE J., TREACY A.M., and CAHAN A. (1963) The application of −Xg^a antiserum to the question of red cell mosaicism in female heterozygotes. *J. Lab. clin. Med.*, 61, 642–649.
16   LEE G.R., MACDIARMID W.D., CARTWRIGHT G.E. and WINTROBE M.M. (1968). Hereditary, X-linked, sideroachrestic anemia. The isolation of two erythrocyte populations differing in Xg^a blood type and porphyrin content. *Blood*, 32, 59–70.
17   COOK I.A., POLLEY MARGARET J. and MOLLISON P.L. (1963) A second example of anti-Xg^a. *Lancet*, i, 857–859.
18   SAUSAIS LAIMA, KREVANS J.R. and TOWNES A.S. (1964) Characteristics of a third example of anti-Xg^a. *Transfusion, Philad.*, 4, 312. (Abstract.)
19   YOKOYAMA M., EITH D.T. and BOWMAN M. (1967) The first example of auto-anti-Xg^a. *Vox Sang.*, 12, 138–139.
20   FISHER NATHALIE (1965) Unpublished observations.
21   SHEPHERD L.P., FEINGOLD ELAINE and SHANBROM E. (1969) An unusual occurrence of anti-Xg^a. *Vox Sang.*, 16, 157–160.

[22] EDWARDS R.G., FERGUSON L.C. and COOMBS R.R.A. (1964) Blood group antigens on human spermatozoa. *J. Reprod. Fert.*, **7**, 153–161.

[23] GAVIN JUNE, NOADES JEAN, TIPPETT PATRICIA, SANGER RUTH and RACE R.R. (1964) Blood group antigen Xgᵃ in gibbons. *Nature, Lond.*, **204**, 1322–1323.

[24] SINISCALCO M., FILIPPI G., LATTE B., PIOMELLI S., RATTAZZI M., GAVIN JUNE, SANGER RUTH and RACE R.R. (1966) Failure to detect linkage between Xg and other X-borne loci in Sardinians. *Ann. hum. Genet.*, **29**, 231–252.

[25] ADAM A., TIPPETT PATRICIA, GAVIN JUNE, NOADES JEAN, SANGER RUTH and RACE R.R. (1967) The linkage relation of Xg to g-6-pd in Israelis: the evidence of a second series of families. *Ann. hum. Genet.*, **30**, 211–218.

[26] BHATIA H.M. (1963) Frequency of sex-linked blood group Xgᵃ in Indians in Bombay. Preliminary study. *Indian J. med. Sci.*, **17**, 491–492.

[27] WONG HOCK BOON, NOADES JEAN, GAVIN JUNE and RACE R.R. (1964) Xg blood groups of Chinese. *Nature, Lond.*, **204**, 1002.

[28] PLATO C.C., CRUZ M.T. and KURLAND L.T. (1964) Frequency of glucose-6-phosphate dehydrogenase deficiency, red-green colour blindness and Xgᵃ blood-group among Chamorros. *Nature, Lond.*, **202**, 728.

[29] GAVIN JUNE, TIPPETT PATRICIA, SANGER RUTH and RACE R.R. (1963) The Xg blood groups of Negroes. *Nature, Lond.*, **200**, 82–83. (In the 6th line of this paper there is a confused heading: it should be 'male' for the first 2 columns of figures and 'female' for the second two.)

[30] OHNO S. (1967) *Sex Chromosomes and Sex-linked Genes.* pp. 192. Springer, Berlin, Heidelberg, New York.

[31] ALLEN F.H. (1967) Personal communication.

[32] SANGER RUTH, TIPPETT PATRICIA and GAVIN JUNE (1971) The X-linked blood group system Xg: tests on unrelated people and families of Northern European ancestry. *J. Med. Genet.*, **8**, 427–433.

[33] METAXAS M.N. and METAXAS-BÜHLER M. (1970) An agglutinating example of anti-Xgᵃ and Xgᵃ frequencies in 558 Swiss blood donors. *Vox Sang.*, **19**, 527–529.

[34] MAYR W.R. (1969) Das Blutfaktorensystem Xg. *Schweiz. med. Wschr.*, **99**, 1837–1844.

[35] HERBICH J., MEINHART K. and SZILVASSY J. (1972) Verteilung 18 verschiedener Blutmerkmalsysteme bei 2440 Personen aus Wien und Umgebung. *Ärztl. Lab.*, **18**, 341–348.

[36] YOKOYAMA M. and McCOY J.E. (1967) Further studies on auto-anti-Xgᵃ antibody. *Vox Sang.*, **13**, 15–17.

[37] TIPPETT PATRICIA and TEESDALE PHYLLIS (1973) Limited blood group tests on samples from two coelacanths (*Latimeria chalumnae*). *Vox Sang.*, **24**, 175–178.

[38] SIMMONS R.T. (1970) X-linked blood groups, Xg, in Australian Aborigines and New Guineans. *Nature, Lond.*, **227**, 1363.

[39] FRASER G.R., STEINBERG A.G., DEFARANAS B., MAYO O., STAMATOYANNOPOULOS G. and MOTULSKY A.G. (1969) Gene frequencies at loci determining blood-group and serum-protein polymorphisms in two villages in Northwestern Greece. *Amer. J. hum. Genet.*, **21**, 46–60.

[40] RATANAUBOL K. and RATANASIRIVANICH P. (1971) Xg blood groups of Thais. *Nature, Lond.*, **229**, 430.

[41] NAKAJIMA H. (1971) The Rh, MNSs, Duffy and Xg blood group frequencies in Japanese—further tests on unrelated people. *J. anthrop. Soc. Japan*, **79**, 178–181.

[42] VALLS A. (1973) Los grupos sanguineos del sistema Xg en espanoles. *Trab. Inst. Bernardino Sahagun Antrop. Etnol.*, **16**, 261–268.

[43] SAHA N. and BANERJEE B. (1973) Xgᵃ blood group in Chinese, Malays and Indians in Singapore. *Vox Sang.*, **24**, 542–544.

[44] TOIVANEN P. and HIRVONEN T. (1973) Antigens Duffy, Kell, Kidd, Lutheran and Xgᵃ on fetal red cells. *Vox Sang.*, **24**, 372–376.

[45] TOIVANEN P. and HIRVONEN T. (1969) Fetal development of red cell antigens K, k, Lu^a, Lu^b, Fy^a, Fy^b, Vel and Xg^a *Scand. J. Haemat.*, **6**, 49–55.

[46] FELLOUS M., BENGTSSON B., FINNEGAN D. and BODMER W.F. (1974) Expression of the Xg^a antigen on cells in culture and its segregation in somatic cell hybrids. *Ann. hum. Genet.*, **37**, 421–430.

[47] COLOMBANI J., D'AMARO J., GABB B., SMITH G. and SVEJGAARD A. (1971) International agreement on a microtechnique of platelet complement fixation. *Transplantation Proceed.*, **3**, 121. (Not seen.)

[48] SANGER RUTH, RACE R.R., TIPPETT PATRICIA, GAVIN JUNE, CLEGHORN T.E. and ROGERS K.L. Quoted by RACE R.R. and SANGER RUTH (1968) *Blood Groups in Man*, 5th ed., p. 576. Blackwell Scientific Publications, Oxford.

[49] BUCKTON KARIN E., CUNNINGHAM CATHERINE, NEWTON MARJORIE S., O'RIORDAN MAUREEN L. and SANGER RUTH (1971) Anomalous Xg inheritance with a probable explanation. *Lancet*, **i**, 371–373.

[50] DAVIDSON R.G., NITOWSKY H.M. and CHILDS B. (1963) Demonstration of two populations of cells in the human female heterozygous for glucose-6-phosphate dehydrogenase variants. *Proc. Nat. Acad. Sci.*, **50**, 481–485.

[51] GARTLER S.M., CHEN S.-H., FIALKOW P.J., GIBLETT ELOISE R. and SINGH S. (1972) *X* chromosome inactivation in cells from an individual heterozygous for two *X*-linked genes. *Nature New Biol.*, **236**, 149–150.

[52] KLINGER R., MIGGIANO V.C., TIPPETT P. and GAVIN J. (1968) Diabete mellito e nanismo ipofisario in chimera XX, XY. *Atti Accad. med. lomb.*, **23**, 1392–1396.

[53] DUCOS J., MARTY YVONNE, SANGER RUTH and RACE R.R. (1971) Xg and X chromosome inactivation. *Lancet*, **ii**, 219–220.

[54] GANDINI E., GARTLER S.M., ANGIONI G., ARGIOLAS N. and DELL'ACQUA G. (1968) Developmental implications of multiple tissue studies in glucose-6-phosphate dehydrogenase deficient heterozygotes. *Proc. Nat. Acad. Sci.*, **61**, 945–948.

[55] FIALKOW P.J., LISKER R., GIBLETT ELOISE R. and ZAVALA C. (1970) *Xg* locus: failure to detect inactivation in females with chronic myelocytic leukaemia. *Nature, Lond.*, **226**, 367–368.

[56] LAWLER SYLVIA D. and SANGER RUTH (1970) Xg blood-groups and clonal-origin theory of chronic myeloid leukaemia. *Lancet*, **i**, 584–585.

[57] FIALKOW P.J., GARTLER S.M. and YOSHIDA A. (1967) Clonal origin of chronic myelocytic leukemia in man. *Proc. Nat. Acad. Sci.*, **58**, 1468–1471.

[58] RACE R.R. (1971) Is the Xg blood group locus subject to inactivation? *Proc. 4th Int. Congr. Hum. Genet.*, Paris, 311–314.

[59] FIALKOW P.J. (1970) X-chromosome inactivation and the Xg locus. *Amer. J. hum. Genet.*, **22**, 460–463.

[60] BUCKTON KARIN E., JACOBS PATRICIA A., RAE LINDA A., NEWTON MARJORIE S. and SANGER RUTH (1971) An inherited *X*-autosome translocation in man. *Ann. hum. Genet.*, **35**, 171–178.

[61] WEATHERALL D.J., PEMBREY M.E., HALL E.G., SANGER RUTH, TIPPETT PATRICIA and GAVIN JUNE (1970) Familial sideroblastic anaemia: problem of Xg and X chromosome inactivation. *Lancet*, **ii**, 744–748.

[62] PASSARGE E. and FRIES ELISABETH (1973) X chromosome inactivation in X-linked hypohidrotic ectodermal dysplasia. *Nature New Biol.*, **245**, 58–59.

[63] KONUGRES ANGELYN A. (1974) Personal communication.

Chapter 29
Xg and X-Chromosome Mapping

Although it is such a struggle to assign loci with certainty to a particular autosome, X-borne loci declare themselves by the characteristic inheritance of their alleles. McKusick[1, 2] in his invaluable compilations 'Mendelian Inheritance in Man' lists more than 150. However, the great majority of these X-linked characters are no use as 'markers' of the X, because the abnormal alleles by which they are recognized are so rare; nevertheless, they provide fine fixed points on the chromosome ready to be themselves plotted.

The markers

Until 1958 the only useful marker was red-green colour blindness, useful because it has a frequency as high as 6% in males. It seems that the two kinds, deutan and protan, do not occupy the same locus, so colour blindness probably involves two loci but so close together that in practice they mark the same point.

Then came the beautiful recognition[3] that glucose-6-phosphate dehydrogenase (G6PD) deficiency is an X-linked condition. This is not a useful marker in northern Europeans for the deficiency is almost unknown amongst them, but in some populations the deficiency is common enough to be really useful—for example in Negroes, oriental Jews and in Greek and Mediterranean people.

Next, in 1962, came the Xg blood groups[4] and this seemed almost the perfect marker system; the two divisions are well distributed in all people so far tested, and in northern Europeans about 45% of females are heterozygotes (the optimal percentage for linkage purposes is 50).

In 1964, Heistö, Harboe and Godal[72] reported an investigation in which the freshly taken serum of about 12% of male donors and about 23% of female donors was found to haemolyse trypsin treated red cells irrespective of the ABO or Rh groups. The male and female frequencies and tests on families virtually established the character as X-linked. But this promising marker got away: intense activity in Oslo[89, 90] failed to find again a trypsin preparation capable of making the red cells respond to an X-borne lytic property of serum. However, the phenomenon should be kept in mind; it may be recaptured some day.

Another very hopeful marker, alas, escaped also: the Xm serum groups (Berg and Bearn[5, 91], 1966, 1968) was obviously going to be very useful, for about 39%

594

of white females were heterozygous. However the rabbit who made the anti-Xm serum died and no subsequent rabbit succeeded in making it. The original supply of serum sufficed to exclude close linkage between *Xm* and *Xg* and to establish linkage between *Xm* and *deutan* before it ran out.

The length of the X

The recognition that the rate of crossing-over in the female is nearly twice that in the male[6, 7] makes the task of establishing linkages between X-borne characters nearly twice as difficult as we had thought it would be: it is only as a result of crossing-over, or not crossing-over, in the female that linkage between two X-borne loci can be detected.

Renwick and Schulze[8] estimate that the length of the X is, in terms of cross-over units, 200 centimorgans, and Edwards[91] increased this to 250 centimorgans. Since in our opinion the limit of measurable X-linkage, from human data likely to be collected, is about 30 centimorgans, it is perhaps not surprising that so few linkages have been demonstrated though so many have been looked for.

Lack of recombination between two loci known to be within measurable linkage distance of each other may mean that no crossing-over has taken place between the two loci or it may mean that crossing-over has happened twice. For purposes of chromosome mapping, formulae are available for converting an observed recombination frequency into a cross-over frequency (Haldane[69], 1919; Kosambi[70], 1944; Carter and Falconer[71], 1951). The cross-over frequency between two loci provides the map distance between them: a cross-over frequency of $0·01 = 1$ centimorgan (1 cM).

Though this distinction between recombination frequency and cross-over frequency is intellectually important it does not, in the present rather rough state of human data, really affect us. This is because the amount of human data that can be collected is limited by time and by expense, and it seems that a recombination frequency of say $0·30$ is the upper limit to the recognition of a linkage on the X. If, then, we can recognize only fairly close linkages a double cross-over is unlikely to happen between the loci involved, and the correction makes little difference: here, for example, are the cross-over frequencies, derived from the three available formulae, for the sort of recombination frequencies we are dealing with:

Recombination frequency	Haldane[69]	Kosambi[70]	Carter and Falconer[71]
0·10	0·11	0·10	0·10
0·20	0·26	0·21	0·20
0·30	0·46	0·34	0·31

So, in the mapping attempts later in the chapter, we are going to use estimates of the recombination rate as if they were the equivalent of the crossing-over rate and consider a recombination rate of, say, $0·20$ as 20 centimorgans.

KNOWN LINKAGES NOT INVOLVING Xg

Colour blindness and haemophilia

This was the first linkage to be found in man: discovered in 1937 by Julia Bell and Haldane[11]. Ten years later Haldane and Smith[12] reviewed the published pedigrees and reestimated the recombination fraction between *deutan* and *haemophilia*. These early recombination estimates are now of mathematical and historical interest only, because the Oxford distinction between haemophilia and Christmas disease had yet to be made. The colour blind loci are now known to be very close to that for haemophilia and far removed from that for Christmas disease[13]; and at least one of the kindred published by Hoogfliet and used by Haldane and Smith in their calculations is now, on revisitation, known to have Christmas disease and not haemophilia (Dr L.N. Went, personal communication).

It was by showing that colour blindness was not linked to Christmas disease that Whittaker, Copeland and Graham[13] demonstrated, in 1962, that haemophilia (factor VIII deficiency) and Christmas disease (factor IX deficiency) were not the expression of alleles, a possibility previously much in mind. This independence of the loci was confirmed when Robertson and Trueman[14] found a family with both haemophilia and Christmas disease and in it a male deficient for both factors.

Colour blindness and G6PD

The locus for G6PD is close to that for deutan and for protan. The linkage with unspecified colour blindness was discovered independently by Adam[15] (1961) in Israel and by Siniscalco and his collaborators[16] (1960) in Sardinia. The probable distance between the loci for deutan and for G6PD was estimated to be 0·05 recombination units, and that between protan and G6PD perhaps somewhat less (Porter, Schulze and McKusick[17, 18], 1962).

Siniscalco, Filippi and Latte[19] (1964) summarized massive Sardinian data which showed the recombination frequency between *G6PD* and *deutan* to be less than 0·04, 'with very narrow confidence intervals' and that between *G6PD* and *protan* to be 0·05 'but with much broader confidence intervals'.

The same authors[19, 28] give details of a Sardinian family showing recombination between *deutan* and *protan*, this together with the family reported by Vanderdonck and Verriest[20] provide all the direct evidence we know of that *deutan* and *protan* occupy separate loci. Indirect support comes from the slightly different recombination frequency of *deutan* and *protan* with *G6PD*, mentioned above.

Colour blindness and Xm

This is the only Xm linkage which could be established before the supply of anti-Xm serum ran out. The recombination fraction between *deutan* and *Xm* is 0·07 with 90% probability limits of 0·04 and 0·27 respectively and the odds on linkage were 186 to 1 (Berg and Bearn[91], 1968).

G6PD and haemophilia (VIII)

Since the locus for G6PD is close to that for deutan which in turn is close to that for haemophilia it was not surprising to hear from Professor Siniscalco (1967, personal communication) that *G6PD* and *haemophilia* are indeed close together: no recombination was observed on 30 occasions when it could have been detected. This was in a survey in Greece.

Electrophoretic variants, A and B, of G6PD are known. The locus responsible (often referred to as the *G6PD* structural locus) is X-borne and has been assumed to be part of, or close to, the locus for G6PD deficiency, and this is borne out by the following sequence. 1. Boyer and Graham[23] studied the variants A and B in three families in which haemophilia was segregating. The families were very informative and point to the *AB* 'structural' locus being very close to the *haemophilia* locus; indeed there was no recombination on the 17 occasions when it could have shown. 2. *Haemophilia* is known to be close to *deutan*. 3. *Deutan* is close to the *G6PD* deficiency locus. 4. Therefore the *G6PD* structural and deficiency genes occupy the same locus or loci close to each other.

A possible: deutan and Becker's muscular dystrophy

In 1969 Emery, Smith and Sanger[92] found a hint of linkage between *deutan* and *Becker* with a most likely recombination fraction of 0·28 but with wide probability limits. The evidence has been somewhat strengthened in the finding by Dr Mayana Zatz[126], of São Paulo, of a slight hint of linkage between *Becker* and *G6PD*. Combining the deutan and G6PD scores results in a most likely recombination fraction of 0·27, but the height of the curve reaches only 13·5.

A condition 'X-linked scapuloperoneal syndrome', was described by Thomas, Calne and Elliott[109] and its likeness to Becker's muscular dystrophy discussed. Interestingly, this family scores well for linkage with *deutan* (3 n-r; z_1 2:0, e_1 2:0) and if it were added to the Becker's calculation would raise the height of the curve to 61 with a most likely recombination fraction of 0·24. (And see Addenda.)

Duchenne's muscular dystrophy, on the other hand, does not appear to be in measurable distance of *colour vision* or *G6PD* as judged by tests on English[92] or Brazilian[126] families.

Another possible: colour blindness and choroideremia

Drs E. Dreisler and Mette Warburg tell us of a hopeful suggestion of linkage between choroideremia and colour vision. The height of the curve is around 28 at $\theta = 0·06$: 27 children scored and there were 3 non-recombinants to 1 recombinant.

20*

SEARCH FOR LINKAGE WITH Xg

In several of the earlier papers on X-linkage the hope was expressed that, once an X-linked marker of useful frequency was found, measured linkages would follow thick and fast. We shared this hope when Xg turned up, but, over the last twelve years our collaborators, who have collected many thousands of family blood samples, and our Unit who had the relatively easy job of grouping them, have learnt how surprisingly hard it is to establish linkage between loci even when they are known to be carried on the same chromosome. The difficulty, we can now see, is largely due to the X being much longer in terms of recombination units than it was thought to be, to the greater recombination rate in the female and to the fact, slowly emerging, that the extent of data likely to be available from human families does not allow the detection of linkage if the recombination fraction is more than, say 0·30. The methods of measurement were those of C.A.B. Smith and Morton as instructed by Maynard-Smith, Penrose and C.A.B. Smith (see Chapter 27). For the mathematical expert the analysis of X-linkage in particular is dealt with by J.H. Edwards[118]—but this, he or she will know already and not need to be told by us innumerates.

An example of one set of data, that for ocular albinism, is given in Table 100.

In Table 101 is summarized all the Xg linkage data we know of, arranged from certain positives through uncertainties to certain negatives, and some comments on this large table now follow.

Linkage with *Xg* established

X-borne ichthyosis

A series of families around Oxford (Kerr, Wells and Sanger[24], 1964) gave the first indication of measurable linkage between *Xg* and the X-borne form of ichthyosis. This stimulated investigations in Israel (Adam, Ziprkowski, Feinstein, Sanger, Tippett, Gavin and Race[25, 27]) in London (Wells, Jennings, Sanger and Race[26]), in the Netherlands (Went, de Groot, Sanger, Tippett and Gavin[22]) and in Sardinia (Filippi and Meera Khan[78]) and each succeeding investigation supported the linkage (Table 101).

The reports on 55 Israeli families[27] and on the very large Dutch kindred[22] each give detailed pedigrees and afford a fine exercise, were it wanted, in applying lod scores. Both series provide overwhelming evidence in favour of linkage: for the Israelis the odds in favour of linkage are 270 thousand million to 1 and for the Dutch 5,422 to 1. There is good agreement about the most likely recombination fraction (θ):

Israelis: $\theta = 0·105$, 90% probability limits 0·06 and 0·16
Dutch: $\theta = 0·115$, 90% probability limits 0·06 and 0·24

Table 100. Ocular albinism and Xg: the proving of a linkage

| | No. of mothers | Scoring children | Phase-known | | Recombination fraction, θ | | | | | | | | |
			n-r	r	0·05	0·1	0·15	0·2	0·25	0·3	0·35	0·4	0·45
Fialkow et al.[29]	11	25	6	1	1·159	2·280	2·622	2·627	2·436	2·110	1·686	1·186	0·623
Pearce et al.[79]	2	9	0	0	0·578	0·703	0·693	0·619	0·512	0·382	0·247	0·123	0·033
Hoefnagel et al.[81]	1	4	3	1	−0·163	0·066	0·168	0·214	0·227	0·216	0·187	0·140	0·078
Pearce et al.[80]	2	7	4	0	1·601	1·447	1·284	1·112	0·932	0·744	0·554	0·363	0·176
Sum of lods					3·175	4·496	4·767	4·572	4·107	3·452	2·674	1·812	0·910
Antilog = relative probability					1,496	31,330	58,480	37,330	12,790	2,831	472	65	8

The higher recombination fraction found in the original Oxford series[24] was evidently due to chance of sampling and can be attributed to one family in which there were three phase-known recombinants and no non-recombinants: the chance of finding such a family must be about one in a thousand.

Ocular albinism

The second reward for a great deal of work came when Fialkow, Giblett and Motulsky[29] (1967) grouped one large and two smaller kindred in which ocular albinism was segregating and found significant evidence of linkage. Subsequent kindred supported the linkage: one English (Pearce *et al.*[69]), one American (Hoefnagel *et al.*[81]) and one Newfoundlander (Pearce *et al.*[80]). The lod scores for the four investigations are set out in Table 100. The height of the antilog curve is nearly 60,000 and corresponds (page 560) to odds in favour of linkage of 16,000 to 1. The estimate of the recombination fraction is $0 \cdot 153$ and the 90% probability limits are $0 \cdot 09$ and $0 \cdot 25$.

The Newfoundland kindred[80] makes a substantial contribution to the linkage information (4 non-recombinants and z_1 3:0) 'but had the Xg groups segregated more informatively the family might have pin-pointed the recombination fraction much more precisely, for no less than 29 living males were found on examination to have ocular albinism and 41 females were ophthalmologically detectable carriers'.

Retinoschisis

This rare eye condition is probably more frequent in Finland than elsewhere: it has been studied by Eriksson, Forsius and their colleagues for more than 10 years. Lod scores pointing to linkage with *Xg* have slowly mounted, see Table 101. The first indication of linkage was reported in 1967 (Eriksson *et al.* [52]): the most likely recombination fraction was $0 \cdot 28$.

Ives and her colleagues[82] found a lower recombination fraction (13 n-r: 3 r) counterbalanced by Dr Went's finding (3 n-r: 4 r). Adding these two series to the vast data of Eriksson gives a recombination fraction of $0 \cdot 27$ and the height of the curve is 1,150 and the odds on linkage 338 to 1.

Linkage with *Xg* probable

Fabry's disease

This is also known as α-galactosidase deficiency and sometimes as angiokeratoma, though the latter trouble is we understand not always present. Six families with this rare condition were Xg grouped and four of them gave linkage information (Opitz *et al.*[49], 1965). The analysis suggested that linkage might prove measurable: the estimate of the recombination fraction was $0 \cdot 27$ but the 90% probability limits were wide ($0 \cdot 16$ and $0 \cdot 44$) and the height of the curve only 8.

Table 101. A synopsis of the search for linkage between Xg and other X-borne characters. (Reference numbers show that the work has been published: lack of a number means that the work has not yet been published. Most of the Xg testing was done at the MRC Blood Group Unit. On a few occasions we have been bold to recalculate the lod scores.)

Loci for	References	Number of scoring children	Non-rec	Rec	Lods at $\theta =$ 0·10	0·30
LINKAGE ESTABLISHED (sum of lods >2 at some value of θ)						
ichthyosis	Kerr et al.[24]	35	9	4	0·069	0·889
	Wells et al.[26]	17	3	0	1·157	0·728
	Adam et al.[27]	115	34	2	12·024	7·060
	Went et al.[22]	34	18	1	4·240	2·838
	Filippi et al.[78]	8	1	1	0·410	0·244
					17·900	11·759
ocular albinism	Fialkow et al.[29]	25	6	1	2·280	2·110
	Pearce et al.[79]	9	0	0	0·703	0·382
	Hoefnagel et al.[81]	4	3	1	0·066	0·216
	Pearce et al.[80]	7	4	0	1·447	0·744
					4·496	3·452
retinoschisis	Eriksson et al.[52]	100	12	5	−1·978	1·775
	Ives et al.[82]	16	13	3	1·218	1·232
	Dr L.N. Went	17	3	4	−1·368	−0·046
	Dr A.C. Bird	3	0	0	−0·305	−0·045
					−2·433	2·916
LINKAGE PROBABLE (sum of lods >1 at some value of θ)						
Fabry's disease	Opitz et al.[49]	35	6	1	−0·699	0·866
	Johnston et al.[85, 86]	6	1	0	0·828	0·503
	Malmqvist et al.[87]	4	0	0	0·865	0·328
	Dr W.B. Bean	6	1	0	−0·632	−0·005
					0·362	1·692
a mental retardation ±hydrocephalus	Fried et al.[88]	10	9	1	1·596	1·092
LINKAGE POSSIBLE (sum of lods positive, but low, at $\theta = 0·3$)						
hypogamma-globulinaemia	Sanger et al.[53]	12	2	3	−1·913	−0·383
	Rosen et al.[54]	8	1	0	0·002	0·202
	Adam et al.[96]	3	2	1	−0·189	0·070
	Dr J.K. Rees	9	0	0	1·196	0·377
					−0·904	0·266

Table 101—*continued*

Loci for	References	Number of scoring children	Non-rec	Rec	Lods at $\theta=$ 0·10	Lods at $\theta=$ 0·30
Lesch-Nyhan syndrome	Shapiro et al.[67, 128]	10	8	2	0·642	0·724
	Newcombe et al.[128]	2	0	0	0·131	0·041
	Nyhan et al.[75]	5	0	1	−0·928	−0·233
	Greene et al.[99]	16	0	0	−0·597	−0·006
	de Bruyn et al.[127]	3	0	0	−0·482	−0·086
					−1·234	0·440
Åland eye disease	Forsius et al.[64]	12	0	0	0·089	0·227
nuclear cataract	Fraccaro et al.[51]	12 either	3	1	0·487	0·718
		or	2	2	−0·101	−0·350
hypophosphatemia	Graham et al.[65]	5	0	0	−0·014	0·043
oligodontia	Erpenstein et al.[74]	8	0	0	−0·295	0·046
deaf-mutism,	Richards[62]	7	0	0	0·030	0·102
congenital deafness	Prof. Fraccaro	3	1	0	−0·085	0·094
	McRae et al.[103]	11	0	0	0·429	0·369
					0·374	0·565
thrombocytopenia	Ata et al.[66]	11	2	3	−1·311	−0·152
	Dr J.M. Opitz	6	0	0	0·276	0·222
					−1·035	0·070
Xm serum groups	Berg et al.[91]	27	6	3	−1·362	0·270
	Prof R. Ceppellini	3	0	0	−0·444	−0·076
					−1·806	0·194
testicular feminization	Sanger et al.[105]	43	1	0	−2·320	0·036
spondyloepiphyseal dysplasia tarda	Bannerman et al.[106]		1	1	−1·146	0·043
mental retardation	Neuhäuser et al.[108]	8	4	0	0·791	0·573
	Prof R.A. Pfeiffer	12	0	0	−1·179	−0·159
	Dr K.D. Zang	3	0	0	−0·482	−0·086
	Dr K. Fried	4	0	0	0·708	0·297
					−0·162	0·625

LINKAGE INFORMATION SLIGHT

Loci for	References	Number of scoring children	Non-rec	Rec	Lods at $\theta=$ 0·10	Lods at $\theta=$ 0·30
keratosis follicularis	Prof S. Borelli	7	2	3	−1·927	−0·426
oral and digital malformation	Dr J. A. Dodge	6	1	3	−2·370	−0·619
dystrophy of the nose	Prof J.H. Edwards	2	0	0	−0·340	−0·052
cerebral sclerosis +Addison's anaemia	Spira et al.[107]	1	0	1	−0·699	−0·222

Table 101—*continued*

Loci for	References	Number of scoring children	Non-rec	Rec	Lods at $\theta =$ 0·10	Lods at $\theta =$ 0·30
pyridoxine responsive anaemia	Elves et al.[60]	3	0	0	−0·482	−0·086
sideroblastic anaemia	Dr R.H. Lindenbaum	3	0	0	−0·482	−0·086
spastic paraplegia	Johnston et al.[61]	2	1	1	−0·444	−0·076
	Dr M. Zatz	2	0	0	−0·340	−0·052
					−0·784	−0·128
chronic granulomatous	Dr P.S. Macfarlane	1	1	0	0·255	0·146
disease (X-linkage in	Prof. J.F. Soothill	1	1	0	0·255	0·146
question)					0·510	0·292
congenital stationary night blindness	Dr L.N. Went	10	3	4	−1·604	−0·290
achromatopsia	Dr J.M. Opitz, Spivey[130]	5	2	3	−1·587	−0·374
choroido-retinal dystrophy	Hoare[57]	6	0	0	−1·239	−0·204
macular dystrophy	Dr A. Adam	4	0	0	−0·911	−0·159
macular degeneration	Dr A.C. Bird	1	1	0	0·255	0·146
microphthalmia	Dr S. Roath	4	0	0	−0·899	−0·152
anophthalmos	Dr N.C. Nevin	6	0	0	−0·667	−0·082
obscure optic atrophy	Went et al.[120]	4	1	1	−0·014	−0·052
deafness, conductive	Thorpe et al.[104]	2	0	0	−0·340	−0·052
Ehlers-Danlos syndrome	Beighton[102]	2	1	1	−0·444	−0·076
Hunter's syndrome	Passarge et al.[129]	1	0	1	−0·699	−0·222

DIRECT LINKAGE UNLIKELY (sum of lods < −2 at $\theta = 0·1$, and between 0 and −2 at $\theta = 0·3$)

Loci for	References	Number of scoring children	Non-rec	Rec	Lods at $\theta =$ 0·10	Lods at $\theta =$ 0·30
low thyroxine binding	Nikolai et al.[68]	12	1	7	−5·549	−1·567
globulin	Bode et al.[95]	5	0	0	−0·899	−0·155
	Grant et al.[119]	5	5	0	1·275	0·730
					−5·173	−0·992
increased thyroxine binding globulin	Fialkow et al.[121]	9	0	2	−2·560	−0·634
hypohidrotic	Dr A. Motulsky	3	0	1	−0·568	−0·181
ectodermal dysplasia	Kerr et al.[56]	2	0	2	−1·398	−0·444
	Dr J.J. van Went	5	0	2	−1·842	−0·520
	Simpson et al.[97]	4	1	3	−1·842	−0·520
	Dr J. André	9	0	0	−1·818	−0·314
	Dr E. Passarge	6	2	1	0·238	0·230
					−7·230	−1·749

Table 101—*continued*

Loci for	References	Number of scoring children	Non-rec	Rec	Lods at $\theta=$ 0·10	0·30
renal diabetes insipidus	Dr A. Motulsky	7	1	0	−0·671	−0·016
	Bode et al.[98]	23	4	1	−2·515	−0·096
					−3·186	−0·112
retinitis pigmentosa	Klein et al.[58]	4	0	0	−0·680	−0·104
	Dr Mette Warburg	2	1	1	−0·444	−0·076
	Prof D. Klein	3	0	0	0·604	0·201
	Prof A. Eriksson	2	0	0	−0·340	−0·052
	Grützner et al.[100]	2	0	0	−0·528	−0·099
	Prof P. Grützner	6	0	2	−0·948	−0·315
					−2·336	−0·445
Norrie's disease	Warburg et al.[55]	11	0	2	−2·324	−0·467
	Nance et al.[101]	10	5	5	−2·220	−0·380
					−4·544	−0·847
Becker's muscular dystrophy	Blyth et al.[48]	10	1	0	−0·557	0·102
	Emery et al.[92]	10	3	5	−2·599	−0·631
	Zatz et al.[126]	6	0	0	−0·581	−0·064
					−3·737	−0·593
choroideremia	Øther[59]	4	2	2	−0·888	−0·152
	Prof D. Klein	3	0	0	−0·482	−0·086
	Dr F.H. Allen	7	1	3	−2·324	−0·606
	Grützner[93]	23	0	0	−2·862	−0·420
	Bell et al.[94]	6	0	0	−1·338	−0·230
	Dr W.G. Pearce	2	0	0	−0·340	−0·052
					−8·234	−1·546
hydrocephalus	Prof J.H. Edwards	3	1	2	−1·143	−0·298
	Dr J.T. Jabbour	6	1	2	−0·678	−0·128
	Dr C. Davison	2	0	0	−0·444	−0·076
					−2·265	−0·502

DIRECT LINKAGE EXCLUDED (sum of lods <-2 at $\theta = 0\cdot30^*$)

G6PD	Adam et al.[31], Sanger et al.[32]	52	6	3	−0·643	1·247
	Fraser et al.[33]	40	4	2	−0·566	0·625
	Siniscalco et al.[36]	193	64	57	−26·951	−3·919
	Adam et al.[38]	92	24	22	−13·160	−1·690
	Fraser et al.[39]	32	19	13	−4·242	−0·112
					−45·562	−3·849

Table 101—*continued*

Loci for	References	Number of scoring children	Non-rec	Rec	Lods at $\theta =$ 0·10	Lods at $\theta =$ 0·30
haemophilia	Davies *et al.*[41]	33	4	1	−3·014	−0·056
(factor VIII)	Harrison[42]	45	4	7	−5·082	−0·739
	Dr Jessica Lewis	43	4	2	−3·956	−0·326
	Dr J.B. Graham	45	8	5	−3·077	0·066
	Woodliff *et al.*[43]	4	3	1	0·066	0·216
	Dr L.N. Went	18	9	3	−0·766	0·476
					−15·829	−0·363
Christmas disease	Davies *et al.*[41]	60	16	18	−11·579	−2·039
(factor IX)	Harrison[42]	6	1	3	−1·711	−0·479
	Dr Jessica Lewis	9	0	2	−2·522	−0·624
	Woodliff *et al.*[43]	2	1	1	−0·444	−0·076
					−16·256	−3·218
deutan colour blindness	Jackson *et al.*[45,8]		9	1	−6·531	−0·556
	Siniscalco *et al.*[36]	152	43	44	−26·603	−4·301
	Davies *et al.*[41]	8	1	1	−0·685	−0·088
	Adam *et al.*[31,32]	20	4	2	−1·772	0·087
	Prof J.H. Edwards	3	1	2	−1·143	−0·298
	Dr L.N. Went	29	14	5	−1·078	−0·148
	Adam *et al.*[27]	7	0	0	−0·879	−0·144
					−38·691	−5·448
protan,	Jackson *et al.*[45,8]		0	1	−4·381	−0·190
colour blindness	Siniscalco *et al.*[36]	31	5	11	−8·895	−2·132
	Fraser *et al.*[33]	6	1	1	−0·528	−0·057
	Adam *et al.*[27]	11	2	4	−2·199	−0·488
	Prof J.H. Edwards	10	6	4	−1·266	−0·012
	Davies *et al.*[41]	5	0	0	−0·886	−0·148
	Dr L.N. Went	7	1	1	−0·795	−0·121
					−18·950	−3·148
Duchenne's muscular	Clark *et al.*[47]	21	2	3	−3·557	−0·566
dystrophy	Blyth *et al.*[48]	29	2	3	−7·461	−1·596
	Filippi *et al.*[73]	7	1	1	−1·332	−0·228
	Zatz *et al.*[126]	23	4	1	−2·288	−0·042
					−14·638	−2·432

Characters clinically indistinguishable from several on this list can be autosomally inherited: to take an extreme example, in only a small minority of families with retinitis pigmentosa is the condition X-linked.

Of the families with Duchenne and Becker muscular dystrophy and with hypogammaglobulin-aemia we have counted only those in which recent mutation could be excluded.

* Haemophilia (viii) excepted, but it is very close to the loci for G6PD and colour blindness, see text.

Further families tested in England[50] and in the States[85] contributed information and analysis of these (Johnston *et al.*[86]), together with the original series, raised the height of the curve to over 30, and it topped 100 when Malmqvist and her colleagues[87] found another informative family (z_1 4:0, e_1 4:0). The only other scoring family we know of is one sent to us by Dr W.B. Bean of Iowa City (z_1 3:2 and 1 n-r). The present position, Table 101, is: most likely recombination fraction 0·23, height of curve about 88, odds on linkage about 32 to 1. The probability limits are however still wide, about 0·16 to 0·35.

A surprisingly long time is being taken to establish the linkage with certainty: we have been sent some excellent families from Holland, Denmark, Germany and England but the Xg segregation has proved tantalizingly uninformative.

A mental retardation

A family with mental retardation, sometimes accompanied by hydrocephalus and sometimes not, is recorded by Fried and Sanger[88] (1973); measurable linkage with *Xg* was considered probable though the analysis was complicated through lack of knowledge of grandparental genotypes. Of course, the difficulty will be recognizing more families with the *same* type of X-borne mental retardation which could support or contradict this linkage, with its present most likely recombination value of 0·11.

Linkage with *Xg* possible

We should, of course, like to test more families with all the conditions in this section of Table 101.

Hypogammaglobulinaemia

Families tested more than 10 years ago in our Unit[53] showed little evidence of measurable linkage with *Xg*. However, subsequent family tests show that the work should continue. We have excluded from the counts in Table 101 some published families[54] in which only one boy was affected and may therefore have been a new mutant.

Lesch-Nyhan syndrome

The linkage information is curious. One kindred[128] gives good positive information which is not supported by other smaller families.

The syndrome is caused by a deficiency in the enzyme hypoxanthineguanine phosphoribosyltransferase, known to the fancy as HGPRT. In Table 101 we have included families with the milder HGPRT deficiency of gout; the large kindred[67, 128] is amongst those showing the full blown Lesch-Nyhan syndrome. Remembering the haemophilias and the muscular dystrophies one wonders whether the genetic background of HGPRT may also be heterogeneous.

Nuclear cataract

A family with this extremely rare form of cataract was investigated by Fraccaro *et al.*[51] (1967). The evidence for linkage with *Xg* is quite hopeful (estimate of recombination fraction 0·17, but with wide confidence limits; height of curve just over 9). However, there is some question whether the cataract of a young boy is of the nuclear type of his relatives; if it is not, then the curve is punctured and subsides to an insignificant height of 2. As the condition is fortunately so rare, it may be a long time before the linkage problem is advanced.

Testicular feminization

This is a rare and interesting condition. People who have it not only pass as females but are said to be particularly attractive examples. However, when their chromosomes come to be counted, probably because of their amenorrhoea, they are found to be cytological males, straightforward XYs. They have a small vagina but no uterus, their gonads are not quite normal testes and are sited in the inguinal canal or in the abdomen.

There was doubt about the manner of inheritance: the condition could have been due to an X-borne gene recessive in effect or to an autosomal gene, dominant in effect, which could express itself only in the male. Usually X-linkage is obvious from pedigrees, and the acid test is that an X-borne character is not handed on from father to son: but this test could not be applied to these infertile XYs.

It was hoped that the Xg groups might settle the problem: if the locus responsible were found to be within measurable distance of *Xg* then testicular feminization would be established as an X-borne character and the rather unlikely alternative would be ruled out. But these hopes were not realized[76], as indicated by the presence of testicular feminization in the 'linkage possible' part of Table 101.

However, the problem was later settled by the finding of the same condition in the mouse and its undoubted X-linkage in that species (Lyon and Hawkes[110]).

Mental retardation

None of the affected members of the eight families which went to make up the list in this section of Table 101 were said to have hydrocephalus as were some members of the mentally retarded family[88] in the 'Linkage probable' section. The eight families may reflect activity at different loci but we thought we would sum their lods just to see what they looked like.

Linkage information slight

Most of the conditions on the list in Table 101 are very rare. A chance to test more families would be welcomed.

Mr James Shields has drawn our attention to a series of papers, from Washington and New York, which suggest that manic-depressive psychosis may be an X-borne dominant character, papers in which some evidence slightly in favour of linkage with Xg is recorded[122, 123]. Evidence, however, is also recorded in favour of linkage with colour blindness[124, 125] which seems incompatible with our present view of the linkage relationship of *Xg* to *colour vision*. Perhaps more clarification of this important subject will have been achieved in time for our Addenda.

Direct linkage with *Xg* unlikely

A few more families with these conditions (Table 101) should really be tested before ruling out measurable linkage. One wonders whether low thyroxine binding globulin may be genetically heterogeneous on seeing 1 non-rec: 7 rec in the family of Nicolai *et al.*[68] and 5 non-rec: 0 rec in that of Grant *et al.*[119].

Direct linkage with *Xg* excluded

Enough families have been tested to exclude the loci for the six conditions in this section of Table 101 from being within direct measurable distance of *Xg*.

G6PD

The linkage relationship of these two loci has been investigated on a scale approaching that of all the other comparisons put together.

Analysis of a series of Israeli families gave evidence that the loci for G6PD and Xg were within measurable distance of each other and the most likely estimate of θ, the recombination fraction, was 0·26 (Adam *et al.*[30, 31], 1962, 1963; Sanger and Adam[32], 1964). In a smaller series of Greek families the estimate of θ was again 0·26 (Fraser *et al.*[33], 1964). Most of the families in these two series were of two generations only, so mathematical tests were required for their analysis.

On the other hand, in a large series of Sardinian families, there was no evidence of measurable linkage between the two loci (Filippi *et al.*[34], 1965; Sanger[35], 1965; and, more definitively, Siniscalco *et al.*[36], 1965). Most of these families were of three generations and the non-recombinants and recombinants could simply be counted.

This discrepancy, evidence of measurable linkage between *G6PD* and *Xg* in Israel and Greece but not in Sardinia, led to the organization of second surveys in Israel (Adam *et al.*[37, 38], 1966, 1967) and in Greece (Fraser *et al.*[39], 1967). All the samples from Israel, Sardinia and Greece, numbering several thousand, were grouped for Xg by members of our Unit.

As a result of this G6PD work we gradually came to realize that the lod score treatment of two generation families could give too low an estimate of the recombination fraction, and we came to pin our faith more and more on the simple counting of non-recombinants and recombinants in phase known, three generation, families. The count for all the G6PD series is given in Table 101: 117 non-recombinants to 97 recombinants, indicating a recombination frequency of 0·45. But this does not differ significantly from 0·5 (that is, no measurable linkage); furthermore, if 0·45 happened to be the true recombination rate an impossibly large increment of families would be needed to prove it. Fraser[39] is of the opinion that inadequacy of the method, rather than chance of sampling, is responsible for the lower recombination fraction derived from the lod scores for two generation families when the loci being surveyed are far apart.

Haemophilia (factor VIII deficiency)

It was quickly realized that the *Xg* locus must be a long way from that for haemophilia (O'Brien *et al.*[40], 1962), and so it proved to be (Davies *et al.*[41], 1963; Harrison[42], 1964 and several unpublished series included in Table 101). Altogether, over 100 families with about 600 children were Xg tested at the Blood Group Unit.

Christmas disease (factor IX deficiency)

Davies *et al.*[41] (1963) tested 20 families involving 331 members. The analysis showed that the two loci were not within measurable distance of each other. One of the families was extraordinary in having 11 recombinants and 1 non-recombinant, and, after the paper was published a further recombinant and non-recombinant were found; we have to suppose this a chance deviation from the 7:7 expected, assuming no linkage, though the probability of it happening in this or in the opposite direction is only 1 in 76.

Incidentally, one of these Christmas disease families, in which Xg and protan were also segregating, provided the first example in man of a double cross-over (Graham *et al.*[46], 1962).

Colour blindness

Jackson, Symon and Mann[44] (1962) showed that *Xg* was not close either to *deutan* or to *protan*. A fuller account[45] (1964) gave details of the informative families amongst the 34 kindred with 544 members who were tested. The results were analysed by Renwick and Schulze[8] using the computer and showed that both *deutan* and *protan* were far away from *Xg*.

A large investigation in Sardinia involving over 2,000 people (Siniscalco *et al.*[36], 1966) showed that linkage was not measurable between *Xg* and *deutan* or between *Xg* and *protan*, and subsequent findings support this (Table 101).

Since the loci for G6PD, colour vision and haemophilia (VIII) are so close to each other we tried pooling their non-recombinant and recombinant counts against *Xg*, and the result is described below, under 'Towards a map of the X'.

Duchenne's muscular dystrophy

Clark, Puite, Marczynski and Mann[47] (1963) tested a series of families with Duchenne's muscular dystrophy: seven were informative and were sufficient to show that the locus responsible was probably not within measurable distance of *Xg*. Blyth *et al.*[48] (1965) came to the same conclusion after testing ten informative families.

It was hoped that linkage relations with *Xg* might decide whether or not the severe Duchenne's type of muscular dystrophy was controlled by the same locus as the benign Becker type: but it seems from Table 101 very unlikely that Xg will settle this question. However it is becoming clearer from the colour vision[92] and G6PD results[126] that the two dystrophies may be controlled from separate loci (page 597).

Searches resulting in no linkage information

Unlucky segregation of the Xg groups has resulted, so far, in there being no linkage information about the relation of *Xg* and the loci for the following conditions:

Hypoplasia of iris with glaucoma   PGK (phosphoglycerate kinase)[111]
Gargoylism (Hurler's syndrome)   Osteodystrophic gerodermia
Lowe's oculo-cerebro-renal syndrome   Alport's syndrome
Scapuloperoneal syndrome   Cerebral palsy
Paroxysmal myoglobinuria   Cleft palate
Partial albinism and deaf mutism   Pure idiocy
Diffuse cerebral sclerosis   Nystagmus
Aldrich syndrome

TOWARDS A MAP OF THE X

We have long pictured the *Xg* locus near the end of the short arm, but our reasons are still frail.

On this crowded chromosome the rather disappointing shortage of proved linkages to *Xg* could be attributed to a terminal position of this marker locus which would there be wasting half its surveying power on thin air. There is, however, some relatively solid evidence that *Xg* is not sited on the distal third of the long arm, so, if indeed it is at an end, it would have to be that of the short arm.

The family upon which this evidence is based was published[105] before the days of banding of chromosomes. Dr P. Pearson subsequently pinpointed the balanced translocation in some members of the family to be between part of the long arm of the X onto the long arm of No. 3. The propositus of the family has a normal X from her father which carries *Xg* and an X lacking the distal third of the long arm from her mother. This maternal X carries the *Xg*^{a} allele yet the Xg^a antigen is perfectly well expressed: ergo the *Xg* locus is not on the distal third of the long arm.

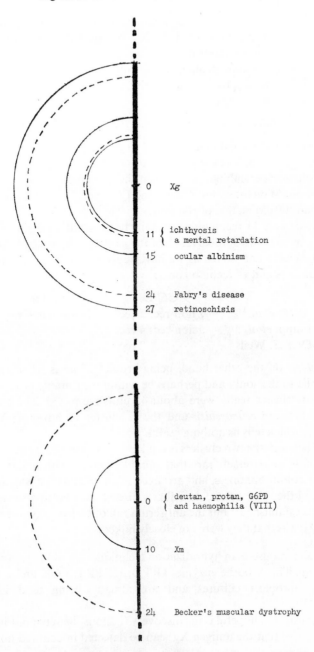

Fig. 39. A tentative map of two parts of the X: the cluster measured from *Xg* and that from *colour vision*. The semicircles indicate uncertainty about the direction of the loci from the two markers. Continuous lines represent established linkages, interrupted lines probable linkages; the numbers represent centimorgans.

There are two clusters of linkages on the X, one around *colour vision* and one around *Xg*, wherever it may be sited (Figure 39); the length of chromosome between the two clusters is unknown.

Since the loci for deutan, protan, G6PD and haemophilia (VIII) are all marking practically the same spot it seemed worth pooling their phase known counts for *Xg* (Table 101) and they come to

236 non-recombinants and 193 recombinants

which represents 0·45 recombination. Expecting 0·5 recombination, no detectable linkage that is, $\chi_1^2 = 4\cdot3$. The lod scores at $\theta = 0\cdot45$ are $+0\cdot798$. We are beginning to wonder whether recombination between the two clusters perhaps is less than 0·5. ($\theta\,0\cdot45 = 50$ cM on the scale of Carter and Falconer, 74 cM on that of Kosambi and more than 100 cM on that of Haldane.)

If *ichthyosis* were 11 recombination units to the south of *Xg* it would still be too far away to be in measurable reach of the *cv* cluster because of the inevitable limit to informative data. Such as we have suggest no linkage, for there are 14 non-recombinants and 14 recombinants:

	G6PD	protan
Adam et al.[27]	7 non-rec: 2 rec	2 non-rec: 6 rec
Filippi et al.[78]	5 non-rec: 4 rec	
Dr R.S. Wells	2 rec	

Retinoschisis on the other hand, being around 27 units from *Xg*, might be expected to lie to the south and perhaps be within measurable distance of the *cv* cluster (if this cluster really were about 45 units from *Xg*). The phase known information between *retinoschisis* and the *cv* cluster is, however, limited to 1 non-rec: 1 rec which tells us nothing useful.

The gap between the two clusters is unlikely to be spanned by ocular albinism, the condition is so extremely rare that suitable families with it and with G6PD deficiency or colour blindness, and arranged in an informative way, may seldom be found; and the same applies to Fabry's disease. *Xm* failed also: its closeness to *deutan* was established[91] but the antiserum ran out when all that could be said of *Xm* and *Xg* was that they were not closely linked.

Before long, mouse-man hybridization techniques should begin to contribute to X-mapping. The X-borne enzymes G6PD, HGPRT, PGK and α-Gal can be detected in fibroblast cultures and are already being used in mapping attempts[111–116].

Most exciting and hopeful is the discovery (Fellous, Bengtsson, Finnegan and Bodmer[117], 1974) that the antigen Xg^a can be detected in cultured fibroblasts.

REFERENCES

[1]   McKusick V.A. (1962) On the X chromosome of man. *Quart. Rev. Biol.*, 37, 69–175.
[2]   McKusick V.A. (1966, 1968, 1971, 1974) *Mendelian Inheritance in Man.* Catalogs of

autosomal dominant, autosomal recessive and X-linked phenotypes. Johns Hopkins Press, Baltimore.

3   CHILDS B., ZINKHAM W.H., BROWNE E.A., KIMBRO E.L. and TORBERT J.V. (1958) A genetic study of a defect in glutathione metabolism of the erythrocyte. *Bull. Johns Hopkins Hosp.*, **102**, 21–37.

4   MANN J.D., CAHAN A., GELB A.G., FISHER NATHALIE, HAMPER JEAN, TIPPETT PATRICIA, SANGER RUTH and RACE R.R. (1962) A sex-linked blood group. *Lancet*, **i**, 8–10.

5   BERG K. and BEARN A.G. (1966) An inherited X-linked serum system in man. The Xm system. *J. exp. Med.*, **123**, 379–397.

6   COOK P.J.L. (1965) The Lutheran-secretor recombination fraction in man: a possible sex difference. *Ann. hum. Genet.*, **28**, 393–401.

7   RENWICK J.H. and SCHULZE JANE (1965) Male and female recombination fractions for the nail-patella: ABO linkage in man. *Ann. hum. Genet.*, **28**, 379–392.

8   RENWICK J.H. and SCHULZE JANE (1964) An analysis of some data on the linkage between Xg and colorblindness in man. *Amer. J. hum. Genet.*, **16**, 410–418.

9   LINDSTEN J., FRACCARO M., POLANI P.E., HAMERTON J.L., SANGER RUTH and RACE R.R. (1963) Evidence that the Xg blood group genes are on the short arm of the X chromosome. *Nature, Lond.*, **197**, 648–649.

10 FERGUSON-SMITH M.A. (1966) X-Y chromosomal interchange in the aetiology of true hermaphroditism and of XX Klinefelter's syndrome. *Lancet*, **ii**, 475–476.

11 BELL JULIA and HALDANE J.B.S. (1937) The linkage between the genes for colour-blindness and haemophilia in man. *Proc. Roy. Soc. B.*, **123**, 119–150.

12 HALDANE J.B.S. and SMITH C.A.B. (1947) A new estimate of the linkage between the genes for colour-blindness and haemophilia in man. *Ann. Eugen., Lond.*, **14**, 10–31.

13 WHITTAKER D.L., COPELAND D.L. and GRAHAM J.B. (1962) Linkage of color blindness to hemophilias A and B. *Amer. J. hum. Genet.*, **14**, 149–158.

14 ROBERTSON J.H. and TRUEMAN ROSEMARY G. (1964) Combined hemophilia and Christmas disease. *Blood*, **24**, 281–288.

15 ADAM A. (1961) Linkage between deficiency of glucose-6-phosphate dehydrogenase and colour blindness. *Nature, Lond.*, **189**, 686.

16 SINISCALCO M., MOTULSKY A.G., LATTE B. and BERNINI L. (1960) Indagini genetiche sulla predisposizione al favismo. II. Dati familiari. Associazione genica con il daltonismo. *Atti Accad. naz. Lincei Rc.*, **28**, 1–7.

17 PORTER I.H., SCHULZE J. and McKUSICK V.A. (1962) Linkage between glucose-6-phosphate dehydrogenase deficiency and colour blindness. *Nature, Lond.*, **193**, 506.

18 PORTER I.H., SCHULZE JANE and McKUSICK V.A. (1962) Genetical linkage between the loci for glucose-6-phosphate dehydrogenase deficiency and colour-blindness in American Negroes. *Ann. hum. Genet.*, **26**, 107–122.

19 SINISCALCO M., FILIPPI G. and LATTE B. (1964) Recombination between protan and deutan genes; data on their relative positions in respect of the g6pd locus. *Nature, Lond.*, **204**, 1062–1064.

20 VANDERDONCK R. and VERRIEST G. (1960) Femme protanomale et hétérozygote mixte (gènes de la protanomalie et de la deutéranopie en position de repulsion) ayant deux fils deutéranopes, un fil protanomal et deux fils normaux. *Biotypologie*, **21**, 110–120. Not seen but quoted by McKusick[1, 2] and by Kalmus[21].

21 KALMUS H. (1962) Distance and sequence of the loci for protan and deutan defects and for glucose-6-phosphate dehydrogenase deficiency. *Nature, Lond.*, **194**, 215.

22 WENT L.N., DE GROOT W.P., SANGER RUTH, TIPPETT PATRICIA and GAVIN JUNE (1969) X-linked ichthyosis: linkage relationship with the Xg blood groups and other studies in a large Dutch kindred. *Ann. Hum. Genet.*, **32**, 333–345.

23 BOYER S.H. and GRAHAM J.B. (1965) Linkage between the X chromosome loci for glucose-6-phosphate dehydrogenase electrophoretic variation and hemophilia A. *Amer. J. hum. Genet.*, **17**, 320–324.

24   KERR C.B., WELLS R.S. and SANGER RUTH (1964) X-linked ichthyosis and the Xg groups. *Lancet*, ii, 1369–1370.

25   ADAM A., ZIPRKOWSKI L., FEINSTEIN A., SANGER RUTH and RACE R.R. (1966) Ichthyosis, Xg blood-groups, and protan. *Lancet*, i, 877.

26   WELLS R.S., JENNINGS M.C., SANGER RUTH and RACE R.R. (1966) Xg blood-groups and ichthyosis. *Lancet*, ii, 493–494.

27   ADAM A., ZIPRKOWSKI L., FEINSTEIN A., SANGER RUTH, TIPPETT PATRICIA, GAVIN JUNE and RACE R.R. (1969) Linkage relations of X-borne ichthyosis to the Xg blood groups and to other markers of the X in Israelis. *Ann. Hum. Genet.*, 32, 323–332.

28   LATTE B., FILIPPI G. and SINISCALCO M. (1965) Genetica della cecità per i colori (Daltonismo): un secondo caso di ricombinazione tra i loci deutan e protan. *Atti Ass. genet. ital.*, 10, 282–295.

29   FIALKOW P.J., GIBLETT ELOISE R. and MOTULSKY A.G. (1967) Measurable linkage between ocular albinism and Xg. *Amer. J. hum. Genet.*, 19, 63–69.

30   ADAM A., SHEBA C., RACE R.R., SANGER RUTH, TIPPETT PATRICIA, HAMPER JEAN and GAVIN JUNE (1962) Linkage relations of the X-borne genes responsible for glucose-6-phosphate dehydrogenase and for the Xg blood-groups. *Lancet*, i, 1188–1189.

31   ADAM A., SHEBA C., SANGER RUTH, RACE R.R., TIPPETT PATRICIA, HAMPER JEAN, GAVIN JUNE and FINNEY D.J. (1963) Data for X-mapping calculations, Israeli families tested for Xg, g-6-pd and for colour vision. *Ann. hum. Genet.*, 26, 187–194.

32   SANGER RUTH and ADAM A. (1964) Xg and 6-g-pd in Israeli families: an addendum. *Ann. hum. Genet.*, 27, 271–272.

33   FRASER G.R., DEFARANAS B., KATTAMIS C.A., RACE R.R., SANGER RUTH and STAMATO-YANNOPOULOS G. (1964) Glucose-6-phosphate dehydrogenase, colour vision and Xg blood groups in Greece: linkage and population data. *Ann. hum. Genet.*, 27, 395–403.

34   FILIPPI G., LATTE B., PIOMELLI S., RACE R.R., RATTAZZI M. and SINISCALCO M. (1965) Mappa del cromosoma X in Sardegna assenza di linkage tra il locus Xg^a e quelli per la g6pd e per la cecità ai colori (deutan e protan). *Atti Ass. genet., ital.*, 10, 279–281.

35   SANGER RUTH (1965) Genes on the X chromosome. *Can. J. Genet. Cytol.*, 7, 179–186.

36   SINISCALCO M., FILIPPI G., LATTE B., PIOMELLI S., RATTAZZI M., GAVIN JUNE, SANGER RUTH and RACE R.R. (1966) Failure to detect linkage between Xg and other X-borne loci in Sardinians. *Ann. hum. Genet.*, 29, 231–252.

37   ADAM A., SHEBA C., SANGER RUTH and RACE R.R. (1966) The linkage relation of g6pd to Xg. *Amer. J. hum. Genet.*, 18, 110.

38   ADAM A., TIPPETT PATRICIA, GAVIN JUNE, NOADES JEAN, SANGER RUTH and RACE R.R. (1967) The linkage relation of Xg to g-6-pd in Israelis: the evidence of a second series of families. *Ann. hum. Genet.*, 30, 211–218.

39   FRASER G.R. and MAYO O. (1968) A comparison of the two-generation and three-generation methods of estimating linkage values on the X chromosome in man with special reference to the loci determining the Xg blood group and glucose-6-phosphate dehydrogenase deficiency. *Amer. J. hum. Genet.*, 20, 534–548.

40   O'BRIEN J.R., HARRIS J.B., RACE R.R., SANGER RUTH, TIPPETT PATRICIA, HAMPER JEAN and GAVIN JUNE (1962) Haemophilia (VIII) and the Xg blood-groups. *Lancet*, i, 1026.

41   DAVIES S.H., GAVIN JUNE, GOLDSMITH K.L.G., GRAHAM J.B., HAMPER JEAN, HARDISTY R.M., HARRIS J.B., HOLMAN C.A., INGRAM G.I.C., JONES T.G., MCAFEE L.A., MCKUSICK V.A., O'BRIEN J.R., RACE R.R., SANGER RUTH and TIPPETT PATRICIA (1963) The linkage relations of haemophilia A and haemophilia B (Christmas disease) to the Xg blood group system. *Amer. J. hum. Genet.*, 15, 481–492.

42   HARRISON J.F. (1964) Haemophilia, Christmas disease and the Xg blood groups. Observations based on the haemophiliacs of Birmingham. *Brit. J. Haemat.*, 10, 115–121.

43   WOODLIFF H.J. and JACKSON J.M. (1966) Combined haemophilia and Christmas disease: a genetic study of a patient and his relatives. *Med. J. Aust.*, 1, 658–661.

44 JACKSON C.E., SYMON W.E. and MANN J.D. (1962) Colour-blindness and blood group Xgᵃ. *Lancet*, **ii**, 512.

45 JACKSON C.E., SYMON W.E. and MANN J.D. (1964) X chromosome mapping of genes for red-green colorblindness and Xg. *Amer. J. hum. Genet.*, **16**, 403–409.

46 GRAHAM J.B., TARLETON H.L., RACE R.R. and SANGER RUTH (1962) A human double cross-over. *Nature, Lond.*, **195**, 834.

47 CLARK J.I., PUITE R.H., MARCZYNSKI R. and MANN J.D. (1963) Evidence for the absence of detectable linkage between the genes for Duchenne muscular dystrophy and the Xg blood group. *Amer. J. hum. Genet.*, **15**, 292–297.

48 BLYTH HELEN, CARTER C.O., DUBOWITZ V., EMERY A.E.H., GAVIN JUNE, JOHNSTON H.A., McKUSICK V.A., RACE R.R., SANGER RUTH and TIPPETT PATRICIA (1965) Duchenne's muscular dystrophy and the Xg blood groups: a search for linkage. *J. med. Genet.*, **2**, 157–160.

49 OPITZ J.M., STILES F.C., WISE D., RACE R.R., SANGER RUTH, VON GEMMINGEN G.R., KIERLAND R.R., CROSS E.G. and DE GROOT W.P. (1965) The genetics of angiokeratoma corporis diffusum (Fabry's disease) and its linkage relations with the Xg locus. *Amer. J. hum. Genet.*, **17**, 325–342.

50 JOHNSTON A.W., WARLAND B.J. and WELLER S.D.V. (1966) Genetic aspects of angio-keratoma corporis diffusum. *Ann. hum. Genet.*, **30**, 25–41.

51 FRACCARO M., MANFREDINI U., MORONE G. and SANGER RUTH (1967) X-linked cataract. *Ann. hum. Genet.*, **31**, 45–50.

52 ERIKSSON A.W., FELLMAN J., VAINIO-MATTILA B., SANGER R., RACE R.R., KRAUSE U. and FORSIUS H. (1967) Studies of X-linked retinoschisis in Finland. *Int. Congr. Neuro-Genet. and Neuro-Ophthal.*, Montreal. Excerpta Med. Int. Cong. Series No. 176. 360–362.

53 SANGER RUTH and RACE R.R. (1963) The Xg blood groups and familial hypogamma-globulinaemia. *Lancet*, **i**, 859–860.

54 ROSEN F.S., HUTCHISON G.B. and ALLEN F.H. (1965) The Xg blood groups and congenital hypogammaglobulinaemia. *Vox Sang.*, **10**, 729–730.

55 WARBURG METTE, HAUGE M. and SANGER RUTH (1965) Norrie's disease and the Xg blood group system: linkage data. *Acta genet., Basel*, **15**, 103–115.

56 KERR C.B., WELLS R.S. and COOPER K.E. (1966) Gene effect in carriers of anhidrotic ectodermal dysplasia. *J. med. Genet.*, **3**, 169–176. (Xg grouping done after this report.)

57 HOARE G.W. (1965) Choroido-retinal dystrophy. *Brit. J. Ophthal.*, **49**, 449–459.

58 KLEIN D., FRANCESCHETTI A., HUSSELS IRÈNE, RACE R.R. and SANGER RUTH (1967) X-linked retinitis pigmentosa and linkage studies with the Xg blood-groups. *Lancet*, **i**, 974–975.

59 ØTHER A. (1968) Choroideremia and the Xg blood group. *Acta Ophth.*, **46**, 79–82.

60 ELVES M.W., BOURNE M.S. and ISRAËLS M.C.G. (1966) Pyridoxine-responsive anaemia determined by an X-linked gene. *J. med. Genet.*, **3**, 1–4.

61 JOHNSTON A.W. and McKUSICK V.A. (1962) A sex-linked recessive form of spastic para-plegia. *Amer. J. hum. Genet.*, **14**, 83–94. (Xg grouping done after this report.)

62 RICHARDS B.W. (1963) Sex-linked deaf mutism. *Ann. hum. Genet.*, **26**, 195–199. (Xg group-ing done after this report.)

63 FORSIUS H., VAINIO-MATTILA B. and ERIKSSON A. (1962) X-linked hereditary retinoschisis. *Brit. J. Ophthal.*, **46**, 678–681. (Xg grouping done after this report.)

64 FORSIUS H. and ERIKSSON A.W. (1964) Ein neues Augensyndrom mit X-chromosomaler Transmission. Eine Sippe mit Fundusalbinis, Foveahypoplasie, Nystagmus, Myopie, Astigmatismus und Dyschromatopsie. *Klin. Mbl. Augenheilk.*, **144**, 447–457; and, A new X-chromosomal ocular syndrome. *Acta ophthal. (Kbh.)*, **42**, 928–929. (Xg grouping done after these reports.)

65 GRAHAM J.B. and WINTERS R.W. (1961) Familial hypophosphatemia: an inherited demand for increased vitamin D? *Ann. N.Y. Acad. Sci.*, **91**, 667–673.

[66] ATA M., FISHER O.D. and HOLMAN C.A. (1965) Inherited thrombocytopenia. *Lancet*, **i**, 119–123.

[67] SHAPIRO S.L., SHEPPARD G.L., DREIFUSS F.E. and NEWCOMBE D.S. (1966) X-linked recessive inheritance of a syndrome of mental retardation with hyperuricemia. *Proc. Soc. exp. Biol., N.Y.*, **122**, 609–611. (Xg grouping done after this report.)

[68] NIKOLAI T.F. and SEAL U.S. (1966) X-chromosome linked familial decrease in thyroxine-binding globulin activity. *J. clin. Endocr. Metab.*, **26**, 835–841.

[69] HALDANE J.B.S. (1919) The combination of linkage values, and the calculation of distances between the loci of linked factors. *J. Genet.*, **8**, 299–309.

[70] KOSAMBI D.D. (1944) The estimation of map distances from recombination values. *Ann. Eugen., Lond.*, **12**, 172–175.

[71] CARTER T.C. and FALCONER D.S. (1951) Stocks for detecting linkage in the mouse and the theory of their design. *J. Genet.*, **50**, 307–323.

[72] HEISTÖ H., HARBOE M. and GODAL H.C. (1965) Warm haemolysins active against trypsin-ized red cells; occurrence, inheritance and clinical significance. *Proc. 10th Congr. int. Soc. Blood Transf.*, Stockholm 1964, 787–789.

[73] FILIPPI G. and MACCIOTTA A. (1967) Xg blood groups in muscular dystrophy. *Lancet*, **ii**, 565.

[74] ERPENSTEIN H. and PFEIFFER R.A. (1967) Geschlechtsgebunden-dominant erbliche Zahn-unterzahl. *Humangenetik*, **4**, 280–293.

[75] NYHAN W.L., PESEK J., SWEETMAN L., CARPENTER D.G. and CARTER C.H. (1967) Genetics of an X-linked disorder of uric acid metabolism and cerebral function. *Pediat. Res.*, **1**, 5–13.

[76] SANGER RUTH, TIPPETT PATRICIA, GAVIN JUNE, GOOCH ANN and RACE R.R. (1969) The problem of the inheritance of the testicular feminization syndrome: some negative linkage contributions. *J. med. Genet.*, **6**, 26–27.

[77] SANGER RUTH and RACE R.R. (1969) Towards mapping the X-chromosome, pp. 241–266 in *Modern Trends in Human Genetics*. Ed. A. E. H. Emery, Butterworths, London.

[78] FILIPPI G. and MEERA KHAN P. (1968) Linkage studies on X-linked ichthyosis in Sardinia. *Amer. J. hum. Genet.*, **20**, 564–569.

[79] PEARCE W.G., SANGER RUTH and RACE R.R. (1968) Ocular albinism and Xg. *Lancet*, **i**, 1282–1283.

[80] PEARCE W.G., JOHNSON G.J. and SANGER RUTH (1971) Ocular albinism and Xg. *Lancet*, **i**, 1072.

[81] HOEFNAGEL D., ALLEN F.H. and WALKER MARY (1969) Ocular albinism and Xg. *Lancet*, **i**, 1314.

[82] IVES E.J., EWING C.C. and INNES R. (1970) X-linked juvenile retinoschisis and Xg linkage in five families. *Amer. J. Hum. Genet.*, **22**, No. 6, 17a–18a (Abstract).

[83] VAINIO-MATTILA BIRGITTA, ERIKSSON A.W. and FORSIUS H. (1969) X-chromosomal reces-sive retinoschisis in the region of Pori. An ophthalmo-genetical analysis of 103 cases. *Acta Ophthalmol.*, **47**, 1135–1148. (Xg groups not included in this report.)

[84] ERIKSSON A.W., FORSIUS H. and VAINIO-MATTILA B. (1972) X-kromosomaalinen retino-skiisi. *Duodecim*, **88**, 43–51.

[85] SPAETH G.L. and FROST P. (1965) Fabry's disease. Its ocular manifestations. *Arch. Ophthal-mol.*, **74**, 760–769.

[86] JOHNSTON A.W., FROST P., SPAETH G.L. and RENWICK J.H. (1969) Linkage relationships of the angiokeratoma (Fabry) locus. *Ann. Hum. Genet.*, **32**, 369–374.

[87] MALMQVIST EVA, IVEMARK B.I., LINDSTEN J., MAUNSBACH A.B. and MÅRTENSSON E. (1971) Pathologic lysosomes and increased urinary glycosylceramide excretion in Fabry's disease. *Lab. Invest.*, **25**, 1–14.

[88] FRIED K. and SANGER RUTH (1973) Possible linkage between *Xg* and the locus for a gene causing mental retardation with or without hydrocephalus. *J. med. Genet.*, **10**, 17–18.

89 HEISTØ H., JENSEN LEILA and KNUDS F. (1971) Studies on trypsin treatment of red cells with special reference to differences between trypsin preparations. *Vox Sang.*, **21**, 115–125.

90 HEISTØ H., JENSEN LEILA and KNUDS F. (1972) Warm haemolysins active against trypsinized red cells. *Vox Sang.*, **22**, 131–136.

91 BERG K. and BEARN A.G. (1968) Human serum protein polymorphisms. A selected review. *A. rev. Genet.*, **2**, 341–362.

92 EMERY A.E.H., SMITH C.A.B. and SANGER RUTH (1969) The linkage relations of the loci for benign (Becker type) X-borne muscular dystrophy, colour blindness and the Xg blood groups. *Ann. Hum. Genet.*, **32**, 261–269.

93 GRÜTZNER P. (1974) In preparation.

94 BELL A.G. and MCCULLOCH J.C. (1971) Choroideremia and the Xg locus: another look for linkage. *Clin. Genet.*, **2**, 239–241.

95 BODE H.H., ROTHMAN K.J. and DANON M. (1973) Linkage of thyroxine-binding globulin deficiency to other X-chromosome loci. *J. clin. Endocrinol. Metab.*, **37**, 25–29.

96 ADAM A., LEVIN S., ARNON A., SADAN N. and KLAJMAN A. (1971) X-linked hypogammaglobulinemia. Additional observations in a previously reported family. *Israel J. Med. Sci.*, **7**, 1280–1285.

97 SIMPSON J.L., ALLEN F.H., NEW MARIA and GERMAN J. (1969) Absence of close linkage between the locus for Xg and the locus for anhidrotic ectodermal dysplasia. *Vox Sang.*, **17**, 465–467.

98 BODE H.H. and MIETTINEN O.S. (1969) Nehprogenic diabetes insipidus: absence of close linkage with Xg. *Amer. J. Hum. Genet.*, **22**, 221–226.

99 GREENE M.L., NYHAN W.L. and SEEGMILLER J.E. (1969) Hypoxanthine-guanine phosphoribosyltransferase deficiency and Xg blood group. *Amer. J. Hum. Genet.*, **22**, 50–54.

100 GRÜTZNER P., SANGER RUTH and SPIVEY B.E. (1972) Linkage studies in X-linked retinitis pigmentosa. *Humangenetik*, **14**, 155–158,

101 NANCE W.E., HARA S., HANSEN A., ELLIOTT J., LEWIS MARION and CHOWN B. (1969) Genetic linkage studies in a Negro kindred with Norrie's disease. *Amer. J. hum. Genet.* **21**, 423–429.

102 BEIGHTON P. (1968) X-linked recessive inheritance in the Ehlers-Danlos syndrome. *Brit. Med. J.*, **3**, 409–411.

103 McRAE K.N., UCHIDA IRENE A. and LEWIS MARION (1969) Sex-linked congenital deafness. *Amer. J. Hum. Genet.*, **21**, 415–422.

104 THORPE P., SELLARS S. and BEIGHTON P. (1974) X-linked deafness in a South African kindred. *S. Afr. med. J.*, **48**, 587–590.

105 CLARKE G., STEVENSON A.C., DAVIES PAMELA and WILLIAMS C.E. (1964) A family apparently showing transmission of a translocation between chromosome 3 and one of the 'X-6-12' or 'C' group. *J. med. Genet.*, **1**, 27–34.

106 BANNERMAN R.M., INGALL G.B. and MOHN J.F. (1971) X-linked spondyloepiphyseal dysplasia tarda: clinical and linkage data. *J. med. Genet.*, **8**, 291–301.

107 SPIRA T.J., ADAM A., GOODMAN R.M. and BERGER A. (1971) Recombination between cerebral sclerosis-Addison's disease and the Xg blood-groups. *Lancet*, **ii**, 820–821.

108 NEUHÄUSER G., ZERBIN-RÜDIN E., PFEIFFER R.A. and KLAR H. (1969) Beobachtungen zum Problem des geschlechtsgebunden-recessiven Schwachsinns. *Arch. Psychiat. Nervkrankh.*, **212**, 207–224. (IV-11 and IV-12, dizygous twins in family We.-Wi. later found to be affected.)

109 THOMAS P.K., CALNE D.B. and ELLIOTT C.F. (1972) X-linked scapuloperoneal syndrome. *J. Neurol. Neurosurg. Psychiat.*, **35**, 208–215.

110 LYON MARY F. and HAWKES SUSAN G. (1970) X-linked gene for testicular feminization in the mouse. *Nature, Lond.*, **227**, 1217–1219.

111 CHEN SHI-HAN, MALCOLM L.A., YOSHIDA AKIRA and GIBLETT ELOISE R. (1971) Phosphoglycerate kinase: an X-linked polymorphism in man. *Amer. J. hum. Genet.*, **23**, 87–91.

[112] MILLER O.J., COOK P.R., MEERA KHAN P., SHIN S. and SINISCALCO M. (1971) Mitotic separation of two human X-linked genes in man-mouse somatic cell hybrids. *Proc Nat. Acad. Sci.*, **68**, 116–120.

[113] MEERA KHAN P., WESTERVELD A., GRZESCHIK K.H., DEYS B.F., GARSON O.M. and SINISCALCO M. (1971) X-linkage of human phosphoglycerate kinase confirmed in man-mouse and man-Chinese hamster somatic cell hybrids. *Amer. J. Hum. Genet.*, **23**, 614–623.

[114] GRZESCHIK K.H., ALLDERDICE P.W., GRZESCHIK A., OPITZ J.M., MILLER O.J. and SINISCALCO M. (1972) Cytological mapping of human X-linked genes by use of somatic cell hybrids involving an X-autosome translocation. *Proc. Nat. Acad. Sci.*, **69**, 69–73.

[115] GRZESCHIK K.H., GRZESCHIK A.M., BENOFF S., ROMEO G., SINISCALCO M., VAN SOMEREN H., MEERA KHAN P., WESTERVELD A. and BOOTSMA D. (1972) X-linkage of human α-galactosidase. *Nature New Biol.*, **240**, 48–50.

[116] SINISCALCO M. (1974) Strategies for X-chromosome mapping with somatic cell hybrids. In *Somatic Cell Hybridization* ed. R.L. Davidson and F. de la Cruz. Raven Press, N.Y., 35–44.

[117] FELLOUS M., BENGTSSON B., FINNEGAN D. and BODMER W.F. (1974) Expression of the Xgᵃ antigen on cells in culture and its segregation in somatic cell hybrids. *Ann. Hum. Genet.*, **37**, 421–430.

[118] EDWARDS J.H. (1971) The analysis of X-linkage. *Ann. Hum. Genet.*, **34**, 229–250.

[119] GRANT D.B., MINCHIN CLARKE H.G. and PUTMAN D. (1974) Familial thyroxine binding globulin deficiency: search for linkage with Xg blood groups. *J. med. Genet.*, **11**, 271–274.

[120] WENT L.N., DE VRIES-DE MOL E.C. and VÖLKER-DIEBEN H.J. (1974) A family with apparently sex-linked optic atrophy. J. med. Genet., in the press.

[121] FIALKOW P.J., GIBLETT ELOISE R. and MUSA B. (1970) Increased serum thyroxine-binding globulin capacity: inheritance and linkage relationships. *J. Clin. Endocr.*, **30**, 66–70.

[122] WINOKUR G. and TANNA V.L. (1969) Possible role of X-linked dominant factor in manic depressive disease. *Dis. nerv. Syst.*, **30**, 89–93.

[123] FIEVE R.R., MENDLEWICZ J. and FLEISS J.L. (1973) Manic-depressive illness: linkage with the Xg blood group. *Am. J. Psychiat.*, **130**, 1355–1359

[124] REICH T., CLAYTON PAULA J. and WINOKUR G. (1969) Family history studies: V. The genetics of mania. *Am. J. Psychiat.*, **125**, 1358–1369.

[125] MENDLEWICZ J., FLEISS J.L. and FIEVE R.R. (1972) Evidence for X-linkage in the transmission of manic-depressive illness. *J. Am. med. Ass.*, **222**, 1624–1627.

[126] ZATZ MAYANA, ITSKAN SUELI B., SANGER RUTH, FROTA-PESSOA O. and SALDANHA P.H. (1974) New linkage data for the X-linked types of muscular dystrophy and G-6-PD variants, colour blindness and Xg blood groups. *J. med. Genet.*, **11**, 321–327.

[127] DE BRUYN C.H.M.M., OEI T.L., GEERDINK R.A. and LOMMEN E.J.P. (1973) An atypical case of hypoxanthine-guanine phosphoribosyltransferase deficiency (Lesch-Nyhan syndrome). II. Genetic studies. *Clin. Genet.*, **4**, 353–359.

[128] NEWCOMBE D.S. and DREIFUSS F.E. (1974) In preparation.

[129] PASSARGE E., WENDEL U., WÖHLER W. and RÜDIGER H.W. (1974) Krankheiten infolge genetischer Defekte im lysosomalen Mucopolysaccharid-Abbau. *Dtsch. med. Wschr.*, **99**, 144–158.

[130] SPIVEY B.E. (1965) The X-linked recessive inheritance of atypical monochromatism. *Arch. Ophthal.*, **74**, 327–333.

Chapter 30
Xg and Sex-Chromosome Aneuploidy

In somatic cells the chromosomes should be present in pairs. If a particular chromosome lacks its partner, or is present in threes or fours or more, the condition is called aneuploidy.

Outstanding accounts of the cytogenetic background and the clinical effects of aneuploidy of the sex chromosomes will be found in the following books: *Les Chromosomes Humains* by Turpin and Lejeune[1], 1965, *Abnormalities of the Sex Chromosome Complement in Man* by Court Brown, Harnden, Jacobs, Maclean and Mantle[2], 1964, and *Chromosomes in Man* edited by J.L. Hamerton[3], 1962. The classical monograph of McKusick[4], 1962, *On the X Chromosome of Man* and two papers by Polani[5, 6], 1965, give excellent general accounts.

This chapter deals with the contribution that Xg can make to defining the particular cell division at which the accident responsible for sex-chromosome aneuploidy has happened. The accident usually occurs at some cell division in the preparation of the gametes, that is, during spermatogenesis or during oogenesis.

At this stage a diagram of normal meiosis as it affects the sex chromosomes seems called for and our attempt is to be found in Figure 40.

It is known that the accident which can cause an abnormal number of sex chromosomes can happen both at the first and at the second division of spermatogenesis. Presumably it can happen at both divisions of oogenesis, it certainly happens at one or the other, but we do not think there is yet proof in man that it can happen at both divisions of oogenesis. There is some convincing evidence that the accident can also happen post-meiotically, on occasion, at an early division of the zygote (see page 539).

The accident, called non-disjunction, is a sticking together of two chromosomes, X to X, at cell division when they should have parted and gone one into each daughter cell: instead they both go into one daughter cell and leave the other daughter cell without a sex chromosome.

When a Y is involved the accident may be that called anaphase lag: at spermatogenesis the Y, not being aligned with the X centromere to centromere like the other chromosome pairs, may be freer to wander off and, on rare occasions, get into the same daughter cell as the X or fail to get into either daughter cell.

Family studies of characters known to be controlled by genes on the X can sometimes show whether the accident, the misdivision, has happened at spermatogenesis in the father or at oogenesis in the mother.

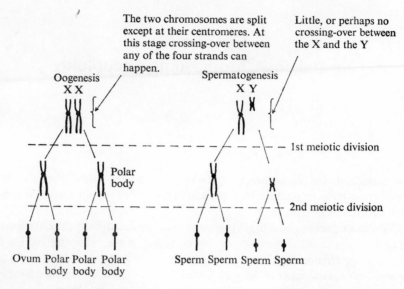

Fig. 40. Diagram of meiosis, showing only the sex chromosomes.

It is not surprising that in sex chromosome upsets the distribution and inheritance of X-linked characters may reflect the abnormality, and sufferers from the syndromes of Klinefelter and Turner serve as examples. Polani, Lessof and Bishop[7] were the first to realize this and, as long ago as 1956, they tested Turner patients for red-green colour blindness and found them to have an incidence of this recessive condition too high for females. Having acknowledged this priority we will go straight on to the subsequent use of the Xg groups for the same purpose: the more useful frequencies of the Xg groups compared with colour vision make the data vastly the more informative.

The tables to follow in this chapter are a summary of the Xg tests on samples sent to our Unit[32] up to the beginning of 1971. (The tables therefore do not include the 16 XO and the 19 XXY Canadian families reported by Soltan[48].) A few of the more interesting of our counts have been brought up to the end of 1973 and it is made clear when this has been done.

The samples came from more than a hundred physicians or cytogeneticists, the majority being sent by Dr A. Frøland and Dr Gudrun Dahl, Copenhagen; Professor M.A. Ferguson-Smith, Glasgow; Professor P.E. Polani, London; Professor J.H. Edwards, Birmingham; Dr A. de la Chapelle, Helsinki; the late Dr W.M. Court Brown, Dr W.H. Price and Dr Marjorie Newton, Edinburgh; Dr J. Lindsten, Stockholm; Professor H. van den Berghe, Louvain and Professor R.A. Pfeiffer, Münster.

We apologise for using in this chapter the old notation XXY rather than 47,XXY and XO rather than 45,X etc.; just for our present purpose it seemed clearer to avoid writing, for example, 395 47,XXY patients.

KLINEFELTER'S SYNDROME

People with the syndrome named after Klinefelter are males with too many X chromosomes. They are infertile. The proportion of patients with the karyotype XXY is certainly higher than would appear from the list in Table 102: samples of blood from many of the more exotic karyotypes below the XXY row were selected for Xg grouping because of their special curiosity.

The karyotype XXY

Superficially one might expect men with two X chromosomes to have the female distribution of an X-linked character such as Xg. But, as may be seen from the XXY row of Table 102, this is not quite so: the observed proportion Xg(a+), 0·848, differs significantly from that expected of females which, based on the 6,784 samples of page 579, is 0·884. (The observed distribution of course differs wildly from that expected of males, 0·659 Xg(a+).)

The difference between the Xg distribution in XXY males and normal females is to be explained in the following way. If one of the two Xs came from the father and one from the mother then the normal female Xg distribution would be expected. When the two Xs come from the mother they may be different Xs in terms of the *Xg* locus, the one she had from her father and the one she had from her mother: XXY males of this origin again would be expected to have the normal

Table 102. Klinefelter's syndrome in Northern European males: distribution of the Xg groups

Karyotype	Total tested	Number Xg(a+)	Proportion Xg(a+)	χ_1^2 comparison with normal males	females
XXY	395	335	0·848	62·87	4·96
XXXY	12	11 ⎫			
XXXXY	33	28 ⎬	0·881	14·57	0·01
XXYY	22	20 ⎭			
XXY/XY	27	25 ⎫	0·957	18·13	2·36
other mosaics*	19	19 ⎭			
expected normal females			0·884		
expected normal males			0·659		

See text for acknowledgment to the physicians and cytogeneticists who sent most of the samples. This table records the results of Xg tests in the MRC Blood Group Unit up to the 7th of January, 1971 (Sanger, Tippett and Gavin[32], 1971). Some of the XXY collection have been published (Frøland et al.[8]; Ferguson-Smith et al.[9]; Court Brown et al.[2]; Race[10, 28, 33]; Race and Sanger[34]; Frøland et al.[11]) and so have some of the rarer karyotypes (XXXXY, Lewis et al.[12]; Frøland et al.[11]; Murken and Scholz[31]; XXYY, de la Chapelle et al.[13]; Pfeiffer et al.[14]. Thus caution will be needed in attempts to pool the data of the table above with other publications.

* XXY/XXYY, 3; XXY/XY/XXYY, 2; XXY/XX, 4; XXY/XXXY, 3; XXY/XXXY/XXXX, 1; XXY/XX/XY, 4; XXY/XO, 1; XXY/XX/XY/XXXY, 1.

21

female distribution of the groups. But, on the other hand, the mother may give to her XXY son two Xs which, again in terms of the *Xg* locus, are simply duplicate copies of one of her Xs, and XXYs of this origin would be expected to show the male distribution of the groups: it is the XXY males of this type that cause the difference between 0·848 and 0·884 Xg(a+).

So, the Xg frequencies alone indicate a heterogeneity of the site of origin of the non-disjunction. But the Xg groups of the parents of Klinefelter patients can be more informative, and it is hoped that when the figures are large enough they will allow an accurate calculation of the relative frequency of non-disjunction at the various stages of gametogenesis.

The Xg groups have already, in some families, given direct evidence about the site of the accident. In Figure 41 the Klinefelter son on the left is Xg(a+) and his mother is Xg(a−); therefore, he must have received his father's X carrying *Xgᵃ*, and his Y must have come from his father too. This fixes the accident of non-disjunction has having happened in the father, an X and a Y having got into one sperm. Further, the pedigree shows that the non-disjunction has been an accident of the first meiotic division: Figure 40 may help to show that if both X and Y are to get into one sperm they must take the false step at the first meiotic division (or perhaps earlier). If non-disjunction had happened at the second meiotic division sperm with two Xs or sperm with two Ys could result, but not sperm with an X *and* a Y.

That XXY could arise through an accident at spermatogenesis had been assumed but had been proved only in one mouse: the Klinefelter son on the left of Figure 41 provided the first proof in man (Frøland *et al.*[8], 1963). We have now tested several such families showing that the accident has happened at spermatogenesis.

The XXY son in the family on the right of Figure 41 has his father's Y but not his father's X, for the father's X carries *Xgᵃ* and the son is Xg(a−). Therefore both Xs of the son are maternal in origin, but it cannot be said at which meiotic division,

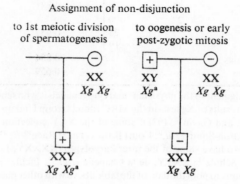

Fig. 41. Information provided by the **Xg** groups in two cases of XXY Klinefelter's syndrome. + = Xg(a+); − = Xg(a−).

first or second, the accident of non-disjunction happened. We have tested thirteen Northern European families in which the Xg groups show that both Xs are maternal.

When both parents of an XXY Klinefelter are available for testing the Xg groups will show whether the extra X is of maternal or paternal origin in about one-seventh of the cases. As will be seen later, it is more difficult to label the extra X of a Klinefelter as paternal or maternal than it is to label the single X of a Turner, though the Xg information about the site of the non-disjunction is more penetrating in the Klinefelter families.

Table 103 shows what is known about the Xg groups of the parents of the 395 XXY males of Table 102. At a stage when the total number of XXY males was less (190) the data were analysed by the formulae devised by Professor G.R. Fraser[17] and also by a computer method worked out by Professor J.H. Edwards at Birmingham. Both methods gave about the same answer to the following question: given the *Xg* gene frequencies for Northern Europeans, what proportions of the XXY males would be expected to have two maternal Xs, the same or different, and what proportion would be expected to have one maternal and one paternal X, to fit the observed frequencies of the Xg groups?

In 1971 Professor Edwards[35] analysed the data for the 395 XXY families in Table 103 with these results:

$$X^M X^P Y \quad 0{\cdot}39$$
$$Xg^{M_1} Xg^{M_2} Y \quad 0{\cdot}44$$
$$\left.\begin{array}{l} Xg^{M_1} Xg^{M_1} Y \\ Xg^{M_2} Xg^{M_2} Y \end{array}\right\} \; 0{\cdot}17$$

(Since, when the two Xs are maternal it is the *Xg* locus and not the whole chromosome which is being tracked, Professor Edwards suggested that in this event *Xg* rather than X should be written.)

Table 103. The extent of the parental data for the 395 XXY Klinefelter males of Table 102

Xg groups of			Source of the		Xg groups of			Source of the	
father	mother	Klinef.	extra X	Obs.	father	mother	Klinef.	extra X	Obs.
+	+	+	undisclosed	69	n.t.	+	+	undisclosed	40
+	+	−	maternal	5	n.t.	+	−	undisclosed	2
+	−	+	paternal	5	n.t.	−	+	paternal	2
+	−	−	maternal	5	n.t.	−	−	undisclosed	4
−	+	+	undisclosed	31	+	n.t.	+	undisclosed	3
−	+	−	undisclosed	4	+	n.t.	−	maternal	3
−		−	undisclosed	6	−	n.t.	+	undisclosed	2
					−	n.t.	−	undisclosed	2
					n.t.	n.t.	+	undisclosed	183
					n.t.	n.t.	−	undisclosed	29
				125					270

See footnote to Table 102.

Dr Côté[36], working with Professor Edwards, analysed a total of 506 XXY made up of the 395 of Table 103, a further 86 from our Unit and 25 from Winnipeg (Chown, personal communication to Côté, 1972): the results were 0.41 ± 0.10, 0.38 ± 0.10 and 0.21 ± 0.06 in the three classes of the last paragraph.

In Sardinia, where glucose-6-phosphate dehydrogenase deficiency is common, Professor Siniscalco and Dr Filippi and their colleagues[18] are studying the Xg groups, G6PD deficiency and colour blindness in the families of men with Klinefelter's syndrome, in the hope of getting evidence of the distance of the three loci from the centromere. Up to the present, 48 families have shown six of the propositi to be $X^M X^P Y$ (four by Xg and two by G6PD) and five propositi to be $X^M X^M Y$ (three by Xg and two by G6PD). These results are not included in Tables 102 or 103 because the frequency of the Xg groups in Sardinia differs from that in Northern Europe.

The karyotype XXXY

As may be seen from Table 102 this karyotype is relatively rare. Since the compilation of that table our total XXXY propositi has reached 16 and both parents of 7 of them were Xg grouped and in two families were informative (Zollinger and Mürset[37]; and Pfeiffer and Sanger[39]). A third informative family is reported by Greenstein et al.[38]

In two families[37, 38] the XXXY son is Xg(a−), the father Xg(a+) and the mother Xg(a−) thus showing that all 3 of the sons' Xs are maternal, and nondisjunction at both the first and second maternal meiotic divisions was assumed to be the most likely cause of the aneuploidy.

In the third family[39] the XXXY son is Xg(a−), his father Xg(a−), his mother Xg(a+); this mother must be heterozygous $Xg^a Xg$ because 2 of her 3 daughters are Xg(a−). Successive non-disjunction at the first and second paternal meiotic division was considered to be much the most likely cause of the aneuploidy.

The karyotype XXXXY

Thirty-three propositi (Table 102) and both parents of 29 of them were grouped in our Unit. Four families were informative (three of them published[12, 31]) and showed that the shower of Xs was all of the mothers' shedding: in each of these families the father was Xg(a+) and the mother and XXXXY son Xg(a−). (We presume that one Xg^a-carrying X would make detectable Xg^a antigen in face of three Xg-carrying Xs, but this is an opinion based only on tests of artificial mixtures of hemizygous Xg(a+) and Xg(a−) cells.) If all four Xs are usually maternal the easiest explanation is that disjunction had failed at the first and the second division of oogenesis, and this fits with the female distribution of the 33 propositi. The female distribution of Xg is, however, compatible with other theoretically possible backgrounds but does show that two post-zygotic non-disjunctions cannot be a frequent cause of the abnormality for, if they were, the Xg distribution would approach that of males: the observed distribution differs significantly from that of males, χ_1^2 being 5·34.

The karyotype XXYY

Twenty-two propositi have been grouped (Table 102) and both parents of 11 of them. In two of the families the groups are informative (de la Chapelle et al.[13] and Pfeiffer et al.[14]): the fathers are Xg(a+), the mothers Xg(a−) and the XXYY sons Xg(a+). The groups therefore show, in both the Finnish and German families, that the father has given an X to his son together with two Ys. Non-disjunction at first and second meiotic divisions in the formation of the sperm that produced the Klinefelter seems the most likely explanation. At the first division the X and Y instead of parting and going into two cells have stuck together and gone both into one cell. At the second division the two X chromosomes have parted correctly but this time the two Ys have stuck together. The sperm with one X and two Ys then fertilized a normal ovum, making an XXYY zygote. The Finnish family provided the first evidence in man that non-disjunction at consecutive meiotic divisions is possible. Such double paternal non-disjunction was later invoked to explain one of the XXXY propositi above.

XXY/mosaics

The Xg groups are giving some rather surprising information about Klinefelters with a mosaic karyotype. Such people all have some cells XXY but they all have other cell lines as well: the commonest mosaic of this sort is XXY/XY. We had supposed that these mosaics arose post-meiotically from non-disjunction at an early mitotic division of the zygote and we assumed that the zygote was straight-forward XY. But if mosaic Klinefelters do result from misdivisions of an XY zygote they would be expected to have a distribution of the Xg groups just that of normal XY men. But they do not: the 46 XXY mosaics of Table 102, mostly patients of Professor Ferguson-Smith, have an Xg distribution which differs very significantly from that of males ($\chi_1^2 = 18\cdot13$) and is indeed slightly ultra-female ($\chi_1^2 = 2\cdot36$). So, these mosaics cannot, except perhaps on rare occasion, result from post-zygotic non-disjunction of an XY zygote: presumably they usually arise from mitotic non-disjunction of an XXY zygote.

XX males

The existence of the very rare XX males has perhaps stimulated more thought than has been given to any other sex chromosome abnormality. The subject was admirably reviewed by de la Chapelle[40] (1972).

The finding of the first and second XX males was reported by de la Chapelle, Hortling, Niemi, Wennström and Johansson[15, 16], 1964, 1965. The Xg groups in each family (one is given in Figure 42) appeared to show that both Xs were

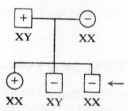

Fig. 42. The Xg groups of the family of the first known XX male. (After de la Chapelle, Hortling, Niemi and Wennström[15], 1964.) Arrow = propositus, + = Xg(a+), − = Xg(a−).

maternal and it was concluded that such people arose from XXY zygotes and that the Y, after initiating male development, became lost. But slowly, as more XX males were tested their Xg distribution began to look like that of XY males and this fitted in with a very attractive idea (Ferguson-Smith[20], 1966), yet to be disproved, about the possibility of interchange between a small part of the tip of the short arm of the X and of the Y. The consequences of such an interchange, were it an occasional possibility, are brilliantly pursued by Professor Polani in a paper which he is at present preparing.

The 45 XX males of Table 104, all Northern Europeans, are the collection of 12 years, but the numbers are still too few to give a decisive answer as can be seen from the analysis at the foot of the table, for which a method devised by Professor C.A.B. Smith was used. When the total was 39 analysis by Côté[36] also pointed slightly in favour of an XXY origin rather than interchange (3·4 to 1).

Table 104. Xg groups of XX males (Blood Group Unit counts to end of 1973)

	Xg(a+)		χ_1^2 comparisons with		
Total tested	number	proportion	males	females	XXY
45	35	0·778	2·83	4·95*	1·72*
Expected, normal males		0·659			
Expected, normal females		0·884			
Observed in 395 XXY		0·848			

* The expected Xg(a−) figures in these two comparisons are rather small for the χ^2 test, but a method of Professor C.A.B. Smith for this situation gives the answer:
The Xg distribution is 1·8 times more likely to be male than female.
The Xg distribution is 2·1 times more likely to be XXY than male.
The Xg distribution is 3·7 times more likely to be XXY than female.

The information we have about the Xg groups of the parents of the XX males is given in Table 105. In six of the families the groups are informative (2++−, 3+−− and 1 nt−− in which the father must have been + for three sisters of the propositus are +) and show both Xs of the XX male to be maternal: this appears to support the XXY origin of at any rate these 6 XX males. However, both Xs are

Table 105. Parental data for the 45 male XX of Table 104

Xg groups of				Xg groups of			
father	mother	XX male	No.	father	mother	XX male	No.
+	+	+	15	+	nt	+	0
+	+	−	2	+	nt	−	0
+	−	+	1	−	nt	+	0
+	−	−	3	−	nt	−	0
−	+	+	6	nt	+	+	6
−	+	−	0	nt	+	−	1
−	−	−	0	nt	−	+	0
				nt	−	−	2
				nt	nt	+	7
				nt	nt	−	2

not always maternal in origin as shown by the $+-+$ family of Table 105 and by a Japanese XX male[41].

TURNER'S SYNDROME

People with the syndrome named after Turner are females but they have various things wrong with their gonads and with other parts of their body. They are infertile and are almost always under five feet in height. Several karyotypes may cause the condition but the basic trouble is usually the lack of the whole of one X or, less commonly, the lack of the short arm of one X.

The proportion of patients with the karyotype XO is probably higher than would appear from Table 106: many of the other examples must have been selected for their special curiosity.

The patients of Table 106 have, as expected, the male Xg distribution. The reason is obvious in the XOs who have a single X in any one of their cells. The distribution to be expected in the XXqi, XO/XXqi, XXp−, and XO/XXp− depends on the answer to two questions—whether the *Xg* locus is involved in the preferential inactivation of a defective X chromosome (Muldal *et al.*,[44] 1963) and whether the *Xg* locus is sited on the short or the long arm of the X. These questions will be discussed below: here it is enough to say that the Xg distribution in the XXqi etc. class is clearly male.

The figures for the XO/XY class are nearly twice as likely to represent a female rather than a male distribution; this is surprising, though the numbers are small.

The Xg groups of other classes of Turner's syndrome are listed by Sanger *et al.*[32]

In one-third of the families the Xg groups make clear whether the single X of a Turner is of maternal or paternal origin, but the groups cannot show, as they may so neatly in Klinefelter's syndrome, just where the causative accident has happened. For example, in Figure 43 the family on the left shows that the sole X

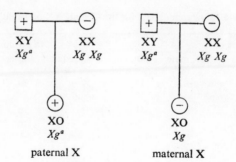

Fig. 43. Source of the single X in Turner's syndrome. (After Lindsten *et al.*[23], 1963.)

possessed by the XO Turner girl is her father's, since she can have inherited her *Xgᵃ* only from him. This family, nearly eleven years ago, provided the first convincing proof that the single X of a Turner can be paternal in origin: belief was mounting that the missing X was always the father's fault, but here the accident has happened to a maternal X. The family on the right of Figure 43 shows that the sole X possessed by the Turner girl is from her mother: the girl cannot have her father's X because it carried *Xgᵃ* and she is Xg(a−).

Table 106. Turner's syndrome in Northern European females: distribution of the Xg groups of patients with one short arm of the X (from Sanger, Tippett and Gavin[32], 1971)

Karyotype	Total tested	Number Xg(a+)	Proportion Xg(a+)	χ_1^2 comparison with normal	
				males	females
XO	326	227	0·696	2·02	111·96
XXqi	37	22 ⎫			
XO/XXqi	66	46 ⎪			
XXp−	7	4 ⎬ 0·649		0·05	61·37
XO/XXp−	4	2 ⎭			
XO/XY	21	17			
	461	318	0·690	1·95	169·51

Recommended cytogenetic notation (Chicago Conference[29], 1966)

The diagonal stroke separates cell lines in describing mosaicism.

Xqi = isochromosome for the long arm of the X, that is an X with no short arm but two long arms (q = long arm of a chromosome).

Xp− = an X chromosome lacking a short arm but without duplication of the long arm (p = short arm of a chromosome).

See page 621 for acknowledgement to the physicians and cytogeneticists who sent most of the samples. This table records the results of Xg tests in the M.R.C. Blood Group Unit up to the 7th of January, 1971. Only a few of the cases have been published (Lindsten *et al.*[23, 24, 25], Court-Brown *et al.*[2], Turpin *et al.*[26, 27], Race[10, 28], Dahl *et al.*[46]) but others no doubt will be. Thus caution will be needed in attempts to pool the data of the table above with those of publications in the future.

Both parents of 324 of the 461 patients of Table 106 were grouped with the results shown in the top part of Table 107. In 102, or about a third of the 324 families, Xg shows whether the single normal X of an XO, XXqi, etc. Turner is paternal or maternal.

The three father-mother-Turner Xg arrangements which can demonstrate a maternal X in the Turner are commoner than the one which can demonstrate a paternal X, so mathematical tests are needed to show what proportion of the normal Xs of XO Turners are indeed maternal and what proportion paternal. Fraser[17] (1963) provided formulae which, when applied to the 234 XO families of Table 107 where father, mother and Turner have been grouped, give the answer that of the XO patients about 77% are X^MO and 23% are X^PO. For computer analysis Professor J.H. Edwards used the same 234 XO families, together with the further 41 XOs of Table 107 with only one parent tested: the answer came out 78% X^MO and 22% X^PO.

Table 107. Parental Xg information about the 461 females with Turner's syndrome listed in Table 106 (from Sanger, Tippett and Gavin[32], 1971)

F	M	T	Source of Normal X	XO	XXqi	XO/XXqi	XXp–	XO/XXp–	XO/XY	Total
+	+	+	?	117	16	24	0	1	2	
+	+	–	maternal	23	4	5	0	1	1	
+	–	+	paternal	3	1	1	0	0	0	
+	–	–	maternal	7	0	1	0	0	0	
–	+	+	maternal	44	2	5	2	0	2	
–	+	–	?	27	4	8	2	0	1	
–	–	–	?	13	5	1	0	1	0	
		Total		234	32	45	4	3	6	324
+	·	+	?	2	0	1	0	0	1	
+	·	–	maternal	1	0	1	0	1	0	
–	·	+	maternal	1	0	0	0	0	0	
–	·	–	?	0	0	0	0	0	0	
·	+	+	?	28	1	9	0	0	3	
·	+	–	?	5	2	2	0	0	0	
·	–	+	paternal	1	0	0	0	0	0	
·	–	–	?	3	0	0	0	0	0	
·	·	+	?	32	2	5	2	0	9	
·	·	–	?	19	0	3	1	0	2	
		Total		326	37	66	7	4	21	461

F = father; M = mother; T = Turner; + = Xg(a+); – = Xg(a–); · = not tested; ? = not disclosed.

22

OTHER ABNORMAL FEMALE KARYOTYPES

XXX females

Such females may be fertile but their intelligence is sometimes impaired.

Were non-disjunction at oogenesis the usual cause of XXX, a series of such women would be expected to show an ultra-female distribution of Xg if either there were recombination between the locus and the centromere, or if non-disjunction were at the first meiotic division. If, on the other hand, non-disjunction at spermatogenesis were the usual cause, a normal female distribution of the groups would be expected.

Samples of blood from 65 XXX women have been sent for Xg grouping, mostly from the MRC Clinical and Population Cytogenetics Unit and from Professor Polani at Guys. All but 3 were Xg(a+): this suggests, but is not significant ($\chi_1^2 = 3\cdot1$) of, an ultra-female distribution.

Both parents of 20 patients have been grouped, but Xg cannot give direct evidence of the source of the extra X in these families.

XXXX females

We have been sent samples of blood from only eight such people. Seven were Xg(a+) and one Xg(a−). The one Xg(a−) girl was reported by de Grouchy et al.[42] (1968); her father was Xg(a+), her mother Xg(a−), and we have nothing to add to the following comment:

(i) There is very good reason to believe that the legal father is the biological father. (ii) We presume that one Xg^a will make its presence felt in the company of three Xg genes (see XXXXY section above). (iii) Assuming that (ii) is correct, then the father has contributed no X to the XXXX daughter, and our guess is that all four Xs were present in the egg-cell nucleus. This could come about by successive non-disjunction at the first and second meiotic divisions at oogenesis. If the father's sperm carried a Y, there is no obvious reason why the Y should be rejected from the nucleus of the zygote, for XXXXYs are relatively common compared with XXXXX, which is an extreme rarity; it may be that five Xs are usually too many for the mitotic divisions of the zygote to cope with and that one is rejected. (Race and Sanger[34], 1969.)

XXXXX females

We have grouped only one such sample sent to us by Dr Larget-Piet, of Angers: the patient was Xg(a+), her father Xg(a−) and her mother Xg(a+) but this does not tell us how many of the Xs are maternal.

Females lacking the long arm of an X

Table 108 shows the Xg groups of such females as we have tested. There is an excess of Xg(a−) propositi, 9 out of 18 (leaving out the one XX/XXq−): this distribution does not differ significantly from that expected of males but does so, very significantly, from that expected of normal females; it is, we think, 1,165 times more likely to represent a male than a female distribution. (If only the 10 XXpi and XXq– are considered then their Xg distribution is 50 times more likely to be male than female.) This category of patients is involved in the question of inactivation of the *Xg* locus to be discussed below.

Table 108 was compiled before grouping the XXpi case of de la Chapelle and his colleagues[47]: the propositus is a remarkably weak Xg(a+), her father is Xg(a+) and her mother Xg(a–).

Table 108. Xg groups of 19 propositi with an X lacking a long arm (from Sanger, Tippett and Gavin[32], 1971)

Karyotype	Father	Mother	Propositus	Identity	Case of
XXpi	−	+	−	U.R.*	Lindsten
	·	·	+	PRU 752/2065*	Polani
XXq–	+	+	+	PRU 126/100*	Polani
	+	+	−	PRU 748/98*	Polani
	−	+	+	Di.	Van Went
	−	+	−	H.F.*	Philip
	+	·	+	Lo.	Richards
	·	·	+	Boy.	Lucas
	·	·	−	17/59*	Court Brown
	·	·	−	Z.C.*	Crawfurd
XO/XXq–	+	+	+	34/62*	Court Brown
	+	+	+	H.L.*	Lindsten
	+	+	+	PRU 4604	Polani
	+	+	+	Le.	de Grouchy
	+	−	−	R.H.*	de la Chapelle
	+	−	−	De.	Ferguson-Smith
	−	+	−	L.P.*	Grove-Rasmussen
	−	+	−	Bog.	Dahl
XX/Xq–	·	−	−	L.H.*	Davidson

+ = Xg(a+); − = Xg(a–); · = not tested.
* The 12 of these cases included in Polani *et al.* (1970).

XY females

Testicular feminization. This rare and interesting syndrome has been mentioned on page 607. These XY females have, as would be expected, a male and not a female distribution of the Xg groups. Indeed the 77 Northern European propositi we have tested have a significantly ultra-male distribution: 41 Xg(a+) and 36 Xg(a–) for which $\chi_1^2 = 5·49$ and the probability 1 in 50, though we cannot bring ourselves to believe that this is significant of anything but chance. (Amongst the 77 propositi are the 7 Polish patients about whom and whose families Boczkowski[19] gave details.)

Pure gonadal dysgenesis. Some females with this condition are XY; we have tested 14 such of whom 9 were Xg(a+).

Other sex abnormalities

The Xg groups in series of other conditions are listed by Sanger *et al.*[32]: conditions such as male pseudo-hermaphroditism, hypospadias, pure gonadal dysgenesis, true hermaphroditism, 'intersex', male Turner's syndrome, Bonnevie-Ullrich syndrome and primary amenorrhoea.

X CHROMOSOME ABNORMALITIES AND THE QUESTION OF Xg INACTIVATION

We have given reasons on page 585 for believing that the *Xg* locus escapes inactivation when carried on a structurally normal X. Sanger, Tippett and Gavin[32] describe the state of affairs when the *Xg* locus is carried on an *abnormal* X as follows:

If because of its behaviour on a normal X we suppose that *Xg* is not subject to inactivation when carried on an *abnormal* X we are faced with a paradox. In Table 107 there are 13 XXqi or XXp− patients, with or without XO cell lines, who are Xg(a−) with Xg(a+) fathers and they would seem to place the *Xg* locus on the missing short arm: in Table 108, on the other hand, there is one XXq− and two XO/XXq− patients who are Xg(a−) with Xg(a+) fathers, and they would seem to place the missing *Xg* locus on the long arm. Polani *et al.*[43] (1970) concluded that this contradiction could only be resolved by assuming that, in the known preferential inactivation of an abnormal X (Muldal *et al.*[44]), the *Xg* locus is also inactivated.

Inactivation of *Xg* would also explain the unquestionably male distribution of Xg in the 114 XXqi, XXp− etc., of Table 107 and the 18 XXq− etc. of Table 108. The evidence provided by the XXp− etc. and XXq− etc. when mosaic with an XO cell line was realized to depend on the proportion of the two cell lines in the marrow of the mosaic[43]. This possible complication was recently illustrated by the family reported by Buckton *et al.*[45] mentioned on page 585. However, excluding the demonstrable mosaics does not alter the picture: in Table 107 the XXp− and XXqi that remain have a male distribution of Xg which differs very significantly from the female; in Table 108 the 10 XXpi or XXq− that remain have an Xg distribution 50 times more like male than female.

The present evidence is therefore that the *Xg* locus is not subject to inactivation when carried on a normal X, and probably is subject to inactivation when carried on a deleted X.

So the Xg groups have made a good contribution to knowledge in the field of sex-chromosome aneuploidy.

REFERENCES

1   TURPIN R. and LEJEUNE J. (1965) *Les Chromosomes Humains*, pp. 535, Gauthier-Villars Paris.
2   COURT BROWN W.M., HARNDEN D.G,. JACOBS PATRICIA A., MACLEAN N. and MANTLE D.J.

(1964) *Abnormalities of the Sex Chromosome Complement in Man*, pp. 239, H.M. Stationery Office, London.

3   BARR M.L., CARR D.H., CLARKE C.M., FORD C.E., FRACCARO M., HAMERTON J.L., HARNDEN D.G., POLANI P.E., SMITHELLS R.W. and SYMONDS N.D. (1962) *Chromosomes in Medicine*, ed. J. L. Hamerton, National Spastics Society and Heinemann, London, pp. 231.

4   MCKUSICK V.A. (1962) On the X chromosome of man. *Quart. Rev. Biol.*, **37**, 69–175 and (1964) American Institute of Biological Sciences, Washington, pp. 141.

5   POLANI P.E. (1965) Sex-chromosome anomalies: recent developments. *Sci. Basis Med. Ann. Review*, 141–163.

6   POLANI P.E. (1965) The sex chromosomes of man and their anomalies. *Proc. R. Instn. Gt. Br.*, **40**, 427–445.

7   POLANI P.E., LESSOF M.H. and BISHOP P.M.F. (1956) Colour-blindness in ovarian agenesis. *Lancet*, **ii**, 118–120.

8   FRØLAND A., JOHNSEN S.G., ANDRESEN P., DEIN E., SANGER RUTH and RACE R.R. (1963) Non-disjunction and XXY men. *Lancet*, **ii**, 1121–1122.

9   FERGUSON-SMITH M.A., MACK W.S., ELLIS PATRICIA M., DICKSON MARION, SANGER RUTH and RACE R.R. (1964) Parental age and the source of the X chromosomes in XXY Klinefelter's syndrome. *Lancet*, **i**, 46.

10 RACE R.R. (1965) Identification of the origin of the X chromosome(s) in sex chromosome aneuploidy. *Can. J. Genet. Cytol.*, **7**, 214–222.

11 FRØLAND A., SANGER RUTH and RACE R.R. (1968) Xg blood group studies on 76 patients with Klinefelter's syndrome and on their parents. *J. med. Genet.*, **5**, 161–164.

12 LEWIS F.J.W., FRØLAND A., SANGER RUTH and RACE R.R. (1964) Source of the X chromosomes in two XXXXY males. *Lancet*, **ii**, 589.

13 DE LA CHAPELLE A., HORTLING H., SANGER RUTH and RACE R.R. (1964) Successive non-disjunction at first and second meiotic division of spermatogenesis: evidence of chromosomes and Xg. *Cytogenetics*, **3**, 334–341.

14 PFEIFFER R.A., KÖRVER G., SANGER RUTH and RACE R.R. (1966) Paternal origin of an XXYY anomaly. *Lancet*, **i**, 1427–1428.

15 DE LA CHAPELLE A., HORTLING H., NIEMI M. and WENNSTRÖM J. (1964) XX sex chromosomes in a human male. First case. *Acta med. scand.*, *Suppl.*, **412**, 25–38.

16 DE LA CHAPELLE A., HORTLING H., WENNSTRÖM J., NIEMI M. and JOHANSSON C.-J. (1965) Two males with female chromosomes. *Acta endocr. Copenh.*, Abstract 58, Suppl. 100, 90.

17 FRASER G.R. (1963) Parental origin of the sex chromosomes in the XO and XXY karyotypes in man. *Ann. hum. Genet.*, **26**, 297–304; and see FRASER G.R. (1966), Corrigenda and addendum. *Ann. hum. Genet.*, **29**, 323.

18 FILIPPI G., ROSSI DE CAPOA A., RACE R.R., SANGER R., SINISCALCO M., VAN WENT J.J. and WENT L.N. (1967) Distribuzione della enzimopemia g-6-pd del Daltonismo e dell'antigene Xgᵃ in un gruppo di Klinefelters Sardi. *Proc. Ital. Genet. Soc.* (Abstract).

19 PENROSE L.S. (1961) *Recent Advances in Human Genetics*, p. 14, Churchill, London.

20 FERGUSON-SMITH M.A. (1966) X-Y chromosomal interchange in the aetiology of true hermaphroditism and of XX Klinefelter's syndrome. *Lancet*, **ii**, 475–476.

21 SANGER RUTH, RACE R.R., TIPPETT PATRICIA, GAVIN JUNE, HARDISTY R.M. and DUBOWITZ V. (1964) Unexplained inheritance of the Xg groups in two families. *Lancet*, **i**, 955–956.

22 NOADES JEAN, GAVIN JUNE, TIPPETT PATRICIA, SANGER RUTH and RACE R.R. (1966) The X-linked blood group system Xg. Tests on British, Northern American, and Northern European unrelated people and families. *J. Med. Genet.*, **3**, 162–168.

23 LINDSTEN J., BOWEN P., LEE CATHERINE S.N., MCKUSICK V.A., POLANI P.E., WINGATE M., EDWARDS J.H., HAMPER JEAN, TIPPETT PATRICIA, SANGER RUTH and RACE R.R. (1963) Source of the X in XO females: the evidence of Xg. *Lancet*, **i**, 558–559.

24 LINDSTEN J., FRACCARO M., POLANI P.E., HAMERTON J.L., SANGER RUTH and RACE R.R.

(1963) Evidence that the Xg blood group genes are on the short arm of the X chromosome. *Nature, Lond.*, **197**, 648–649.

[25] LINDSTEN J., FRACCARO M., IKKOS D., KAIJSER K., KLINGER H.P. and LUFT R. (1963) Presumptive iso-chromosomes for the long arm of X in man. Analysis of five families. *Ann. hum. Genet.*, **26**, 383–395.

[26] TURPIN R., LEJEUNE J. and SALMON C. (1965) Discussion de l'origine paternelle de l'X d'un s. de Turner XO, protanope et Xg(a–). *C.R. Acad. Sc., Paris*, **260**, 369–372.

[27] TURPIN R., LEJEUNE J. and SALMON C. (1965) Discussion de l'origine paternelle de l'X d'un syndrome de Turner XO, protanope et Xg(a–). Nouvelle estimation numérique. *C.R. Acad. Sc., Paris*, **261**, 1381–1383.

[28] RACE R.R. (1965) Contributions of blood groups to human genetics. *Proc. Roy. Soc.*, B, **163**, 151–168.

[29] Chicago Conference: Standardization in human cytogenetics (1966) *Birth Defects Original Article Series*, **2**, 1–21.

[30] NANCE W.E. and UCHIDA IRENE (1964) Turner's syndrome, twinning, and an unusual variant of glucose-6-phosphate dehydrogenase. *Amer. J. hum. Genet.*, **16**, 380–392.

[31] MURKEN J.-D. and SCHOLZ W. (1968) Serologische Klärung der Herkunft der überzähligen X-Chromosomen beim XXXXY-Syndrom. *Blut*, **16**, 164–168.

[32] SANGER RUTH, TIPPETT PATRICIA and GAVIN JUNE (1971) Xg groups and sex abnormalities in people of Northern European ancestry. *J. Med. Genet.*, **8**, 417–426.

[33] RACE R.R. (1970) The Xg blood groups and sex-chromosome aneuploidy. *Phil. Trans. R. Soc.* **259**, 37–40.

[34] RACE R.R. and SANGER RUTH (1969) Xg and sex-chromosome abnormalities. *Brit. Med. Bull.*, **25**, 99–103.

[35] EDWARDS J.H. (1971) On the distribution of phenotypes in XXY males and their parents. *J. Med. Genet.*, **8**, 434–437.

[36] COTÉ G.B. (1973) On the origin of 46,XX and 47,XXY males, 46,XY females and the position of the Xg locus. *Ann. Hum. Genet.*, **37**, 21–30.

[37] ZOLLINGER H. and MÜRSET GERTRUD (1969) Personal communication cited in references 34, 32 and 39.

[38] GREENSTEIN R.M., HARRIS D.J., LUZZATTI L. and CANN H.M. (1970) Cytogenetic analysis of a boy with the XXXY syndrome: origin of the X-chromosomes. *Pediatrics*, **45**, 677–686.

[39] PFEIFFER R.A. and SANGER RUTH (1973) Origin of 48,XXXY: the evidence of the Xg blood groups. *J. Med. Genet.*, **10**, 142–143.

[40] DE LA CHAPELLE, A. (1972) Nature and origin of males with XX sex chromosomes. *Amer. J. Hum. Genet.*, **24**, 71–105.

[41] MORI Y., MIZUTANI S., SONODA T. *et al.* (1969) XX-male: a case report. *Jap. J. Urol.*, **60**, 279–285. (Not seen. Cited by de la Chapelle[40].)

[42] DE GROUCHY J., BRISSAUD H.E., RICHARDET J.M., REPÉSSÉ G., SANGER RUTH, RACE R.R., SALMON C. and SALMON DENISE (1968) Syndrome 48,XXXX chez une enfant de six ans transmission anormale du groupe Xg. *Annls. Génét.*, **11**, 120–124.

[43] POLANI P.E., ANGELL ROSLYN, GIANNELLI F., DE LA CHAPELLE A., RACE R.R. and SANGER RUTH (1970) Evidence that the Xg locus is inactivated in structurally abnormal X-chromosomes. *Nature, Lond.*, **227**, 613–616.

[44] MULDAL S., GILBERT C.W., LAJTHA L.G., LINDSTEN J., ROWLEY J. and FRACCARO M. (1963) Tritiated thymidine incorporation in an isochromosome for the long arm of the X chromosome in man. *Lancet*, i, 861–863.

[45] BUCKTON KARIN E., CUNNINGHAM CATHERINE, NEWTON MARJORIE S., O'RIORDAN MAUREEN L. and SANGER RUTH (1971) Anomalous Xg inheritance with a probable explanation. *Lancet*, i, 371–373.

[46] DAHL G. and ANDERSEN H. (1972) Chromosome studies in 30 children with Turner's syndrome. *Acta paediat. scand.*, **61**, 17–23.

[47] DE LA CHAPELLE A., SCHRÖDER J. and PERNU M. (1972) Isochromosome for the short arm of X, a human 46,*XXpi* syndrome. *Ann. Hum. Genet.*, **36**, 79–87.

[48] SOLTAN H.C. (1968) Genetic characteristics of families of XO and XXY patients, including evidence of source of X chromosome in 7 aneuploid patients *J. Med. Genet.*, **5**, 173–180.

[49] BOCZKOWSKI K. (1968) Genetical studies in testicular feminization syndrome. *J. Med. Genet.*, **5**, 181–188.

Distribution of χ^2

n	Probability													
	·99	·98	·95	·90	·80	·70	·50	·30	·20	·10	·05	·02	·01	·001
1	·0^{3}157	·0^{3}628	·00393	·0158	·0642	·148	·455	1·074	1·642	2·706	3·841	5·412	6·635	10·827
2	·0201	·0404	·103	·211	·446	·713	1·386	2·408	3·219	4·605	5·991	7·824	9·210	13·815
3	·115	·185	·352	·584	1·005	1·424	2·366	3·665	4·642	6·251	7·815	9·837	11·341	16·268
4	·297	·429	·711	1·064	1·649	2·195	3·357	4·878	5·989	7·779	9·488	11·668	13·277	18·465
5	·554	·752	1·145	1·610	2·343	3·000	4·351	6·064	7·289	9·236	11·070	13·388	15·086	20·517
6	·872	1·134	1·635	2·204	3·070	3·828	5·348	7·231	8·558	10·645	12·592	15·033	16·812	22·457
7	1·239	1·564	2·167	2·833	3·822	4·671	6·346	8·383	9·803	12·017	14·067	16·622	18·475	24·322
8	1·646	2·032	2·733	3·490	4·594	5·527	7·344	9·524	11·030	13·362	15·507	18·168	20·090	26·125
9	2·088	2·532	3·325	4·168	5·380	6·393	8·343	10·656	12·242	14·684	16·919	19·679	21·666	27·877
10	2·558	3·059	3·940	4·865	6·179	7·267	9·342	11·781	13·442	15·987	18·307	21·161	23·209	29·588
11	3·053	3·609	4·575	5·578	6·989	8·148	10·341	12·899	14·631	17·275	19·675	22·618	24·725	31·264
12	3·571	4·178	5·226	6·304	7·807	9·034	11·340	14·011	15·812	18·549	21·026	24·054	26·217	32·909
13	4·107	4·765	5·892	7·042	8·634	9·926	12·340	15·119	16·985	19·812	22·362	25·472	27·688	34·528
14	4·660	5·368	6·571	7·790	9·467	10·821	13·339	16·222	18·151	21·064	23·685	26·873	29·141	36·123
15	5·229	5·985	7·261	8·547	10·307	11·721	14·339	17·322	19·311	22·307	24·996	28·259	30·578	37·697
16	5·812	6·614	7·962	9·312	11·152	12·624	15·338	18·418	20·465	23·542	26·296	29·633	32·000	39·252
17	6·408	7·255	8·672	10·085	12·002	13·531	16·338	19·511	21·615	24·769	27·587	30·995	33·409	40·790
18	7·015	7·906	9·390	10·865	12·857	14·440	17·338	20·601	22·760	25·989	28·869	32·346	34·805	42·312
19	7·633	8·567	10·117	11·651	13·716	15·352	18·338	21·689	23·900	27·204	30·144	33·687	36·191	43·820
20	8·260	9·237	10·851	12·443	14·578	16·266	19·337	22·775	25·038	28·412	31·410	35·020	37·566	45·315

This table is reprinted (abridged) from Table IV of Fisher and Yates: *Statistical Tables for Biological, Agricultural and Medical Research*, published by Oliver & Boyd Ltd., Edinburgh, by permission of the authors and publishers.

n = number of degrees of freedom.

Addenda

Chapter 2. The ABO Groups

Attention should be drawn to *Blood Group Substances: Their Nature and Genetics*, a recent review by Winifred M. Watkins. It deals with ABO, Lewis, MNSs, P_1 and Rh (D). It is Chapter 7 in *The Red Blood Cell*, volume 1, 2nd edition, 1974, Ed. D. MacN. Surgenor, Academic Press Inc., New York and London.

A family of Finnish extraction with a dominant B variant is reported by Zelenski *et al.* (1974, *Vox Sang.*, **26**, 189–193). It seems to us that this variant could possibly be squeezed into the rather broad first category of page 19, depending on whether salivary B could be demonstrated when the test system was anti-B with the person's own weak B cells as indicator.

At the 17th Annual Meeting of the American Association of Blood Banks two families were reported in which several members were $A_2 + O$ mosaics; an allele at the *ABO* locus was thought to be the most likely cause (Marsh *et al.* 1974, *Transfusion, Philad.*, **14**, 506, Abstract). We wonder whether this could be an echo of the Japanese family described by Furuhata *et al.* (Cited on page 18, Chapter 2).

For the *ABO* and for the *P* genes we wish we had used the symbols A^1 and A^2 rather than A_1 and A_2, and P^1 and P^2 rather than P_1 and P_2.

Chapter 3. The MNSs Blood Groups

On page 42 we gave references to conflicting opinions whether or not the MNSs antigens were present on leucocytes. Marsh *et al.* (1974, *Transfusion*, **14**, 462–466) find that neutrophil leukocytes have U but lack M, N, S and s.

Stoltz *et al.* (1974, *Vox Sang.*, **26**, 467–469) measured the effect of anti-M on the electrophoretic mobility of the lymphocytes of 34 donors. Slowing of mobility was shown only by the samples from M and MN donors. The authors concluded 'our results indirectly demonstrate the fixation of antibodies on the lymphocyte membrane and consequently the corresponding antigen'.

A hopeful source of anti-N lectin is described by Moon and Wiener (1974, *Vox Sang.*, **26**, 167–170): an extract of the leaves of *Vicia unijuga* from Korea. The extract needs to be absorbed with M cells.

Chapter 4. The P Blood Groups

During 1974, chemical knowledge of the antigens of the P system was greatly increased and before long a more firmly based genetical pathway scheme should take the place of previous attempts (see page 161 *et seq.*).

Naiki and Marcus (1974, *Biochem. Biophys. Res. Commun.*, **60**, 1105–1111) working with red cell extracts identified the P antigen as the glycosphingolipid globoside, βGalNAc(1 → 3)αGal(1 → 4)βGal(1 → 4)Glc-cer, and the P^k antigen as ceramide trihexoside, αGal(1 → 4)βGal(1 → 4)Glc-cer.

Cory, Yates, Donald, Watkins and Morgan (1974, *Biochem. Biophys. Res. Commun.*, **61**, 1289–96) working with sheep hydatid cyst fluid find the P_1 determinant to be D-galactosyl-α(1 → 4)-D-galactosyl-β(1 → 4)-N-acetyl-D-glucosamine.

Chapter 5. The Rh Blood Groups

After the printing of Table 38 (pages 211–12) we were told of two more families with $-D-/-D-$ members, one by Miss Marjory Stroup of Raritan and the other by Dr G. Reali of Genoa. Both the white American and the Ligurian family add to two counts of such families which have for long puzzled us: the highly significant excess of consanguinity in the parents of the propositi and the excess of homozygous $-D-/-D-$ amongst the sibs of the propositi (page 214). The parents of the American propositus (Z.C.) were double first cousins, and 2 of her 4 sibs were $-D-/-D-$: of the Ligurian propositus (I.M.) the parents were first cousins, and 4 of her 6 sibs were $-D-/-D-$. The excessive consanguinity was already very highly significant, but the addition of these two families now make the sibship count significant ($\chi_1^2 = 6\cdot8$) even excluding C^wD- and $cD-$ homozygotes.

Spielmann *et al.* (1974, *Vox Sang.*, **27**, 473–477) report the finding of anti-ce (anti-f) in a $CDe/cD-$ mother of a haemolytic disease child, the first time anti-ce has been found in a person of this genotype.

The difficult problem of the specificity of the antibodies anti-V, −VS etc. (see pages 206 *et seq.*) was investigated by Tregellas and Issitt (1974, *Transfusion, Philad.*, **14**, 506. Meeting abstract); and no doubt a full account will soon be published.

A second example of anti-D^w (pages 193–4) was recently identified by Miss G. Kaczmarski and by our Unit in a serum containing other Rh antibodies.

Chapter 7. The Kell Blood Groups

More information about the relationship of the Kell system to chronic granulomatous disease (pages 296–8) is to be found in Marsh *et al.* (1975, *Brit. J. Haemat.* **29,** 247–262). 'Lack of red cell Kx is associated with the McLeod pheotype, lack of leucocyte Kx is associated with chronic granulomatous disease.'

Chapter 8. Secretors and Non-secretors

Using precipitin tests Napier *et al.* (1974, *Vox Sang.*, **27**, 447–458) demonstrated two distinct lectin specificities in *Lotus tetragonolobus* seed extracts. This may have a bearing on certain difficulties in using this extract as an anti-H reagent (see page 316).

Chapter 10. The Duffy Blood Groups

Another example of anti-Fy3 has been found in Fy(a–b–) transfused patient (pages 356–7), but this time the patient *is* a Negro (Oberdorfer *et al.*, 1974, *Transfusion, Philad.*, **14**, 608–611).

Chapter 23. Some Other Antigens

A 'new' antigen called In^a with a frequency of about 2 to 4% in Bombay was reported by Badakere *et al.* (1973, *Ind. J. med. Res.*, **61**, 563 and 1974, *Vox Sang.*, **26**, 400–403). A convincing case for the existence of the antithetical antibody, anti-In^b, was made by Giles (1975, *Vox Sang.*, in the press), and the controlling locus was shown to be independent of *ABO, MNSs, Kidd* and of X and Y.

Chapter 26. Blood Groups in Twins and Chimeras

A further twin chimera pair (see Table 92, pages 522–4) is recorded in a paper on automatic grouping (Garretta *et al.*, 1974, *Vox Sang.*, **27**, 141–155): C. Mer., male, A 33%, B 67%, sec. A and H; C. Mer. female, A 21%, B 79%, sec. B and H.

Chapter 27. Blood Groups and Mapping of the Autosomes

To the list of autosomal blood group loci and their linkages (Table 95, page 561) can be added another 'probable'. The lod score for *P* and *reinclusion of molar 1*, at $\theta = 0.0$, amounts to +2·14, not far off significance (Nijenhuis *et al.*, *Cytogenetics and Cell Genetics*, 1975, in press).

The enzyme UMPK (uridine monophosphate kinase) was shown to be polymorphic (Giblett *et al.*, 1974, *Amer. J. hum. Genet.*, **26**, 627–635). The evidence for linkage between the *UMPK* and *Rh* loci is impressive but not yet quite significant; there is a fainter hint of linkage also with the *Sc* locus (Giblett *et al.*, *Cytogenetics and Cell Genetics*, 1975, in press).

Chapter 29. Xg and X-Chromosome Mapping

There is more information about the possible *deutan:Becker* muscular dystrophy linkage (Skinner, Smith and Emery, 1974, *J. med. Genet.*, **11**, 317–320); this when added to the figures given on page 597 reduces the most likely recombination fraction from 0·24 to 0·22 and increases the height of the probability curve from 61 to 135. So the linkage now seems to be established.

Index

A antigen of red cells   8–18
  A_1 and A_2 9–12
  A_3 14–15, 29
  A_{bantu} 18
  A_{el} 18
  A_{end} 17–18
  A_{finn} 17–18
  A_h and A_m^h 24–7, 29
  A_{hel} or A_{HP}, A_{HH} 58
  A_{int} 17
  A_m 15–17, 25, 27–8, 29–31
  A^p 44
  A_x, A_4, A_5, A_z, A_0 15–17, 28
  A_1Le^b 337–8, 529
  'intermediate'   17
  number of sites   38–9
  other weak A   18
  quantitative measurements   35–6, 38–9
A substance   39–40, 59–63, 311
  caught by O cells   40–1
  chemistry   59–63
  in animals   39, 44
  in cyst fluids   40, 59
  in saliva   311–12
  in serum   40–1
  other sites   39, 43
  secretion of   311–22
ABO (A_1A_2BO) groups   8–91
  A, B and H substances   39–43, 59–63
    secretion of   311–22
  A and *B* in *cis*   33–5
  acquired B   31–2
  age effects   31
  agglutinins, in cervical secretion   45
    in cord blood   45, 48
    in chickens   46
    in fish   58–9, 166–7
    in milk   45
    in saliva   45
    in salmon caviar   58
    in seeds   54–8
    in snails   58–9
    in tears   46
    missing   15–20, 27–8, 45, 526–7
    seasonal variation   45

  see also antibodies
    'suppressed'   53
  A_h phenotype   24–7, 29
  A_m^h phenotype   24–7
  an anti-D susceptible to   53
  and acquired tolerance   47, 526–7
  and anthropology   11
  and environment   29–32
  and I groups   53, 452–3, 457–8
  and leukaemia   29–31
  and serum alkaline phosphatase   44
  and *Hh* genes   20–4, 59–63
  and *Yy* genes   27–8
  antibodies   45–53 *see also* Anti-A, -B, -H,
      -O
    auto   53
    cross-reacting   48–50
    development of   45–7
    'immune'   46–7
    in cord blood   45, 48
    in body fluids   45–6
    in saliva   45
    in seeds   54–8
    in snails   58–9
    origin   46
  antigens   8–33
    acquired   31–33, 519
    adsorption of A by O cells   40–1
    development of   37–8
    in amnion cells   41, 43
    in cancer cells   43
    in cornea   41
    in epidermal cells   42
    in epithelial cells   42–3
    in normoblasts   41
    in platelets   42
    in saliva   311–22
    in serum   40–1
    in spermatozoa   43
    in tissue culture   41
    in white cells   42
    number of sites   38–9
    quantitative measurements   35–6, 38–9
    weak A and B   15–32
  B^h phenotype   24–7

641

Anti-N—*cont.*
made in rabbits 124
reaction with M cells 120–1
Anti-N^A 118
Anti-Ny^a 114–5, 127
'Anti-O' 50–2, 452
reaction with cord blood 38
Anti-Or 434
Anti-Ot 475
Anti-P 157, 167–8
and PCH 171
Anti-p 155
Anti-P$_1$ 139, 166–7
Anti-P^k 157 168
Anti-PP$_1$P^k (anti-Tj^a) 157, 167
and abortions 169–70
Anti-Pr 486
Anti-Pt^a 434
'Anti-Q' 165
Anti-R in sheep 328
Anti-$\bar{R}^N$ 204–6
Anti-Rd 434
Anti-Re^a 434
Anti-Rh, discovery 178
Anti-Rh^A, −Rh^B, etc. 190–3
Anti-Rh$_0$, *see* Anti-D
Anti-Rh33 203–4
Anti-Rh35 206
Anti-rh', *see* Anti-C
Anti-rh", *see* Anti-E
Anti-rh$_1$ 200–1
Anti-Ri^a 114, 126
Anti-Rl^a 435
Anti-Rm 441
Anti-S 92–3, 125
Anti-s 125
Anti-Sc1 406, 408
Anti-Sc2 406, 409
Anti-Sd^a 395, 401, 403
Anti-Sf^a 478
Anti-Sj 108, 125
Anti-Skjelbred 442
Anti-Sm (Sc1) 406, 408
Anti-Sp$_1$ 486
Anti-St^a 114, 126
Anti-Stobo 440
Anti-Sul 115, 127
Anti-Sw^a 435
Anti-T 486–8
Anti-'T' (Le^a) 323
Anti-Tj^a 149, 157, 167
and abortion 169–70
Anti-Tk 488
Anti-Tm 108, 125
Anti-Tn 488–91
Anti-To^a 435
Anti-Tr^a 435
Anti-Ts 442
Anti-U 100, 125

Anti-Ul^a 290, 304
Anti-V 206–8
Anti-Vel 415–6
Anti-Ven 441
Anti-Vr 114, 126
Anti-VS 197, 208–9
Anti-Vw 112, 126
Anti-Wb 435
Anti-Wiel 193–4, 638
Anti-Wk^a 291, 304
Anti-Wk^b 291, 304
Anti-Wr^a 436, 439
Anti-Wr^b 439
Anti-Wu 436
Anti-Yk^a 478
Anti-Yt^a 379, 381
Anti-Yt^b 381
Anti-X, *see* Anti-Le^x
Anti-Xg^a 578, 588
Anti-Zd 210, 442
Arachis hypogaea 487
Ascitic fluid, antibodies in 45, 240, 381
At^a (August) antigen 411–12, 423–4
Au^a antigen 383–5
Auberger groups 383–5
antibody 383
association with Lutheran 384–5
development 383
frequencies 383
immunization 383
independence 267–71, 384
inheritance 384
inhibition by *In(Lu)* 267–71, 384–5
Auto-antibodies 232, 239–40, 447, 451–7
and abortion 169–71
and α-methyldopa 240
and Kell 298
and PCH 171
anti-A, -B, -H 53
anti-e 239–40
anti-LW 232
anti-I 447, 451–2, 456–7
anti-i 453
anti-Tj^a 169
in acquired haemolytic anaemia 239–40
Autosomes 6, 547–9

B antigen 8–11
acquired B 31–2
B$_2$, B$_3$, B$_m$, B$_w$, B$_x$ 19–20, 33–5
B$_h$ and B$_m^h$ 24–7
number of sites 38–9
quantitative measurements 35–6, 39
weak B 19–20, 33–5
B substance 39, 59–63, 311
chemistry 59–63
in animals 39, 44
in saliva 311